UROLOGY

UROLOGY

SECOND EDITION

John Blandy

CBE, MA, DM, MCh, FRCS, FACS (Hon) FRCSI
Emeritus Professor of Urology
University of London
at the London Hospital Medical College,
Consulting Urologist, St Peter's Hospital

Christopher Fowler

BSc, MRCP, FRCS, FRCS (Urol)
Consultant Urological Surgeon
to the Royal Hospitals NHS Trust
and Newham Healthcare NHS Trust
Tutor to the Minimal Access
Therapy Training Unit,
The Royal College of Surgeons of England

b
**Blackwell
Science**

© 1996 by
Blackwell Science Ltd
Editorial Offices:
Osney Mead, Oxford OX2 0EL
25 John Street, London WC1N 2BL
23 Ainslie Place, Edinburgh EH3 6AJ
238 Main Street, Cambridge
  Massachusetts 02142, USA
54 University Street, Carlton
  Victoria 3053, Australia

Other Editorial Offices:
Arnette Blackwell SA
  224, Boulevard Saint Germain
75007 Paris, France

Blackwell Wissenschafts-Verlag GmbH
  Kurfürstendamm 57
  10707 Berlin, Germany

  Zehetnergasse 6
  A-1140 Wien
  Austria

First published 1976
Second edition 1996
Reprinted 1996

Set by Setrite Typesetters, Hong Kong
Printed and bound in Great Britain
by The Bath Press, Bath, Avon

The Blackwell Science logo is a
trade mark of Blackwell Science Ltd,
registered at the United Kingdom
Trade Marks Registry

DISTRIBUTORS

  Marston Book Services Ltd
  PO Box 269
  Abingdon
  Oxon OX14 4YN
  (*Orders*: Tel: 01235 465500
          Fax: 01235 465555)

USA
  Blackwell Science, Inc.
  238 Main Street
  Cambridge, MA 02142
  (*Orders*: Tel: 800 215-1000
          617 876-7000
          Fax: 617 492-5263)

Canada
  Copp Clark, Ltd
  2775 Matheson Blvd East
  Mississauga, Ontario
  Canada, L4W 4P7
  (*Orders*: Tel: 800 263-4374
          905 238-6074)

Australia
  Blackwell Science Pty Ltd
  54 University Street
  Carlton, Victoria 3053
  (*Orders*: Tel: 03 9347-0300
          Fax: 03 9349-3016)

A catalogue record for this title
is available from the British Library

ISBN 0-632-03679-6

Library of Congress
Cataloging-in-Publication Data

Blandy, John P. (John Peter), 1927-
  Urology/John Blandy, Christopher Fowler. — 2nd ed.
      p.   cm.
  Rev. ed. of: Urology/edited by John Blandy. 1976.
  Includes bibliographical references
  and index.
  ISBN 0-632-03679-6
  1. Urology. I. Fowler, Christopher, 1950–   . II. Title.
III. Title: Urology. IV. Title: Blandy and Fowler's urology.
  [DNLM: 1. Urogenital Diseases.
WJ 100 B642b 1996]
RC871.U76 1996
616.6 — dc20

Contents

Preface to the Second Edition

Since the first edition the battle to establish urology as a separate specialty in the British Isles has been won and today it is accepted that Higher Surgical Training in the specialty should begin as soon as the young surgeon has finished Basic Training in the Common Trunk of Surgery-in-General. So the young urologist of tomorrow should be able to start with a clear-cut scheme of education whose content and syllabus are clearly set out, whose training programme is regularly inspected, and whose completion will be formally tested by the Intercollegiate Specialty Fellowship Examination in Urology. It is for the young urologist starting out on this second phase of training that this book has been entirely rewritten.

This second edition departs from many of the conventions of the usual multi-author text. Our aims have been, first, to provide a solid foundation of common ground upon which new knowledge may be built, and against which new developments may be evaluated. Few other branches of surgery have changed and will continue to change so quickly as urology — where technical innovations succeed each other with bewildering speed.

Secondly, as other considerations increasingly shoulder out the traditional undergraduate education in the basic sciences we have attempted to provide an integrated refresher course in the basic sciences of anatomy, embryology, physiology and pathology that are relevant to urology.

Our purpose has not been to provide a huge encyclopaedia, but rather a workaday handbook to be a friendly companion in the ward and the operating theatre which will make each day more interesting and more fun.

Many of the contributors to the first edition have kindly permitted us to re-use their illustrations, and for this we thank Dr Elizabeth Courtauld, Mr Philip Clark, Dr David Evans, Professor Aziz Fam, Mr J. G. Gow, Mr Herbert Johnston, Dr Frank Marsh, Dr J. K. Oates, Mr Kenneth Owen, Dr Roger Pugh, Mr, Peter Riddle, Professor Tom Sherwood, Mr Manmeet Singh, Mr Joe Smith, Mr Gerald Tresidder, Dr Peter Trott, Mr Robert Whitaker and Mr John Wickham.

In addition we are very grateful to the Editor of the *British Journal of Urology* and Messrs Basil Page and David Jones for illustrations from their classic studies on the anatomy of the prostate, and Mr Patrick Keane for his picture of calcification on a ureteric stent. We thank Dr A. K. Sharma and the Editor of the *North India Journal of Surgery* for his illustration of malignant fungus testis, Mr Govindar Ravi and Dr S. W. Attwood for the illustrations of hydatid disease and bilharziasis, Mr Henry Yu and Professor Mya Thaung for the radiographs of filariasis.

We are specially grateful to Dr Suhail Baithun for all the trouble he has taken to obtain new photomicrographs, to Professor J. D. Williams for the micrographs of the hooklets of hydatid and *Treponema pallidum*, Dr George Lindop and the Editor of *Histopathology* for the microphotographs of a renin-secreting tumour, Dr J. Newman for the electron micrographs of normal and malignant urothelium, and to Dr Connie Parkinson for her help in the quest for these images.

We are exceedingly grateful to Drs Otto Chan, Robert Dick, William Hately, Janet Husband, Mike Kellett, and Miss Leela Kapila who kindly provided us with so many new radiographs, Dr Neil Garvie and Robert Whitaker for the radio-isotope images, Miss Mary Salamon for her help with the flow studies and cystometrograms, and our colleagues Messrs Andrew Paris and David Badenoch for allowing us to use illustrations of their cases and their equipment from the Department of Urology at the Royal London Hospital. We are also most grateful to David Gardner for the reproduction of all the medical illustrations and to Rebecca Huxley and her colleagues in Blackwell Science for all their painstaking work.

Preface to the First Edition

This book has been written for the surgeon intending to make urology his specialty, and for the established general surgeon who would like to keep up to date with recent developments in urological practice. In part, it is also an answer to the question — What is so different about urology that it needs to be regarded as a special field on its own, when by tradition it has always belonged to the main core and body of surgery? In recent years there have been so many changes and developments in urology that the man in training needs a secure base from which to make his forays into the confused jungle of the urological literature, and while there are many and excellent textbooks available from North America they write in a different surgical tradition and a different context of training and practice. Many of the changes in urology have come about as the result of developments in other fields, notably in radiology and nuclear medicine, optical and electrical engineering, endocrinology and genetics, immunology and nephrology, and the style of modern urology reflects its close working association with these other disciplines. Today, urology covers a wide field ranging from tumours to transplants, from histocompatibility to hypertension. To do it justice has meant a long book, even when we have omitted those introductory sections on normal anatomy and physiology which tradition often assigns to such a textbook and most of the operative surgical detail except where recent developments have occurred, or where older methods have been undeservedly neglected. To keep each chapter up to date has called for repeated revisions at every stage, a labour for which the editor is glad to thank his collaborators, as well as Mrs Sue Simpson and Mr John Staunton of Oxford Illustrators for drawing and redrawing some thousand or more illustrations; the staff of Blackwells, especially Mr John Robson and Mrs Diana Porter, for their friendly and ever cheerful guidance; and Mr Per Saugman, for having faith.

PART 1
ARMAMENTARIUM

Chapter 1: Urological technology

Urological endoscopes

History

An endoscope needs a light to illuminate an object within a body cavity and an optical system to transmit to the observer an image of the illuminated object. The cystoscope invented by Nitze in 1876, and used with modification through the first half of the twentieth century was lit by a heated platinum wire at its distal end [1]. The wire was soon replaced by Edison's electric lamp. The telescope, originally made as an integral part of the instrument, was later constructed so as to be removable from a separate sheath through which the instrument could be irrigated. To transmit the image the telescope had glass lenses and prisms separated by spaces of air (Fig. 1.1).

There are still a few elderly urologists who were brought up with these instruments and remember their imperfections. The Bijou lamp kept burning out, casting the operating field into darkness. It was difficult to grind the tiny lenses with accuracy: stray images occurred from their unbloomed surfaces so that the image was degraded by peripheral blurring, ghost images and poor contrast [2]. The annular metal spacers which held the lenses in place reduced the effective internal diameter of the telescope and restricted light transmission.

In 1957 Mr J.G. Gow approached Professor Harold Hopkins with a view to improving this inefficient system [2]. Hopkins responded with a series of innovations which were to transform the design of urological telescopes and make possible all the advances in endoscopy, not only of the urinary tract, which were to follow.

Hopkins' rod-lens telescope

In this rod-lens telescope, the old arrangement of glass lenses with air spaces between was reversed so that there were effectively air lenses separated by spaces of glass (Fig. 1.2).

Changing the main transmission medium from air to glass doubled the light which could pass through a system of given diameter. A second doubling of light transmission resulted from omission of the metal spacers which were no longer needed to position the lenses — the rods could be mounted without them — and light transmission through an optical system was proportional to the fourth power of its diameter.

What is more, the refractive surfaces of the rods were technically easier to grind with precision so that they could be manufactured to a high degree of optical accuracy. Hopkins complemented these improvements by making use of modern glasses, sophisticated computer-aided design and multilayer lens blooming. The latter minimized internal reflections within the sys-

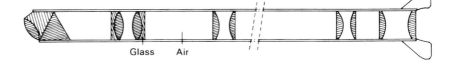

Fig. 1.1 Diagram of conventional cystoscope. The glass lenses are held in place by metal spacers and separated by air spaces.

Glass   Air

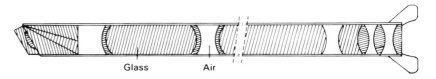

Fig. 1.2 Rod-lens telescope, with 'lenses' of air, separated by 'spaces' of glass, with no need for metal spacers (courtesy of Professor H.H. Hopkins).

Glass   Air

tem, improved light transmission and suppressed stray images [3].

The result of these improvements has been a family of telescopes, each with good optical resolution through an angle of field of 70° or more, with the image quality of a microscope. The angle of view can be varied by incorporating a prism behind the objective lens. The traditional 30° 'fore-oblique' optic is a throwback to the days of distal illumination and may soon give way to the more rational forward viewing (0°) telescope for urethroscopy and resection (Fig. 1.3). Some urologists like to use a retroviewing 120° telescope to see clearly the more distal parts of the anterior bladder wall (Fig. 1.4). This is seldom necessary, particularly now that the flexible cystoscope gives a much better antegrade view of the bladder neck (Fig. 1.5). Because the light transmission through a rod-lens telescope is so good, instruments of small diameter can be made for paediatric endoscopy and for viewing the ureter.

Fibreoptics

The basis of fibreoptics is the passage of light along glass fibres by a process of total internal reflection (Fig. 1.6). J.L. Baird (1927) [4] conceived the idea of using an array of fibres to transmit an image, but it was Hopkins who constructed the first working fibrescope [5]. Fibrebundles are now used in endoscopy in two main ways. Coordinated fibrebundles, in which the arrangement of fibres at the exit face is identical with that at the entry face, are used as the image relay system of flexible fibrescopes. Uncoordinated bundles are used in endoscopic illumination systems to transmit light from an external source.

Apart from the arrangement of the fibres, the two types of fibrebundles are similar. The fibres of a viewing bundle, where small fibres give better resolution, may be as fine as 8 nm in diameter. Illumination bundles often have slightly larger fibres. As there may be up to 10^4 internal reflections over a 1 m length of fibres, even a small light loss at each one would cause a catastrophic fall-off in the efficiency of light transmission. For this reason the glass core of each fibre has a cladding of glass with a lower refractive index. Reflections occur at the interface between the two glasses. The cladding protects the surface of the fibre core from damage and

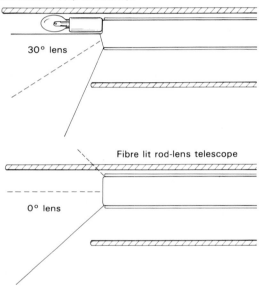

Conventional lamp lit telescope

30° lens

Fibre lit rod-lens telescope

0° lens

Fig. 1.3 Comparison between the angle of view offered by the conventional 30° 'fore-oblique' optic and the forward viewing 0° telescope.

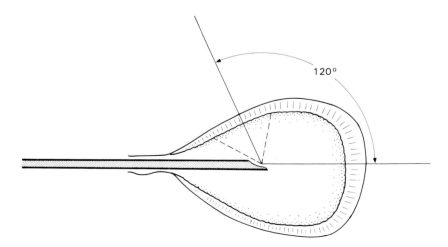

120°

Fig. 1.4 The retroviewing 120° telescope allows the bladder neck and anterior bladder wall to be seen.

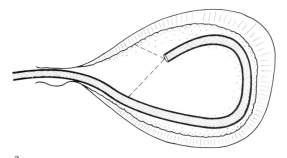

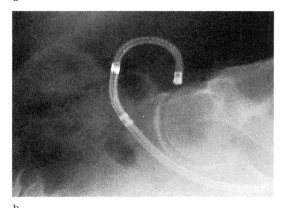

Fig. 1.5 A better view of (a) the anterior bladder wall and bladder neck is provided by (b) the flexible cystoscope.

Fibrelighting

The illumination system of a rod-lens telescope is in two parts. A fibrebundle built into the telescope transmits light to its distal tip. Light from an external light source is focused onto one end of a second flexible fibreoptic bundle (the light guide) which connects with the integral bundle by a screw-fitting at the light post. This arrangement allows the telescope and light guide to be sterilized separately. Its disadvantage is that a major loss of light occurs where the two bundles meet — a loss which is much increased when the connector is dirty.

Fibrelighting replaced the unreliable Bijou bulb. Today's endoscopist uses a simple low power external light source which rarely causes problems. A bonus of fibrelight illumination is that very high intensity light sources can also be used. Quartz halogen filament lamps and xenon arc sources provide the very high levels of light needed for endoscopic television and photography. These very high power sources are used with 'cold' mirrors whose surfaces are made of multilayer thin films which reduce the amount of infrared emission sent down the light guide. Despite this, the heat which reaches the distal end of the guide is quite enough to ignite surgical drapes or burn the patient (Fig. 1.7). High intensity lighting should not be used for direct viewing because of the risk of retinal damage.

Fibrescopes

Fibrescopes were relatively slow to catch on in

contamination which would otherwise interfere with internal reflection. Light losses of 50% or less over a 1 m light path can be achieved with these clad fibres.

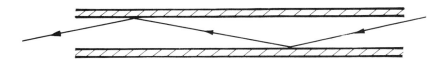

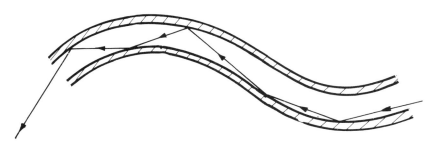

Fig. 1.6 Total internal reflection permits light to travel along a flexible glass fibre.

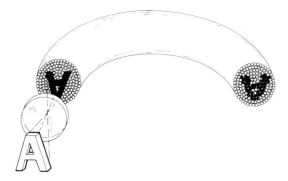

Fig. 1.8 The glass fibres of a fibrescope are bonded at each end, but loose in between, making the bundle flexible.

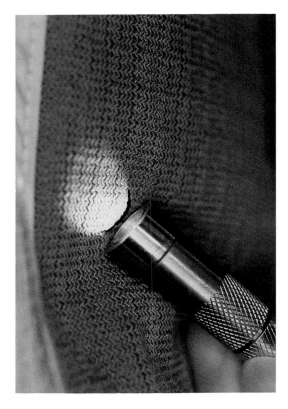

Fig. 1.7 The heat reaching the distal end of the light-guide may ignite surgical drapes and burn the patient.

urology because the granular fibrescopic image was less satisfactory than that of the rod-lens telescope. The increased popularity of these instruments is partly due to improvements in manufacture and design. The size and quality of the image of small calibre instruments has improved. More important has been a reappraisal of the advantages of flexible instruments. The flexible cystoscope is used in the outpatient clinic because it can be passed under topical urethral anaesthesia in both sexes with little discomfort — the instrument adapts its shape to the patient's anatomy [6,7]. Fibreoptic nephroscopes can improve access within the renal collecting system and the fibreoptic ureteroscope offers the promise, as yet only partly fulfilled, of atraumatic transurethral endoscopy of the upper urinary tract.

A modern fibrescope viewing bundle has about 40 000 fibres of approximately 8 nm diameter with a square section of about 2.2 mm at each face. The fibres are bonded together at each end of the bundle but in between they are loose (Fig. 1.8). This makes the bundle very flexible. Since only the core of each fibre traps and conducts light, light falling between the cores is lost

by absorption into the periphery of the bundle. Each fibre traps light from a tiny part of the object. As it passes along the fibre this light is scrambled. When it emerges from the eyepiece end, it is a uniform spot of light from which all detail of colour and intensity of the segment of the object from which it derived have been lost. It is this loss of detail which determines the theoretical limit of resolution of a fibrescope (Fig. 1.9).

Endoscopic television

Full size three tube television cameras used for endoscopic teaching have given way first to single tube and then to 'chip' cameras. As miniaturization proceeded, it became possible to attach the camera directly to the eyepiece of the rod-lens telescope with no need for a cumbersome optical connector to hamper the operator. Video endoscopy has health and safety benefits for the endoscopist as well as making operations more interesting and instructive for theatre staff. Sitting upright, there is no need for the contortions which have damaged many urologists' necks, and working farther from the patient means less liability of contamination with body fluids. It takes very little practice to convert from direct vision to video endoscopy, and most urologists use a beam splitter which allows the possibility of both.

The beam splitter has an important role in orientating the television image. If the chip camera is attached directly in line with the rod-lens, rotation of the telescope produces a rotation of the image on the screen. To avoid this the beam splitter, which deflects light to the camera at a right angle to the axis of the telescope, needs to be mounted on a freely movable cuff. Gravity

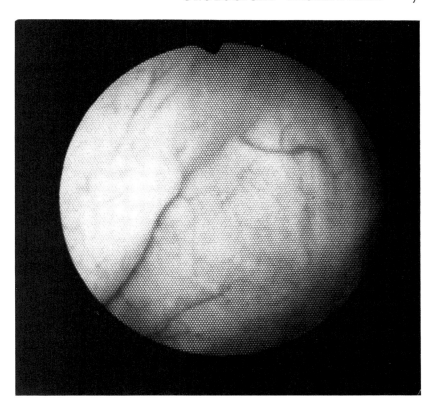

Fig. 1.9 The resolution of a fibrescope is determined by the number of fibres.

keeps the camera hanging downwards so that the screen image rotates with the telescope.

The problem of orientation is particularly important with the development of cameras which are small enough to go on the distal end of the telescope, making a separate rigid or flexible image transmission system unnecessary. Flexible endoscopes of this type are already available for bronchoscopy. The minute camera requires relatively low levels of light. Red, green and blue light are flashed in sequence from the light source and the black and white images returned by the camera are processed by a computer to give a colour picture. The future of endoscopy lies with electronic image transmission and computer processing.

Diathermy

Surgical diathermy exploits the heat generated when an alternating current passes through a conductor. When there is a large density of electrical current passing through tissue, the temperature rise can be enough to give a useful surgical effect. In monopolar diathermy, the surgeon uses a small active electrode to give a high current density and a large heating effect at the operative site. Since the current density, near the large return electrode which completes the circuit, is small, it produces little heat. In bipolar diathermy the thermal effect occurs in tissue held between two small active electrodes.

Nerves and muscles are stimulated by alternating current of low frequency (faradism) but this faradic effect does not occur when the frequency exceeds a certain value. A low frequency current as small as 1 mA can stimulate the myocardium to fatal dysrhythmia, but at radiofrequency (500–5000 kHz) currents as high as 2 A used in surgical diathermy are passed through the body without dangerous neuromuscular effects.

The surgeon uses diathermy for cutting and coagulation. Cutting occurs when sufficient heat is applied to tissue to cause an explosive vaporization of intracellular water with cell destruction. To achieve a temperature above 100°C requires a very high current density. For coagulation, a less violent heating effect leads to cell death by dehydration and protein denaturation. The dead tissue is shrunken and desiccated *in situ* — distortion of the walls of blood vessels, coagulation of plasma proteins and stimulation of the clotting mechanism all act to check bleeding. Ideally, intracellular temperatures do not reach 100°C so there should be no unwanted cutting.

Older diathermy machines gave currents whose waveform was determined by the components used to produce them. These 'valve' and 'spark-gap' devices have been replaced by modern solid-state electronics which allow the designer to provide current which has been tailored to the needs of the surgeon. The desired surgical effect is achieved by varying the amplitude and waveform of the current to cause cutting, coagulation or a combination of the two.

Contact diathermy

In contact diathermy, the main impedance (resistance) to current flow is at the interface between the electrode and tissue, where it is influenced by the type of tissue and its state of hydration. The impedance of fat is high compared to muscle, and contact diathermy works badly on adipose tissue. As diathermy proceeds, the tissue in contact with the electrode dries and impedance rises. Eventually, the current flow is insufficient to produce further heating and the surgical effect ceases. This limits the depth of penetration of diathermy applied to one spot. The effect of contact diathermy also depends on the size and shape of the active electrode. A ball electrode with a large surface area held in contact with tissue will tend to apply current at a relatively low density giving a coagulating effect, but the depth of tissue coagulated is proportional to the square of the diameter of the ball. Contact cutting by point diathermy is mainly by physical disruption of tissue softened by coagulation and is usually less effective than non-contact cutting.

Non-contact cutting

Contact with tissue is necessary in bipolar diathermy but most urological diathermy is monopolar and non-contact. For current to cross a gap between a resectoscope loop and the prostate it must be driven by a sufficient electromotive force to ionize the intervening medium and produce a spark. (A spark is a less sustained discharge than an 'arc'.) Once established, a spark produces the very high temperatures needed for cutting. However, most of its energy is dissipated near the tissue surface and little is available to give the gentler heating needed for deeper coagulation and haemostasis.

The cutting current is a continuous simple sine wave. The peak voltage provided is enough to give short, intense sparks which produce enough local heat to explode cells into steam

(Fig. 1.10). There is little coagulation and the cut is 'pure'. For coagulation, the electrical energy must be applied more slowly so that the heat to which it is converted has time to spread below the surface of the tissue, i.e. the power supplied must be reduced.

In contact diathermy, so long as the effective voltage is sufficient to overcome the impedance of the contact interface, coagulation can be obtained by reducing the voltage of the sine wave current. Alternatively, the current density can be reduced by increasing the contact surface of the electrode.

A high voltage is essential to drive the spark in non-contact diathermy and a different method must be used for coagulation. The total current supplied in a given time, hence the rate of heating is reduced by applying the current in bursts. In the gap between the bursts, no current flows. Because the coagulation current is turned off most of the time, it can have large peak voltages and currents but actually deliver much less power than a continuous cutting current. Fulguration (literally flashing like lightning) is provided by a current with an interrupted waveform. This has a high peak voltage but the effective power can be the same as a cutting current with a much lower voltage peak. The resulting sparks are longer and there is more sustained tissue heating leading to coagulation and haemostasis. The high peak voltage can drive current through the high impedance of desiccated tissue: thus fulguration can continue until carbonization or charring occur.

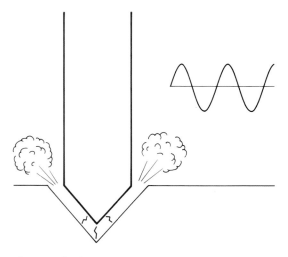

Fig. 1.10 Cutting current: a continuous sine wave provides short intense sparks with explode cells into steam, but there is little heating below the surface, and so little coagulation.

In summary, the 'cut' current is typically a continuous sine wave, producing sparks whose heat explodes intracellular water to steam. The 'coag' current is a sine wave current supplied in bursts, which allows the sustained heating in depth needed for coagulation (Fig. 1.11). Peak voltage and mean power output can be varied by adjusting the duration of bursts of current to give a combination of cutting and coagulation — this is known as 'blended' current.

Surgical diathermy generators differ widely and there is little relationship between the output settings of one machine and another. The setting recommended by the manufacturer is on a scale which is meaningless to the surgeon. An interesting development is the diathermy generator which monitors the changes in electrical impedance that occur as diathermy proceeds. The feedback adjusts the output current to the increased load. This device probably heralds a generation of fully computerized diathermy machines from which the surgeon can demand a precisely controlled tissue effect.

Dangers

Electrocution

Diathermy machines are manufactured to national and international safety standards which minimize the risk of any part of the machine becoming live with mains current. As with any electrical device, servicing must be regular and expert.

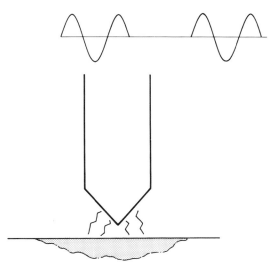

Fig. 1.11 Coagulating current: short bursts of sine waves provide localized heating leading to coagulation.

Fire and explosion

Ignition of alcohol-based solutions used for skin preparation is a well-recognized complication of diathermy which is still reported each year by the medical defence societies. It occurs when the flammable fluid is allowed to pool on or under the patient. The surgeon must take care that all excess spirit is removed before using diathermy. Better still, disinfecting fluids containing alcohol should be avoided if a suitable aqueous alternative is available. Thankfully, explosive gases are rarely used in modern anaesthesia. If they are, diathermy is an unnecessary hazard and should be avoided.

Burns

Burns are the most common type of diathermy accident. They occur when the diathermy circuit is completed in some way other than that intended by the surgeon — usually an unauthorized flow of current to earth. Most monopolar generators are ground referenced by earthing the patient plate side of the output transformer via the metal case of the device (Fig. 1.12). If the active electrode is touched to any earthed object, current will flow. When the system works properly, heating occurs only at the tip of the active electrode. The current passes through the patient's body and escapes safely via the return electrode. Unfortunately, this long current path offers opportunities for alternative unwanted passage of current to earth. If the patient electrode is incorrectly attached, there is a danger that the circuit might be completed by a small earthed contact point. If the current density at this point is sufficient, the patient will be burned.

Most devices monitor the attachment of the patient plate and sound an alarm when contact is inadequate. A simple method is to attach the plate by two wires through which a small current flows: if a wire breaks, the current is interrupted and the diathermy can be automatically inactivated. This checks the integrity of the connection of the plate to the diathermy machine. It does not guarantee that the plate itself is properly attached to the patient. Another safety device uses a small direct current which, in passing through the active electrode, the patient and the patient electrode, monitors the integrity of the whole diathermy circuit. Other machines have even more sophisticated safety measures: however, it remains the surgeon's duty to ensure that

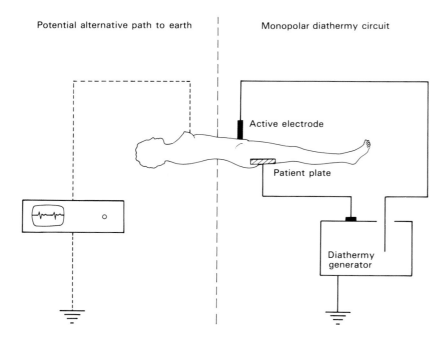

Potential alternative path to earth | Monopolar diathermy circuit

Active electrode

Patient plate

Diathermy
generator

Fig. 1.12 Monopolar diathermy generators are ground referenced by earthing the patient plate to the metal case of the device. There is a risk of a burn if the patient plate is incorrectly attached, and there is contact with any other earthed point, e.g. patient monitoring equipment.

an appropriate plate is used and to supervise its attachment to the patient.

Unfortunately, burns may still occur at small earthed contact points where current will flow at the expense of even a correctly attached return plate. All patient monitoring equipment should be isolated from the earth wherever this is possible. Electrocardiograph electrodes should be well gelled and of large enough area to disperse the current. Needle electrodes should never be used. As a general rule, the return pad should be sited as near to the operation area as possible so that the main current path will be distant from other potential routes that the current might take to ground.

Pressure on the footswitch of most machines leads to activation of all the active electrodes which are connected. Any devices which are not in use must not be in contact with the patient. An unused electrode should be safely stored in an insulated quiver where it will be safe if the footswitch is inadvertently activated.

The surgeon and assistants are also liable to suffer burns when using diathermy equipment because they constitute a very effective alternative path to earth. Such burns are particularly likely in the practice of 'touching' the live electrode onto another metal instrument such as tissue forceps grasping a bleeding vessel. Surgical gloves are not effective insulation against diathermy current — especially if they are holed. The person holding the instrument, often an unfortunate assistant, may receive a small but deep and painful burn.

Bipolar diathermy is intrinsically safer than monopolar diathermy because current passes between two small electrodes on the same handpiece. Secondary currents induced by the main radiofrequency may leak to ground, but they are too small to cause trouble. Unfortunately, in most urological applications, bipolar diathermy is not as useful as monopolar diathermy.

Neuromuscular stimulation — the 'obturator twitch'

Although the high frequency current used for surgical diathermy does not cause neuromuscular stimulation, the sparks which it induces may invoke secondary currents which can do so. The sparks make random electrical 'noise' in the midst of which are alternating frequencies able to induce a faradic effect. Such currents can be electronically suppressed by capacitors in the circuit. However, they may be sufficient to cause trouble in the special conditions of diathermy in the region of the ureteric orifices close to the course of the obturator nerve and the psoas muscle. The problem is seen with both 'cut' and 'coag' currents and can usually be abolished by full chemical neuromuscular blockade.

Pacemakers and diathermy

Implanted pacemakers are not uncommon in elderly patients who come to urological surgery. Diathermy currents can interfere with the working of pacemakers with possible danger to the patient. This was more of a problem with some of the earlier fixed-rate devices which could be fooled into delivering stimulation at such a high rate that dangerous dysrhythmias could result. Modern pacemakers are designed instead to be inhibited by high frequency interference so that the patient may receive no pacing stimulation at all while the diathermy is in use. Some demand pacemakers revert to a fixed rate of pacing and it is essential to have a magnet available so that they can be reset if necessary.

A number of additional precautions are wise in these patients. First, if monopolar diathermy is to be used, the patient plate should be sited so that the current path does not pass through the heart or the pacemaker. Second, the heartbeat should be monitored throughout the operation. Lastly, a defibrillator should be on hand in case a dangerous dysrhythmia develops through malfunction of the pacemaker.

Urological diathermy

Transurethral resection requires high power monopolar diathermy currents which must be handled with great care. There is an almost inevitable leakage of diathermy current from the loop to the metal instrument which poses a potential danger to both the surgeon and the patient. Most resectoscopes now have an all-metal design with an insulated beak so that current which travels into the instrument is free to leak from it into the urethra. This is not usually a problem because the area of contact with the urethra is sufficient to make a burn unlikely. However, if through some fault, the loop comes into direct contact with the sheath, the full diathermy output will be applied to the urethra. Hopefully, however, the surgeon will notice the problem before damage occurs.

A fully insulated sheath might be expected to give protection against this hazard: unfortunately, this has dangers of its own. Damage to the insulating layer will lead to unpredictable leakage into the patient or the surgeon. If the loop should break and make contact with the metal frame of the instrument, a very large current could flow to ground via the surgeon's body. Such currents are usually prevented by the return fault circuit of the machine, but small and significant currents may pass to ground during fulguration. Such currents are usually conducted harmlessly away to the surgeon's hands, but the possibility of leakage to the eye makes it imperative that all resectoscope eyepieces should be insulated.

Conducting lubricating gels should be used with all metal resectoscopes to avoid the possibility of preferential conduction at sites where the gel is thin or absent. By contrast, petroleum jelly or mineral oil, which do not conduct electricity, must be used only with an insulated sheath because these lubricants cannot provide an alternative path between the loop and the urethra; and they always end up smearing the lens.

Laser

Photons are packets of electromagnetic radiation whose energy is directly related to the frequency and wavelength of the radiation: photons of the same energy have the same wavelength. They can be released when a particle changes from a higher to a lower energy state in the process which Einstein called 'spontaneous emission of radiation' (Fig. 1.13). Such changes can only occur in discrete jumps or 'quanta' whose size is fixed by the medium in which they occur. Thus the photons produced by spontaneous emissions in a given medium will all have the same energy and hence the same wavelength.

In stimulated emission of radiation the photon release is itself precipitated by the impact of an identical photon. Both the impacting and the emitted photon have the same wavelength, and because they are discharged together, they are also in phase. Because two photons emerge where there had been one, a twofold amplification occurs: this is the basis of light amplification by stimulated emission of radiation, i.e. laser (Fig. 1.14).

The laser device

A working laser consists of a laser active medium confined in a chamber between two parallel mirrors (Fig. 1.15). Particles within the medium can exist at one or more 'excited' states at which they have higher energy levels but the process of spontaneous emission ensures that few particles are normally at a higher level at a given time. When the device is switched on, energy is 'pumped' into the laser medium from an adjacent

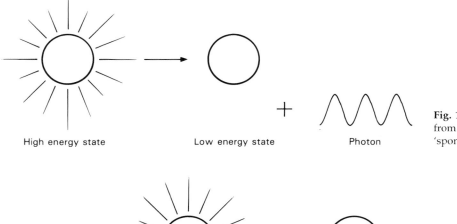

Fig. 1.13 Photons are emitted when a particle changes from a higher to a lower energy state — Einstein's 'spontaneous emission of radiation'.

High energy state   Low energy state   Photon

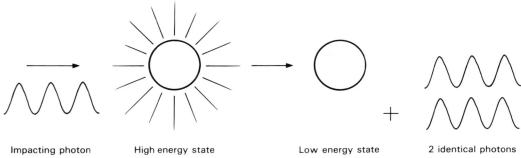

Impacting photon   High energy state   Low energy state   2 identical photons

Fig. 1.14 Laser — light amplification by stimulated emission of radiation. Both the impacting and emitted photon have the same wavelength and are discharged in phase — two photons emerge where only one went in.

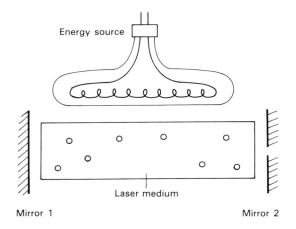

Fig. 1.15 Diagram of a working laser. The active laser medium is contained between mirrors. Energy is pumped into the laser medium from a power source to propel more particles into a higher energy state.

high power source to propel more particles into a higher energy state. With more particles in the excited state (a 'population inversion'), the opportunities for stimulated emission and amplification increase.

The active laser medium is confined between mirrors in the optical cavity in an arrangement called the resonator. Photon emissions produced by stimulated emission will radiate in all directions, but the small proportion which are exactly parallel to the axis of the laser cavity are reflected by the mirrors so that the major amplification occurs along that axis. The other emissions escape from the sides of the cavity and their energy is lost as heat. While the rear mirror of the resonator is 100% reflective, the front mirror is designed to transmit a fraction of the energy built up within the cavity which emerges as the laser beam (Fig. 1.16).

A laser beam has three important characteristics which result from the way it is generated. It is monochromatic, i.e. of a single wavelength dependent on the type of laser medium. It is coherent (in phase) and since only the light reflected between the mirrors is amplified there is very little divergence of the beam. An enormous amount of energy can therefore be focused onto a tiny area providing very high power densities at the point of action.

Lasers in urology

The most common types of medical lasers and their characteristics are shown in Table 1.1. The wavelength of the carbon dioxide, argon and neodymium-yttrium aluminium garnet (YAG) lasers are all fixed, but the dye laser is tunable within a band of wavelengths. Lasers have been used in urology in three main ways [8].

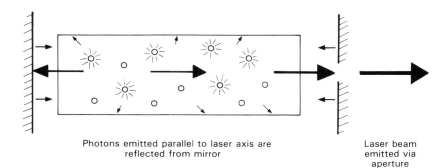

Fig. 1.16 In stimulated emission, photons radiate in all directions. Only those which are parallel to the axis of the laser cavity emerge through the front mirror as the laser beam.

Photons emitted parallel to laser axis are reflected from mirror

Laser beam emitted via aperture

Table 1.1 Physical properties and characteristics of surgical lasers

	Type of laser			
	CO_2	Argon	KTP	Neodymium-YAG
Wavelength (µm)	10.6	0.458–0.515	0.532	1.064
Colour	Infrared	Blue-green	Green	Infrared
Delivery	Air or endoguide	Fibre	Fibre	Fibre
Absorption	All tissues and fluids	Colour dependent	Colour dependent	Colour dependent
Pass through fluids	No	Yes	Yes	Yes
Cutting	Excellent	Good	Good	Good
Coagulation	Fair	Good	Good	Excellent

Tissue destruction

The neodymium-YAG laser produces infrared laser light which can be directed down a quartz fibre using the principle of total internal reflection. When it hits tissue, the beam is substantially transmitted forward so that its energy is dissipated below the surface to give heating in depth. In open surgery an operating handpiece, the laser scalpel, is used to guide the fibre. In endoscopic use, a 400–600 nm quartz fibre is passed down a rigid or flexible cystoscope. The laser scalpel has not proved as popular as expected: though it is haemostatic and gives rise to little postoperative scarring, it is terribly slow [9]. The expense and complexity of the equipment are also significant deterrents. Endoscopic laser tissue destruction of bladder tumours and benign prostatic hypertrophy have yet to be fully accepted for the same reasons [10,11].

Laser lithotripsy

Short pulses of laser light of an appropriate wavelength can be used to disintegrate calculi (see below).

Photodynamic therapy

In photodynamic therapy, the patient with malignancy is pretreated with an agent which is preferentially absorbed by tumour. Laser light is used to induce a photochemical change in the sensitizing agent which releases a tumoricidal metabolite. Photodynamic therapy using haematoporphyrin derivative (HPD) and other photosensitizers has been used to treat both exophytic bladder tumours and urothelial carcinoma *in situ* [12].

Despite its intellectual attractions as a 'magic bullet' and early reports of success, photodynamic therapy has been associated with unacceptable damage to the bladder with fibrosis and ureteric reflux. It seems unlikely that it will find a place in urological practice without major improvement in the specificity of the sensitizing agents.

Lithotriptors

Since its first clinical application in 1980 [13] extracorporeal shockwave lithotripsy (ESWL) has quickly taken over modern stone management, and open surgery for calculi has become a rarity. Endoscopic lithotripsy, which enjoyed a brief heyday before the irresistible rise of ESWL still has a place as an adjunct to ESWL, and for stones which for any reason are inaccessible to ESWL.

Endoscopic lithotripsy

Stones in the urinary tract can usually be approached by retrograde ureterorenoscopy or percutaneous antegrade nephroscopy. Small calculi can be retrieved intact by grasping forceps or basket, but larger calculi must be disintegrated before they can be extracted. In endoscopic lithotripsy stones are broken by applying a mechanical force which disrupts their relatively brittle crystalline structure. Adjacent soft tissue, being pliable and elastic, is relatively immune from injury.

Lithoclast

The Swiss lithoclast uses a mechanical percussive force on the same principle as a jackhammer which is applied to the stone via a more or less flexible metal probe (Fig. 1.17). It is simple and effective and has the added advantage of being relatively cheap.

Ultrasonic lithotripsy

The ultrasonic lithotriptor has a transducer which generates high frequency mechanical oscillations from an electrical input controlled by a foot-switch. These vibrations are transmitted to a rigid metal tube whose toothed tip is in contact with the calculus (Fig. 1.18). When the ultrasound generator is activated the toothed tip grinds the stone into powder which is sucked out through the lumen of the probe. Larger fragments are extracted with grasping forceps.

The ultrasound probe is currently the most widely used endoscopic lithotriptor. It works on a simple mechanical principle, is reliable and comparatively cheap. Inadvertent contact with tissue will cause bleeding and perforation, but in skilled hands it is safe. Its main drawback is its slowness, especially with hard stones, a slowness particularly marked when a long probe is used with the rigid ureteroscope. At present the ultrasound probe cannot be used with a fibrescope.

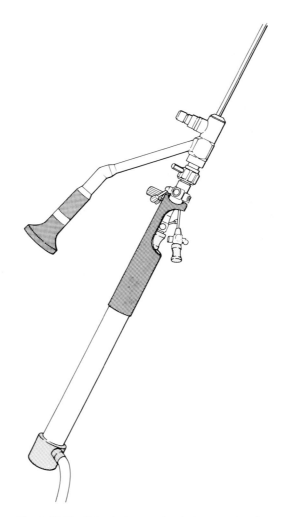

Fig. 1.17 The lithoclast: a mechanical percussive force is applied to the stone through a metal probe which works on the principle of the jackhammer.

Electrohydraulic lithotripsy

The principle of electrohydraulic lithotripsy was discovered by a Russian mining engineer. The discharge of a high voltage capacitor across two electrodes held under water causes a huge spark. The high temperature produced by the spark leads to a short-lived but explosive vaporization of water to steam, which generates a shockwave. When the shockwave is applied to a crystalline solid such as a calculus, it is reflected from surfaces within, leading to comprehensive and tensile forces which break the stone into fragments.

For urological use, the electrohydraulic discharge is usually applied to two electrodes mounted in a flexible wire, either side by side or concentrically. The probes can be made small enough to pass through the tiny instrument

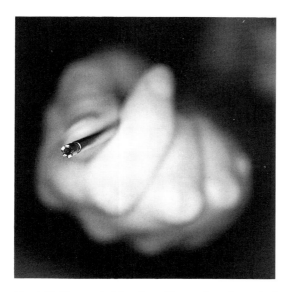

Fig. 1.18 Ultrasonic lithotripsy. The teeth at the end of the hollow probe oscillate at ultrasonic frequency and grind the stone into powder which is aspirated through the lumen of the probe.

channel of a flexible ureteroscope. It tends to produce stone fragments somewhat larger than those made by the ultrasonic lithotriptor and for this reason is quicker to use. It can be valuable for stones which can only be reached with flexible instruments.

Electrohydraulic endoscopic lithotripsy is less popular than ultrasound, perhaps because some of the early machines were liable to perforate the ureter and electrocute the surgeon. Modern versions are much safer.

Laser lithotripsy

The laser lithotriptor uses pulses of laser light to pump bursts of electromagnetic energy into the calculus, causing an explosion of steam which breaks up the crystalline structure of the stone. The first and so far most successful of laser lithotriptors uses a tunable dye laser which is 'Q-switched' to give short, high intensity pulses which are delivered to the stone though a fine flexible quartz fibre that can go through the finest instrument channel.

This device is particularly useful for ureteric stones in the middle and lower third of the ureter which are difficult to treat *in situ* with ESWL and cannot be pushed back into the kidney. Because the pulses of energy are short, the likelihood of damage to soft tissue is decreased. They are very expensive: the indication for using them is relatively rare.

ESWL

ESWL has been claimed as the most exciting advance in urology since transurethral resection. It has altered the management of urinary stone disease, and has saved thousands of people from major surgery. The first device for clinical use was built by Dornier in Munich. Their idea, of generating shockwaves outside the body, and focusing them on a calculus has now been modified in many smaller and cheaper second- and third-generation lithotriptors.

The idea of ESWL arose from a chance observation in Dornier's physics laboratory that shockwave energy could pass through the soft tissues of a human body without injury. There followed a long series of experiments *in vivo* and *in vitro* before the first patient was treated. The first Dornier ESWL machine used the electrohydraulic principle to generate the shockwaves: the high voltage discharge was placed at one focus of a semi-ellipsoid mirror so that the shockwaves converged at the second focus. The patient was manoeuvred under X-ray control until the second focus coincided with the calculus. The continuous fluid path for the shockwaves was obtained by immersing electrodes and patient in a bath of de-ionized water. By aiming two ellipsoids at the stone a very large disrupting force could be deployed.

The size of the pioneer Dornier machine was daunting — the patient had to be lowered into the water by a cumbersome crane — and installing the water-bath, its cranes and X-ray equipment was very expensive. The electrodes required frequent replacement. But the idea was brilliant, and soon imitated and improved upon: a range of ESWL machines using the same principle, but with a simpler fluid path that needed no immersion of the patient. Other machines generated the shockwave not by an electrohydraulic spark, but by piezo-electric generators assembled as a tightly packed matrix on a hemispherical dish, while the stone was put into position using ultrasound rather than X-ray devices (Fig. 1.19).

Every year sees an improved ESWL instrument, so that today the surgeon is offered a choice of X-rays or ultrasound to target the stone.

ESWL is remarkably safe. The shockwaves are timed to coincide with the refractory phase of the cardiac cycle to minimize the risk of inducing arrhythmia.

Pain was proportional to the density of the shockwave passing through skin and soft tissue, which depended on the strength of the source.

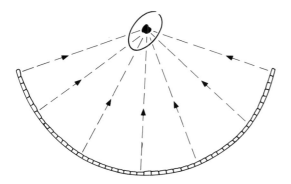

Fig. 1.19 Piezo-electric pulse generators mounted on the inside of a hemispherical dish discharge a pressure wave directed at the centre of the sphere.

When this came from the first focus of an ellipsoid, the skin was struck twice, first by the direct shock, and second by the reflected shock from the ellipsoidal mirror. The piezo-electric array mounted in the spherical basin avoided this twofold shock. There is no doubt that ESWL does produce soft tissue damage: haematuria is common. It is possible that microtrauma may be followed by fibrosis and late hypertension. For larger stones it is now usual to debulk the stones by means of percutaneous nephrolithotripsy, and to help the little fragments pass down the ureter it is usual to put a double-J stent up the ureter (see p. 227).

If a stone overlies the pelvic bones it may be protected from the shockwave.

Bacteria are regularly liberated from stones during fragmentation and if the system is obstructed there is a danger of septicaemia; it is essential to decompress the kidney by percutaneous nephrostomy or a ureteric catheter before dealing with an impacted obstructing stone in the ureter, and antibiotic prophylaxis is essential.

Sterilization

Heat

Autoclave

The autoclave is an extremely efficient method of sterilization because steam penetrates well and the high temperatures kill bacterial spores as well as vegetative forms. It also kills viruses. Heat is ideal for sterilizing all metal parts of instruments such as sheaths, biopsy forceps and handpieces. Unfortunately, the full autoclave cycle is time-consuming, and only the most lavishly equipped urological unit will have sufficient sets to make use of an autoclave in the hospital sterile supply department.

Instruments used in open surgery are sterilized in this way, but the endoscopes used for a busy list must be disinfected in some other way, necessitating a compromise for which urologists have attracted criticism from microbiological purists.

Pasteurization

Boiling for 2 min destroys vegetative organisms, but killing spores takes much longer. By heating instruments to 70°C for 10 min it is possible to kill vegetative organisms and viruses. The small 'pasteurizer' introduced by Francis [14], which is found in most urological theatres, attracts microbiological disdain because it does not deal with spores. However, the heat does reach crevices in taps and hinges and spore-bearing infection is exceedingly rare in urological practice. For want of anything better urologists are likely to continue to use the pasteurizer especially now that rod-lens telescopes are available that can be pasteurized.

Low temperature steam

At pressures below atmosphere, steam forms at a lower temperature: by adding formalin, steam at 80°C will kill spores and will effectively disinfect cystoscopes [15]. In practice, the equipment failed so often that the method fell into disrepute.

Chemical disinfection

Methods of disinfection which use high temperatures are unsuitable for delicate telescopes, and two types of chemical disinfection are regularly used in urology.

Vapour sterilization

Ethylene oxide gas forms an explosive mixture with air unless it is mixed (as is now usual practice) with 12% carbon dioxide. It is highly toxic, and when hot (80°C) and humidified, it is lethal to bacteria, spores and viruses. But its use is limited by the expenses which arise from the need to handle it safely: the cost of the plant and its supervision can be justified only by working in large batches, which extends the 'turn-around' time [16]. Because the gas dissolves in plastics these must be ventilated for 24 h to remove toxins. For practical purposes ethylene oxide is irrelevant when instruments must be rapidly reused or cannot withstand being exposed to a temperature of 80°C.

Liquid chemical immersion

Although other chemical disinfectants are available, 2% activated glutaraldehyde (Cidex) is the most widely used and will serve as an example. It is active at low temperatures against bacteria, fungi and spores. It is relatively harmless to delicate endoscopes whether rigid or flexible. A brief exposure will kill viruses, e.g. the human immunodeficiency virus (HIV) and hepatitis. A much longer time (1 h) is needed to kill *Mycobacterium tuberculosis* — but crossinfection to the urinary tract by *M. tuberculosis* has never been reported. In practice, endoscopes are immersed for only 10 min.

Chemical disinfection can only work on surfaces that are free from contamination with biological debris. Telescopes must be washed thoroughly before immersion — this in itself removes over 99% of organisms. Activated glutaraldehyde can only work on the parts it reaches — all taps, valves and internal cavities must be taken apart or filled with the chemical.

Glutaraldehyde is toxic to living tissues, including the surgeon's eye. It must be carefully washed away with sterile water before the instrument is used. Properly used, activated glutaraldehyde is effective and safe: it has come under scrutiny because of potential dangers to staff in contact with it. In the first edition of this book, Gow reported circumferential irritation of his own eye, perhaps the earliest example of contact irritation, now frequently reported. Respiratory sensitivity may make it impossible for staff to work when there is glutaraldehyde present, and may lead to the introduction of expensive ventilation systems whose expense could perhaps have been better deployed in research into better methods of sterilizing equipment [17].

Radiation

Many urological disposable items are sterilized by gamma radiation. Expense means that this is only suitable on a massive scale. Even then radiation will darken the glass of lenses and fibrebundles.

References

1 Nitze M (1877) Verander an meinen electroendoskopishen Instrumenten zur Untersuchung der mamilischen Harnblase. *Illustr Monantschrt Artzl Polytech* 9: 59.
2 Gow JG (1976) Urological technology, in: Blandy JP (ed.) *Urology*, vol. 1, pp. 3–5. Oxford: Blackwell Scientific Publications.
3 Hopkins HH (1977) *British Patent Specification No. 954629*. London: HM Patent Office.
4 Baird JL (1927) *British Patent Specification No. 20969/27* London: HM Patent Office.
5 Hopkins HH, Kapany NS (1954) A flexible fibrescope using static scanning. *Nature* 173: 39.
6 Fowler CG, Badenoch DF, Thakar DR (1984) Practical experience with flexible cystoscopy in outpatients. *Br J Urol* 56: 618.
7 Davies AH, Mastorakou I, Dickinson AJ *et al.* (1991) Flexible cystoscopy compared with ultrasound in the detection of recurrent bladder tumours. *Br J Urol* 67: 491.
8 Anson K, Seenivasagam K, Miller R, Watson G (1994) The role of lasers in urology. *Br J Urol* 73: 225.
9 Kodama K, Doi O, Higashiyama M, Tatsuta M, Iwanaga T (1991) Surgical management of lung metastases: usefulness of resection with the neodymium: yttrium-aluminum garnet laser with median sternotomy. *J Thorac Cardiovasc Surg* 101: 901.
10 Costello AJ (1993) Treatment of prostatic obstruction with neodymium-YAG laser. *Br J Urol* 71: 71.
11 Turek PJ, Malloy TR, Cendron M, Cariniello VL, Wein AJ (1992) KTP-532 laser ablation of urethral strictures. *Urology* 40: 330.
12 Ruston MA, Fowler CG (1991) Lasers in the treatment of bladder cancer. *Br J Urol* 67: 449.
13 Riehle RA, Newman RC (eds) (1987) *Principles of Extracorporeal Shock Wave Lithotripsy*. New York: Churchill Livingstone.
14 Francis AE (1961) The use of a pasteurising water bath for disinfection of cystoscopes. *J Urol* 86: 679.
15 Alder VG, Brown AM, Gillespie WA (1966) Disinfection of heat sensitive material by low-temperature steam and formaldehyde. *J Clin Pathol* 19: 83.
16 Kelsey JC (1961) Sterilisation by ethylene oxide. *J Clin Pathol* 14: 59.
17 Cooke RPD, Feneley RCL, Ayliffe G, Lawrence WT, Emmerson AM, Greengrass SM (1993) Decontamination of urological equipment: interim report of a working group of the Standing Committee on Urological Instruments of the British Association of Urological Surgeons. *Br J Urol* 71: 5.

Chapter 2: Wound healing in the urinary tract

Healing of urothelium

If the urinary tract is divided and sewn together the edges will be bonded with fibrin, which will be invaded by small blood vessels to form granulation tissue, and gradually replaced by fibrous tissue which matures to form a scar in the course of the next few weeks. There are some unusual features about the process of healing in the urinary tract, because of the techniques used by urologists in making incisions, certain peculiarities of the tissues making up the urinary tract and because of the presence of urine.

Different methods of making surgical incisions

In urological operations alternatives to the classical scalpel are often required because so many operations are performed through endoscopes and there is a special need for perfect haemostasis. Such devices include diathermy, the neodymium-yttrium aluminium garnet (YAG) laser [1] and the 'ultrasonic scalpel' [2]. The price always paid for better haemostasis is more tissue damage, more wound induration and more infection [3,4].

When an ulcer in the skin heals the raw surface of granulations is covered by an advancing film of epithelium pushed in from all sides by mitotic activity at the edges of the defect [5]. The process is different in urothelium which always has abundant mitoses in every layer. This unexpected finding was first reported by Brauer [6] but was largely ignored until confirmed nearly 30 years later by Johnson and McMinn [7] who found that healing in the biliary tree, the salivary ducts and the urinary tract followed a different pattern to that of skin or intestinal mucosa. In the bladder, a defect is filled with the usual granulation tissue, but over this there rapidly spreads a thin film of urothelium in which mitoses are abundant in the growing edge, in contrast to skin and bowel where mitoses are only found some distance away from the edge (Fig. 2.1).

The original inwardly migrating thin film of epithelium becomes thicker and eventually takes on the features of normal urothelium. This has two important implications: (a) any cavity (such as a urinoma) which is in communication with the urinary tract may be relined with urothelium;

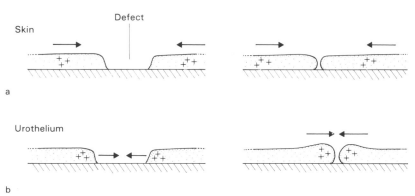

a

b

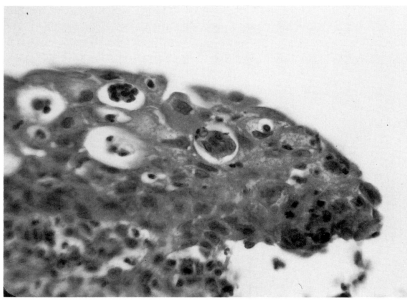

c

Fig. 2.1 (a) In skin and most epithelia mitosis only takes place behind the growing edge. (b) In urothelium there is active mitosis. (c) Photomicrograph of the growing edge showing numerous mitoses.

18

and (b) so rapid and effective is the regeneration of urothelium that it can cover over and bury little islands of the original damaged urothelium.

von Brunn's nests and metaplasia

A century ago von Brunn [8] described how these buried islands of urothelium would form cysts or 'nests'. Over a decade later Giani [9], studying the healing of transitional epithelium in dogs, observed every stage between burying of fragments of epithelium, the development of von Brunn's nests and full-blown cystitis cystica, and was able to create similar nests by implanting vesical epithelium.

Similar epithelial downgrowths caused by healing may occur in the skin where they give rise to innocent implantation dermoids [10] but in the urinary tract they are peculiarly dangerous. The little nests become progressively thicker until they actually form columnar epithelium (Figs 2.2 & 2.3).

Eventually, an area of cystitis cystica may be replaced by a patch of intestinal mucosa. In other mammals such patches of columnar mucosa are normal [11] but in man they are potentially malignant, and are followed by the development of adenocarcinoma [12−15].

Squamous metaplasia

Repeated inflammation and healing can lead to squamous metaplasia when there is chronic irritation or infection, e.g. with a calculus or bilharziasis, and upstream of a urethral stricture. The transitional urothelium changes into stratified squamous epithelium which forms keratin and comes to resemble the skin and, in the presence of urine, changes into a characteristic white plaque — leukoplakia (Fig. 2.4) — which is a precursor of cancer. It must be distinguished from the innocent 'vaginal metaplasia' which is a normal feature of the trigone [16]. The risk of malignant transformation probably varies from one site to another [17,18].

Heterotopic ossification

A graft of urothelium placed in contact with almost any type of connective tissue may induce the formation of heterotopic bone [7,19−21] (Fig. 2.5) which is most likely to be laid down in the vicinity of a foreign body such as a suture [22] but may be found whenever urothelium grows in an unusual site or is used as a graft, e.g. around the track of a chronic urinary fistula or around a urinoma or pseudocyst [23,24].

Regeneration of smooth muscle in the urinary tract

For many years it was believed that smooth muscle could regenerate across a gap in the bladder or the ureter. This was the basis for the intubated ureterotomy of Davis [25] where a stricture in the ureter was incised and a splint was left in for 6 weeks which became surrounded by fibrous tissue, lined with a film of urothelium,

Loss of urothelium

Cells buried under healing urothelium

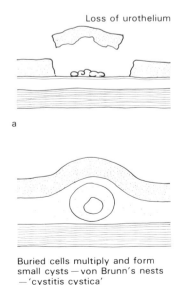

a

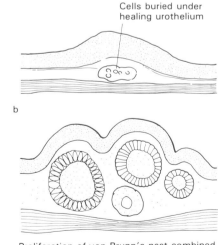

b

Buried cells multiply and form small cysts — von Brunn's nests — 'cystitis cystica'

Proliferation of von Brunn's nest combined with change from urothelium into mucus-secreting columnar epithelium — cystitis glandularis

Fig. 2.2 (a−d) A nest of cells may become buried under the healing urothelium.

c

d

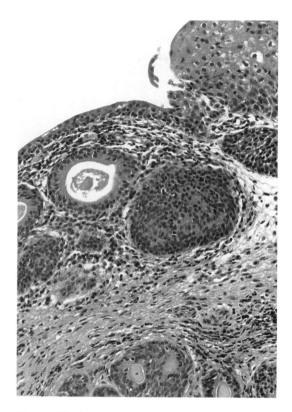

Fig. 2.3 The buried cells may form cysts (von Brunn's nests) under the urothelium, which then undergo metaplasia to form columnar epithelium.

and finally enclosed in smooth muscle. The same principle lay behind the idea that the bladder could regenerate after cystectomy, especially if a mould of plastic was left for it to grow over [26]. Today, it is believed that muscle does not truly

regenerate but spreads in from the cut margin of the urethra [27].

Particular effects of urine

The presence of urine modifies the normal process of healing in the urinary tract in the following three ways.

Necrosis

Urine may lead to necrosis of tissue. The most obvious example is the loss of skin and subcutaneous tissue that can follow extravasation of urine after injury to the perineal urethra when the entire skin of the penis, scrotum and lower abdomen may slough. It is not yet clear why urine should cause this necrosis but when such massive loss of tissue is seen other factors are usually present, e.g. hyperosmolarity, an alkaline pH or secondary infection. The subcutaneous injection of almost any fluid that is markedly hypertonic, acid or alkaline is well known to give rise to pain and inflammation and in practice even if infection is not present at first, it inevitably follows.

Necrosis associated with extravasation of urine is not confined to the skin and subcutaneous tissues. In the abdomen, extravasated urine from a leak after a cystectomy causes widespread necrosis of omentum.

Contracture

More important is the effect that urine has upon

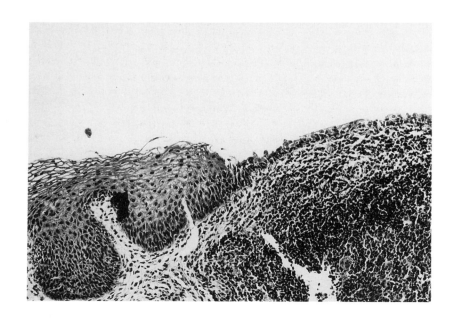

Fig. 2.4 Normal urothelium may undergo metaplasia into squamous epithelium.

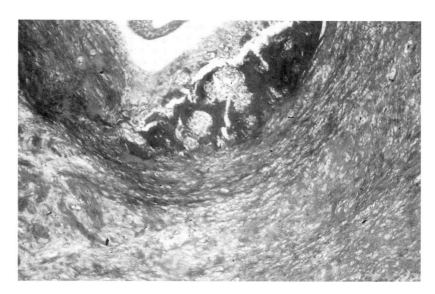

Fig. 2.5 Urothelium may induce the formation of heterotopic bone near connective tissue.

the contracture of scar tissue. All scars contract to some extent and contracture in scars which cross joints is a common problem for the plastic surgeon. In the urinary tract, shrinkage at the site of an anastomosis tends to lead to a stricture. Urine exacerbates the tendency for scars to contract and in the rat if urine is diverted from the site of an injury to the urethra the formation of a stricture may be prevented [28,29]. Avoiding this contracture calls for considerable ingenuity in planning anastomoses in the urinary tract. They are usually designed in the form of a long ellipse, so that even after contracture has taken place there will still be an adequate lumen (Fig. 2.6).

Calculus formation

Any stagnant pocket of undrained urine will encourage the formation of a stone. If in the vicinity of such a pocket there is also a foreign body, e.g. a knot of suture material or a fragment of necrotic tissue, then small stones are almost inevitable which may prevent the healing of a fistula.

Suture materials, splints, meshes and films

Suture materials

Some suture materials are absorbable, being digested by phagocytes or hydrolysed without any residue. Others are non-absorbable: though they may eventually break up they always leave foreign matter in the tissue. This may protect microorganisms from phagocytosis or the action of antimicrobial agents and perpetuate infection in the wound or the urinary tract. They also act as a nucleus for the formation of a stone.

Non-absorbable sutures are often the cause of a persistent sinus. Hence, whenever the urinary tract is to be opened, and especially when there has been infection in the urine, non-absorbable sutures are avoided even when ligating the renal artery and vein at nephrectomy, e.g. for pyonephrosis or an infected calculus. A sinus after nephrectomy caused by non-absorbable ligatures on the stump of the renal vessels will persist until the offending ligatures are removed, which can be both difficult and dangerous.

When other factors make it essential to use a non-absorbable suture, one must bear in mind that monofilament sutures have the advantage over braided or twisted ones in having a smaller surface area and no interstices in which bacteria may linger, so that the hazard of infection is reduced, though not eliminated.

Calculus formation is inevitable if a non-absorbable suture is left exposed to the urinary tract — even absorbable sutures such as plain catgut or polydioxanone may occasionally give rise to stones [30,31]. One near exception to the general rule that foreign material will form calculi is gold — used until recently as radioactive gold grains or radon seeds, but even this is not completely inert. Stone forms on the gold-plated wire used in prostatic spirals [32]. Even the most inert of other metals, e.g. haemostatic clips, can cause stones to form [33].

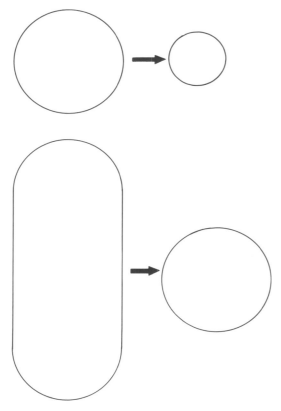

Fig. 2.6 To avoid stenosis, all anastomoses in the urinary tract are designed as an ellipse so that there will still be an adequate lumen even after contracture has taken place.

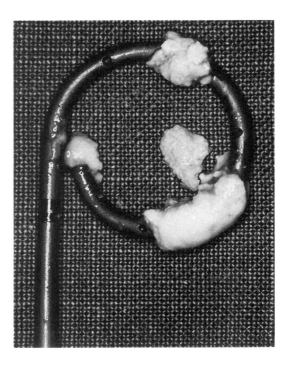

Fig. 2.7 Calculus formation on a double-J splint left in the ureter (courtesy of Mr P.F. Keane and the Editor *British Journal of Urology*).

Sutures placed right outside the urinary tract may, in the course of time, work their way like a cheesewire through living tissue until they come to lie within the urinary tract [34].

The tendency to form calculi does not seem to be related to the amount of histological reaction generated in the tissues. Even the most histologically inert plastics, e.g. silicone elastomer, may give rise to stone formation, sometimes with disastrous results when it occurs on a double-J splint left in the ureter [35,36] (Fig. 2.7).

A new generation of polymers made by joining acrylic acid to polyethylene, polytetrafluoroethylene or polypropylene by irradiation, to form cationic hydrogels have the advantage of swelling up with the absorption of water, but unfortunately even these are not immune from stone formation [37].

Catgut

Catgut is made from intestine from which the mucosa and muscle have been stripped, leaving only the collagen scaffold of the blood vessels of the muscularis mucosae. The oldest sewing material known to primitive man, who used it for bowstrings as well as in clothing, it is strong because it is virtually pure collagen. Its advantages were recognized by John Hunter's American disciple, Philip Syng Physick [38,39]. Its great drawback was that because it came from the intestine, it was likely to be contaminated with *Clostridia* spores and for a long time the problem of how to make it sterile defied the pioneers of antiseptic and aseptic surgery until Bulloch showed that even spores could be sterilized with 1% aqueous iodine [40]. Today, it is sterilized by gamma irradiation. Tanning the catgut with chromium salts makes it more slowly absorbed.

Catgut, being a foreign protein, is treated as such by the tissues of the body, which attack it with a classical inflammatory response, so that any anastomosis sewn with catgut is inevitably succeeded by swelling and some degree of granuloma.

Synthetic absorbable suture materials

Less inflammation is provoked by synthetic absorbable suture materials made of polyglycolic acid (PGA) or polyglactin (a copolymer of glycolide and lactide). These materials disappear because of the chemical action of hydrolysis rather than biological phagocytosis. These newer sutures are relatively strong for their size and keep their strength long after the healing tissue has reached its maximum tensile strength [41–42]. In the urinary tract they have two possible disadvantages: (a) since the knot is suspended in urine, it may take so long for the loop of the suture to hydrolyse that there will be time for a calculus to form; and (b) experimentally, it seems that urine may accelerate the hydrolysis of the suture material, especially in the presence of *Proteus* infection [43–44]. It is also possible that these sutures may be weakened by Renacidin [45].

Clearly the lesson is that the surgeon should choose the suture needed for the job. If it is only necessary that tissues must be held together for 3 or 4 days, and there is no tension, and no particular risk of leakage from a suture line or an anastomosis, then a rapidly disappearing material which gives rise to minimal inflammation has obvious advantages. Where there is a particular risk of leakage, and the tissues need to be held together for at least 10 days, then the advantage of using traditional chromic catgut may still outweigh the disadvantage of an increase in the tissue reaction.

Meshes and films

It is easy to weave a fabric from any of the materials listed above, and these have some useful surgical applications [46–48] but the same rules apply to them, i.e. non-absorbable material in contact with urine will form a stone, infection will persist so long as the foreign body is present and a sling or tape originally placed away from the urinary tract may migrate through the tissues. Most notorious for this are the slings used to support the neck of the bladder, which can work their way into the bladder to cause inflammation and calculi.

Absorbable mesh, film and sponge has been devised from collagen as well as the newer suture materials and used to reconstitute various parts of the urinary tract [49]. Lyophilized human dura mater offered a very strong sheet which was free of the disadvantages of non-absorbable materials and was used with enthusiasm [50–52] until it became apparent that it could carry the virus associated with Jakob–Creutzfeldt disease [53] and was abandoned. For extra strength collagen

films may be reinforced with a backing of silicone, omentum or polyglactin [54–55].

Other materials

Synthetic substitutes for bladder and ureter

The principles which apply to suture material in the urinary tract also apply to substances used to replace parts of the urinary tract, especially the bladder, urethra and ureter. There is a long history of attempts to remove the bladder and replace it with a hollow bag. In its most simple form it was a bag made of the patient's own collagen — in the form of the connective tissue thrown up around an acrylic mould [56] which later became lined with urothelium growing from the ends of the ureters and trigone. Since then, virtually every new suture material has been used experimentally to provide a substitute for the bladder or ureter [57] but so far without success: connective tissue contracts and synthetic materials lead to stones and infection.

Metal staples and clips

Staples of stainless steel or titanium are widely used for ligating vessels and for anastomosing intestine and creating non-refluxing nipples and valves. Stones do form upon them, but perhaps because the staples in question are small most of these stones pass without difficulty and this, so far, seems to have caused little trouble [58].

Injected Teflon and collagen paste

Teflon is a commercial product made of tetrafluoroethylene which does not become wet or stick to other substances, hence its widespread use in cooking utensils and as a coating for catheters and sutures. A stiff paste of Teflon particles in glycerine may be injected to provide bulk where it is needed, e.g. in plastic surgery, under the ureterovesical orifice to prevent reflux [59,60], and around the bladder neck to prevent incontinence [61]. Fine particles of Teflon have been found to migrate to the brain and lung [62] and it is not known whether or not they do any harm there though this has led to misgivings about its use to correct reflux in children with a long life expectancy.

A product with similar putty-like properties capable of giving bulk to a tissue has been prepared from a paste of glutaraldehyde crosslinked collagen which is reputedly equally useful in preventing reflux, without the possible risks of harmful particles migrating elsewhere [63].

References

1 Beisland HO, Sander S (1990) Neodymium YAG laser irradiation of stage T2 muscle-invasive bladder cancer: long-term results. *Br J Urol* 65: 24.

2 Boddy SAM, Ramsay JWA, Carter S StC, Webster P, Levinson DA, Whitfield HN (1987) Tissue effects of an ultrasonic scalpel for clinical surgical use. *Urol Res* 15: 49.

3 Madden JE, Edlich RF, Custer JR, Panek PH, Thul J, Wangensteen OH (1970) Studies in the management of the contaminated wound IV. Resistance to infection of surgical wounds made by knife, electrosurgery, and laser. *Am J Surg* 119: 222.

4 Edlich RF, Rodeheaver GT, Thacker JG, Edgerton MT (1977) *Fundamentals of Wound Management in Surgery: Technical Factors in Wound Management.* New Jersey: Cirurgecom Inc.

5 Billingham RE, Medawar PB (1955) Contracture and intussusceptive growth in the healing of extensive wounds in mammalian skin. *J Anat* 89: 114.

6 Brauer A (1927) The regeneration of transitional epithelium. *Anat Rec* 33: 137.

7 Johnson FR, McMinn RMH (1956) Transitional epithelium and osteogenesis. *J Anat* 90: 106.

8 von Brunn A (1893) Ueber drusenahnliche Bildungen in der Schleimhaut der Nierenbeckens, des Ureters, und der Harnblase beim Menschen. *Archiv Mikroscop Anat* 41: 294.

9 Giani R (1907) Neuer experimenteller Beitrag zur Entstehung der Cystitis Cystica. *Beitr Path Anat* 42: 1.

10 Gillman T, Penn J, Bronks D, Roux M (1953) Reactions of healing wounds and granulation tissue in man to auto-Thiersch, autodermal and homodermal grafts. *Br J Plast Surg* 6: 153.

11 Johnson FR (1957) Some proliferative and metaplastic changes in transitional epithelium. *Br J Urol* 29: 112.

12 de la Pena A, Oliveros M, Tamames JM, Mintz S (1959) Metaplastic and malignant changes of the urothelium. *Br J Urol* 31: 473.

13 Lin JI, Tseng CH, Choy C, Yong HS, Sarsidi PS, Pilloff B (1988) Diffuse cystitis glandularis. *Urology* 15: 411.

14 Cea PC, Ward JW, Lavengood RW, Gray GF (1977) Mesonephric adenocarcinomas in urethral diverticular. *Urology* 10: 58.

15 Navarre RJ, Loening RW, Gray GF (1977) Nephrogenic adenoma: a report of nine cases and review of the literature. *J Urol* 127: 775.

16 Roberts M, Smith P (1976) Disorders of the female urethra, in: Blandy JP (ed.) *Urology*, vol. 2, pp. 963–79. Oxford: Blackwell Scientific Publications.

17 Morgan RJ, Cameron KM (1980) Vesical leukoplakia. *Br J Urol* 52: 96.

18 O'Flynn JD, Mullaney J (1974) Vesical leukoplakia progressing to carcinoma. *Br J Urol* 46: 31.

19 Huggins CB, McCarroll HR, Blocksom BH (1936) Experiments on the theory of osteogenesis: the influence of local calcium deposits on ossification: the osteogeneic stimulus of epithelium. *Arch Surg* 32: 915.

20 Johnson FR, McMinn RMH (1955) The behaviour of implantation grafts of bladder mucosa. *J Anat* 89: 450.

21 Blandy JP, McDonald JH (1961) Heterotopic ossification in uroepithelial regeneration on grafts of ileum and colon. *Surg Forum* 12: 498.

22 Blandy JP (1963) *Substitutes for the urinary bladder*, 2: Appendix C. DM thesis, University of Oxford.

23 Hall BK, Van Exan RJ (1982) Induction of bone by epithelial cell products. *J Embryol Exp Morphol* 69: 37.

24 Segen JC, Mahadeva P (1986) Heterotopic bone formation near a ligated ureter. *J Urol* 135: 124.

25 Davis DM (1943) Intubated ureterotomy: a new operation for ureteral and uretero-pelvic strictures. *Surg Gynec Obstet* 76: 513.

26 Bohne AW, Osborn RW, Hettle PJ (1955) Regeneration of the urinary bladder in the dog following total cystectomy. *Surg Gynecol Obstet* 100: 259.

27 Swinney J, Tomlinson BE, Walder DN (1961) Urinary tract substitution. *Br J Urol* 33: 414.

28 Singh M, Scott TM (1975) The ultrastructure of human male urethral stricture. *Br J Urol* 47: 871.

29 Singh M, Blandy JP (1976) The pathology of urethral strictures. *J Urol* 115: 673.

30 Norris MA, Toquri AG, Waquespack B (1982) Calcification on chromic suture. *Urology* 20: 172.

31 Morris MC, Baquero A, Redovan E, Mahoney E, Bannett AD (1986) Urolithiasis on absorbable and non-absorbable suture materials in the rabbit bladder. *J Urol* 135: 602.

32 Holmes SAV, Miller PD, Crocker PR, Kirby RS (1992) Encrustation of intraprostatic stents: a comparative study. *Br J Urol* 69: 383.

33 Miedema EB, Redman JF (1982) Radiolucent urethral calculus with hemostatic clip nidus. *Urology* 19: 328.

34 Ehrenpreis MD, Alarcon JA, Firfer R (1986) Case profile: large bladder calculus post cervical cirlage. *Urology* 27: 366.

35 Antoine JA (1986) Case profile: double-J catheter encrustation. *Urology* 28: 436.

36 Keane PF, Bonner MC, Johnston SR, Zafar A, Gorman SP (1994) Characterization of biofilm and encrustation on ureteric stents *in vivo*. *Br J Urol* 73: 687.

37 Ford TF, Parkinson MC, Fydelor FJ, Ringrose BJ, Wickham JEA (1985) A preliminary *in vivo* assessment of acrylic acid graft-copolymers in the urinary tract. *J Urol* 133: 141.

38 Physick PS (1795) cited in: Kuss R, Gregoir W (1795) *Histoire Illustree de l'Urologie*, p. 214. Paris: Dacosta.

39 Adams J (1817) *Memoirs of the Life and Doctrines of the Late John Hunter.* London: Callow.

40 Bulloch W (1929) The preparation of catgut for surgical use. *Special Report Series No. 138.* London: Medical Research Council.

41 Miller HC (1973) Reaction of polyglycolic acid sutures in the urinary tract. *Urology* 2: 47.

42 Osterhage HR, Grun BR, Judmann G, Wunsch HP (1988) Experimenteller Vergleich von Maxon und Chrom-Catgut bei der Naht der Harnblase. *Urologe (A)* 27: 61.

43 El-Mahrouky A, McElhaney J, Bartone FF, King L

(1987) *In vitro* comparison of the properties of polydioxanone, polyglycolic acid and catgut sutures in sterile and infected urine. *J Urol* 138: 913.

44 Crocker RH Jr, Lage AL, Parsonnet J, Richie JP (1988) The physical properties of polyglactin 910 (Vicryl) chromic gut and polydioxanone (PDS) in sterile and infected canine urine. *J Urol* 139: 337A.

45 Sarnacki CT, Satrom KD, Foster CD, Jackson WG, Novicki DE (1986) Effect of Renacidin on suture material. *Urology* 28: 391.

46 Lowe DH, Ho PC, Parsons CL, Schmidt JD (1982) Surgical treatment of Peyronie disease with Dacron graft. *Urology* 19: 609.

47 Clark-Pearson DL, Soper JT, Creasman WT (1988) Absorbable synthetic mesh (Polyglactin 910) for the formation of a pelvic 'lid' after radical pelvic resection. *Am J Obstet Gynecol* 158: 158.

48 Schoenenberger A, Mattler D, Roesler H *et al.* (1985) Surgical repair of the kidney after blunt lesions of intermediate degrees using a Vicryl mesh: an experimental study. *J Urol* 134: 804.

49 Tachibana M, Nagamatsu GR, Addonizio JC (1985) Ureteral replacement using collagen sponge tube grafts. *J Urol* 133: 866.

50 Kelami A (1981) Transposition of polar vessels of kidney using lyophilized human dura. *Urology* 18: 187.

51 Kelami A (1980) Peyronie disease and surgical treatment. *Urology* 15: 559.

52 Serrallach N, Gutierrez R, Serrate R *et al.* (1985) Renal allograft rupture: surgical treatment by renal corsetage with lyophilized human dura. *J Urol* 133: 452−5.

53 Masullo C, Pocchiari M, Macchi G, Alema G, Piazza G, Panzera MA (1989) Transmission of Creutzfeldt−Jakob disease by dural cadaveric graft. *J Neurosurg* 71: 954.

54 Diamond DA, Ransley PG (1986) Bladder neck reconstruction with omentum, silicone and augmentation cystoplasty — a preliminary report. *J Urol* 136: 252.

55 Gorham SD, Monsour MJ, Scott R (1987) The *in-vitro* assessment of a collagen/vicryl (Polyglactin) composite film together with candidate suture materials for use in urinary tract surgery I. Physical testing. *Urol Res* 15: 53.

56 Bohne AW, Urwiller KL (1957) Experience with urinary bladder regeneration. *J Urol* 77: 725.

57 Holmes SAV, Kirby RS, Whitfield HN (1993) Urinary tract prostheses and their biocompatibility. *Br J Urol* 71: 378.

58 Brenner M, Johnson DE (1985) Ileal conduit calculi from stapler anastomosis: a long term complication? *Urology* 26: 537.

59 O'Donnell B, Puri P (1986) Endoscopic correction of primary vesicoureteric reflux. *Br J Urol* 58: 601.

60 Dodat H (1990) Treatment of vesicoureteral reflux in children by endoscopic injection of Teflon. Review of 2 years experience. *Eur Urol* 17: 304.

61 Harrison SCW, Brown C, O'Boyle PJ (1993) Periurethral Teflon for stress urinary incontinence: medium term results. *Br J Urol* 71: 25.

62 Aaronson IA (1995) Current status of the 'Sting': an American perspective. *Br J Urol* 75: 121.

63 Waxman SW, Webster GD (1994) Open surgery versus minimally invasive alternatives in the management of stress incontinence. *Curr Opinion Urol* 4: 63.

Chapter 3: Principles of urological oncology

Mitotic cycle

Some cells continue to divide throughout the normal lifespan of the individual, others (e.g. in the central nervous system) never divide once the adult stage has been reached. Cells divide at very different rates, some rapidly, others slowly, but they all follow a cycle which is governed in part by the limitations on the size of any cell whose nutrients must diffuse across the cell membrane.

The cell turnover rate can be measured by how much tritiated thymidine is taken up by its DNA, and this technique identifies four phases in the cycle (Fig. 3.1). First, there is a relatively long gap (G_1) after the previous cell division when the newly divided cell seems to be resting. Mitosis takes about 1 h, and cells may live for hours or years — and the difference depends on the duration of this first gap (G_1).

The next phase of protein synthesis (S) is switched on by some signal, and DNA is now rapidly synthesized until its original quantity has been exactly doubled when a second signal switches off the process of synthesis. There follows a second relatively short gap (G_2) between the completion of DNA synthesis and the beginning of mitosis.

Increasingly the genes controlling these signal substances (chalones) are being identified, e.g. in tissue culture of human skin extracts of epidermis will stop further mitosis [1].

A different kind of inhibition is seen in tissue culture, when the growing edge of one film of cells bumps into another — contact inhibition. Interestingly, in cultures of cancer tissues this contact inhibition is no longer present.

Hormones may influence the cycle of cell division, either by affecting the activity of RNA proliferase which controls protein synthesis, or the interaction between it and DNA.

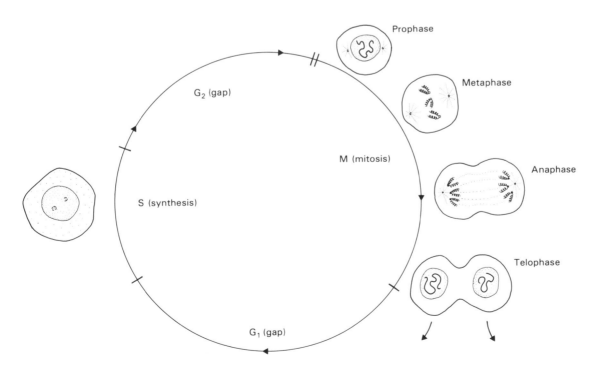

Fig. 3.1 Mitotic cycle.

Tumour growth and the Gompertzian curve

Tumour doubling time (DT) depends upon the difference between the rates of cell division and cell death (apoptosis). In growing tissues and in cancer the rate of cell division outstrips that of apoptosis but even in cancer, cell division does not continue indefinitely at a uniform rate: as it enlarges the growth of a tumour is slowed down — the Gompertzian effect (Fig. 3.2).

When tumours are small the doubling time is more or less constant. Imagine a single cell which has undergone some crucial genetic change making it no longer answerable to the normal controls over cell growth. After 20 DTs there will be 10^6 cells in the clone — only about 1 mg of tumour — far too small to be detected by any known diagnostic method. After another 10 DTs the resulting 10^9 cells will weigh 1 g and still be detectable only on the face or in the bladder.

After another 10 DTs the tumour will now have 10^{12} cells and weigh 1 kg [2]. Such a large tumour would have slowed its rate of growth to follow the Gompertzian curve (Fig. 3.3).

We can never really measure tumour DT, but it seems to vary greatly with different cancers — from weeks to years. In terms of DT, the tiny tumour which seems 'early' to the surgeon has already been present for two-thirds of its possible natural life.

Carcinogenesis

Three important activities distinguish malignant from normal tissue: (a) the capacity to continue to grow without regard to the normal constraints of the body; (b) the ability to invade adjacent normal tissue; and (c) the ability to metastasize.

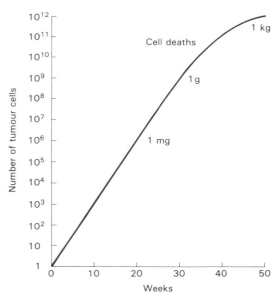

Fig. 3.2 The Gompertzian curve — cell division slows down as the tumour enlarges.

For each of these three activities, so essential to the 'success' of the tumour in killing its host, certain enzymes are deployed by the tumour.

Unlimited growth. The lizard's tail illustrates this central enigma of biology. John Hunter [3] observed that if the lizard's tail is cut off, a new one grows from the stump until it has reached the length of the old one — no more and no less (Fig. 3.4). Among the factors responsible for this tissue regeneration are the growth factors and the vascular neogenesis factor [4].

Invasion. To invade adjacent normal tissue cancers deploy enzymes, e.g. hyaluronidase and metalloproteinases, which dissolve intercellular

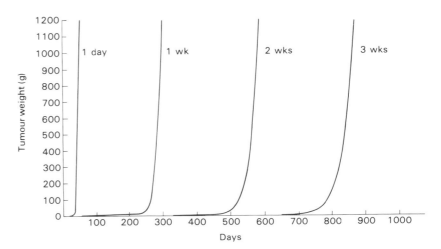

Fig. 3.3 Theoretical weight of tumours of different doubling times (1 day–3 weeks). Whatever its inherent rate of growth, the small tumour that seems 'early' to the surgeon has already been present for at least two-thirds of its natural life.

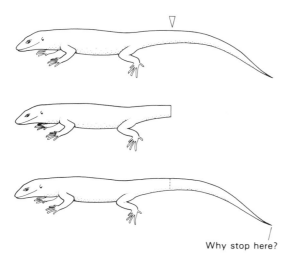

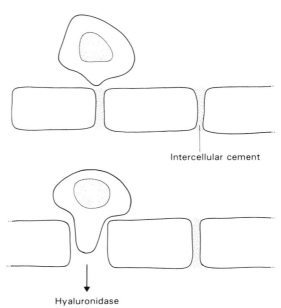

Why stop here?

Fig. 3.4 Normal healing is limited, e.g. a lizard's tail regenerates to its former length. In cancer the natural limiting factors are absent.

Intercellular cement

Hyaluronidase

Fig. 3.5 To invade adjacent tissues a cancer must produce enzymes, e.g. hyaluronidase, which dissolve intercellular cement.

cement (Fig. 3.5). Cancers go on producing these enzymes long after the normal switch-off signals that regulate cell growth and repair [5].

Metastases. When clusters of 'abnormal' cells escape into the circulation, the HLA (human leucocyte antigen) antigens on their cell surface are recognized by the killer T cells which exert local growth controls. Many cancers fail to express these HLA antigens and so escape immune surveillance.

Oncogenes

For every enzyme there is one gene. Genes are helices of DNA strung together in the chromosomes which coil and uncoil in different phases of mitosis. In prophase they are coiled in tight, brittle lengths which are apt to break and stick to each other so that there may be crossing over of whole lengths of a chromosome during mitosis (Fig. 3.6).

Sometimes whole chromosomes are entirely duplicated. Sometimes quite small lengths — even single genes — can become inserted into an adjoining chromosome. This is made use of in modern gene technology which exploits the circular lengths of DNA found in some bacteria. These resemble a bracelet with a snap: the snap is opened by one enzyme (restriction endonuclease) and shut by another (DNA ligase) (Fig. 3.7).

While the snap is open a passenger length of DNA can be inserted, and the snap then closed to produce recombinant DNA. By choosing an

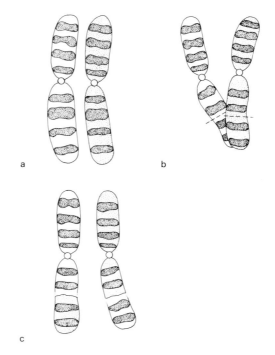

Fig. 3.6 (a–c) In prophase parts of chromosomes may stick to each other or become exchanged.

appropriate length of DNA known to make the desired protein the host bacteria can be farmed and the appropriate protein harvested.

In some diseases there is a similar defect in a single enzyme controlled and inherited by a single gene. Alcaptonuria is a good example:

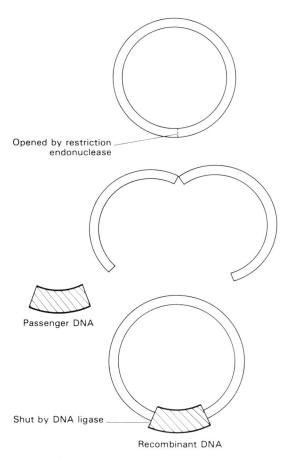

Opened by restriction
endonuclease

Passenger DNA

Shut by DNA ligase

Recombinant DNA

Fig. 3.7 The circular DNA of some bacteria may be 'snapped' open by restriction endonuclease allowing a passenger length of DNA to be inserted. The snap is then closed by DNA ligase.

lack of a single gene leads to deficiency of the enzyme homogentisic oxidase [6].

Oncogenes and viruses

Some RNA viruses have amino acid sequences which are almost but not exactly the same as those of a natural gene. If such a virus also possesses the enzyme reverse transcriptase it can create a copy of itself in DNA, which will be taken up into the DNA of the nucleus, like a kind of genetic cuckoo, where it may perform some of the functions of the normal protooncogene, but no longer respond to the appropriate switch-off signals. DNA from a human bladder cancer cell line was put into normal mouse fibroblasts which promptly underwent malignant transformation (in tissue culture this means losing the property of contact inhibition and no longer undergoing senescence). This DNA was similar to an oncogene in cells infected with mouse sarcomavirus,

and it was later found in about 10% of new human bladder tumours [7].

Today, there is a growing list of factors involved in tumour growth and invasion which can be assigned to specific oncogenes. For many others the controlling gene has yet to be identified. The bogus genes all fail to respond to the switch-off signals when growth or repair has reached the appropriate limit.

Sometimes the difference between the normal protooncogene and the lethal oncogene may be as trivial as one misplaced amino acid in a sequence of many hundreds [8,9]. The replacement of a single peptide in the alpha chain of haemoglobin can result in the lethal sickle-cell haemoglobin (HbS) of sickle-cell disease [10].

Two categories of RNA tumour viruses are recognized according to how quickly they work — slow and acutely transforming retroviruses. Slow viruses must first react with the host genome to produce an acutely transforming retrovirus. The acutely transforming retroviruses actually carry the alien oncogenes.

Some of these viruses are widespread. Human papillomavirus, which may be important in the aetiology of cancer of the cervix, vagina and vulva, is present in about half of men with warts and in another third who seem to have normal penile skin. One in five normal urethral biopsies were found to harbour oncogenic papillomaviruses though not in serum or urine [11].

It is in the brittle stage of prophase between G1 and S that the chromosomes are most vulnerable to outside influences. Ionizing radiation may cause short chains of genetic material to fall out of the DNA strand. Missing nucleotides are rapidly cemented back into position by the polynucleotide ligase enzyme, but not always in the correct order: and the wrong sequence may act either as a faulty gene or cause malfunction of genes on each side of it (Fig. 3.8). Such a bogus gene — a lookalike oncogene — may function normally for nearly all the time but fail to respond to a switch-off signal [10]. (The normal gene that has been replaced by the bogus one is called a protooncogene.)

An alkylating agent can insert a single pair of bases into a chromosome during the S phase and this trivial alteration could lead to a mutation [12].

The genes responsible for the growth factors can be altered by crossing over or reduplication of whole lengths of chromosomes during normal mitosis. One example of this is the Philadelphia chromosome present in the bone marrow of patients with chronic myelogeneous leukaemia

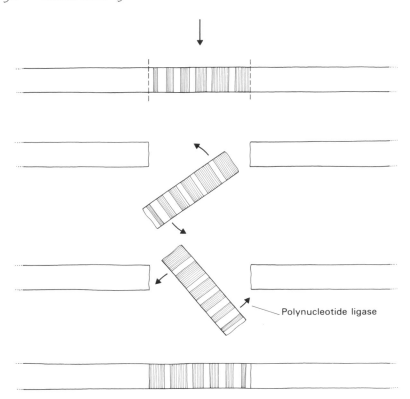

Polynucleotide ligase

Fig. 3.8 Ionizing radiation may dislodge short lengths of genetic material which may be cemented back in the wrong sequence.

[13]. Here part of the long arm of chromosome 22 has stuck to the long arm of chromosome 9. As the disease progresses the chromosomes becomes increasingly bizarre: duplicates appear for the Philadelphia chromosome as well as for chromosomes 8 and 17.

Other examples are retinoblastomas where there is loss of a specific segment of chromosome 13, and in certain lymphomas where is a specific abnormality of chromosome 14 [10].

It is not yet known how many protooncogenes there are in the human genome, nor how many of these factors are involved in carcinogenesis. Whatever the ultimate number, if there is one protooncogene for each factor concerned with each step in the processes of growth, invasion and metastasis, then it follows that tumours become progressively more malignant in a series of steps [14].

Growth factors

Growth factors are polypeptide sequences released by many cells [4]. Several of them can be detected in human bladder cancer cell lines especially in the more invasive tumours. Not all growth factors lead to proliferation of cells but some such as the tumour growth factor beta (TGFβ) have the opposite effect and inhibit cell

division [15]. Failure to respond to a normal switch-off signal could result from changes in the genes expressing growth factor, their receptors or an inhibitory factor [8]. Oncogenes may affect malignant transformation in other ways, e.g. *fos*, *myc* and *jun* speed up the transcription of some of the genes needed for cell proliferation [16].

In urological cancer the *ras* oncogene is present in many bladder tumours as well as in the prostate and kidney, though its function is unknown [17]. The oncogene *c-myc-p62* (*c-myc*) is found in superficial bladder tumours though not in invasive ones [18]. A defective *meg* oncogene leaves cells able to repair damage caused by radiation, but not by alkylating agents [19]. So efficient are the repair mechanisms within the nucleus that although many things can damage DNA, neoplastic change is the exception. Many cells may undergo early premalignant changes but only a few go through to the final changes [20].

Tumour angioneogenesis factor

A tumour that is more than 2 mm in diameter can no longer rely on the diffusion of oxygen and nutrients through the tissues. To survive it has to be able to attract new blood vessels towards it (Fig. 3.9). William Harvey realized this ingrowth

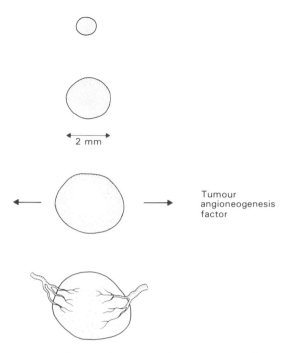

Fig. 3.9 Diffusion of oxygen and nutrients can only supply a tumour < 2 mm in diameter, to grow bigger it must attract ingrowth of capillaries by tumour angioneogenesis factor.

of new blood vessels to be a factor which was just as necessary to the growth of cancers as it was to the growing embryo of the chick [21]. Tumours attract this ingrowth of new blood vessels by secreting tumour angioneogenesis factor [22]. It is switched off in resting cells.

Initiation and promotion

In the experimental animal there are two distinct phases in starting off a cancer — initiation and promotion. Giving a mouse benzopyrine may, in time, give rise to cancer, but if other substances are added, which by themselves only cause inflammation (e.g. croton oil), the onset of the cancer may be greatly accelerated. This gives rise to the concept of initiation, where presumably the genome is changed, and promotion, whereby another set of genes are attacked to speed up the neoplastic process. Substances which cause this synergistic promotion, are sometimes called cocarcinogens. This is particularly relevant for cancer of the bladder where many factors — infection, obstruction, the presence of a calculus — can all act as promotors to the initiating factor which may be an industrial carcinogen or smoking.

Immune factors and tumour spread

The evidence for immunological control of tumour growth and metastasis is tantalizingly patchy and disjointed. Mice may be immunized against one form of leukaemia by an inoculum of irradiated leukaemia cells. In another form of mouse leukaemia, a missing antigen can be put back into the cells by a vaccine, making them benign again [20].

Tumours flourish when the immune system is suppressed. A tumour which usually does not metastasize may do so with immunosuppression. A surgical operation may itself be immunosuppressive and accelerate tumour growth in experimental animals, explaining why tumours sometimes seem to explode with metastases shortly after an operation. In the cervix oncogenic human papillomaviruses types 16 and 18 are associated with a reduction in the numbers of Langhans' cells [23,24].

The importance of the immune response to cancer can be exploited, nowhere with more success than in human bladder cancer, where intravesical bacille Calmette–Guérin (BCG) appears to activate killer T cells to destroy cancers usually resistant to their attack (Fig. 3.10). Less remarkable has been the success of interferon in Kaposi's sarcoma and renal cell carcinoma [25].

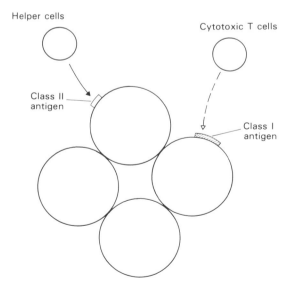

Fig. 3.10 Usually killer T cells will recognize foreign class I antigens on the cell surface. This recognition fails to occur in cancer, but may be stimulated by bacille Calmette–Guérin (BCG).

Metastasis

Specific clones of malignant cells home to a specific organ and tumours appear to be programmed by their HLA antigens to metastasize to certain end organs — a phenomenon first demonstrated in tumours of the bladder and testis [26–28].

If cells invaded by alien oncogenes continue to replicate despite signals to stop, they express fewer and fewer HLA antigens and so progressively escape immune surveillance.

Chemotherapy

Most drugs used against cancer act by inhibiting cell division, but there are a few which act regardless of the mitotic cycle. Some work only at one phase of mitosis; others throughout. Most chemotherapeutic regimes have been arrived at empirically, and efforts to rationalize their action by referring to a supposed point of action have been disappointing. In general, tumours with the quickest mitotic cycle are the most sensitive to chemotherapy.

The effectiveness of chemotherapy, i.e. response and survival, is related to the patient's performance status measured by the Karnofsky scale (Table 3.1) as well as tumour sensitivity to treatment [29].

Because most chemotherapeutic agents act against dividing cells, those cells in the body which normally divide most quickly, e.g. the mucosa of the bowel and the bone marrow, are susceptible to chemotherapy. Because of their action on the bone marrow, immunity against infection is also depressed.

Radiotherapy

The ability of radiation to penetrate tissues is related to radiation energy: the greater the energy the deeper the penetration [30].

The old measure of ionizing radiation, the röntgen, was related to the number of ionizations produced by radiation in air. Later this was replaced by the radian, which was defined in terms of the energy absorbed during the interaction of radiation with tissue (1 gray = 100 rad).

There are certain differences in the effect upon tissues of radiation from sources with different energy. This is particularly important in skin and bone. With conventional 240 kV X-rays most of the absorption is at the surface of the skin; for gamma rays emitted by cobalt$_{60}$ the maximum

Table 3.1 Karnofsky performance scale

Normal: no complaints: no evidence of disease	100
Able to carry on normal activity: minor signs or symptoms of disease	90
Normal activity with effort: some signs or symptoms of disease	80
Cares for self: unable to carry on normal activity or do active work	70
Able to care for most self needs: requires occasional assistance	60
Requires occasional considerable assistance and frequent medical care	50
Disabled: requires special care and assistance	40
Severely disabled: hospitalization is indicated although death not imminent	30
Very sick: hospitalization necessary: active supportive treatment is necessary	20
Dead	0

absorption is about 5 mm below the surface; and with 8 MeV linear accelerator megavoltage the maximum absorption is about 20 mm below the skin surface, hence the considerably lessened damage to the skin with megavoltage radiation (Fig. 3.11).

In bone, lower energy radiation produces a higher absorbed dose, compared with that from megavoltage irradiation. In order to achieve a high dose in the cancer and the least possible in the surrounding healthy tissue radiotherapists use multiple ports of entry. The crossfire builds up the appropriate dose in the target while minimizing surface damage (Fig. 3.12). Today, the calculation of the correct distribution of radiation — the radiation isodose curve — is carried out by means of a computer linked to the image of the tumour in the computerized tomography (CT) scanner.

The early morbidity after radiotherapy results from three processes: (a) acute inflammation; (b) the death of stem cells; and (c) the vascular response. The early changes are most marked in the skin and the bowel where cell turnover is most rapid, but because enough stem cells remain, these epithelia usually recover.

Late morbidity results from the aftermath of the inflammatory process — fibrosis and the late consequences of the changes within the small blood vessels which lead to ischaemia and, at its worst, necrosis. At any one time relatively few cells are at the most vulnerable stage when the long G1 gap is giving way to the S phase frenzy of DNA synthesis — the tiny window in time when they are most affected by ionizing radiation.

Radiation treatment schedules are designed

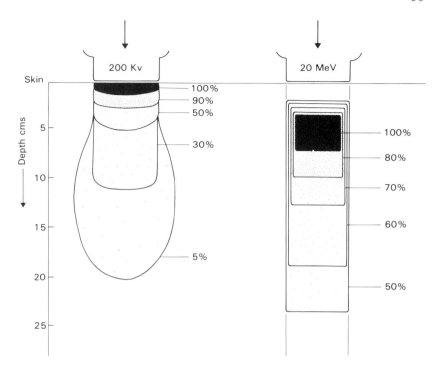

Fig. 3.11 With higher energy radiation there is less absorption at the skin level.

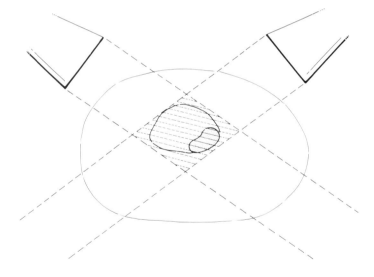

Fig. 3.12 Using multiple ports of entry crossfire builds up the dose of radiation to the deeply seated target, e.g. a bladder cancer, while sparing the surrounding tissues.

empirically though they may be based on model systems (e.g. the cell survival curves of tissue cultures) which suggest the advantage of giving the radiation in repeated fractions. Nevertheless, the design of courses of treatment continues to be largely an empirical art in which clinical judgement and experience continues to be of crucial importance. It is hard-won experience which has taught the lesson that small volume irradiation is tolerated better than large [30]. Radiosensitivity varies with oxygen tension.

More radiation is needed to kill anoxic cells and all tumours contain hypoxic cells in their centres which may remain viable at low oxygen tensions. After radiation these hypoxic cells seem to become reoxygenated — another reason for fractionation.

There have been immense efforts to improve the results of radiation therapy by giving the irradiation under hyperbaric oxygen. Two trials have however shown only equivocal results [31,32].

Radiosensitizing agents

Much effort has been spent on increasing the differential effect of radiation on cancer and normal tissues. Oxygen was the first to be used, on the principle that anoxic tissues were radioresistant but in practice it was of no value [31,32]. One group of drugs mimic the radiosensitizing effect of oxygen on hypoxic cells. These included metronidaxone and misonidaxone, but clinical trials with these compounds revealed an unacceptable level of neurotoxicity [33].

The agent 5-fluorouracil has been used as a cytotoxic agent which is incorporated into the cell during the S phase. It had an additive effect in combination with radiation. The closely related agent, 5-bromodeoxyruridine (5-BUDR) is a true sensitizer but sensitizes normal as well as tumour tissues and has no therapeutic value. These drugs are only incorporated into the cell during the S phase.

Radiosensitivity of the kidney

The normal kidney is exceedingly sensitive to radiation. A dose of 2300 rad within 5 weeks will give rise to an 'acute nephritis' appearing after 6—12 months to be followed shortly afterwards by malignant hypertension. Clinically, there is albuminuria and hypertension. Histologically, there is perinephric fibrosis; thickening of the renal capsule; interstitial oedema, capillary dilatation, swelling of glomerular endothelial cells and thickening of tufts leading inexorably to fibrosis; hyaline obliteration and fibrinoid necrosis in glomeruli and the other features of end-stage renal disease. This is prevented by careful shielding of the kidney.

Bladder side effects

In the bladder, the aftermath of radiation is of considerable clinical importance. Its severity varies from one patient to another, and is largely unpredictable. At first, there is an acute 'radiation cystitis' resembling ordinary bacterial cystitis, and often made worse by coexisting infection [34]. This is succeeded 6 months to a year later by chronic radiation cystitis. The patient has more or less severe frequency and often haematuria. Cystoscopically, the bladder is diffusely red and injected. Biopsy shows typically hyaline changes in the submucosal tissue. Essentially the process is ischaemic and it continues to get slowly worse. In severe forms it is complicated by ischaemic necrosis of the tissue leading to a fistula into the rectum or vagina or both.

Phototherapy

For many years the fluorescence of malignant tissues with tetracycline and other dyes was used as an aid in the diagnosis of tumours in the larynx and to some extent for carcinoma *in situ* in the bladder. Experimentally, it was found that when enough light was used of the right wavelength, tissues stained with these dyes could be destroyed, because the absorbed light produced singlet oxygen which was cytotoxic.

Kelly *et al.* [35] found that a derivative of haematoporphyrin could sensitize human bladder tumours grown in nude mice, and later confirmed this in human bladder cancers [36,37]. It was not long before a more active fraction of haematoporphyrin was isolated (dihaematoporphyric ether — DHE or Photofrin II). This was used for treatment of bladder tumours [38].

These agents were given systemically, so that all tissues were stained, and the effect of light depended on the cancers taking up more of the dye than normal tissues. The original light source was mercury vapour, emitting ultraviolet light. Later a more accurate wavelength was provided by a tuneable dye laser. The systemic photosensitizing agents made the patient sensitive to light, and for 6—8 weeks after treatment they had to stay in the shade or else they would develop severe sunburn.

Because there was such a small margin between the uptake by cancer and normal tissues, in practice the deeper layers of the bladder wall were damaged, muscle being replaced by fibrous tissue, which contracted to leave a small bladder with ureteric reflux [39—41]. Nevertheless, the bladder tumours did respond, the more so when there had been previous irradiation [42].

The search continues for agents that are taken up by tumour tissue and not by normal tissue, and that can be given intravesically so as to avoid systemic sensitization. Chloro-aluminium sulphonated phthalocyanine shows promise in animal studies [43]. Until this, or some similar agent, becomes available for clinical use, the method is unlikely to have more than a very limited application, especially considering the cost of the tuneable dye laser light source.

References

1 Blunt MJ (1981) Development — growth and ageing, in: Burnett W (ed.) *Clinical Science for Surgeons*, pp. 23—34. London: Butterworths.

2 Forbes JT (1981) Neoplasia, in: Burnett W (ed.) *Clinical Science for Surgeons*, pp. 74—86. London: Butterworths.

3 Hunter J (1861) in: Owen R (ed.) *Essays and Observations on Natural History, Anatomy, Physiology and Geology*. London: Van Hoorst.

4 Mydlo JH, Macchia RJ (1992) Growth factors in urological tissues: detection, characterization and clinical applications. *Urology* 40: 491.

5 Aznavoorian S, Murphy AN, Stetler-Stevenson WG, Liotta LA (1993) Molecular aspects of tumor cell invasion and metastasis. *Cancer* 71: 1368.

6 La Du BN, Zannoni VG, Laster L, Seegmiller JE (1958) The nature of the defect in tyrosine metabolism in alkaptonuria. *J Biol Chem* 2130: 251.

7 Yoshida O, Habuchi T, Ogawa O (1994) Recent advances in the molecular genetics of urogenital tumors. *Int J Urol* 1: 1.

8 Brewster SF, Simons JW (1994) Gene therapy in urological oncology: principles, strategies and potential. *Eur Urol* 25: 177.

9 Feig LA, Bast RC Jr, Knapp RC, Cooper GM (1984) Somatic activation of *ras K* gene in a human ovarian carcinoma. *Science* 223: 698.

10 Kerr JFR, Winterford CM, Harmon BV (1994) Apoptosis: its significance in cancer and cancer therapy. *Cancer* 73: 2013.

11 Katelaris PM, Cossart YE, Rose BR *et al.* (1988) Human papillomavirus: the untreated male reservoir. *J Urol* 140: 300.

12 Loveless A (1969) Possible relevance of *O*-6-alkylation of deoxyguanosine to the mutagenicity and carcinogenicity of nitrosamines and nitrosamides. *Nature* 223: 206.

13 Rowley JD (1973) A new consistent chromosomal abnormality in chronic myelogeneous leukaemia identified by quinacrine fluorescence and Giemsa staining. *Nature* 243: 290.

14 Land H, Parada LF, Weinberg RA (1984) Cellular oncogenes and multistep carcinogenesis. *Cancer Surv* 3: 183.

15 Klein G (1987) The approaching era of the tumor suppressor genes. *Science* 238: 1539.

16 Tiniakos DG, Mellon K, Anderson JJ, Robinson MC, Neal DE, Horne CHW (1994) *c-jun* oncogene expression in transitional cell carcinoma of the urinary bladder. *Br J Urol* 74: 757.

17 Viola MV, Fromowitz F, Oravez S *et al.* (1986) Expression of *ras* oncogene p21 in prostate cancer. *New Engl J Med* 314: 133.

18 Masters JRW, Vesey SG, Munn CF, Evan GI, Watson JV (1988) *c-myc* oncoprotein levels in bladder cancer. *Urol Res* 16: 341.

19 Douglas BF, Fowler JF (1976) The effect of multiple small doses of X-ray on skin reactions in the mouse and a basic interpretation. *Radiation Res* 66: 401.

20 Banster SF, Simon T (1944) Gene therapy in urological oncology. *Eur Urol* 25: 177.

21 Harvey W (1651) *Exercitationes de Generatione Animalium Exercit 19. Quinta Ovi Inspectio*. London: Wellcome Historical Medical Library.

22 Fox SB, Dickinson AJ, Westwood M *et al.* (1994) Angiogenic growth factor expression in bladder carcinoma. Presented at BAUS July 1, 1994.

23 Hawthorn RJS, Murdoch JB, MacLean AB, MacKie RM (1988) Langerhans' cells and subtypes of human papillomavirus in cervical intraepithelial neoplasia. *Br Med J* 297: 643.

24 Noel JC, Peny MO, Thiry L *et al.* (1994) Transitional cell carcinoma of the bladder: evaluation of the role of human papillomaviruses. *Urology* 44: 671.

25 Prummer O (1993) Interferon-alpha antibodies in patients with renal cell carcinoma treated with recombinant interferon-alpha-2A in an adjuvant multicenter trial. *Cancer* 71: 1828.

26 Eisenbach L, Hollander N, Greenfield L, Yakor H, Segal S, Feldman M (1984) The differential expression of H-2K versus H-2D antigens, distinguishing high-metastatic from low-metastatic clones, is correlated with the immunogenic properties of the tumor cells. *Int J Cancer* 34: 567.

27 Oliver RTD, Atkinson A, Bodmer J, Bodmer HF (1985) Possible involvement of HLA in determining clinical behaviour of germ cell tumours of the testicle. *Proc Am Assoc Cancer Res* Abstr. 222.

28 Iles RK, Chard T (1991) Human chorionic gonadotrophin expression by bladder tumors. *J Urol* 145: 453.

29 Karnofsky DA (1965) Problems and pitfalls in the evaluation of anticancer drugs. *Cancer* 18: 1517.

30 Bleehen NM (1982) Radiotherapy, in: Chisholm GD, Innes Williams DI (eds) *Scientific Foundations of Urology*, pp. 616—23. London: Heinemann.

31 Cade IS, McEwen J, Dische S *et al.* (1978) Hyperbaric oxygen and radiotherapy: a Medical Research Council trial in carcinoma of the bladder. *Br J Radiol* 1: 876.

32 Plenk HP (1972) Hyperbaric radiation therapy. Preliminary results of a randomised study of cancer of the urinary bladder and review of the oxygen experience. *Am J Roentgenol* 114: 152.

33 Bleehen NM (1973) Combination therapy with drugs and radiation. *Br Med Bull* 29: 54.

34 Stewart FA, Denekamp J, Hirst DG (1980) Proliferation kinetics of the mouse bladder after irradiation. *Cell Tissue Kinetics* 13: 75.

35 Kelly JF, Snell ME, Berenbaum MC (1975) Photodynamic destruction of human bladder carcinoma. *Br J Cancer* 31: 237.

36 Kelly JF, Snell ME (1976) Hematoporphyrin derivative: a possible aid in the diagnosis and therapy of carcinoma of the bladder. *J Urol* 115: 150.

37 Dougherty TJ, Boyle DG, Weishaupt KR *et al.* (1983) Photoradiation therapy — clinical and drug advances, in: Kessel D, Dougherty TJ (eds) *Porphyrin Photosensitization*, pp. 3—15. New York: Plenum Press.

38 Benson RC (1986) Integral photoradiation therapy of multifocal bladder tumors. *Eur Urol* 12 (Suppl 1): 47.

39 Harty JI, Amin M, Wieman TJ, Tseng MT, Ackerman D, Broghamer W (1989) Complications of whole bladder dihematoporphyrin ether photodynamic therapy. *J Urol* 141: 1341.

40 Prout GR, Lin C, Benson R *et al.* (1987) Photo-dynamic therapy with hematoporphyrin derivative in the treatment of superficial transitional cell carcinoma of the bladder. *New Engl J Med* 317: 1251.

41 Windahl T, Lofgren LA (1993) Two years' experience with photodynamic therapy of bladder carcinoma. *Br J Urol* 71: 187.

42 O'Hallewin MA, Baert L, Marijnissen JPA, Star WM (1992) Whole bladder wall photodynamic therapy with *in situ* light dosimetry for carcinoma *in situ* of the bladder. *J Urol* 148: 1152.

43 Rachor R, Flotte TJ, Scholz M, Dretler S, Hasan T (1992) Comparison of intravenous and intravesical administration of chloro-aluminum sulfonated phthalocyanine for photodynamic treatment in a rat bladder cancer model. *J Urol* 147: 1404.

PART 2
KIDNEY AND
URETER

Chapter 4: Kidney and ureter — anatomy

Comparative anatomy

Life began in the primeval oceans and the main function of the most simple renal system — the excretory vacuole of the amoeba — was to regulate osmolarity. During the long process of evolution a wide variety of kidneys evolved, capable of dealing with life in the water — whether fresh or saline — or on land in extremes of climate which ranged from swamp to desert, and in the air [1–3].

The basic unit of the mammalian kidney is the renal pyramid. It is arranged like a bunch of flowers in a vase. The flowers are the glomeruli; the stalks are the collecting tubules; the vase is the calix (Fig. 4.1).

In the adult human kidney the pyramids are compressed so that the external surface is smooth but the original lobulation can be seen in the fetal kidney where it resembles a bunch of grapes and this is still the norm in aquatic mammals such as porpoises, whales and otters [4]. Some mammals like the rabbit have only one large calix. Others like the pig and man have about a dozen calices. In man, the design of the normal pyramid is important in preventing reflux of urine up into the renal parenchyma (see p. 53).

Embryology

The earthworm's kidney consists of a segmental pronephros with nephrostomes (Fig. 4.2). There is some dispute as to whether any trace of the pronephros can be found in the human embryo but that nephric ducts once opened into the coelomic cavity is echoed in the way the fallopian tube opens into the peritoneal cavity. It is believed that the structures of the inner ear are vestiges of pronephric nephrostomes [2,5–9].

The amphibian mesonephros (Fig. 4.3) can be identified in the 4-week-old (10 mm) human embryo. There are a pair of sausage-shaped swellings on the posterior abdominal wall on either side of the mesentery — the genitourinary ridges — and a faint groove demarcates each ridge into a medial gonadal and a lateral nephrogenic part — the mesonephros (Fig. 4.4).

Lateral to the mesonephros is the long Wolffian

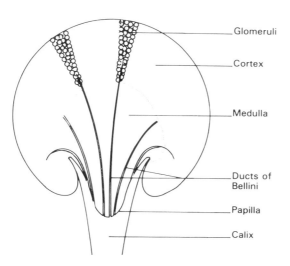

Fig. 4.1 The basic unit of the mammalian kidney is the pyramid which is arranged like a bunch of flowers in a vase.

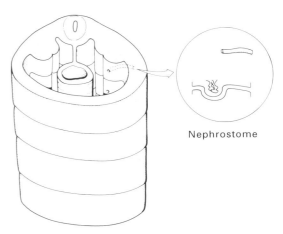

Fig. 4.2 In segmented earthworms, the kidney (the pronephros) consists of a set of nephrostomes (one per segment) which let fluid pass from the coelom to the exterior.

duct which drains into the cloaca at the caudal end of the embryo. The Wolffian duct induces the formation of glomeruli in one segment after another as it grows down towards the tail of the embryo.

The most caudal end of the nephrogenic ridge will form the metanephros. As the tail end of the fetus curls up, the hind-gut is curled with it and so are the nephrogenic ridges and their Wolffian ducts which twist upwards and inwards. Branches from the most caudal part of the Wolffian ducts enter the metanephros. These are the ureteric buds (Fig. 4.5).

The ureteric bud subdivides, and induces the formation of glomeruli in the mesenchyme of the metanephros. The branches of the ureteric bud grow peripherally into the cortex. The first four or five generations of dividing ureteric branches become dilated and incorporated in the eventual renal pelvis. The remaining four or five generations form the calices and collecting tubules [10] (Fig. 4.6). This process of branching out and induction of more glomeruli continues after birth — the numbers of glomeruli increasing threefold in the first 100 days of childhood [11].

As the tail end of the fetus curls up and bends the hind-gut into a U, mesoderm grows down into the gap between the future rectum and

bladder. This forms the urorectal septum. The Wolffian ducts lie in this wedge-shaped septum, and grow down with it. They also become bent into a loop, and take the ureteric buds with them [12] (Fig. 4.7).

Part of the septum is incorporated into the bladder to form the trigone (Fig. 4.8) and because of the pronounced loop of the Wolffian duct, the ureteric bud comes to open into the bladder cephalad to the Wolffian duct. In males the Wolffian duct will become the vas deferens and seminal vesicle [12]. The tail end of the fetus at this stage is barely a centimetre long, and the small space between the stumpy tail and the relatively large umbilical cord is filled by the cloacal membrane, on either side of which are two small genital tubercles (Fig. 4.9).

The cloacal membrane is made of only two thin layers — ectoderm and endoderm. As it dissolves the genital tubercles come together to form the united phallic tubercle.

While all this is taking place, the mesonephros is withering away, but as it vanishes the Wolffian duct generates a second duct parallel and lateral to it — the Müllerian duct. As the urogenital ridge twists round, so the Müllerian ducts approach each other, meet in the midline in front of the Wolffian ducts, and burrow down in the urorectal

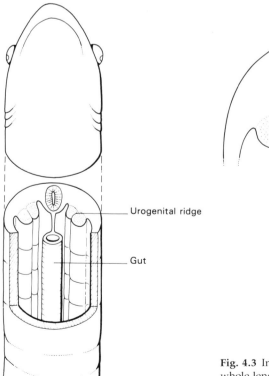

Urogenital ridge

Gut

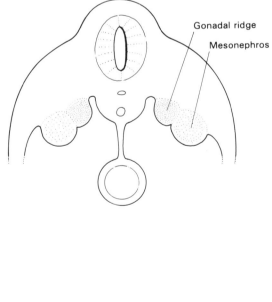

Gonadal ridge

Mesonephros

Fig. 4.3 In amphibia the mesonephros runs along the whole length of the animal on the lateral side of the genitourinary ridge.

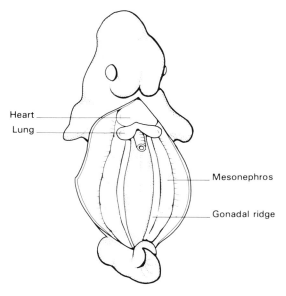

Heart
Lung
Mesonephros
Gonadal ridge

Fig. 4.4 The amphibian type of mesonephros can be identified in the 4-week-old human embryo.

septum (Fig. 4.10). The urorectal septum is partially absorbed into the trigone, and the Müllerian ducts open into the urethra medial to, and in front of, the Wolffian ducts.

The subsequent fate of the Wolffian and Müllerian ducts is determined by the X and Y chromosomes. Until the fourth week the urogenital ridge is neuter. At 4 weeks it is invaded by gonadal cells which migrate by amoeboid movements from the yolk sac across the coelom and burrow into the gonadal ridge (Fig. 4.11). By 6 weeks it is estimated that there are about 60 000 gonadal cells in each gonadal ridge. The male ones are active at once: the female gonadocytes stay dormant for another 2 weeks.

The male gonadal cells have a Y chromosome, carrying the HY gene whose product is a simple chemical which is common to all mammals. It does two things one after the other.

1 It makes the gonadocytes differentiate into Sertoli cells which secrete another simple polypeptide — the Müllerian duct-inhibiting factor. This has a dramatic effect: the entire Müllerian duct system disappears within a single day, leaving behind only the tiny vestige of the utriculus masculinus in the verumontanum (Fig. 4.12).

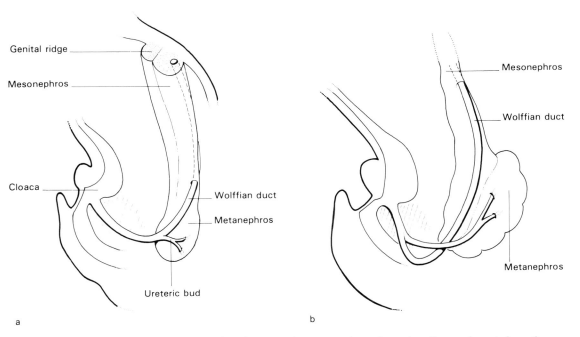

Genital ridge
Mesonephros
Cloaca
Wolffian duct
Metanephros
Ureteric bud

a

Mesonephros
Wolffian duct
Metanephros

b

Fig. 4.5 (a) The caudal part of the mesonephros becomes the metanephros. It receives its own branch from the mesonephric (Wolffian) duct — this is the ureteric bud. (b) As the fetus curls up, the Wolffian duct and ureteric bud are bent round.

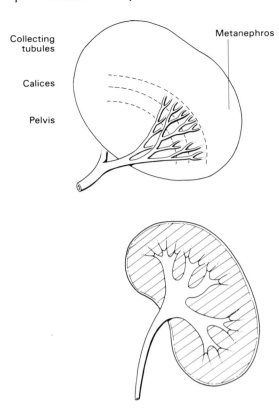

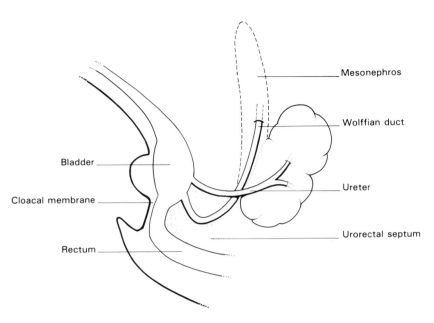

Fig. 4.7 The urorectal septum grows down between the future bladder and rectum.

Fig. 4.6 As the ureteric bud approaches the metanephros it branches repeatedly. The branches induce the formation of glomeruli. The first four or five generations of branches become incorporated into the renal pelvis.

2 About 1 week later, the HY gene causes the gonadocytes to form Leydig cells which make testosterone which is activated by the enzyme 5-alpha reductase to 5-alpha dihydrotesto-sterone. This active substance reacts with a cytosol receptor in the phallic tubercles and Wolffian ducts to secrete growth factors which result in the two changes necessary to convert the neuter fetus into the male. The cytosol receptor factor is a product of one of the genes in the X chromosome.

The phallic tubercle elongates and becomes a penis, while the genital folds on either side of it roll in together and fuse along the midline to carry the urethra to the tip of the penis (Fig. 4.13).

The simple drainpipe of the Wolffian duct becomes the muscular canal of the vas deferens, the reprocessing plant of the epididymis, and the ejaculatory system of the seminal vesicles (Fig. 4.14).

Topographical anatomy

The kidneys lie protected from injury by the spine, ribs and a thick packing of fat. The right kidney is a little smaller than the left [13] and lies very slightly lower down, perhaps because the right lobe of the liver is so much bigger than the left. As a rule the vertical length of each kidney should roughly equal 2.5 times the height of a vertebral body.

Anatomical relations

Posterior to each kidney are the 12th rib, 12th subcostal and ilio-inguinal nerves, quadratus lumborum and psoas muscles (Fig. 4.15), lateral to which there is the entire thickness of the abdominal wall made up of the transversus, internal and external oblique muscles. Behind the 12th rib lies the broad sweep of the latissimus dorsi and the trivial slips of serratus posterior inferior. Perhaps the most important of the posterior relations of the kidney is that of the pleura, which crosses about the middle of the 12th rib [14].

Medial to the kidney are the great vessels — on the right side the inferior vena cava, on the left the aorta.

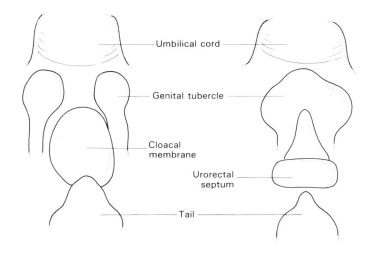

Fig. 4.8 The cloacal membrane disappears.

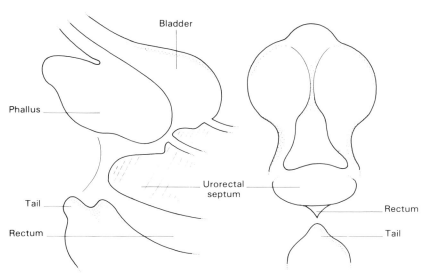

Fig. 4.9 The phallic tubercles meet in the midline.

Anteriorly, each kidney is overlain by bowel: on each side a part of the duodenum, as well as the colon, which must be reflected when approaching the kidney from the front (Fig. 4.16).

Renal fasciae

There is a loose packing of fat around the kidney (Zuckerkandl's fascia) contained within a thin firm envelope (Gerota's fascia). Outside this, and separating the kidney from the peritoneum is more or less fatty tissue [14] (Fig. 4.17).

Macroscopic appearances

A cut section of the kidney shows two distinct parts — cortex and medulla. The cortex contains the glomeruli. The medulla is divided into an inner and outer zone according to the pres-

ence of long or short loops of Henle (Fig. 4.18). Between each pyramid is a portion of cortex — the column of Bertin (Fig. 4.19).

Arterial supply

The pattern of the arterial supply of the kidney was established by Graves [15] using injection-corrosion casts of the renal vessels. He found that there were five main renal segments arranged like the fingers of the hand, and each had its own artery (Fig. 4.20). This basic pattern makes it more easy to interpret angiograms, but not every kidney displays such a clear-cut pattern. Variations are common and one or more of the segmental arteries may spring independently from the aorta.

When the kidneys are in unusual places, such as the pelvic kidney, their segmental arteries

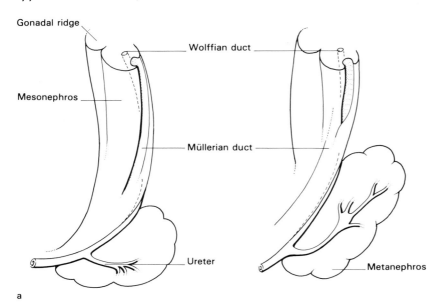

a

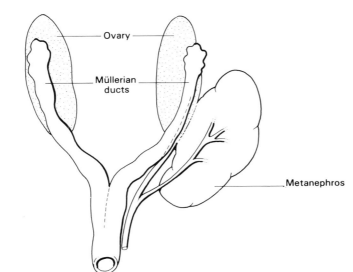

b

Fig. 4.10 (a) A second (Müllerian) duct forms on the lateral side of the mesonephros. (b) The Müllerian ducts roll towards each other, meet in the midline in front of the Wolffian ducts and burrow down into the urorectal septum to form (in the female) the future uterus and fallopian tubes.

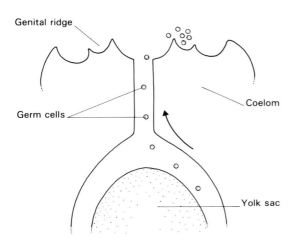

Fig. 4.11 Migration of the germ cells from the yolk sac to the genital ridge.

may arise from any of the nearby vessels, e.g. the aorta, lumbar, common or internal iliac arteries.

Each renal artery supplies a discrete segment of the kidney, so that occlusion of one branch will lead to total infarction of a complete segment of parenchyma. These segments do not correspond to the pattern of the calices and pyramids, as in the bronchopulmonary segments, which makes it more difficult to plan a partial nephrectomy. It does however make it possible to carry out any operation on the kidney in a virtually bloodless field once the main renal artery has been occluded; the only slight loss of blood is from the veins.

Each segmental artery divides into smaller

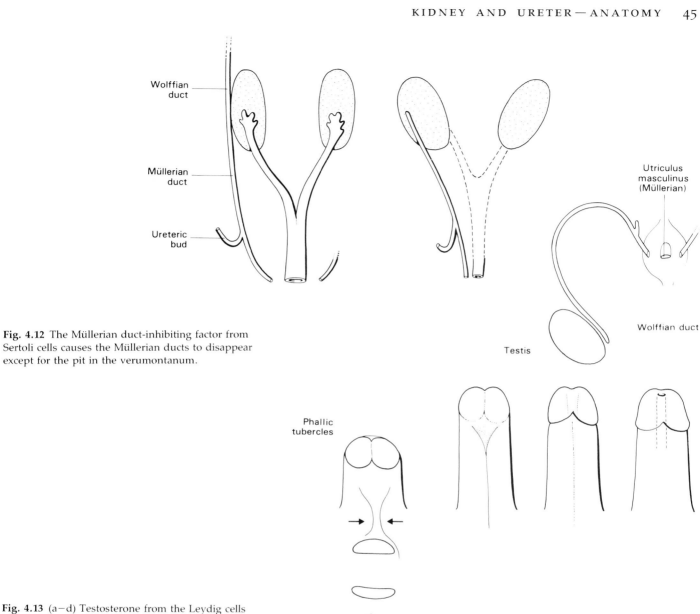

Fig. 4.12 The Müllerian duct-inhibiting factor from Sertoli cells causes the Müllerian ducts to disappear except for the pit in the verumontanum.

Fig. 4.13 (a–d) Testosterone from the Leydig cells causes the phallus to grow and the urethra to roll in from either side.

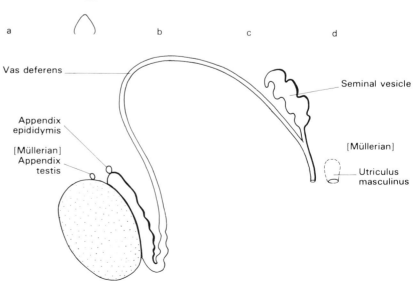

Fig. 4.14 In males the Wolffian duct becomes the vas deferens, epididymis and seminal vesicles.

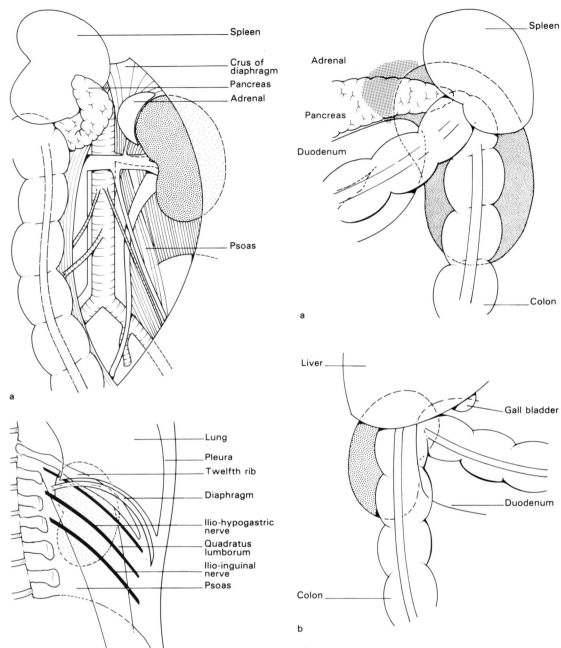

Fig. 4.15 (a & b) Posterior relations of the kidney showing the 12th rib, 12th subcostal and ilio-inguinal nerves, quadratus lumborum and psoas muscles.

Fig. 4.16 Anterior relations of the kidney showing (a) on left duodenum and colon, (b) on the right side and (c) gallbladder and liver (Fig. 4.16 continued on p. 47).

branches which run towards the cortex where they give off the arcuate arteries, from which every glomerulus receives its afferent arteriole (Fig. 4.21). Emerging from the glomerulus, the efferent arteriole runs among the proximal and distal tubules. The efferent arteries from the innermost row of glomeruli (juxtaglom-erular) send long straight branches down into the papilla, among the collecting tubules and the long loops of Henle. These vasa recta are believed to be of importance in the counter-current mechanism which concentrates the urine (see p. 58).

The vasa recta open into wide thin-walled

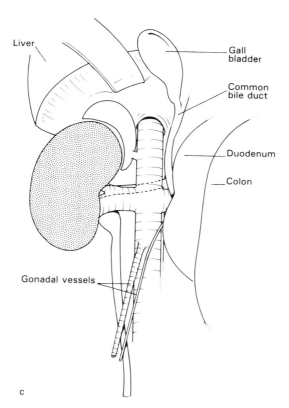

Liver

Gall bladder

Common bile duct

Duodenum

Colon

Gonadal vessels

c

Fig. 4.16 (Continued) (c) gallbladder and liver.

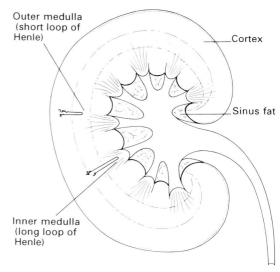

Outer medulla (short loop of Henle)

Cortex

Sinus fat

Inner medulla (long loop of Henle)

Fig. 4.18 Diagrammatic section through the kidney. The medulla is divided into an inner and outer zone.

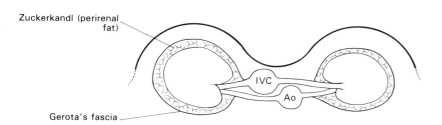

Zuckerkandl (perirenal fat)

IVC

Ao

Gerota's fascia

Fig. 4.17 The fasciae surrounding the kidney. Note that Gerota's fascia is tough enough to tamponade haemorrhage from the ruptured kidney. Ao, aorta; IVC, inferior vena cava.

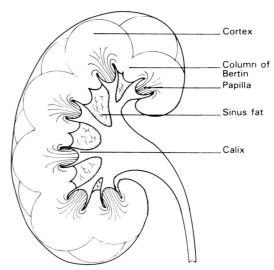

Cortex

Column of Bertin

Papilla

Sinus fat

Calix

Fig. 4.19 The portions of cortex between each pyramid form the columns of Bertin: when these are exceptionally large they can be mistaken for a tumour.

capillaries in the tip of the renal papilla, which ramify among the ascending loops of Henle and collecting tubules.

Renal veins

The renal veins communicate freely with each other (Fig. 4.22). Tributaries from each renal pyramid drain into larger veins around the pyramid which end in the main renal vein. Emissary veins emerge from the cortex and enter veins in the fat around the kidney. These are usually quite small, but when the main renal vein is blocked by thrombosis or tumour, they are sufficient to prevent infarction.

Usually there is only one large renal vein. On the left side it receives the adrenal vein and gonadal vein before crossing in front of the aorta to enter the inferior vena cava. On the right side the renal vein is much shorter and the adrenal and gonadal veins usually enter the inferior vena cava directly.

It is common to find more than one renal vein on the right side; on the left the renal vein often

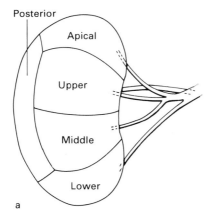

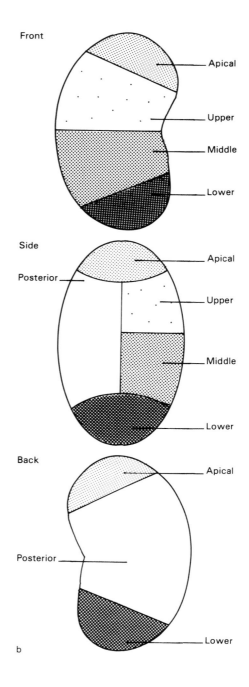

Fig. 4.20 (a) The basic pattern of the segmental arterial supply to the kidney. (b) Each of the five main end arteries supplies a distinct segment of the kidney.

divides to encircle the aorta; while on either side large lumbar veins often enter the renal vein from behind and may cause formidable bleeding if they are inadvertently torn during nephrectomy.

Lymphatics

The kidney has a profuse lymphatic drainage system. The lymphatics follow the course of the arcuate arteries towards the renal hilum where they form three or four main trunks which run medially into the cisterna chyli. When the ureter is obstructed these lymphatics act as a very efficient safety-valve [15,16].

Innervation of the kidney

'With the exception of the adrenal gland the kidney is the richest innervated organ per unit of tissue mass' [11]. Small unmyelinated nerve fibres form a main renal plexus in the hilum of the kidney with secondary plexuses around the renal artery, but their function is little under-

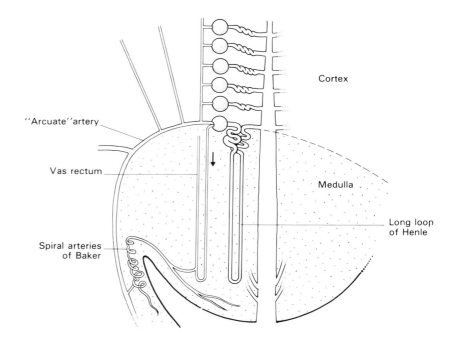

Fig. 4.21 Branches of the segmental arteries within the kidney. The renal papilla is supplied by the vasa recta as well as the spiral arteries of Baker.

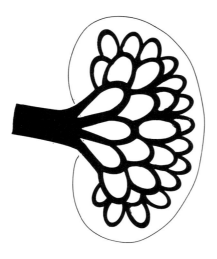

Fig. 4.22 The renal veins communicate freely with each other. Not shown are the many small emissary veins from the cortex to the perirenal fat which prevent the kidney from becoming infarcted when the main renal vein is obstructed.

stood. The branches of these nerves ramify among the tubules, glomeruli and vasa recta. They are common in the region of the juxtaglomerular apparatus. Ever since the classic experiments of Claude Bernard in 1858, it has been known that section of the splanchnic nerve in the dog causes a diuresis in the ipsilateral kidney which can be reversed by stimulating the nerve. It has also been shown that dividing the sym-

pathetic nerves reduces the rate of tubular fluid reabsorption from the proximal tubules without altering the renal blood flow [17].

It has been shown that stimulation of the nerves in the renal hilum gives pain. Despite this rich nerve network, all measurable functions of the kidney continue in renal transplants whose nerve supply has been completely cut off [17].

Nephron

The human nephron is the basic unit of the kidney. It consists of two parts: (a) the glomerulus where water and solutes are filtered from the blood; and (b) the tubules where the filtrate is processed.

Glomerulus

The glomerulus consists of a convoluted arteriole which is invaginated into Bowman's capsule on a stalk — the mesangium [18] (Fig. 4.23). At the base of the stalk the afferent arteriole is surrounded by endothelial cells containing granules which are the precursors of renin — the macula densa. This juxtaglomerular body is a pressure-sensing mechanism, responding to the blood pressure in the afferent arteriole (Fig. 4.24). It also contains beta adrenergic receptors.

The endothelium of the arteriole of the glomerulus and the epithelium lining Bowman's capsule are separated by a basement membrane

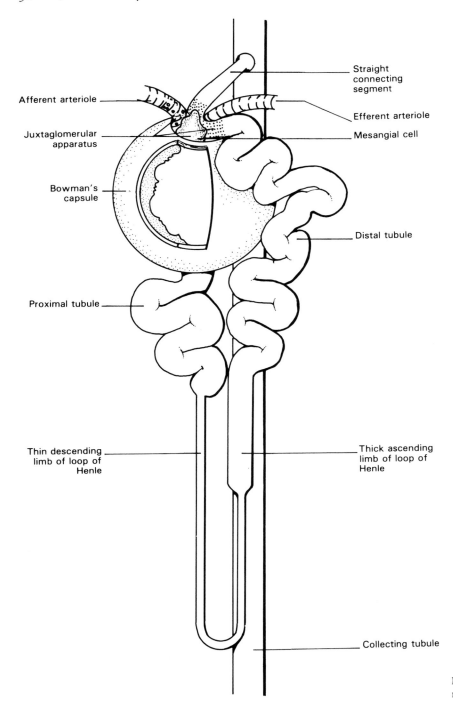

Fig. 4.23 Diagram of the nephron.

Labels on figure:
- Afferent arteriole
- Juxtaglomerular apparatus
- Bowman's capsule
- Proximal tubule
- Thin descending limb of loop of Henle
- Straight connecting segment
- Efferent arteriole
- Mesangial cell
- Distal tubule
- Thick ascending limb of loop of Henle
- Collecting tubule

which serves as a filter to retain cells and proteins of the blood [18] (Fig. 4.25).

The basement membrane rests on a grid formed by the interlocking foot-processes of the epithelial cells (podocytes) of Bowman's capsule, rather as filter paper is supported on a metal grid in the laboratory [18] (Fig. 4.26).

The endothelium of the glomerular arteriole is perforated in a regular pattern of holes so that blood is in direct contact with the basement membrane (Fig. 4.25) (see p. 57).

The Bowman's capsule drains into the proximal tubule — a thick-walled metabolically active structure whose brush border increases the surface area offered to the glomerular filtrate (Fig. 4.27). It is these cells of the proximal tubule

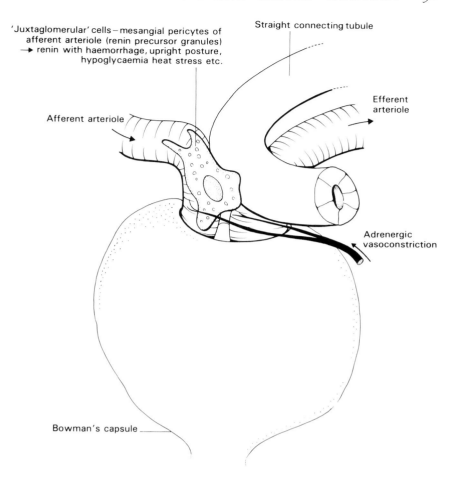

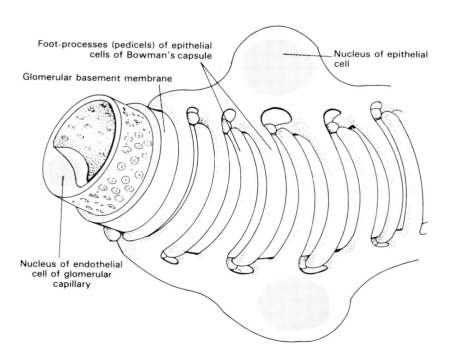

Fig. 4.24 The juxtaglomerular body is sited on the stalk of the mesangium, to monitor pressure in the afferent arteriole.

Fig. 4.25 The basement membrane lies between the endothelium of the glomerular arteriole and the epithelium of Bowman's capsule.

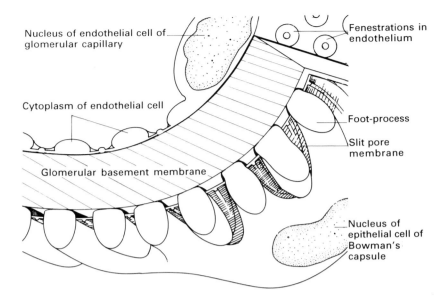

Nucleus of endothelial cell of glomerular capillary

Fenestrations in endothelium

Cytoplasm of endothelial cell

Foot-process

Slit pore membrane

Glomerular basement membrane

Nucleus of epithelial cell of Bowman's capsule

Fig. 4.26 The basement membrane is supported by the grid of foot-processes of the epithelial cells.

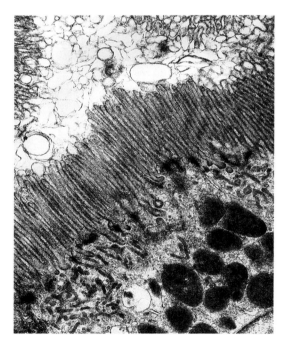

Fig. 4.27 The cells of the proximal tubule are lined with a brush border.

which do most of the metabolic work involved in reabsorption of salt and water. They also give rise to renal cell carcinomas.

From the proximal tubule the processed glomerular filtrate flows into the loop of Henle. Some of these loops of Henle are short; others — notably those from the innermost row of nephrons next to the medulla — are long and reach the tip of the papilla. The long loops have a thick metabolically active segment.

From the loop of Henle, the filtrate enters the distal convoluted tubule, which also has thick metabolically active cells, but no brush border. Finally, the filtrate enters the collecting tubule which receives the filtrate from 10–15 nephrons and descends through the medulla to open on the tip of the papilla. The collecting tubule is thin-walled and its cells metabolically inert.

Collecting system and ureter

Each renal papilla is composed of collecting tubules, loops of Henle, the vasa recta and veins. The papilla protrudes into the calix, and the collecting tubules open through a series of oblique slits along the sides of the papilla in such a way that when the pressure is increased inside the papilla, the collecting tubules are occluded, and urine is not forced up into the parenchyma of the kidney (Fig. 4.28).

Not all papillae are perfectly formed. In the upper and lower poles, compound papillae are a common congenital anomaly, where two or three papillae are clustered together, with the result that the collecting tubules at the site of fusion open straight into the calix and there is no valvular mechanism to prevent urine being forced back into the renal tissues (Fig. 4.29). This malformation is important in reflux nephropathy [19] (see p. 146).

The blood supply of the renal papilla is two-fold: (a) via the vasa recta which loops down from the efferent arterioles of the glomeruli; and (b) via the smaller arteries entering at the

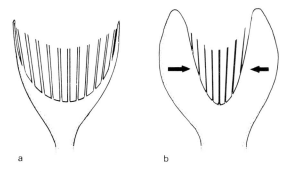

Fig. 4.28 (a & b) The normal valvular arrangement of collecting tubules in the renal papilla, which prevents intrarenal reflux when pressure rises in the calix.

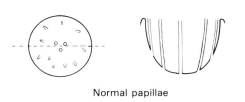

Normal papillae

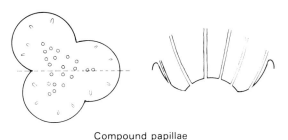

Compound papillae

Fig. 4.29 Congenitally deformed papillae — 'compound papillae' — may permit intrarenal reflux and so cause reflux nephropathy.

base of each papilla from the rim of the calix (see Fig. 4.21).

Each papilla is covered with a single layer of cuboidal cells, perforated for the openings of the collecting tubules. The calix is lined with transitional epithelium (urothelium), outside which there is a layer of smooth muscle.

Calices and pelvis

There are about 12 calices in each kidney, grouped in twos and threes, which drain through a common channel into the renal pelvis. The same pattern of smooth muscle lined with transitional epithelium is continued from the calices along the entire length of the ureter.

For the smooth muscle to act efficiently as a pump it must be free to contract, expand and move up and down (Fig. 4.30). The renal pelvis is

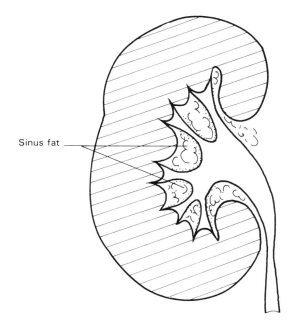

Sinus fat

Fig. 4.30 The sinus fat allows free movement for the contraction and expansion of the renal pelvis and calices.

surrounded with a slippery layer of fascia, which is easily stripped off when operating for hydronephrosis. Outside this is a thick packing of sinus fat. As the ureter descends behind the peritoneum, its slippery coat allows it to writhe behind the peritoneum with each wave of peristalsis and to move freely up and down with respiration.

Anatomical relations of the ureter

The ureter on each side descends anterior to the psoas muscle and the ilio-inguinal nerves, just anterior to the tips of the lumbar transverse processes. It crosses in front of the bifurcation of the common iliac artery, and curves medially towards the bladder whose wall it perforates through an oblique tunnel (Fig. 4.31).

In its course from kidney to bladder the ureter lies behind the second part of the duodenum and caecum, appendix and ascending colon on the right side, and the duodenojejunal flexure and descending colon on the left side.

About half way down, the ureter is crossed anteriorly by the gonadal vessels. In its lower third the ureter passes behind the superior vesical branch of the internal iliac artery which is continued upwards as the 'obliterated hypogastric artery' (obliterated in name, but seldom in practice).

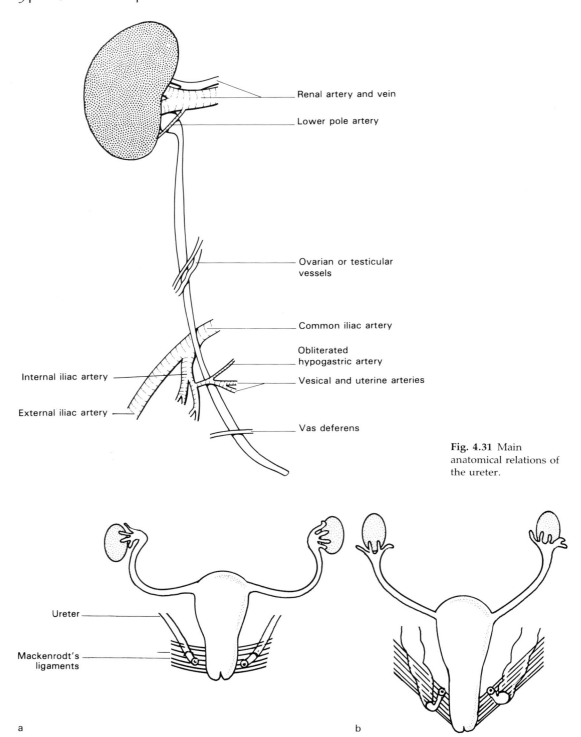

Renal artery and vein

Lower pole artery

Ovarian or testicular vessels

Common iliac artery

Obliterated hypogastric artery

Internal iliac artery

Vesical and uterine arteries

External iliac artery

Vas deferens

Fig. 4.31 Main anatomical relations of the ureter.

Ureter

Mackenrodt's ligaments

a   b

Fig. 4.32 (a) In females, the ureter runs through the fibrous tissue of the ligaments of Mackenrodt on either side of the pelvis. (b) In prolapse of the uterus this may cause obstruction.

To find the ureter at operation the surgeon's most useful landmark is the bifurcation of the common iliac artery. In operating on the lower third of the ureter it is helpful first to ligate and divide the superior vesical artery.

In males, the ureter passes under the vas deferens just where it approaches the bladder.

In females, the ureter runs through a stiff band

of fibrous tissue (the ligament of Mackenrodt) on either side of the uterine cervix as it approaches the bladder; here it is easily damaged during operations on the uterus (Fig. 4.32).

Blood supply

The blood supply of the renal pelvis is profuse and comes from branches of all the main segmental arteries which communicate freely with each other in the muscle of the pelvis. This makes it possible to use long flaps of renal pelvis in repairing hydronephrosis without fear of necrosis [20].

The ureter is supplied by a single longitudinal artery (Fig. 4.33) which runs inside the slippery sheath of connective tissue. This artery arises from the inferior segmental branch of the renal artery, and although it is reinforced at intervals along its course by branches from the lumbar arteries, these are small and unreliable. The next important tributary comes upwards from the superior vesical artery. If the longitudinal artery of the ureter is pulled on, it becomes even more narrow, hence in any operation on the ureter it is essential to avoid tension.

Nerve supply

Small unmyelinated nerve fibres reach the ureter from the autonomic system. The function of some of them is to transmit pain which is experienced in a segmental manner. They are not necessary for ureteric peristalsis, since this continues perfectly well in the completely denervated transplanted kidney. Ultramicroscopic examination of the ureter shows a rich plexus of fine nerves in its muscular wall [20]. The wave of peristalsis is carried by direct excitation from one cell to another through close junctions.

The entry of the ureter into the bladder is along an oblique tunnel, which provides a non-return valve preventing vesicoureteric reflux [21] (Fig. 4.34). This valve can be congenitally defective, or put out of use by injury or disease. Many congenital deformities of this oblique tunnel are seen in association with duplex kidney and ureterocele (see p. 92).

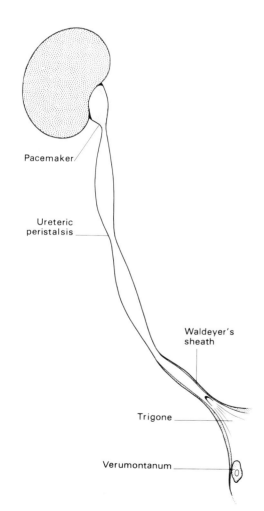

Fig. 4.34 The antireflux ureterovesical valve.

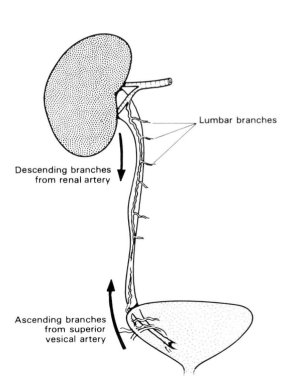

Fig. 4.33 Blood supply of the ureter.

References

1 Smith HW (1953) *From Fish to Philosopher*. Boston: Little, Brown.

2 Dantzler WH (1992) Comparative physiology of the kidney, in: Windhager EE (ed.) *Handbook of Physiology 8*, vol. 1 *Renal Physiology*, pp. 415–74. Oxford: Oxford University Press.

3 Fraser EA (1950) The development of the vertebrate excretory system. *Biol Rev* 25: 159.

4 Harrison RJ, Tomlinson JDW (1956) Observations on the venous system in certain *Pinnipedia* and *Cetacea*. *Proc Zool Soc Lond* 126: 205.

5 Vaughan ED, Middleton GW (1975) Pertinent genitourinary embryology: review for the practising urologist. *Urology* 6: 139.

6 Marshall FF (1978) Embryology of the lower genitourinary tract. *Urol Clin North Am* 5: 3.

7 Keith A (1948) *Human Embryology and Morphology*, 6th edn. Baltimore: Williams & Wilkins.

8 Frazer JES, Baxter JS (1953) *Manual of Embryology: the Development of the Human Body*, 3rd edn. Baltimore: Williams & Wilkins.

9 Allan FD (1960) *Essentials of Human Embryology*. Oxford: Oxford University Press.

10 Osathanondh V, Potter EL (1964) Pathogenesis of polycystic kidney: survey of results of microdissection. *Arch Pathol* 77: 502.

11 Spitzer A, Schwartz GJ (1992) The kidney during development, in: Windhager EE (ed.) *Handbook of Physiology 8*, vol. 1 *Renal Physiology*, pp. 474–544. Oxford: Oxford University Press.

12 Stephens FD (1982) Embryopathy of malformations. *J Urol* 127: 13.

13 Blandy JP, Pead J (1967) Normal and abnormal variation in the dimensions of pairs of kidneys. *Br J Urol* 39: 536.

14 Dixon JS, Gosling JA (1990) Fundamentals of renal anatomy, in: Chisholm GD, Fair WR (eds) *Scientific Foundations of Urology*, 3rd edn, pp. 1–10. Oxford: Heinemann.

15 Graves FT (1971) *The Arterial Anatomy of the Kidney: the Basis of Surgical Technique*. Bristol: John Wright.

16 Kriz W, Dieterich HJ (1970) The lymphatic system of the kidney in some mammals. Light and electron microscopic investigations. *Z Anat Entwickungsgesch* 131: 111.

17 Moss NG, Colindres RW, Gottschalk CW (1992) Neural control of renal function, in: Windhager EE (ed.) *Handbook of Physiology 8*, vol. 1 *Renal Physiology*, pp. 1061–128. Oxford: Oxford University Press.

18 Kanwar YS, Venkatachalam MA (1992) Ultrastructure of glomerulus and juxtaglomerular apparatus, in: Windhager EE (ed.) *Handbook of Physiology 8*, vol. 1 *Renal Physiology*, pp. 3–40. Oxford: Oxford University Press.

19 Ransley PG, Risdon RA (1981) Reflux nephropathy: effects of anti-microbial therapy on the evolution of the early pyelonephritic scar. *Kidney Int* 20: 733.

20 Gosling JA, Dixon JS, Humpherson JR (1982) *Functional Anatomy of the Urinary Tract*. London: Gower Medical Publishing.

21 Thomson AS, Dabhoiwala NF, Verbeek FJ, Lamers WH (1994) The functional anatomy of the ureterovesical junction. *Br J Urol* 73: 284.

Chapter 5: Kidney and ureter — physiology

Glomerulus

Filtration

One-fifth of the cardiac output flows through the 2.5–3 million glomerular arterioles, losing about 170 l of plasma water per day, completely recycling it every 30 min and the whole body water four times a day [1].

The fenestrations of the capillary give the plasma direct access to the basement membrane whose effective mesh has been measured with molecules of known molecular weight, e.g. dextrans and peroxidases, and found to be about 40 000 mol. wt, i.e. the glomerular filtrate is plasma minus its proteins [1].

Filtration depends not only on the size of the molecule but also on its electrical charge. The proteins of the glomerular basement membrane carry a negative charge which repels negatively charged protein molecules, e.g. albumen. The blood pressure within the glomerular arteriole is about 60 mmHg. The plasma oncotic pressure is about 25 mmHg, so that there is a filtration pressure of about 35 mmHg (Fig. 5.1).

Measurement of glomerular filtration rate (GFR)

The GFR can be measured by several methods [2]. The gold standard is inulin clearance. Inulin is filtered by the glomerulus but neither absorbed nor secreted in the renal tubule. In this test inulin is infused intravenously until a steady-state is reached. Its concentration is measured in blood and urine collected over a carefully timed period. The formula

$$\frac{UV}{P}$$

where U = urine concentration, V = volume of urine per minute and P = plasma concentration gives the volume of blood cleared of inulin per minute. In practice inulin is tedious to measure (even though today there is an automated method) and inulin clearance is only used in laboratory studies.

The usual clinical method is creatinine clearance. This presupposes that creatinine is neither excreted nor reabsorbed in the tubule, and is produced in the body at a constant rate. These premises are not quite true. Up to 40% of creati-

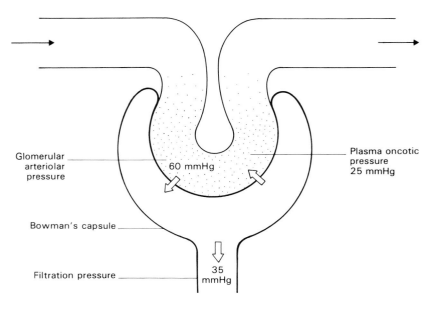

Glomerular arteriolar pressure

Plasma oncotic pressure 25 mmHg

60 mmHg

Bowman's capsule

Filtration pressure

35 mmHg

Fig. 5.1 Filtration in the glomerular arteriole.

nine can be excreted in the proximal tubule, and the endogenous production of creatinine is not constant but varies with the intake of meat in the diet. When GFR is very low, measured creatinine clearance can exceed true inulin clearance by 50–100% [2].

In practice, there is a more important practical drawback to the measurement of creatinine clearance in a busy surgical ward: it demands an exactly timed collection period. Usually, the patient passes urine before going to sleep and notes the time. In the morning the bladder is emptied and the time is noted again: the overnight urine specimen plus a blood sample taken early in the morning is sent to the laboratory [3,4]. This system only works when the patient is reasonably well and cooperative which is not always the case in the uraemic patient.

Isotopic methods for measuring GFR are much more efficient and accurate, though more expensive. Chelating compounds, e.g. ^{51}Cr-ethylenediaminetetra-acetic acid (EDTA), diethylenetriaminepenta-acetic acid (DTPA) labelled with [140]La or [99]technetium, make it possible to measure their rate of disappearance from the blood with a gamma camera [2,4].

Disorders of glomerular filtration

Glomerular filtration may be impaired in underperfusion from dehydration, septicaemia, cardiac failure, the syndrome of hepatorenal failure and drugs such as cyclosporine or angiotensin-converting enzyme inhibitors.

Renal tubules

Tubular function

As the glomerular filtrate passes through the proximal tubules 80% of the excess water is reabsorbed along with sodium, glucose, phosphate and amino acids. Most common diuretics act on the proximal tubule and reduce sodium and water reabsorption.

Regulation of urine concentration

Tissue sodium chloride concentration and osmolality increase towards the tip of the renal papilla. According to the countercurrent hypothesis [5,6], an active metabolic mechanism in the thick segment of the ascending loop of Henle pumps out sodium in exchange for potassium, reducing the sodium concentration and osmo-

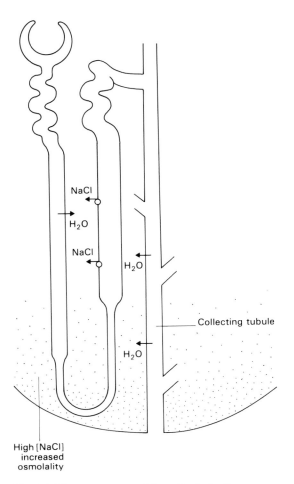

Fig. 5.2 The countercurrent hypothesis for the formation of hyperosmotic urine.

lality of the filtrate, and increasing them in the interstitial fluid (Fig. 5.2).

The filtrate which flows down the descending limb starts off being isoosmotic with systemic plasma and glomerular filtrate. As it descends through the hyperosmotic zone, water diffuses out and the filtrate becomes more concentrated. As it rises up through the thick limb of the loop of Henle, it brings a high concentration of sodium chloride to the active sodium/potassium exchange pump, and sodium is pumped out into the interstitial tissue, raising its osmolality still further. The ability of the sodium pump in the thick segment of the ascending limb of the loop of Henle to establish a modest concentration difference across the wall of the ascending limb is augmented by countercurrent flow to achieve a large difference in osmolality [6].

Surgeons who find the countercurrent theory difficult to believe can take comfort in the knowledge that it is still the subject of dispute among physiologists: 'how the inner medulla concentrates urine is one of the major unsolved problems of renal physiology' [7].

Several control mechanisms are involved in this process of water conservation. Two are of special importance. The pituitary antidiuretic hormone, arginine vasopressin, is the most important of these. Receptors for arginine vasopressin are found along the entire length of the renal tubule although it is thought that its principal action is to control the permeability of the cells of the collecting ducts [6].

The atrial natriuretic peptide is a polypeptide secreted by the human atrium which causes diuresis and loss of sodium. It is of interest to urologists because it is secreted whenever obstruction of urine is relieved [8]. It may play a part in the diuresis which occurs when the bladder is catheterized for chronic retention. Both proximal and distal tubules take part in this postobstructive diuresis [9].

Diuretics which prevent reabsorption of sodium in the proximal tubule mean that more sodium reaches the distal tubule to be exchanged for potassium, hence the hypokalaemia seen after prolonged administration of diuretics.

Acid–base balance

The renal tubules play an important part in regulating acid–base balance (Fig. 5.3). H^+ ions are exchanged with sodium in $NaHCO_3$ and Na_2HPO_4 by means of carbonic anhydrase in the proximal tubule. In the distal tubule glutaminase forms ammonia from glutamine which combines with H^+ to form ammonium:

Glutamine = glutamic acid + NH_3 (glutaminase)

$NH_3 + H^+ = NH_4^+$.

Tests of tubular function

It is possible to measure the acidifying power of the renal tubules by giving the patient a load of ammonium chloride but the test is very unpleasant and the results seldom satisfactory [4].

It is equally possible to measure the ability of the tubules to concentrate urine by depriving the patient of water or by giving them arginine vasopressin by injection. Normal active people may concentrate their urine to the maximum extent, and dehydration by either means may be dangerous in renal failure, diabetes and myeloma

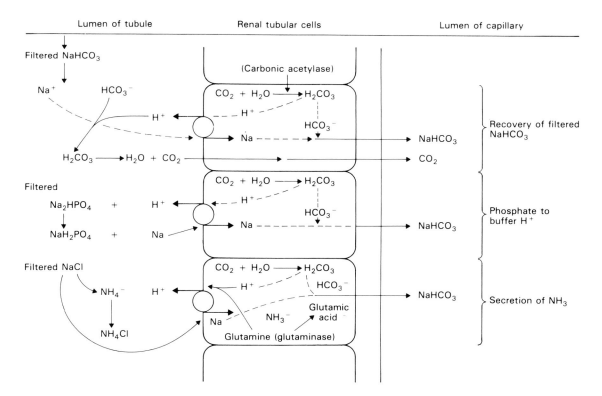

Fig. 5.3 Diagram showing the mechanisms involved in regulating acid–base balance in the renal tubule.

[10]. For routine purposes [99m]Technetium dimer-captosuccinic acid uptake is used to measure tubular function [12].

Disturbed renal tubular function

Obstructive uropathy

The most common and most important disturbance of renal tubular function occurs in obstruction when, for whatever cause, the pressure rises in the urinary tract.

In the multicaliceal human kidney, unlike the unicaliceal kidney of many experimental animals, acute obstruction is not immediately followed by atrophy. For a short time, about 1−2 h, the pressure rises inside the renal pelvis until the filtration pressure is exceeded and filtration ceases. Then the pressure suddenly falls: an isotope placed inside the renal pelvis suddenly enters the bloodstream at this moment. It has been shown that the lymphatics fill before the veins, and before the fornices split [11−14].

The mechanism appears to be splitting of the renal tissue, most marked at the edge of each calix, which allows urine to enter the renal lymphatics and veins [15,16]. Pyelograms taken during acute obstruction by a calculus often show the contrast medium in the perirenal tissues, so that the splits obviously extend not only into the lymphatics and veins but also into the tissues around the kidney.

There are two practical implications of this phenomenon. First, microorganisms in the upper tract can gain immediate access to the bloodstream, i.e. obstruction complicated by infection is easily followed by septicaemia.

The second is that when urine finds its way into the lymphatics or veins of the kidney, the pressure inside the lumen of the renal pelvis will fall, and filtration will start again. Thanks to this safety-valve mechanism acute obstruction in the human kidney does not mean that the kidney ceases to function. An apparently non-functioning kidney may recover completely after the obstruction has been relieved (Fig. 5.4). Indeed, it may be possible to retrieve useful function even after several years; the author has seen useful function return after pyeloplasty in a kidney that had been obstructed for 6 years.

A more important consequence of obstruction, whether continued or intermittent, is the development of hydronephrosis which destroys the medulla rather than the renal cortex. This has the selective effect of reducing the tubular functions of the kidney, whilst leaving filtration relatively undamaged.

The hydronephrotic kidney continues to make urine, but is unable to process the glomerular filtrate properly. The hyperosmolar renal papillae have disappeared. The glomerular filtrate emerges with a fixed osmolarity, a specific gravity of 1010, and the kidney is no longer able to regulate extracellular volume or control acid−base bal-

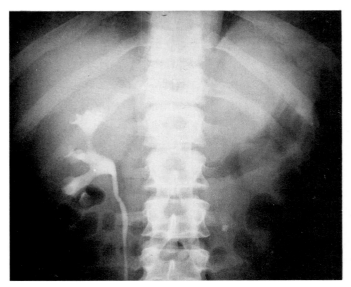
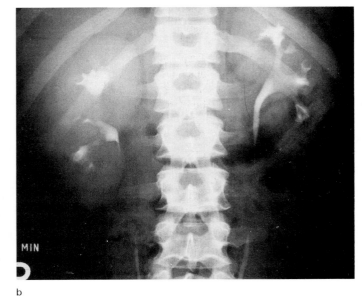

a   b

Fig. 5.4 (a) Urogram taken during a period of obstruction by a calculus showing apparent non-function in the kidney. (b) Urogram after removal of the stone: there was a complete recovery of function.

ance. The patient passes a large volume of urine, develops acidosis, loses salt and becomes dehydrated. The clinical picture is made worse by anaemia. It should be noted that there can be considerable atrophy of the renal medulla before conventional measures of glomerular filtration detect anything wrong.

Special disorders of renal tubules

A number of specific diseases arise from disorders of the renal tubules.

Cystinuria is inherited as a Mendelian recessive autosomal gene which leads to a deficiency in enzymes that transport four amino acids across the bowel and renal tubular cells [17].

The other amino acids — arginine, ornithine and lysine — are of little consequence, but if cystine is not reabsorbed in the proximal tubule, its concentration in the urine easily exceeds its low solubility (see p. 223) and stones are formed.

Hartnup's disease. Here the deficiency involves the transport of tryptophane across the renal tubule and bowel wall. The loss of tryptophane in the urine is not important, but the want of uptake from the bowel results in deficiency of nicotinamide, resulting in cerebellar ataxia and pellagra [18].

Fanconi's syndrome. The proximal tubule is converted into a short, thin functionless tube. As a result there is failure of absorption of glucose, several amino acids and phosphate. There is usually proteinuria and acidosis [18].

Renal glycosuria. There may be incomplete reabsorption of glucose from the filtrate — resulting in 'renal glycosuria' which is harmless, but must be distinguished from diabetes [18].

Renal tubular acidosis. If the distal tubule cannot pump out hydrogen ions in exchange for sodium and potassium, the urine remains alkaline and the plasma bicarbonate remains low. There is loss of phosphate. With a low plasma bicarbonate, less calcium remains bound to protein and consequently escapes in the glomerular filtrate to be precipitated in the collecting tubules to form speckled calcifications called 'nephrocalcinosis'. The continual loss of calcium may drain the bone reserves and result in osteomalacia [18].

Nephrogenic diabetes insipidus. Here a sex-linked Mendelian recessive gene in males makes the collecting tubules resist the antidiuretic hormone. As a result there is a continual diuresis. This may be so severe as to lead to dehydration and brain damage in a baby; it also can lead to a striking dilatation of the entire urinary tract which at first view can be mistaken for that caused by obstruction [18].

Endocrine functions of the kidney

Renin

Renin is secreted by cells in the zona glomerulosa, situated on the afferent arteriole of the glomerulus, in response to a fall in blood pressure [1,19]. It is an enzyme which splits angiotensinogen (a globulin) into angiotensin I (a decapeptide) which in turn is converted to angiotensin II (a potent pressor). Angiotensin II causes an increased cardiac output and constriction of the peripheral arterioles, as well as stimulation of the secretion of aldosterone to conserve sodium and increase the total extracellular fluid volume.

Erythropoietin

This is a polypeptide hormone which is secreted by kidneys containing cysts or tumours, and has the property of stimulating red cell production in the bone marrow. In renal failure lack of erythropoietin results in anaemia, but fortunately synthetic erythropoietin, made by recombinant DNA technology is available for patients on dialysis [20].

Transport of urine

When the urine reaches the renal calix the muscular wall of the calix responds by contraction. Earlier observers suggested that there may be a pacemaker system in the wall of the renal calices, but this is misleading, since it suggests that there is some system analogous to the pacemaker mechanism in the heart, and there is none.

The fine structure of the ureter shows a system whereby one muscle cell approaches or interdigitates with another. It is thought that these allow the wave of contraction to pass from cell to cell. Nerve fibres are scanty, but have been shown to be of at least three kinds, those containing acetylcholinesterase, noradrenergic nerves or 'substance P' [21,22].

The ureter transports urine perfectly well after

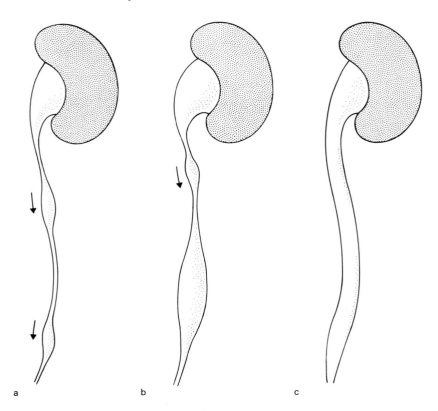

Fig. 5.5 In diuresis the ureter dilates (a), the peristaltic contractions become less occlusive (b) until eventually the ureter acts as an open pipe (c).

transplantation in the absence of any innervation, so the part that its nerve fibres play in normal peristalsis is unknown.

With diuresis the frequency of the peristaltic contractions in the calices, pelvis and ureter increase in frequency and force. The lumen of the ureter enlarges until its walls no longer come together to form a bolus of urine, and the ureter serves as a simple pipe or conduit [23] (Fig. 5.5).

The special valvular anatomical arrangement of the renal calices which prevents intrarenal reflux, and the equally important valve which prevents vesicoureteric reflux are discussed elsewhere (see pp. 53 and 146).

Measurements of ureteric function

A common dilemma is posed by the finding of ureteric dilatation in an ultrasound scan or a urogram. Often the dilatation is caused by obstruction, but from time to time, and especially in children, a 'wide' ureter may not be obstructed, and it may be very important to distinguish between the two entities.

The classic technique is that of Whitaker [24] by which water or saline is run into the ureter at a rate calculated to be greater than the maximum urine flow in diuresis, while at the same time the

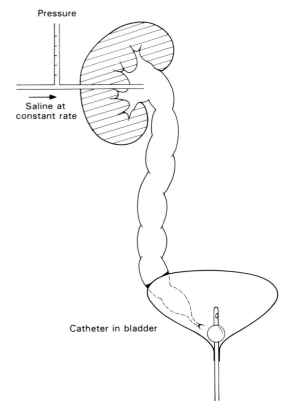

Fig. 5.6 Whitaker's test. Saline or water is infused into the renal pelvis through a percutaneous cannula while the pressure is monitored.

pressure is measured in the system (Fig. 5.6). This suffers from the disadvantage that it is necessary to pass a fine needle and cannula into the dilated renal pelvis. Attempts have been made to obtain equally useful information from radionuclide studies [25].

References

1 Kanwar YS, Venkatachalam MA (1992) Ultrastructure of glomerulus and juxtaglomerular apparatus, in: Windhager EE (ed.) *Handbook of Physiology 8*, vol. 1 *Renal Physiology*, pp. 3–40. Oxford: Oxford University Press.

2 Levinsky NG, Lieberthal W (1992) Clearance techniques, in: Windhager EE (ed.) *Handbook of Physiology 8*, vol. 1 *Renal Physiology*, pp. 227–47. Oxford: Oxford University Press.

3 Brown SCW, O'Reilly PR (1995) Glomerular filtration rate measurement a neglected test in urological practice. *Br J Urol* 75: 296.

4 Reynolds TM, Burgess N, Matanhelia S, Brain A, Penney MD (1993) The frusemide test: simple screening test for renal acidification defect in urolithiasis. *Br J Urol* 72: 153.

5 Burckhardt G, Greger R (1992) Principles of electrolyte transport across plasma membranes of renal tubular cells, in: Windhager EE (ed.) *Handbook of Physiology 8*, vol. 1 *Renal Physiology*, pp. 639–57. Oxford: Oxford University Press.

6 Jamison RL, Gehrig JJ (1992) Urinary concentration and dilution: physiology, in: Windhager EE (ed.) *Handbook of Physiology 8*, vol. 2, pp. 1219–79. Oxford: Oxford University Press.

7 Stephenson JL (1992) Urinary concentration and dilution, in: Windhager EE (ed.) *Handbook of Physiology 8*, vol. 2, pp. 1349–408. Oxford: Oxford University Press.

8 Glumi FA, Mooppan UMM, Chou S-Y, Kim H (1989) Atrial natriuretic peptide in patients with obstructive uropathy. *J Urol* 142: 268.

9 Jones DA, Atherton JC, O'Reilly PH, Barnard RJ, George NJR (1989) Assessment of the nephron segments involved in post-obstructive diuresis in man, using lithium clearance. *Br J Urol* 64: 559.

10 Tryding N, Berg B, Ekman S, Nilsson J-E, Sterner G, Harris A (1988) DDAVP test for renal concentration capacity. *Scand Med Assoc J* 139: 753.

11 Gillenwater JY *et al*. (1975) Renal function after release of chronic unilateral hydronephrosis in man. *Kidney Int* 7: 179.

12 Chibber PJ *et al*. (1982) ^{99m}Technetium DMSA and the predication of recovery in obstructive uropathy. *Br J Urol* 53: 492.

13 Cuttino JT, Clark RL, Fried FA, Stevens PS (1978) Microradiographic demonstration of pyelolymphatic backflow in the kidney. *Am J Roentgenol* 131: 501.

14 Murphy JJ, Myint MK, Rattner WH, Klaus R, Shallow J (1958) The lymphatic system of the kidney. *J Urol* 80: 1.

15 Dominguez R, Adams RB (1960) Pyelovenous communications: a functional study, in: Quinn EL, Kass EH (eds) *Biology of Pyelonephritis*, p. 189. Boston: Little, Brown.

16 Gottschalk CW (1960) Observations on the intrarenal pressure, in: Quinn EL, Kass EH (eds) *Biology of Pyelonephritis*, p. 183. Boston: Little, Brown.

17 Kachel TA, Vijan SR, Dretler SP (1991) Endourological experience with cystine calculi and a treatment algorithm. *J Urol* 145: 25.

18 Brenton DP (1985) Tubular function and its disturbance in disease, in: Marsh FP (ed.) *Postgraduate Nephrology*, pp. 151–79. London: Heinemann Medical Books.

19 Goldfarb DA, Novick AC (1994) The renin–angiotensin system: revised concepts and implications for renal function. *Urology* 43: 572.

20 Cotes PM (1988) Erythropoietin: the developing story. *Br Med J* 296: 805.

21 Gosling JA, Dixon JS, Humpherson JR (1983) *Functional Anatomy of the Urinary Tract*. London: Gower Medical Publishing.

22 Notley RG (1971) The structural basis for normal and abnormal ureteric motility. *Ann Roy Coll Surg Engl* 49: 248.

23 Struthers NW, Constantinou CE (1992) Ureteric physiology. *Curr Opinion Urol* 2: 310.

24 Whitaker RH (1976) Equivocal pelvi-ureteric obstruction. *Br J Urol* 47: 771.

25 Whitaker RH, Buxton-Thomas M (1984) A comparison of pressure flow studies and renography in equivocal upper urinary tract obstruction. *J Urol* 131: 446.

Chapter 6: Renal failure

Acute renal failure

Aetiology

Acute renal failure has many causes but there are three underlying pathological processes [1].

Underperfusion of the kidney. Pre-renal renal failure from underperfusion of the kidney is seen when there is hypovolaemic shock from blood loss, major injury, septicaemia, burns, diarrhoea and vomiting. It is a major cause of delayed function when there is delay in perfusing a transplant kidney or delay in putting it into the recipient. In its most extreme form it occurs when the main renal artery is occluded by a dissecting aneurysm or embolism.

Renal tubular toxins. A number of substances selectively poison the renal tubules, e.g. mercury, phenol, carbon tetrachloride, glycol and the exotoxin of *Clostridium welchii*. Similar damage to the nephron occurs in acute glomerulonephritis (see p. 134). If the injury affects the cells of the tubules it does not always obstruct them, and acute renal failure may occur in the absence of oliguria [2].

Postrenal obstruction. The obstruction may occur anywhere in the urinary tract. The renal tubules may be blocked by myoglobin in the crush syndrome, by bilirubin in severe jaundice, by haemoglobin in haemolysis of any cause, by crystals of sulphonamide if given in the presence of oliguria, and uric acid in the catabolism of bulky tumours in response to chemotherapy.

The ureter may be obstructed by calculi or accidental surgical occlusion; the bladder outflow may be obstructed by the prostate. Surgical obstruction is probably the most common cause of acute renal failure.

Pathology

The naked eye appearance of the kidney in acute renal failure varies slightly according to the cause, but it is usually large, oedematous and pale. Cross-section shows a congested medulla and a pale cortex. Histological section shows tubules choked with cellular debris giving the appearance of necrosis — hence the common term acute tubular necrosis. In fact the cells of the tubules are not usually necrotic, and the condition is often reversible if normal circulation can be restored.

When renal failure is due to underperfusion, blood is often shunted from the cortex to the medulla via arteriovenous anastomoses and the cortex may become so ischaemic that it dies [3]. After about 10 days calcification appears at the inner and outer borders of the dead cortex — tramline calcification. This is a sure sign that the renal damage is irreversible (Fig. 6.1).

Clinical features

The overriding clinical features of the case may be dominated by the condition that has given rise to renal failure, e.g. trauma or septicaemia, and it is not easy to discern those that are due to the onset of renal failure.

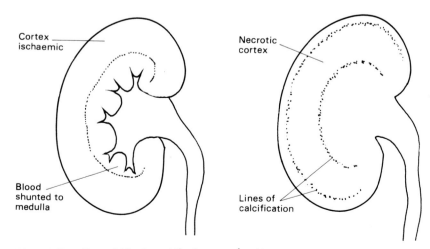

Fig. 6.1 Tramline calcification at the inner and outer borders of the renal cortex signifying irreversible damage.

There are usually three phases in an episode of acute renal failure: prodromal, anuria or oliguria, and recovery.

Prodromal. Whatever the cause of the acute renal failure it is usual for some glomerular filtration to continue at first. The urine which is formed is clouded, dark in colour, and full of debris and casts. This can be helpful in distinguishing between renal failure and complete obstruction where no urine is formed at all.

Anuria or oliguria. After the prodromal phase the formation of urine may cease altogether, gradually or suddenly. In cases without oliguria the urine volume has a fixed specific gravity of 1010. The plasma urea and creatinine rise steadily, the rise is related to the amount of tissue which is being broken down by infection or trauma.

Recovery. Unless the renal cortex has become irreversibly ischaemic there will be recovery. The first urine to appear is of low specific gravity. Then there follows a diuresis, as the tubules are unblocked, and the glomeruli start to filter large volumes of filtrate. During this phase many litres of fluid may have to be given intravenously to keep the patient hydrated and blood volume replenished.

Investigations

It is essential that the diagnosis is made as a matter of urgency [4–6]. The most important possibility to rule out is surgical obstruction: it is easy to check whether there is dilatation of the bladder or ureters with an ultrasound scan and a suspicion of obstruction can be confirmed by catheterizing the bladder or percutaneous nephrostomy. If acute glomerulonephritis is suspected a renal biopsy may be urgently needed in case the condition is one of those which is likely to be reversed by immunosuppressive treatment.

The urea, creatinine and electrolytes will show acidosis and elevated creatinine and urea.

When there is the suspicion that the kidneys are underperfused, a challenge with a water load is part of the investigation. Physiological saline 500 ml or 20% mannitol 125 ml are infused, and the urine output monitored over the next hour or two. Whatever the cause of the renal failure, dehydration must be treated, adding dopamine 1–5 µg/kg/min if the blood pressure remains low.

Management

When renal failure occurs that is likely to be reversible, the objective used to be to keep the patient alive pending natural recovery which could take as long as 6 weeks [7]. During this time there was a danger that giving too much water would overload the circulation and lead to heart failure, and too much protein would exacerbate the rise in urea and creatinine. Only as much water was given as had been lost in sweat and respiration plus what little urine was passed. To minimize unnecessary protein catabolism about 4200 J (1000 cal) a day were given. Potassium was removed by giving glucose and insulin and ion-exchange resins. With this regime the patient suffered torments from thirst.

Today the patient is dialysed from the outset, either with intermittent peritoneal dialysis (see below) or haemodialysis. Since haemodialysis is likely to be for a short time only, there is no need for a shunt or a fistula, and a double-lumen catheter is inserted into the subclavian vein. Dialysis is performed daily or on alternative days according to the catabolic rate.

Chronic renal failure

In some cases the rate of deterioration of renal function is very slow, e.g. in polycystic disease. Here for a time the patient can be kept well by a diet low in protein: even with a creatinine clearance as little as 20 ml/min the plasma creatinine can be halved by limiting the protein in the diet to 40 g/day, and by restricting it to 20 g/day the patient can be relatively healthy with a creatinine clearance of only 5 ml/min. To a large extent these measures are used because of a shortage of facilities for dialysis and transplantation. The quality of life provided by either of the latter is far better than existence on a fluid and protein-restricted diet.

Clinical features

Itching and pigmentation of the skin can be a distressing feature of renal failure. Anaemia varies with the erythropoietin produced by the remaining renal tissue, and may be relieved by injections of artificial erythropoietin [8]. To prevent anaemia the failing kidneys are kept *in situ* for as long as possible, but they must be removed if they harbour infection or are secreting so much renin that hypertension becomes uncontrollable.

There is also a new disease entity which is being seen increasingly often in patients maintained on all forms of treatment for end-stage kidney disease — acquired polycystic disease of the kidneys — in about 16% of whom multicentric carcinomas will develop [9].

Neuropathy occurs in end-stage renal disease because of loss of myelin from peripheral nerves and results in paraesthesiae, weakness and loss of sensation, most marked in the feet [10].

Mental changes may be difficult to detect: want of cooperation and forgetfulness may not be noticed until dialysis restores the patient to normal. In children there is a failure to grow, and in these cases both the children and their parents need considerable help and support [11].

Hypertension is often present, and may be accompanied by retinal changes.

Pericarditis is a potentially lethal complication of uraemia which occurs if the creatinine has been allowed to rise too high. This should be prevented by dialysis.

Two important changes occur to bone metabolism in renal failure. First, the bowel becomes less sensitive to vitamin D and less calcium is absorbed, as a result growing bone is imperfectly calcified, and ostoid forms around each trabecula rather than true bone. The bone becomes weak and prone to fracture (osteomalacia).

Second, the accumulation of phosphate with renal failure lowers the plasma calcium, stimulating hypertrophy of the parathyroids (secondary hyperparathyroidism) which leads to loss of calcium and thinning of the bony trabeculae (osteoporosis). A biopsy of the bone will show typically thinned-out trabeculae covered with a thick seam of osteoid.

The calcium added to the blood from the bony trabeculae is deposited in soft tissues. In the joints of the middle ear this causes deafness. In the edges of the intervertebral discs the stripes of calcification contrast with the osteoporotic vertebral body to give a 'rugger jersey spine'. (Fig. 6.2). Bizarre complications of heterotopic calcification have involved the heart, lungs, skin and small vessels where it may lead to ischaemia [12] (Fig. 6.3).

Other unusual features are seen in patients with long-term renal failure. Carpal tunnel syndrome can occur as a result of the deposit of a type of amyloid [13]. It tends to occur in the arm where a shunt has been set up, and usually requires release of the median nerve.

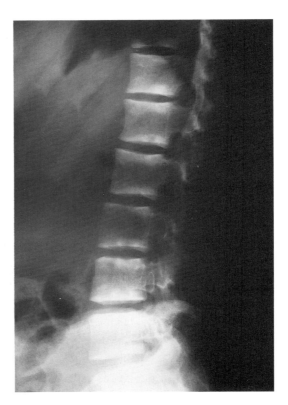

Fig. 6.2 'Rugger jersey spine' — heterotopic calcification in the edges of the intervertebral discs contrasts with rarefaction of the osteoporotic vertebral bodies.

Dialysis

The chief causes of chronic end-stage renal failure requiring dialysis or transplantation are chronic glomerulonephritis (54%), chronic pyelonephritis (12%) and polycystic kidney (5%).

Continuous ambulant peritoneal dialysis (CAPD)

A silicone rubber Tenckhoff catheter [14,15] (Fig. 6.4) is inserted into the peritoneal cavity. Its end lies in the pelvis (Fig. 6.5). Two litres of fluid are run into the peritoneal cavity and left for up to 4 h while the patient can walk about and lead a relatively normal life. The fluid is then run out, taking with it the products of nitrogenous metabolism, and is then replaced. Patients learn to do this themselves. Predictably, the main complications are peritonitis and adhesion formation [15].

It seems to matter less where the catheter lies, and more whether the omentum is able to occlude its openings. Fluid drains as easily from

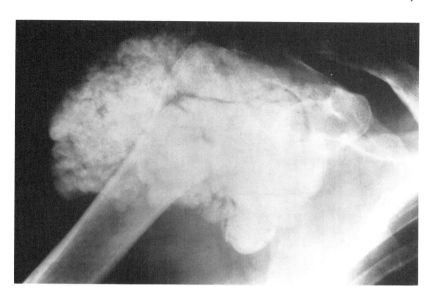

Fig. 6.3 Metastatic calcification around the shoulder joint in renal failure in a patient on haemodialysis for 4 years (courtesy of Dr D.V. Evans).

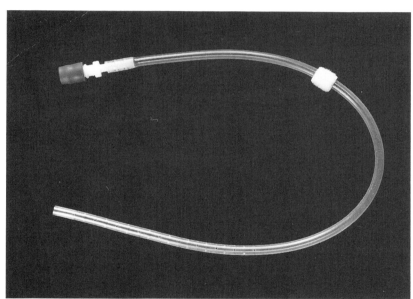

Fig. 6.4 Tenckhoff catheter for CAPD.

the top as from the bottom of the abdomen. The reason why catheters placed in the pelvis do better is probably because the omentum does not reach there.

For temporary dialysis, e.g. in acute renal failure, catheters are available that are introduced on a stylet but if more permanent dialysis is required then a Tenckhoff-type catheter with one or two dacron cuffs is inserted through a short surgical incision (Fig. 6.6). The dacron cuffs stimulate the formation of a ring of granuloma which protects the silastic stalk of the catheter from becoming infected. Even so about 4% of patients with CAPD need treatment for infection every year. The half-life of a given Tenckhoff catheter is about 18 months [15]. There have been many modifications: the shaft may be preformed into an S shape [16], made of polyurethane, or provided with a large flat disc on the peritoneal aspect, which is relatively free from the risk of being clogged by omentum (Fig. 6.7). When inserting these cannulae it is possible to check that the position is correct by peritoneoscopy.

Complications of CAPD

1 Pain on inflow soon after placing the catheter may mean that it is not correctly placed in the peritoneal cavity, but may be from the effect of

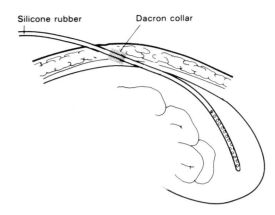

Fig. 6.5 In CAPD a cannula is placed in the pelvis and 2 l quantities of dialysate are run into the peritoneal cavity, left there for 4 h, and run out again.

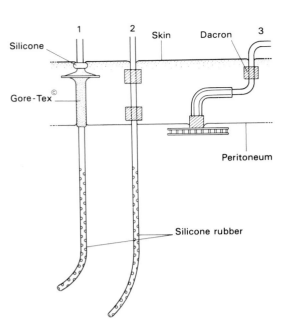

Fig. 6.7 Various types of peritoneal cannulae: (1) Gore-Tex (C. Gore Ass. Inc.); (2) Lifemed C (Division of Vernitron); (3) Lifecath C (Physiocontrol Co).

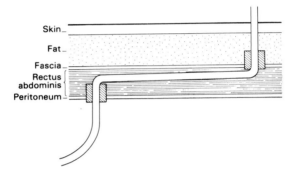

Fig. 6.6 For more permanent peritoneal dialysis a cannula is placed through a long oblique track. The two dacron cuffs provoke barriers of granulation tissue which help to prevent infection.

the inflow through the fine tip of the catheter. Pain is said to be less with the disc type of cannulae.

2 Perforation of the bowel is rare and seals spontaneously in most patients but if there is any deterioration a small laparotomy is necessary to allow the hole to be oversewn.

3 Leakage of fluid tends to occur in the first few weeks, so that if one can delay the instillation of fluid it may be prevented.

4 Blocked cannulae can sometimes be unblocked by instilling streptokinase or urokinase and heparin.

5 Infection: if there are more than three episodes of peritonitis it is usually necessary to replace the cannula and site it elsewhere. The underlying cause is the biofilm of protein that always coats the silicone catheter, through which some organisms, e.g. staphylococci, can invade the surface of the silicone catheter [15].

Haemodialysis

Blood from the patient flows over a thin membrane separating it from the dialysis fluid (Fig. 6.8). There are a number of different artificial kidneys which make this possible, but the underlying principle is the same. As a rule, the management of the haemodialysis falls to our nephrologist colleagues, but the urological surgeon is often involved in the crucial matter of vascular access [17,18].

The chief problem in haemodialysis is vascular access. Cannulae tied into the radial artery and vein were used at first but these soon became thrombosed. Later they were replaced by permanent silicone rubber cannulae emerging through the skin — the Scribner shunt [19] (Fig. 6.9).

If a small arteriovenous fistula (Cimino—Breschia fistula) [20] is created between two peripheral vessels (Fig. 6.10), varicosities soon form on the venous side which make it possible for needles to be inserted at regular intervals. Usually, one needle is inserted for outflow of blood and a second for inflow of blood. In some systems a single needle is used with a two-way intermittent flow.

The creation of a fistula or the insertion of a shunt can usually be performed under brachial plexus block or local anaesthesia. External shunts are still used for acute renal failure, or as tem-

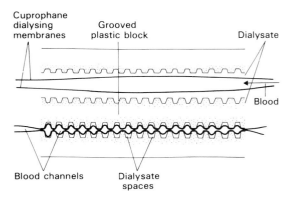

Fig. 6.8 Principle of haemodialysis: blood flows over a thin semipermeable membrane which separates it from the dialysis fluid.

porary measures which give time for varicosities to develop from a fistula.

The classical site for a Cimino fistula is between the radial artery and a vein near the wrist. Alternatives include the radial artery to a dorsal vein in the anatomical snuff-box, a transpalmar anastomosis between the ulnar artery and vein (provided careful tests are performed beforehand to ensure that this will not lead to ischaemia) and between the brachial artery and cephalic vein at the elbow.

By using a valve stripper it is possible to turn a length of vein into an 'artery', much increasing the length of vein available for needling [18].

Many types of graft have been used to create fistulae. The best is the saphenous vein, but it may be ruled out in patients for whom coronary artery bypass surgery is being contemplated. A length of saphenous vein is used to form a bridge between the brachial artery and a forearm vein. Bovine carotid artery has been used, but is prone to aneurysm formation. Grafts made from PTFE, e.g. Gore-Tex, carry a special risk of infection and thrombosis.

A cannula introduced on a guide-wire into the subclavian or femoral vein will give satisfactory access for dialysis in the short term.

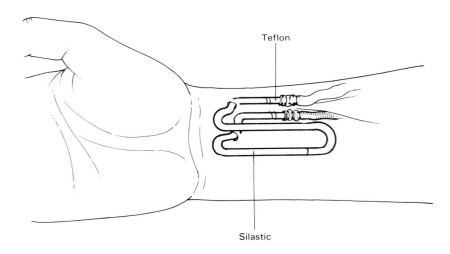

Fig. 6.9 Scribner shunt. Cannulae are placed through an oblique subcutaneous tunnel into the radial artery and vein.

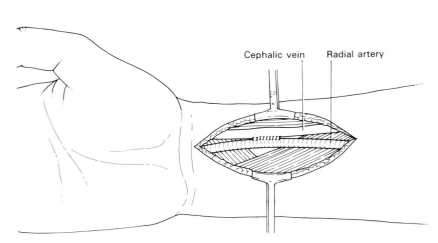

Fig. 6.10 Principle of the Cimino–Breschia fistula.

Complications of fistulae

1 Haemorrhage may occur usually through incorrect management of needles at the time of dialysis.

2 Aneurysms may form in the venous side.

3 Embolism is rare, and arises if a clot is dislodged downstream from the needled site.

4 Infection may occur in and around the fistula, and even necessitate CAPD for a time until the infection can be controlled.

5 Venous hypertension in the hand, often coupled with venous ischaemia gives rise to the 'sore thumb syndrome'. A fistulogram may show that the cause is a stenosis of the proximal draining vein: if so this can be excised and corrected.

6 Arterial steal: claudication and muscle wasting may be seen together with paraesthesiae in the distribution of the median nerve.

7 High output cardiac failure is a rare complication. Like the arterial steal, it can usually be corrected by banding the fistula.

References

1 Nortman DF, Franklin SS (1984) Therapy and management of acute renal failure, in: Suki WN, Massry SG (eds) *Therapy of Renal Diseases and Related Disorders*, pp. 47–62. Dordrecht: Martinus Nijhoff.

2 Dixon BS, Anderson RJ (1985) Nonoliguric acute renal failure. *Am J Kidney Dis* 6: 71.

3 Trueta J, Barclay AE, Daniel PM, Franklin KJ, Pritchard MML (1947) *Studies of the Renal Circulation*. Oxford: Blackwell Scientific Publications.

4 Corwin HL (1987) Prediction of outcome in acute renal failure. *Am J Nephrol* 7: 8.

5 Smithies MN, Cameron JS (1989) Can we predict outcome in acute renal failure? *Nephron* 51: 297.

6 Warren DJ (1987) Acute renal failure: diagnosis of cause needed within hours. *Br Med J* 294: 1569.

7 Kerr DNS (1979) Treatment of acute renal failure with artificial kidneys. *Br Med J* 2: 250.

8 Cotes PM (1988) Erythropoietin: the developing story. *Br Med J* 296: 805.

9 Grantham JJ, Levine E (1985) Acquired cystic disease: replacing one kidney disease with another. *Kidney Int* 28: 99.

10 Tenckhoff HA, Boen FST, Jebsen RH, Sriegler JH (1965) Polyneuropathy in chronic renal insufficiency. *J Am Med Assoc* 192: 1121.

11 Winterborn MH (1987) Growing up with renal failure. *Br Med J* 295: 870.

12 Ashouri OS, Perez RA (1986) Vascular calcification presenting as necrosis of penis in patient with chronic renal failure. *Urology* 28: 420.

13 Zamora JL, Rose JE, Rosario V, Noon GP (1985) Hemodialysis-associated carpal tunnel syndrome. A clinical review. *Nephron* 41: 70.

14 Tenckhoff H, Schechter H (1968) A bacteriologically safe peritoneal access device. *Trans Am Soc Artif Intern Organs* 14: 181.

15 Ash SR, Carr DJ, Diaz-Buxo JA (1990) Peritoneal access devices, in: Nissenson AR, Fine RN, Gentile DE (eds) *Clinical Dialysis*, 2nd edn, pp. 212–39. London: Prentice-Hall International.

16 Twardowski ZJ, Nolph KD, Khanna R *et al.* (1985) The need for a 'swan neck' permanently bent arcuate peritoneal dialysis catheter. *Perit Dial Bull* 5: 219.

17 Lumley JSP (1984) Vascular aspects of haemodialysis. *Br J Hosp Med* 32: 244.

18 Bell PRF, Veitch PS (1990) Vascular access for hemodialysis, in: Nissenson AR, Fine RN, Gentile DE (eds) *Clinical Dialysis*, 2nd edn, pp. 26–44. London: Prentice-Hall International.

19 Scribner BH, Caner JEZ, Buri R, Quinton W (1960) The technique of continuous haemodialysis. *Trans Am Soc Artif Intern Organs* 6: 88.

20 Breschia MJ, Cimino JE, Appel K *et al.* (1966) Chronic hemodialysis using venipuncture and a surgically created arteriovenous fistula. *New Engl J Med* 275: 1089.

Chapter 7: Renal transplantation

Most patients with end-stage renal failure are suitable for transplantation; patients with primary oxalosis, which inexorably destroys the graft, are not. Glomerulonephritis and interstitial nephritis are the most common underlying conditions. About 10% of recipients have polycystic disease and a steadily increasing number of diabetics survive to suffer from renal failure.

Preparation of the recipient

Because there is a shortage of donor organs most patients have been on dialysis for some time before they are offered transplantation. During this time they are vulnerable to the complications of chronic renal failure and the complications of dialysis. The condition of a recipient at the time of transplantation will depend on the skill of his or her nephrologist but anaemia, abnormalities of calcium metabolism and some degree of general debility are common. Previous blood transfusion may raise antibodies which can cause hyperacute rejection. These preformed antibodies will be detected in the crossmatching procedure. In general previous transfusion appears to improve graft survival [1].

Although profound long-standing anaemia may alarm the anaesthetist, peroperative transfusion may cause metabolic difficulties until the graft begins to function. So long as adequate tissue oxygenation is maintained by attention to the inspired oxygen concentration and there is no unexpected haemorrhage, fluid volume replacement by clear fluid is probably preferable.

Native kidneys are rarely removed before transplantation. Even when they lack excretory function they may continue to have a role in haemopoiesis and calcium metabolism which will be important if the transplant fails and is removed. Exceptionally, bilateral nephrectomy may precede transplantation when the native kidneys are the seat of persistent sepsis. Kidneys that are causing uncontrollable hypertension are usually small and contracted and embolization may be a less invasive alternative to nephrec-

tomy. Polycystic kidneys are seldom so large that there is no room for a donor kidney — and even then only one needs to be removed.

Transplantation is occasionally considered for patients who have had bilateral nephrectomy for upper tract tumours. A period of dialysis is useful to allow presentation of clinically silent metastases which would cause trouble when the patient is immunosuppressed.

Kidneys from cadaver donors

The condition of an ischaemic kidney deteriorates quickly unless it is cooled. After 1 h of warm ischaemia there will be a significant loss of function and soon after that the kidney is useless. By contrast, kidneys have been successfully transplanted after being packed in ice for 24 h or more. The main criteria for selecting a donor kidney are that the kidney should be relatively normal in structure and function and that it should be perfused with blood until it can be cooled or installed in a recipient. In practice this means that almost all donor kidneys come from 'beating-heart' cadavers or living donors.

Nearly all suitable kidneys over the age of 2 years can be transplanted so long as there is no evidence of infection or cancer (other than tumours of the brain). Serological tests are performed to make sure the donor does not carry the human immunodeficiency virus (HIV) or hepatitis B viruses.

The kidneys are not used when there is evidence of systemic sepsis, and this excludes some patients whose terminal illness has been managed with indwelling lines for a week or more. If in doubt, the evidence of recent negative blood cultures may make it possible to use the donor kidney. Urinary sepsis is not an absolute bar unless the upper tracts are involved. In older kidneys one must be especially careful to note small renal cell carcinomas and severe atheroma in the donor renal artery [2].

In practice most donor kidneys are provided from patients with head injuries or subarachnoid haemorrhage, who have been maintained on ventilators. Unfortunately, there are too few of these to meet the current demand for donor organs [3].

Strict rules have been agreed to establish that the donor is brain dead [4]. This diagnosis is made by the team responsible for the overall care of the donor and the transplant surgeon has a clear duty to make sure that the appropriate criteria have been used. Once the potential donor is declared brain dead (or strictly, brain stem dead), concern for the feelings of bereaved relatives and the need to release scarce intensive care unit (ICU) resources dictate that the organs should be harvested as quickly as possible.

The use of organs from dead people raises social and ethical problems. It helps if the deceased person carried a donor card, or had discussed the prospect of kidney donation with relatives. Great tact is needed when asking relatives for consent, and a trained transplant coordinator will have the necessary skills to present this as an opportunity for good amidst tragedy. It is inadvisable to go against the wishes of the relatives even if the potential donor carried a card offering organs after death.

Until the diagnosis of death is made the clinical needs of the donor must not be compromised. Good hydration and preservation of renal perfusion by the use of intravenous inotropes will minimize renal damage and a good urine output provoked by frusemide and mannitol is reassuring.

With increasing frequency the donor is used as the source of multiple organs [5], and arrangements must be made for the use of the heart, lungs, liver and possibly pancreas, and to organize the recipient operation for a time when the most experienced transplant team is available.

Kidneys from living donors

Potentially, organs from living donors could make up the shortage of cadaveric kidneys and in some countries, not necessarily those in which the use of organs from the dead is taboo, most kidney transplants are from living donors. Because the donor and recipient operations can be planned in advance, the ischaemia time can be minimized and there is no need for the kidney to be preserved or transported. If the donor and recipient are related, it is possible to select the donor most genetically like the recipient so that there is less chance of rejection. These factors combine to make renal transplantation from living donors highly successful.

Unfortunately, transplanting organs from one living person to another raises a number of ethical problems which may never be fully resolved. There is a danger that the rights of the potential donor will be threatened by emotional, social and even financial pressure. Though life expectancy is not seriously impaired after kidney donation, the operation has morbidity and a small mortality, and there may be psychological sequelae whether or not the transplant is successful. Against this background, the transplant surgeon has a duty to see that donors are effectively selected and counselled and that the surgery is carried out with the greatest technical skill. The donor work-up will include split renal function studies, intravenous urograms and renal arteriograms as well as a thorough search for malignancy or sepsis which would contraindicate organ donation.

Immunology of rejection

Grafts from an identical twin are not rejected, nor is there any rejection if a kidney is taken from the loin and placed in the pelvis of the same patient (an autograft). The antigens responsible for initiating rejection are found on the surface of most cells in the body, but since they were first studied in white cells, they are called human leucocyte antigens (HLAs) [6–8].

The HLA antigens are glycoproteins which are expressed by a group of genes on the short arm of chromosome 6 which make up the human major histocompatibility complex (MHC). There are other minor histocompatibility factors which can lead to graft rejection between siblings even when all the known antigens of the MHC have been correctly matched.

The antigens coded for by the genes of the MHC are classified in two groups according to the position of the genes on chromosome 6. Class I antigens are coded for by genes at the A, B and C loci; class II antigens by those at DP, DQ and DR. For each locus up to 25 different antigens can be identified [7] (Fig. 7.1).

The HLA antigens each have two polypeptide chains. The class I antigens have one chain coded on chromosome 6 (which gives it antigen specificity) while the other is ordinary $beta_2$ microglobulin (from chromosome 15). Both chains of the class II antigens are coded for by genes on chromosome 6. The differences between the

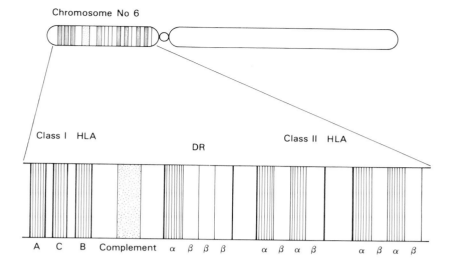

Fig. 7.1 Diagram of chromosome 6.

various HLA antigens are due to variations in the sequence of amino acids.

Nearby on the sixth chromosome are other important genes coding for the 21-hydroxylase enzyme and some of the complement components [7].

Sera with which to identify these antigens are obtained from women who have had multiple pregnancies or who are the recipients of multiple blood transfusions. More recently some monoclonal antibodies to HLA antigens have been synthesized.

When lymphocytes from unrelated people are cultured together in mixed lymphocyte culture (MLC) they will swell up and divide, a reaction determined by human lymphocyte-activating determinants (LADs). These provoke division and activation of both T and B lymphocytes.

There is very good evidence that the outcome of renal transplantation is best when the tissue type of the recipient resembles that of the donor. The A, B and C antigens are detected by serological tests which take an hour or two. Mixed lymphocyte culture is used to detect the D and D-related antigens which are now thought to be of equal or greater importance: this takes up to 10 h using donor lymphocytes recovered from spleen and mesenteric lymph nodes and peripheral lymphocytes harvested from the recipient's blood.

Donor and recipients must also be of the same ABO blood group. The shortage of A donors means that recipients with this group may have a long wait for a kidney, especially if they are rhesus negative.

The immune response

The antigens on the transplant are taken up by macrophages or dendritic cells, and carried to the helper T cells which produce lymphokines such as interleukins 2 and 4, and gamma interferon. Interleukin 2 converts the cytotoxic T cell precursor into the mature cytotoxic T cell, and acts on interleukin 2 receptors (IL2R) present in T and B cells and macrophages (Fig. 7.2). Interleukin 4 turns B lymphocytes into plasma cells that produce antibodies. Gamma interferon induces the appearance of class II HLA antigens in tissues including the graft [6−9]. Activated T lymphocytes are mobilized to mount a cell-mediated immune response against these antigens.

Four main types of rejection are important in kidney transplantation. Preformed antibodies raised by previous exposure to appropriate antigens (by pregnancy, transfusion or transplantation) cause hyperacute rejection: the kidney swells and infarcts within minutes of its circulation being restored. Antibodies are deposited, attract complement and leucocytes, and the vessels thrombose. Likewise, accelerated rejection is mediated by antibodies produced in response to an antigen encountered previously — a similar effect on the graft occurs a day or two after transplantation as the antibody is manufactured by activated plasma cells. Acute rejection occurs at any time after transplantation, though the graft is particularly susceptible at about 1 week postoperatively. This is a manifestation of cell-mediated immunity. The graft is infil-

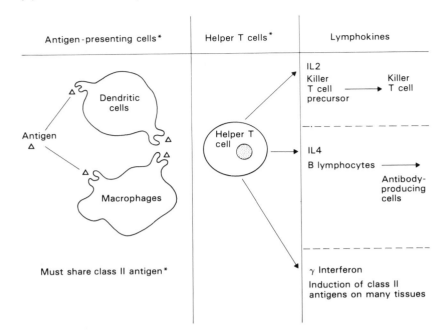

| Antigen-presenting cells* | Helper T cells* | Lymphokines |

Fig. 7.2 The immune response. Antigens from the transplant are taken up by macrophages and dendritic cells which present them to the helper T cells which produce lymphokines such as interleukins 2 and 4 and gamma interferon.

trated by large numbers of aggressive activated T cells. Typically, the transplanted kidney swells, becomes tender and its function declines. The patient often suffers systemic symptoms with pyrexia and profound malaise. Acute rejection can often be aborted by massive doses of intravenous steroids but remains the main cause of graft loss in the first year after transplantation. Chronic rejection causes a steady decline of transplant function months or years after successful grafting. It is associated with deposition of immunoglobulin M (IgM) which clogs the glomeruli. It is difficult to treat and is a cause of late graft loss.

Immunosuppression

The following methods are used to suppress the immune rejection response [10].

Cyclosporin A

Cyclosporin A is the most effective and least toxic of the various agents available [11]. It is an 11 amino acid polypeptide which is insoluble in water. It has now been synthesized. Its principal action is to prevent the T helper lymphocytes from producing lymphokines. By preventing the production of interleukin 2 it stops their precursors from turning into cytotoxic T cells, and may also inhibit the induction of class II HLA antigens in the kidney by gamma interferon, i.e. make the graft less antigenic.

By stopping the production of cytotoxic T cells cyclosporin encourages the proliferation of suppressor T lymphocytes which help prolong graft survival.

In the early trials of cyclosporin it was found to give effective immunosuppression with low doses of steroids or none at all, but it was soon found to be nephrotoxic, though this could be reduced by reducing the dose of cyclosporin.

Several different regimes have been used. In some the patient starts off with cyclosporin, and then changes over to azathioprine and steroids after 3 months, with the great advantage of reducing the high cost of cyclosporin. In others the patient is maintained on cyclosporin alone, reserving steroids for the treatment of rejection episodes. Other centres use combinations of drugs, e.g. three (cyclosporin, azathioprine and steroids) or four (azathioprine, steroids, anti-lymphocyte globulin at first, followed by cyclosporin after about 2 weeks when good renal function has been established).

Cyclosporin has special advantages in children, those over 55, diabetics and those who have been sensitized by previous graft rejection. It is probably not necessary in living related HLA identical transplants, but useful in non-HLA identical living donor transplants. It has also made it possible to achieve good results with unrelated living donor transplants, e.g. between spouses.

Nephrotoxicity from cyclosporin takes three forms. Early nephrotoxicity is seen especially when there has been a prolonged warm ischaemic time. Interim nephrotoxicity appears to be related to high serum levels, and to improve with a lowered dose. The mechanism is thought to be vasospasm of the glomerular afferent arterioles, and it responds to withdrawing the cyclosporin. In practice it may be difficult to distinguish from rejection, and fine needle aspiration or biopsy may be required. Delayed nephrotoxicity takes the form of interstitial fibrosis, and is perhaps concomitant with chronic rejection.

Hepatotoxicity which may progress to cirrhosis occurs in high doses or patients who start off with abnormal liver function.

Lymphoma and carcinoma of the skin may occur with any form of immunosuppression, and is not special to cyclosporin.

Some drug interactions are of potential importance in the event of urological complications: aminoglycosides, sulphonamides, and trimethoprim can all increase the nephrotoxicity of cyclosporin.

Azathioprine and steroids

The oldest effective immunosuppressant, azathioprine, may work by blocking the production of interleukin 2. Steroids affect T lymphocytes and monocytes but their true effect on immunosuppression — which is complementary to azathioprine — is little understood [11]. The usual dose of the combination is azathioprine 2–3 mg/ kg/day as a single dose, plus a high initial dose of prednisolone dropping to 10–15 mg/day after 6 months. Units do not agree over these doses: the initial high dose varies from 20 to 30 mg/kg/ day, but if lower doses of steroids are given, then higher doses of azathioprine are needed.

The complications of azathioprine include bone marrow suppression, anaemia and impaired liver function. The side effects of steroids include stunting of growth, poor wound healing, osteoporosis, Cushingoid features, cataracts, diabetes and peptic ulceration. On the combined regime patients are more susceptible to infections including tuberculosis and cytomegalovirus.

Antilymphocyte globulin (ALG)

By immunizing horses with human lymphocytes sera were obtained which were shown to be effective in treating graft rejection but the sera were so heterogenous that they proved to be of limited value. When cell hybridization was discovered monoclonal antibodies were developed which could suppress T cells and their subsets.

Randomized trials have given inconsistent results when comparing azathioprine–steroid with ALG as the method of immunosuppression, but consistent success when used for rejection [12]. Different monoclonal antibodies, e.g. OKT3, CBL1 and WT32, are undergoing trials which suggest that they may be very valuable in reversing rejection when conventional high dose prednisolone has failed. Their side effects include fever, asthma and pulmonary oedema [13].

Total lymphoid irradiation

Radiation was used in the early days of transplantation as a means of immunosuppression and was reintroduced when a method developed for treating Hodgkin's disease was found to be an effective immunosuppressant, and to diminish the absolute number and response of T cells for as long as 10 years [14]. The proportion of T suppressor cells increased at the expense of T helper cells. It was used in patients who had frequently rejected previous transplants, but cyclosporin A was found to be easier and more reliable in use. However, when used in combination with ALG or cyclosporin the method appears to hold out the promise of inducing tolerance that can be indefinitely prolonged [15].

Inheritance of MHC

Chromosome pairs are split at meiosis, so each child must receive one half of its MHC antigens from the father, the other half from the mother. Siblings and parents must therefore have half their antigens in common (Fig. 7.3). The results of transplantation improve if more antigens are identical, so that living donor transplants from parent to child, or one sibling to another, tend to do very well. For the same reason living unrelated donor transplants do no better than kidneys from unrelated cadavers [6,16].

In larger families there will always be one or two siblings with identical HLA antigens and the results of transplantation begin to approach that seen in identical twins but not quite, for there are always minor transplantation antigens to be reckoned with.

In cadaveric transplantation the chance of finding an HLA identical recipient means that it is necessary to organize a large pool of recipients, and have their HLA status kept on a central register. The kidneys are sent to the best matched

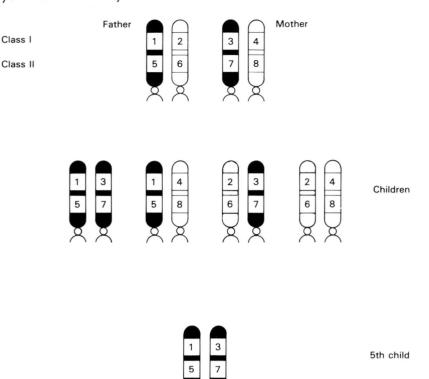

Father

Mother

Class I

Class II

Children

5th child

Fig. 7.3 Inheritance of class I and II HLA antigens.

available recipient. These schemes require immense effort and goodwill and in the past were opposed by many who felt that the benefit achieved did not justify the extra trouble and expense. Today, it is quite clear that a good HLA match greatly improves the long-term survival of the graft [16,17].

Technique of removal of the donor kidney

Cadaver donor

Once the decision has been made that the cadaver is brain dead and permission has been given to proceed [4], steps are taken to restore the dead patient's blood volume by infusion of intravenous saline, mannitol and inotropes to relax intrarenal vessels [18,19].

The technique for removing the cadaver kidneys aims to preserve the renal vessels, all the fat in the renal hilum and the fine vessels that supply the ureter. In modern conditions, with a beating heart donor, there is no need for haste, and the overriding consideration must be to make sure the kidneys are well preserved and undamaged.

If the decision has been made to remove only the kidneys for transplantation, a long midline incision is made, enlarged if necessary by an additional transverse incision (Fig. 7.4). A careful but rapid search is made for evidence of malignancy or sepsis.

The ascending colon and small bowel are completely mobilized by incising their peritoneal reflections, and placed on the chest (Fig. 7.5). The superior mesenteric and coeliac arteries are divided between ligatures, allowing access to the aorta well above the renal vessels (Fig. 7.6). The aorta and vena cava are taped just above the bifurcation. A clamp is placed on the aorta at the level of the coeliac artery. A Foley catheter is inserted into the aorta and secured with a strong ligature (Fig. 7.7). Ice-cold preservative solution (see below) is run in to perfuse and cool the kidneys *in situ*. After about 500 ml have been run in the kidneys will be seen to have become cold and pale. The perfusion is continued at a slower rate until the effluent from the renal veins is quite clear.

The aorta and vena cava are now removed *en bloc* with the kidneys and the upper two-thirds of the ureters, clipping and dividing each pair of lumbar arteries (Fig. 7.8). The block of

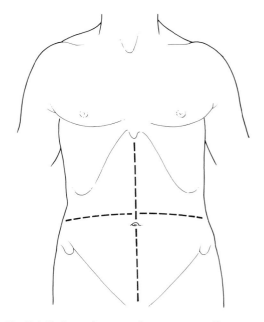

Fig. 7.4 Cadaver donor nephrectomy: cruciform incision.

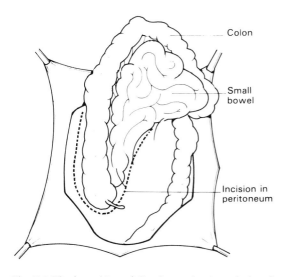

Fig. 7.5 The bowel is mobilized completely and placed on the chest.

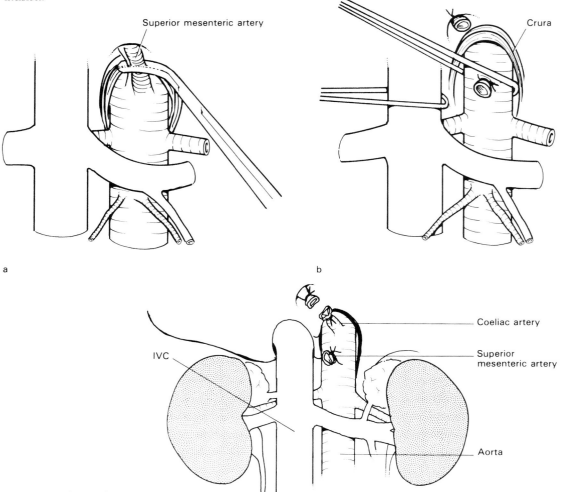

Fig. 7.6 (a & b) The superior mesenteric and (c) coeliac arteries are divided between ligatures.

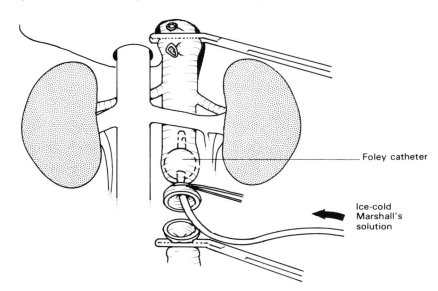

Fig. 7.7 Perfusion of the kidneys through a foley catheter in the aorta.

kidneys, vena cava and aorta is now removed and placed in a bowl of ice-cold perfusion fluid, where it can be examined at leisure. The aorta and vena cava, are slit open in the midline (Fig. 7.9) and careful note is made of the presence of more than one vessel on each side, for the information of the team who are to use the kidneys later on. One or two lymph nodes and a 3 cm portion of spleen are removed for the purposes of tissue typing and placed with each kidney attached to its half of the vena cava and aorta and put in a pair of sterile nylon bags inside a polystyrene container containing ice chips. The wound is closed with a continuous suture.

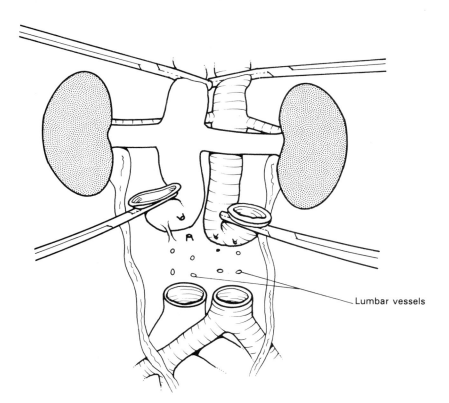

Fig. 7.8 The aorta and vena cava are removed *en bloc* with the kidneys and upper two-thirds of the ureters; the lumbar vessels are clipped and divided.

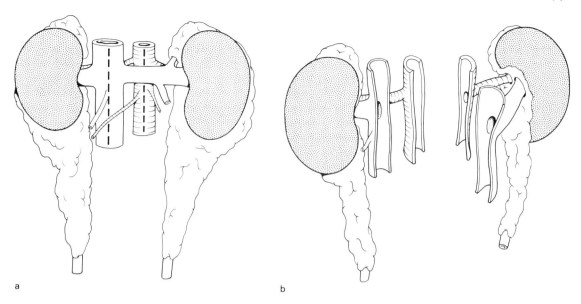

Fig. 7.9 (a & b) The aorta and vena cava are slit open in the midline, carefully noting if more than one renal artery is present on either side.

Living donor

Every volunteer living donor must receive a most careful investigation to make sure that the remaining kidney is perfect, and that there is no unsuspected serious disorder that would make the operation unsafe. The wise surgeon will make absolutely sure that the potential donor understands the sacrifice he or she is to make, and has not been unduly persuaded to give the kidney.

The courage and generosity of the living donor elicits the utmost respect and places a heavy burden upon the surgeon: there is no operation so stressful to the surgeon than removing a perfectly good kidney from a perfectly healthy individual [20]. It is helpful to be able to explain to the donor that the operation is very safe, and that there is a normal life expectancy with only one kidney [21]. The facts are that there have been about 20 deaths in more than 40 000 living donor transplants or 0.05% (most of them from pulmonary embolism) [21].

The preliminary investigations include a bilateral angiogram. It is easier and safer to use a kidney with a single artery. The left renal vein is longer than the right and easier to put in.

An adequate exposure is provided by a 12th rib bed approach. It is not necessary to remove the rib or open the pleura. The renal artery is dissected and taped, and the renal vein carefully cleaned (Fig. 7.10). On the left side take great

care that there is not a circumaortic left renal vein, or a large lumbar vein entering the left renal vein posteriorly. If this is present and recognized it is divided between ligatures, but if not noticed and torn by mistake there can be considerable haemorrhage.

Great care is taken not to disturb the hilar fat and risk injuring the small vessels that supply the ureter [19].

When the message is received from the other operating theatre that everything is ready for the donor operation, the ureter is gently dissected out and divided, the artery and vein are ligated and divided and the kidney placed in a bowl of ice-cold perfusing solution, where the renal artery is perfused with ice-cold perfusing solution in the usual way, until the effluent from the vein is entirely clear (Fig. 7.11). The wound is closed without drainage.

Preservation of the kidney

Over the last 25 years methods of preserving the donor kidney have steadily improved [22]. Prolonged graft survival was first achieved when the kidney was perfused with a solution [23,24] whose composition was intended to resemble that of the intracellular fluid. A modification of Collins solution without the magnesium was widely adopted in Europe ('Euro-Collins'). More recently, the Wisconsin University solution which includes a synthetic colloid hydroxyethyl starch

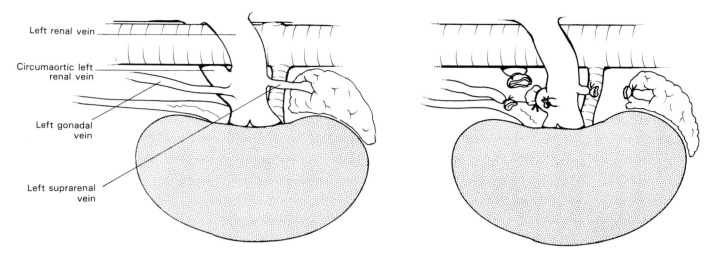

Fig. 7.10 Living donor nephrectomy. On the left side beware of a circumaortic renal vein, or a large lumbar vein entering the renal vein at this point.

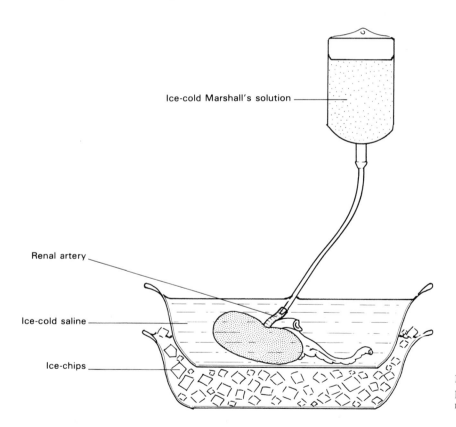

Fig. 7.11 The donor kidney is irrigated with ice-cold preserving fluid until the fluid emerging from the renal vein is seen to be clear.

was introduced for the preservation and transport of livers with conspicuous success. In renal transplantation it has been shown to give 23% delayed graft function (compared with 33% for Euro-Collins) and a 6% better graft function at the end of the first year [25]. Using these fluids, and keeping the kidney in a sterile ice-cold container makes it possible to use the kidney even after 3 days. The critical factors are the delay, causing warm ischaemia time, between death and removal of the kidney, and between taking the kidney out of its ice-box and sewing it into the recipient. This warm-up time can be minimized by keeping the kidney in a cool jacket [19].

Inserting the kidney

Whether the kidney comes from a cadaver or a living donor, the technique of renal transplantation is virtually the same.

Through an oblique groin incision, or the pararectal incision of Alexandre (Fig. 7.12), the inferior epigastric vessels are divided and the peritoneum is reflected off the common iliac vessels and bladder (Fig. 7.13). Unless the arteries show evidence of much atheroma, it is usual to join the donor renal artery onto the internal iliac artery, but to prevent it from being kinked the common and external iliac arteries are cleaned and mobilized as well (Fig. 7.14). Care is taken to ligate the lymphatics in the connective tissue sheath of the arteries and veins to prevent the subsequent formation of a lymphocele. The common and external iliac veins are now cleaned and all their posterior tributaries ligated and divided so as to mobilize them thoroughly.

The internal iliac artery is irrigated with heparinized saline and anastomosed end to end to the donor renal artery using 6-o monofilament prolene (Fig. 7.15). The vessels are flushed with heparinized saline to expel the air before the suture is tied.

If the internal iliac is found to be very atheromatous it may need endarterectomy, or the donor

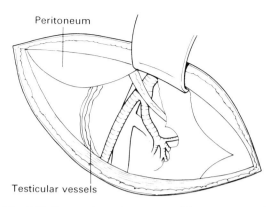

Fig. 7.13 Extraperitoneal exposure of the common and internal iliac vessels.

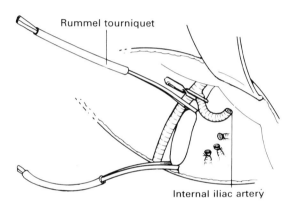

Fig. 7.14 Preparation of the internal iliac artery.

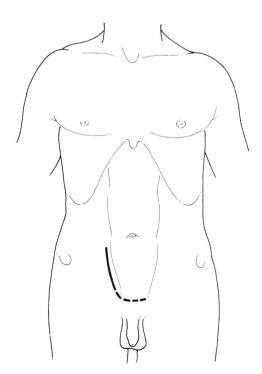

Fig. 7.12 The pararectal incision of Alexandre.

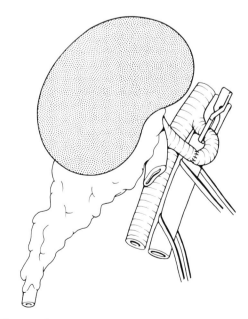

Fig. 7.15 End to end anastomosis of the internal iliac artery to the donor renal artery.

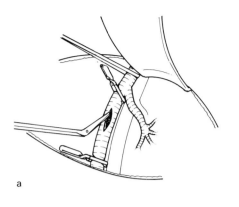

a

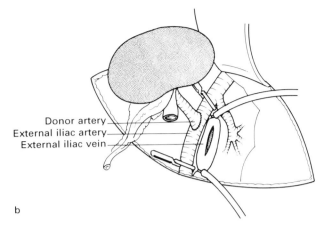

b

Donor artery
External iliac artery
External iliac vein

Fig. 7.16 (a) Preparation of the external iliac artery for end to side anastomosis of the donor renal artery to the external iliac artery. (b) External iliac vein prepared for anastomosis.

renal artery can be anastomosed end to side to the external iliac artery (Fig. 7.16). When there is more than one renal artery one may anastomose each one to a branch of the internal iliac, or sew a Carrel patch onto the side of the external iliac artery (Fig. 7.17).

The donor renal vein is anastomosed end to side to the recipient external iliac vein (Fig. 7.18). The venous clamps are removed first, any small leak being controlled by gentle pressure or a recovery suture. The arterial clamps follow and the kidney is seen to expand, throb and turn from white to a healthy pink.

The technique of ureterovesical anastomosis varies from one centre to another. In many units the standard Leadbetter–Politano technique is used as for vesicoureteric reflux (see p. 152). In other centres the ureter is placed in a submucosal tunnel on the anterior presenting part of the bladder (Fig. 7.19). With either technique a mucosa–mucosal anastomosis is made after spatulating the ureter, and reflux is prevented by a submucosal tunnel. Opinions vary amongst transplant surgeons as to the advantages of splinting the anastomosis with a suitable catheter for a few days.

Diagnosis of rejection

There are four types of rejection [25].

Hyperacute rejection occurs when there are donor-specific HLA class I antibodies. Sometimes within minutes of taking off the vascular clamps the kidney becomes flabby and blue and stops making urine. This may be noticed on the operating table, or within an hour or so of the transplant.

At this early stage the differential diagnosis lies between hyperacute rejection, acute tubular

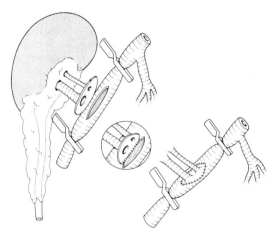

Fig. 7.17 Where there is more than one renal artery a Carrel patch of donor aorta is sewn onto the side of the external iliac artery.

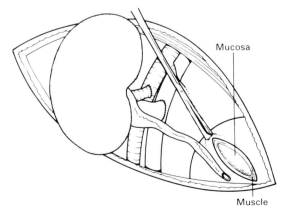

Mucosa

Muscle

Fig. 7.18 The vascular anastomoses are completed, and the submucosal tunnel is then prepared in the bladder for the ureter.

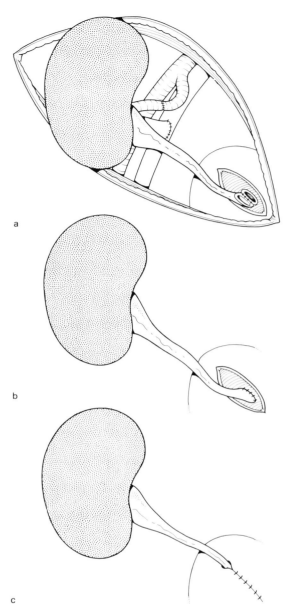

Fig. 7.19 (a & b) A wide elliptical anastomosis is made between the ureter and bladder mucosa. (c) The terminal 5 cm of ureter are buried in a loose tunnel of bladder muscle.

necrosis, renal arterial thrombosis or ureteric obstruction. A renogram or Doppler studies will show that perfusion has stopped. An ultrasound scan will rule out ureteric obstruction. It may still be difficult to be sure whether the kidney is rejected or undergoing tubular necrosis, and a biopsy may be necessary.

Accelerated rejection is comparable to the 'second set' rejection and occurs in a patient who has been sensitized to the graft by a previous transplant or pregnancy. After a period of 2 or 3 days after the transplant operation the creatinine rises, the patient has a fever and the graft becomes swollen and tender.

An ultrasound scan will show whether there is ureteric obstruction. A biopsy may be necessary to make certain that rejection is taking place, but fine needle aspiration, which will show lymphoblasts and macrophages in the aspirate may enable the diagnosis to be made at once.

Acute rejection occurs between 1 and 8 weeks after transplantation, and with conventional immunosuppression with azathioprine and steroids the clinical picture is identical to accelerated rejection described above. When cyclosporin is used the picture is less florid and it is very difficult to be sure that the rising creatinine is not caused by cyclosporin nephrotoxicity. Fever, a fall in urine output and a low serum level of cyclosporin suggest rejection. Fine needle aspiration cytology will show blast cells and macrophages in rejection. A biopsy with the Biopty needle may be the only way to make sure by showing the dense cellular infiltration and oedema of rejection. Biopsies can give rise to arteriovenous fistulae, but these are usually small and need no treatment. Acute rejection can take place years after an apparently successful transplant, perhaps precipitated by inadvertent failure to take the drugs, infection or a blood transfusion [26–28].

Chronic rejection may take place at any time after transplantation. It is marked by a gradual deterioration in renal function which does not improve when the dose of steroids is increased. A biopsy shows interstitial fibrosis and intimal fibrosis of arteries with hyalinization of glomeruli. The differential diagnosis from cyclosporin nephrotoxicity is difficult even with a biopsy.

References

1 Black RM, Poppel DM, Khauli RB (1991) Blood transfusions and renal transplantation — are pretransplant blood transfusions still needed in the cyclosporine era? *Urology* 38: 397.

2 Foster MC, Wenham PW, Rowe PA *et al.* (1988) Use of older patients as cadaveric kidney donors. *Br J Surg* 75: 767.

3 Gore SM, Hinds CJ, Rutherford AJ (1989) Organ donation from intensive care units in England. *Br Med J* 299: 1193.

4 Smith R, Barnes AD, Bessey GS *et al.* (1983)

Cadaveric Organs for Transplantation: a Code of Practice Including the Diagnosis of Brain Death. London: DHSS.

5 Odom NJ (1990) Organ donation 1. Management of the multiorgan donor. *Br Med J* 300: 571.

6 Hayes JM (1993) The immunobiology and clinical use of current immunosuppressive therapy for renal transplantation. *J Urol* 149: 437.

7 Ting A, Simpson E (1989) Major and minor histocompatibility antigens, in: Brent L, Sells RA (eds) *Organ Transplantation: Current Clinical and Immunological Concepts*, pp. 1–18. London: Baillière Tindall.

8 Jordan ML (1993) Immunosuppressive therapy and results of renal transplantation. *Curr Opinion Urol* 3: 126.

9 Strom TB (1989) Immunosuppression in tissue and organ transplantation, in: Brent L, Sells RA (eds) *Organ Transplantation: Current Clinical and Immunological Concepts*, pp. 39–56. London: Baillière Tindall.

10 Morris PJ (1988) Cyclosporine, in: Morris PJ (ed.) *Kidney Transplantation: Principles and Practice*, pp. 285–317. Philadelphia: WB Saunders.

11 Walker RG, d'Apice AJF (1988) Azathioprine and steroids, in: Morris PJ (ed.) *Kidney Transplantation: Principles and Practice*, pp. 319–42. Philadelphia: WB Saunders.

12 Waer M, Strober S (1988) Total lymphoid irradiation (TLI), in: Morris PJ (ed.) *Kidney Transplantation: Principles and Practice*, pp. 371–82. Philadelphia: WB Saunders.

13 Cosimi AB (1988) Antilymphocyte globulin and monoclonal antibodies, in: Morris PJ (ed.) *Kidney Transplantation: Principles and Practice*, pp. 343–69. Philadelphia: WB Saunders.

14 Salaman JR, Griffin PJA, Johnson RWG *et al.* (1993) Controlled trial of RS-61443 in renal transplant patients receiving cyclosporine monotherapy. *Transplant Proc* 25: 695.

15 Opelz G (1989) Renal transplantation in Europe, in: Brent LS, Sells RA (eds) *Organ Transplantation: Current Clinical and Immunological Concepts*, pp. 185–93. London: Baillière Tindall.

16 Waltezer WC, Shabtal M, Malinowski K, Rapaport FT (1994) Current status of immunological monitoring in the renal allograft recipient. *J Urol* 152: 1070.

17 Nicol DL (1995) Urologic aspects of renal transplantation. *Current Opinion in Urology* 5: 86.

18 Forsythe JLR, Dunnigan PM, Proud G, Lennard TWJ, Taylor RMR (1989) Reducing renal injury during transplantation. *Br J Surg* 76: 999.

19 Cosimi AB (1988) The donor and donor nephrectomy, in: Morris PJ (ed.) *Kidney Transplantation: Principles and Practice*, pp. 93–121. Philadelphia: WB Saunders.

20 Merrill JP, Murray JE, Harrison HH, Guild WR, Boston MD (1956) Successful homotransplantation of the human kidney between identical twins. *J Am Med Assoc* 160: 277.

21 Najarian JS, Chavers BM, McHugh LE, Matas AJ (1992) 20 years or more of follow-up of living kidney donors. *Lancet* 340: 807.

22 Belzer FO, Southard JH (1988) Principles of solid-organ preservation by cold storage. *Transplantation* 45: 673.

23 Ploeg RJ (1990) Kidney preservation with the UW and Euro-Collins solutions. *Transplantation* 49: 281.

24 Ploeg RJ, van Bockel JH, Langendijk PTH *et al.* (1992) Effect of preservation solution on results of cadaveric kidney transplantation. *Lancet* 340: 129.

25 Morris PJ (1989) The clinical and laboratory diagnosis of graft rejection, in: Brent L, Sells RA (eds) *Organ Transplantation: Current Clinical and Immunological Concepts*, pp. 57–69. London: Baillière Tindall.

26 Jordan ML, Shapiro R, Vivas CA *et al.* (1994) FK506 'rescue' for resistant rejection of renal allografts under primary cyclosporine immunosuppression. *Transplantation* 57: 860.

27 Laskow DA, Deierhoi MH, Hudson SL, Orr CL, Curtis JJ, Diethelm AG (1994) The incidence of subsequent acute rejection following the treatment of refractory renal allograft rejection with Mycophenolate Mofetil (RS61443). *Transplantation* 57: 640.

28 Merkus JWS, Seebregts CJAM, Hoitsma AJ, van Asten WNJC, Koene RAP, Skotnicki SH (1993) High incidence of arteriovenous fistula after biopsy of kidney allografts. *Br J Surg* 80: 310.

Chapter 8: Kidney and ureter — congenital abnormalities

Ectopia, aplasia, etc.

To understand the many congenital anomalies in the site and position of the kidney, it is necessary to recall that the two metanephroi arise in the caudal end of the embryo where they are close to each other, and if the two lumps of amorphous mesenchyme touch, they can easily fuse together [1]. As the caudal part of the fetus enlarges, pelvic organs such as the metanephros are carried upwards.

Most of the anomalies in position of the kidney occur either because the two metanephroi fuse together, or because they fail to rise.

Rotated kidney

The metanephros is a lump of mesenchyme slightly caudal and lateral to the tail end of the nephrogenic ridge, and the ureteric bud enters on its anterior aspect (Fig. 8.1). With the development of the caudal end of the fetus the metanephros not only rises up but it also rotates. The kidney may fail to rotate, although it may reach the normal position in the loin. It gives an unusual urogram but is otherwise of no significance (Fig. 8.2). In a sense it should be called an 'unrotated kidney'.

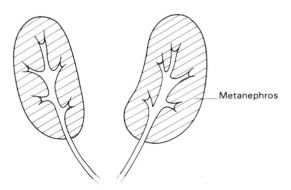

Fig. 8.1 The ureteric bud starts by entering the anterior aspect of the metanephros; if this persists it gives rise to the 'rotated kidney'.

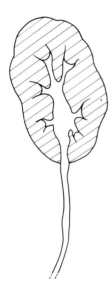

Fig. 8.2 Appearance of a 'rotated kidney'. Note the medially facing calices.

Pelvic kidney

Here the kidney fails to rise and remains unrotated in the pelvis (Figs 8.3 & 8.4). Its segmental arteries arise from the aorta, and common, internal and external iliac arteries. Pelvic kidneys seldom cause obstruction in labour, but as one anomaly is often accompanied by another, they often cause trouble when there is a coexisting obstruction at the pelviureteric junction or reflux.

Fused kidneys

If the two metanephroi touch each other and fuse, several variations occur. The most common is the horseshoe kidney where the metanephroi fuse at their lower poles. As the caudal part of the embryo enlarges, and the kidneys rise up the fused kidney rises until it is held up — usually by the superior mesenteric artery but sometimes by the inferior mesenteric artery (Fig. 8.5).

Horseshoe kidneys occur in 0.1% of births and seldom cause any trouble unless associated with

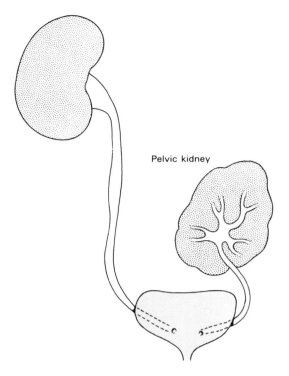

Fig. 8.3 If the kidney remains in the pelvis it stays 'rotated'.

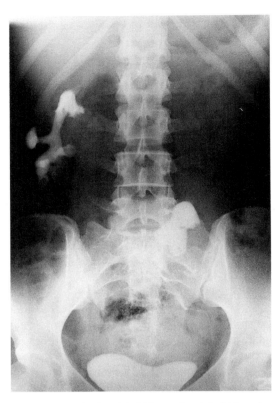

Fig. 8.4 IVU of left pelvic kidney; the right kidney is 'rotated'.

some other anomaly such as pelviureteric junction obstruction. This obstruction has nothing to do with the isthmus though in the past mis-

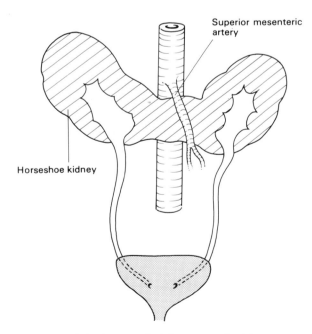

Fig. 8.5 If the lower end of the metanephroi fuse together, they remain 'rotated' and their course up the abdomen is held up by the superior or, rarely, the inferior mesenteric arteries.

guided attempts were often made to cure hydronephrosis by dividing the isthmus.

Horseshoe kidneys may be found by chance in the course of operations for aortic aneurysms. The isthmus may be divided in the midline which is usually bloodless. Small veins crossing the mid-line may need to be secured with suture ligature.

The intravenous urogram (IVU) in a horseshoe kidney has a typical appearance with a pair of medially facing calices. The renogram shows the junction of the two kidneys (Figs 8.6 & 8.7).

Crossed renal ectopia

If the metanephroi meet and fuse, one may follow the other across the midline to result in crossed renal ectopia (Fig. 8.8). Cystoscopy shows both ureteric orifices in their normal position. Radiographic appearances are characteristic (Fig. 8.9).

Cake kidney

Sometimes fused kidneys do not rise up, but remain in the pelvis where they form a large amorphous mass in front of the sacrum (Figs 8.10

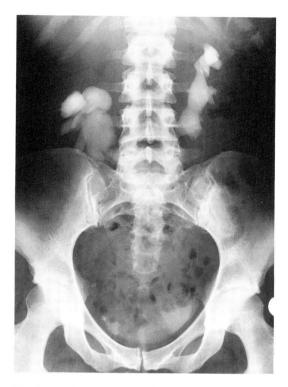

Fig. 8.6 IVU showing typical appearance of a horseshoe kidney.

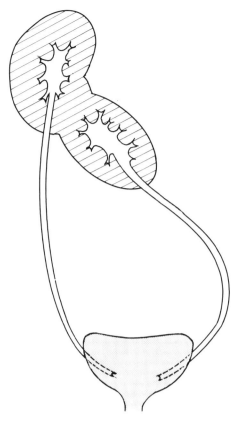

Fig. 8.8 Diagram of crossed renal ectopia.

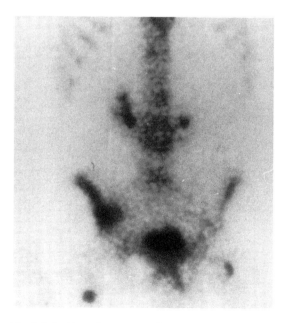

Fig. 8.7 Incidental renogram obtained in the course of a bone scan shows fused lower poles of a horseshoe kidney (courtesy of Dr Neil Garvie).

& 8.11). They have a bizarre but profuse blood supply [2].

These anomalous kidneys only cause trouble if they are associated with some other condition —

usually pelviureteric junction obstruction, infection or stones. There is, however, one major hazard: they may be discovered by chance in the course of abdominal palpation, ultrasonography, computerized tomography (CT) scanning or at laparotomy. If the condition is not suspected the mass may be mistaken for a neoplasm. Biopsy may be followed by severe bleeding and several cases are on record where removal of the 'mass' has resulted in fatal anuria.

To expose any of these variations on the theme of a fused kidney, a generous abdominal incision should be made to give room to mobilize the right colon and terminal ileum. The inferior colic artery may need to be divided. Whatever needs to be done to the kidney, e.g. removal of a stone or pyeloplasty for pelviureteric junction, is completed and the bowel is then replaced. A transabdominal approach makes it easy to see and control the unusual arterial supply.

Thoracic kidney

The thoracic kidney is caused not by any fault in the embryogenesis of the kidney, but by an error

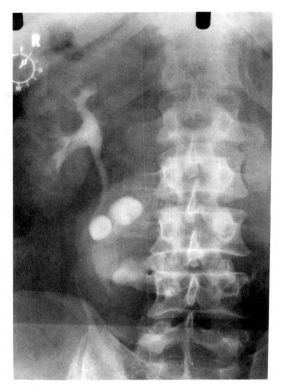

Fig. 8.9 IVU showing crossed renal ectopia.

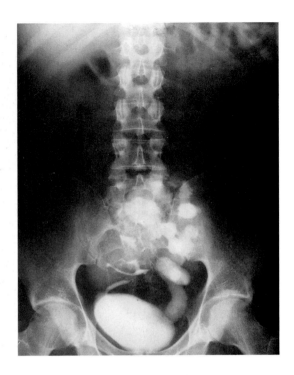

Fig. 8.11 Urogram of a 'cake kidney'.

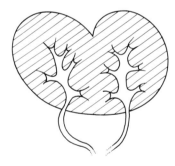

Fig. 8.10 When the two metanephroi fuse and fail to ascend, they form a 'cake kidney'.

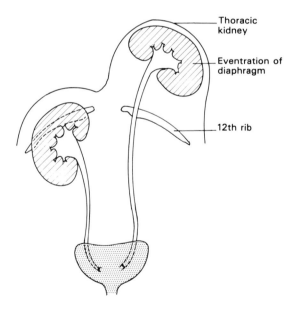

Fig. 8.12 When there is a herniation of the diaphragm the kidney may be seen in the chest, but it is not truly an ectopic kidney.

in the formation of the diaphragm, resulting in herniation of some of the abdominal contents into the chest. The usual cause is a persistent foramen of Bochdalek. Thoracic kidneys are exceedingly rare, and are detected by chance in an X-ray of the chest [3] (Figs 8.12 & 8.13).

Retrocaval ureter

A retrocaval ureter is due not to an embryological defect in the kidney or ureter but to persistence of the right subcardinal vein. As a result the bogus 'vena cava' lies in front of the ureter instead of behind it (Fig. 8.14). It was for retro-caval ureter that Anderson and Hynes devised their operation for hydronephrosis [4]. It is only present on the right side.

Patients have pain in the right loin or urinary infection. Investigation shows a hydronephrosis,

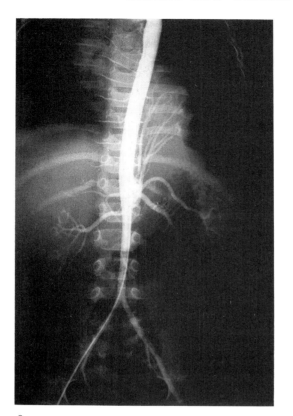

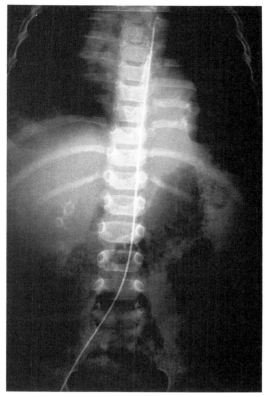

a

b

Fig. 8.13 Radiograph of a 'thoracic kidney':
(a) angiogram,
(b) pyelogram (courtesy of Miss Leela Kapila).

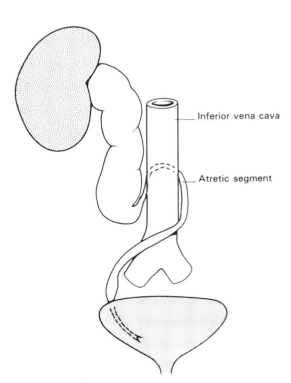

Inferior vena cava

Atretic segment

Fig. 8.14 Diagram of retrocaval ureter.

with a very characteristic shape to the upper part of the dilated ureter (Fig. 8.15).

The section of ureter lying behind the vena cava is useless and not worth attempting to get out. Through a generous transverse or vertical mid-line incision the right colon and duodenum are reflected medially to expose the vena cava, kidney and ureter. The dilated upper part of the ureter is mobilized, and the inferior part freed up to where it disappears behind the vena cava where the ureter is cut across. A long oblique anastomosis is then made between the baggy upper ureter and the normal lower part (Fig. 8.16).

Errors in development of the metanephros

Agenesis

If there is absence of the entire nephrogenic ridge, or of the Wolffian duct [5], then there can be none of the structures derived from either the gonadal or the nephrogenic ridges, or their Wolffian or Müllerian ducts. On the affected side, there will be neither kidney, testis nor vas

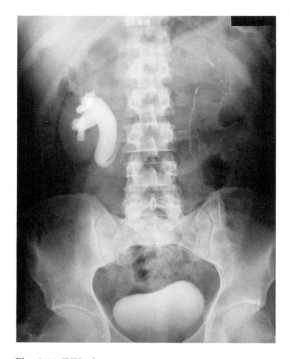

Fig. 8.15 IVU of a retrocaval ureter.

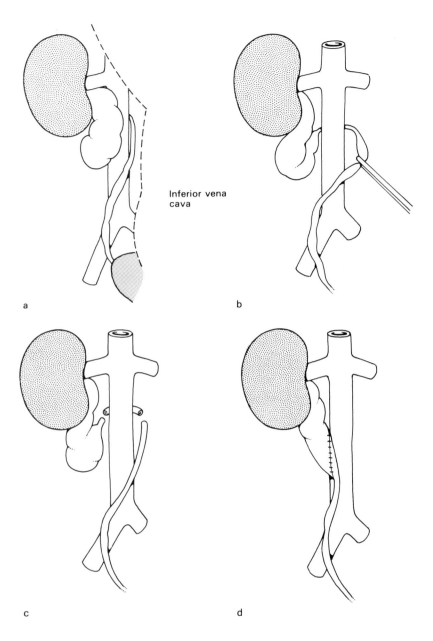

Fig. 8.16 (a−d) Operation for a retrocaval ureter: there is no need to remove the narrow segment of ureter from behind the vena cava. A long elliptical anastomosis is made between the redundant pelvis and the ureter.

deferens in the male, and no fallopian tube and only one half of the uterus in the female. Half the trigone will be missing (Fig. 8.17).

Clinically, no kidney is found in an intravenous urogram (IVU) or abdominal ultrasound. Cystoscopy will show a ureteric orifice only on one side, and the interureteric bar disappears in the midline (Fig. 8.18).

Defects in the ureteric bud

Aplasia and dysplasia

Although the genital ridge is formed, and the Wolffian duct forms a normal vas deferens and seminal vesicle, the ureteric bud fails to meet the metanephros and cause it to differentiate. This is called aplasia and it occurs in various degrees.

Sometimes the ureteric bud does find the metanephros, but fails to produce a completely differented kidney — this is dysplasia.

In aplasia no kidney can be seen in the IVU. Sometimes a nubbin of tissue may be suspected on the CT scan. Cystoscopy shows a complete trigone and both ureteric orifices. A retrograde urogram will outline a thin ureter. The pyelogram may show a tiny kidney on one side.

There may be some need to explore the

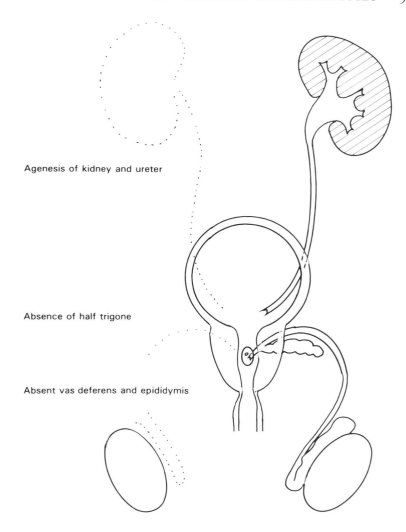

Agenesis of kidney and ureter

Absence of half trigone

Absent vas deferens and epididymis

Fig. 8.17 Absence of one nephrogenic ridge results in absence of all Wolffian or Müllerian structures.

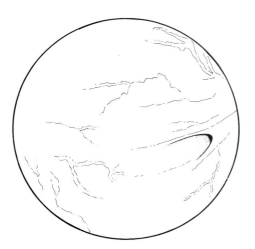

Fig. 8.18 Cystoscopic findings in agenesis: there is no ureter on one side.

kidney — for pain or hypertension — and a small cystic lump may be found (Fig. 8.19) which on histological section may show primitive tubules resembling epididymis, a curious fetal stroma resembling that of the nephrogenic ridge, and odd structures which resemble the proglomeruli of amphibians (Fig. 8.20). Muscle and cartilage are sometimes present. Cysts are common, and sometimes there are nests of nodular renal blastema — perhaps a precursor of Wilms' tumour [6]. Renal dysplasia is commonly associated with other congenital anomalies, e.g. Turner's syndrome, scoliosis and congenital dislocation of the hip [7].

Cystic dysplasia

Small cysts are often present in dysplastic kidneys, sometimes they are multiple (Fig. 8.21).

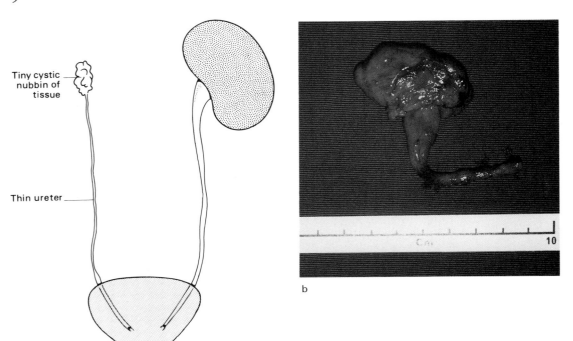

Tiny cystic
nubbin of
tissue

Thin ureter

a

b

Fig. 8.19 Dysplasia: (a)
a tiny, often cystic
nubbin of tissue is
found at (b) the upper
end of a thin ureter.

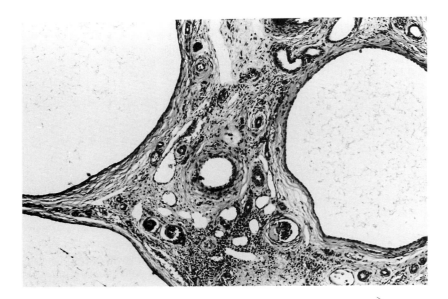

Fig. 8.20 Histology of dysplasia of the kidney showing
fetal tissues.

There is a more important, though fortunately
rare, condition in which a localized mass forms
in the kidney — mimicking in every way cystic
degeneration in a renal cell cancer. This is a
variation on the theme of dysplasia in which
there are cysts and elements of nephrons [8].

Duplex kidney

Like all the ducts associated with the nephrogenic ridge the ureteric bud tends to duplicate

itself. At the lower end of the ureter there are
often several short blind-ending ducts running
parallel with the ureter (Fig. 8.22). They never
reach the metanephros and there is never any
kidney associated with them [1].

Less often, one division of the ureteric bud
finds the metanephros and induces development
of a normal kidney while the other branch ends
blindly. This blind stump may engender infection and cause pain. It can be diagnosed with a
retrograde urogram (Figs 8.23 & 8.24).

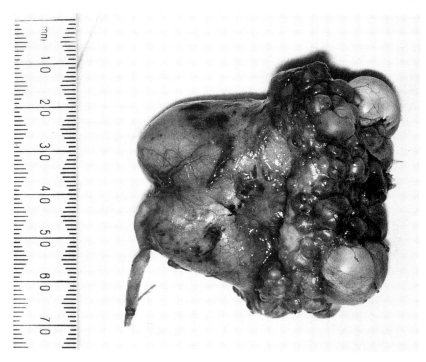

Fig. 8.21 Multiple cysts are often present in dysplasia.

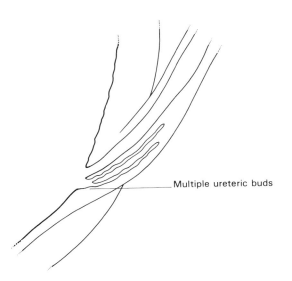

Fig. 8.22 At the lower end of the ureter there are often a number of blind-ending ducts, presumably attempts at formation of ureteric buds.

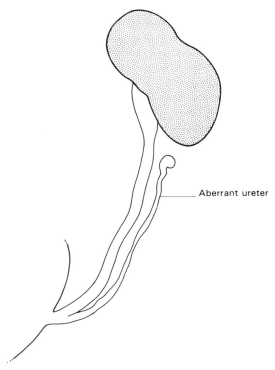

Fig. 8.23 An aberrant ureter may end in a blind-ended pouch.

Most often, the early divisions of the ureter reach the metanephros and give rise to the common duplex kidney. The two parts of a duplex kidney are always joined at a slight waist. The upper part is smaller, with only two major calices; the lower moiety has three (Fig. 8.25).

Occasionally, a patient will have pain in the loin caused by the flow of urine from the larger lower half-kidney flushing back up and distending the upper half-kidney, and thus engendering pain — so-called yo-yo or see-saw reflux.

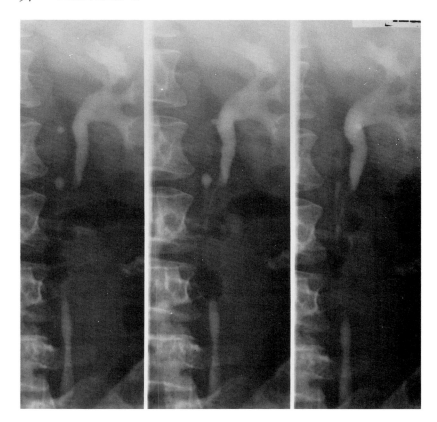

Fig. 8.24 Retrograde urogram of a blind-ending aberrant ureter, the cause of loin pain and repeated urinary tract infections.

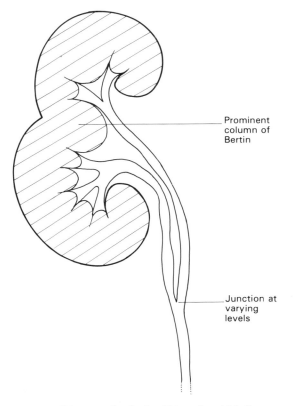

Fig. 8.25 Diagram of a duplex kidney in which the ureters divide about half way up to the kidney.

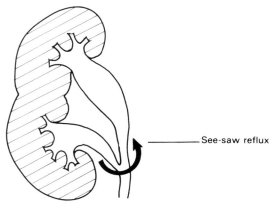

Fig. 8.26 Diagram of see-saw reflux: the urine from the lower moiety of the duplex kidney passes up to the upper calix causing distension and pain.

It is diagnosed by a retrograde ureterogram under fluoroscopic control [9] (Figs 8.26 & 8.27).

When both ureters enter the bladder separately the ureter from the upper half-kidney always enters the bladder caudal to the ureter from the lower half (Fig. 8.28).

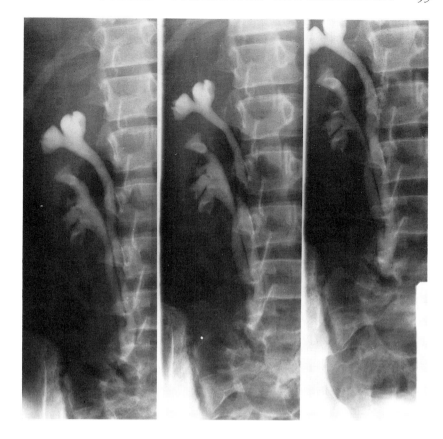

Fig. 8.27 Retrograde urogram showing see-saw reflux (courtesy of Mr G.C. Tresidder).

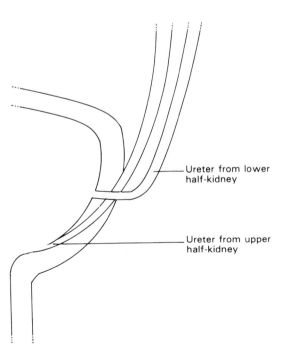

Ureter from lower half-kidney

Ureter from upper half-kidney

Fig. 8.28 When there is complete duplication, the ureter from the upper half-kidney always enters the bladder caudal to the ureter from the lower half.

Malformation of the urorectal septum

Another common anomaly is found, alone or in association with duplex, where the urorectal septum may be imperfectly absorbed and form a thick balloon-like covering for the ureteric orifice. If associated with duplex this anomaly always affects the ureter from the upper half-kidney — a ureterocele (Figs 8.29 & 8.30). Small ureteroceles are very common and cause no trouble. In larger ones a calculus may form and occasionally the ureteric opening may be so narrow as to cause obstruction.

In the female, the ureterocele may be pushed right through the internal urethral orifice and present as a lump at the external meatus with acute obstruction of urine (Fig. 8.31).

The ureter from the upper half-kidney may open below the sphincter, causing incontinence, and occasionally the ectopic opening can be seen in the vagina (Fig. 8.32).

The ureter from the lower half-kidney opens cephalad to the other ureter and its layer of uro-rectal septum is often nearly completely absorbed

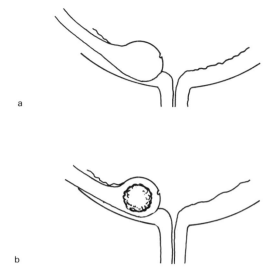

a

b

Fig. 8.29 A ureterocele may cause (a) obstruction and (b) the formation of a calculus.

so that there is an insufficient valve causing vesicoureteric reflux.

Duplex is often associated with one or more of these other anomalies, and it is not uncommon to have bilateral reflux as well as bilateral ureteroceles.

Ureter entering the seminal vesicle

The ureteric bud is an offshoot of the Wolffian duct which is to become the vas deferens and seminal vesicle. An error in the absorption of the lower ends of the Wolffian duct may result in the ureter opening into the seminal vesicle (Fig. 8.33). Usually the ureteric bud is poorly developed on that side, and any kidney it has tried to induce is dysplastic and does not show in a urogram.

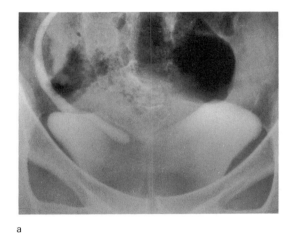

a

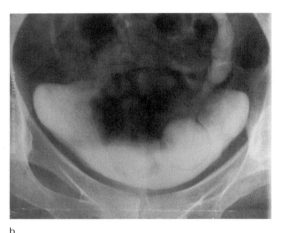

b

Fig. 8.30 (a) Small and (b) large ureteroceles.

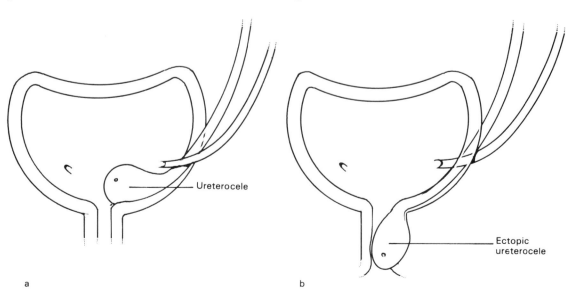

a

b

Fig. 8.31 (a & b) A ureterocele may prolapse through the urethra and cause obstruction.

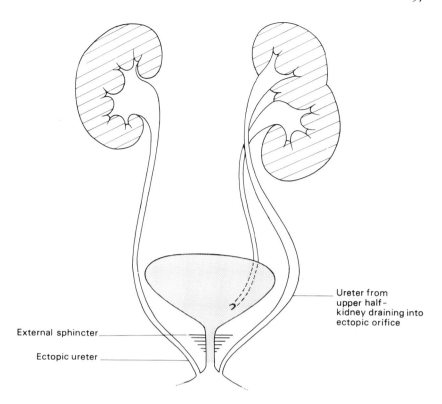

Fig. 8.32 The ureter from the upper half-kidney may open into the vagina below the sphincter and cause incontinence.

Ureter from upper half-kidney draining into ectopic orifice

External sphincter

Ectopic ureter

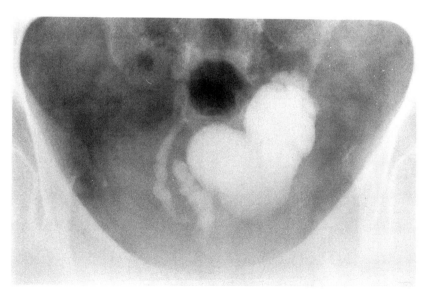

Fig. 8.33 Urogram showing ureter opening into the seminal vesicle.

Cysts of the kidney

The pathogenesis of most cysts of the kidney is still a matter of controversy. The prevailing idea that branches of the ureteric bud fail to meet the developing nephron, which therefore blows up to form cysts, is a misinterpretation of the early microdissection studies which were performed by steeping kidneys in caustic soda and then teasing apart the individual nephrons. This separation is very delicate, and the slightest clumsiness was apt to break a nephron, whereupon its ends would appear to seal up, giving the appearance that one end of a tubule was blind ending, and never joined up with the other [10].

Aware of this artefact, the original investigators found no single instance where a tubule failed to join up with a nephron. On the contrary, in all the examples of cystic disease which they studied, the reverse was the case — the tubules were grossly dilated from one end to the other and the cause still remains a mystery [10] (Fig. 8.34).

Congenital multicystic disease

The studies of Osathanondh and Potter [10], important as they are, refer entirely to congenital cystic disease — the strange condition found in babies who are born with one or both kidneys grossly enlarged, and converted into something resembling a sponge. If both kidneys are affected the fetus can make no urine, i.e. amniotic fluid, and without amniotic fluid the fetus is compressed and deformed — Potter's facies (Fig. 8.35).

Only in one form of this disease are the ureters obliterated and form mere fibrous cords, and in this type the cystic changes are probably secondary to obstruction (Fig. 8.36).

Polycystic diseases of the kidney

Five types of this condition are now recognized, the first four usually occurring in childhood, the fifth mostly in adults [11,12]. The childhood polycystic diseases are in general inherited by recessive genes, the adult form by an autosomal dominant gene.

Childhood polycystic disease

It is not yet clear whether the first four forms of this disease are merely variations in severity or truly distinct entities. These are inherited by recessive genes. The four recognized forms are:
1 Perinatal. These babies are born with huge kidneys, which are today detected by antenatal ultrasound [13]. The child dies at birth or shortly afterwards from renal failure, with 90% of the tubules affected. There is no hepatic fibrosis (Fig. 8.37).
2 Neonatal. These present in the first month with large kidneys, with 60% of the tubules affected. Uraemia leads to death in the first year, and there is little hepatic fibrosis.
3 Infantile polycystic disease. These children present at 3–6 months with uraemia and large kidneys, with 25% of tubules affected. There is hepatosplenomegaly, systemic and portal hypertension and death occurs in childhood.
4 Juvenile polycystic disease. These children present in later childhood. About 10% of their tubules are affected. They may survive into their teens before dying from portal and systemic hypertension [14,15].

Adult polycystic disease

This is much more common, and is inherited by an autosomal dominant gene on chromosome 16

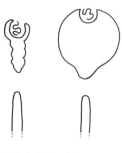

Tubule fails to join nephron

a

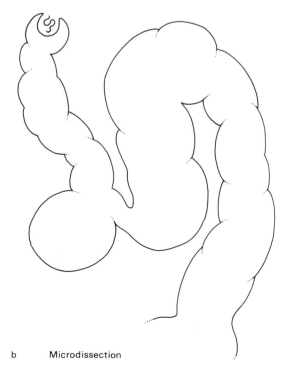

b   Microdissection

Fig. 8.34 (a) It was formerly believed that cysts were the result of failure of a tubule to join a glomerulus. (b) In fact Potter and her colleagues found that in cystic disease the nephrons were always dilated throughout their entire length.

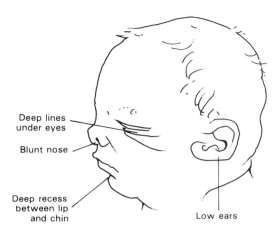

Fig. 8.35 In congenital multicystic disease, without amniotic fluid, the fetus is compressed and the face deformed — Potter's facies.

which is situated near the genes for alpha globin and phosphoglycolate phosphatase [16] which has promise as a marker for those likely to develop the condition.

Although the adult form of polycystic disease may appear in children [11,15] it usually appears in those carrying the gene in their thirties and forties, at first with one or two little cysts which cannot at this stage be distinguished from simple cysts. They are detected by ultrasound or in a pyelogram performed for haematuria.

As the disease progresses more and more cysts appear in one or both kidneys, and sometimes in other organs as well such as the liver, pancreas and spleen. Gradually, hypertension appears and there is a slow deterioration in renal function leading to dialysis and transplantation. About 10% of those needing treatment for end-stage renal failure have polycystic disease [12].

Eventually, one or both kidneys are transformed into a mass of cysts, resembling a bunch of grapes of unequal size (Fig. 8.38). The renal tissue is so tightly squeezed between the adjacent cysts that it is difficult to find any identifiable parenchyma.

Occasionally, one or more of the cysts become infected from blood-borne bacteria and require drainage.

In the past, attempts were made to puncture the cysts in the hope that this would relieve pressure on the remaining parenchyma. In practice, the operation (named after Rövsing) is both impossible and futile: the cysts extend right through the entire substance of the kidney, and as often as one layer of cysts are punctured, another layer offers itself to the needle. It is futile because careful studies of renal function show that this procedure does not improve renal function.

Rarely, patients are in pain due to the very large cysts and occasionally cysts will compress

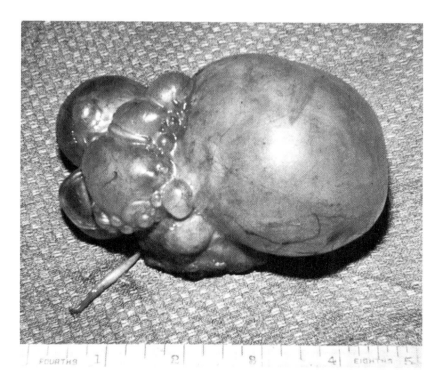

Fig. 8.36 In the form of congenital multicystic disease where there is atresia of the ureters, the cystic changes are thought to be secondary to obstruction.

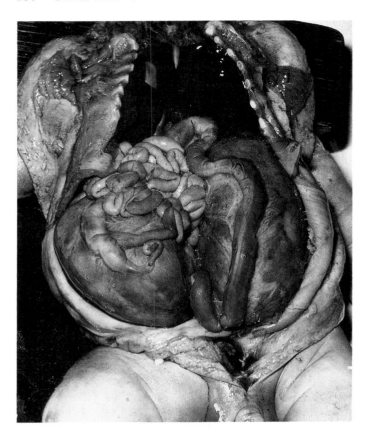

Fig. 8.37 Perinatal form of polycystic disease (courtesy of Mr J.H. Johnston).

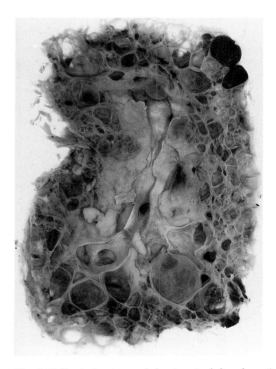

Fig. 8.38 Typical autosomal-dominant adult polycystic disease.

the neck of a calix. This can be relieved by percutaneous aspiration directed by means of a CT scan or ultrasound.

The management of these patients calls for great tact. When the diagnosis is first made, e.g. by ultrasound scanning for some unrelated symptom, it is impossible to know how rapidly the condition will progress. The best advice is to follow the patient carefully with annual measurements of creatinine and an occasional ultrasound. Eventually, hypertension or the features of slow deterioration in renal function will call for more active treatment by dialysis or transplantation. Until then, there is nothing the patient can do to postpone his or her fate.

Genetic counselling

A urologist would be wise to refer a patient for counselling with an expert clinical geneticist. Clearly some kind of advice must also be given to other family members when it is discovered that a relation has polycystic disease.

In the recessive variety, seen in childhood, a first child has about a 0.2% chance of developing the disease; if one child has already developed the disease, subsequent children born to that family have a 33% chance of developing it.

If the gene is dominant — as in the adult type of polycystic disease — any child of a parent with the disease has a 50% chance of developing it, though not always so severely that it will cause symptoms or shorten life.

Caliceal cysts

Caliceal cysts are sometimes seen in children but more often are detected in adults with recurrent urinary infection. There is no known embryological explanation. They present with pain and fever. In an IVU one may detect a missing calix, but this is usually missed until a retrograde urogram reveals a distended hydrocalix (Fig. 8.39). The treatment is simple: the 'cyst' is unroofed. It is logical (and easy) to ligate the offending calix (Fig. 8.40), but in practice simple unroofing of the cysts is not followed by fistula [17].

Simple cysts

Simple cysts are common at any age, from the

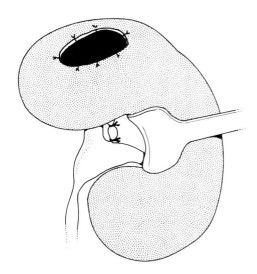

Fig. 8.40 Caliceal cyst. The relevant calix may be ligated by dissecting in the renal sinus, but simple unroofing is seldom followed by a fistula.

3-month-old fetus into adult life. The microdissection studies of Osathanondh and Potter suggested that they were probably diverticula of the collecting tubules [10], but no reason has ever been advanced for the formation of such diverticula. They can be of any size, single or multiple.

If they compress the pelvis or a calix against a branch of the renal artery they may give rise to obstruction or infection. They sometimes cause pain in the loin. They may become infected, giving rise to pyrexia, and pain in the loin, but the urine is free from organisms. A CT scan may reveal a cyst with a greater Hounsfield number than that of the usual cyst. Aspiration will yield pus and if antibiotics do not lead to rapid resolution it is best to drain and deroof the abscess.

Simple renal cysts are commonly found during routine urography (Fig. 8.41) or ultrasound scanning (Fig. 8.42). In a former generation they presented the diagnostic problem of a space-occupying lesion of the kidney, and the question was always how to be sure the 'mass' was not a cancer. The complete freedom of echoes within the cyst in ultrasound is sufficient evidence of its innocent nature. If there is any remaining doubt, the cyst may be aspirated and its fluid examined for malignant cells.

If cysts recur after aspiration or if they cause symptoms, they can be cured by removing a small window from their wall (Fig. 8.43). There is no need to remove the inner part of the wall of the cyst: this only provokes unnecessary bleeding.

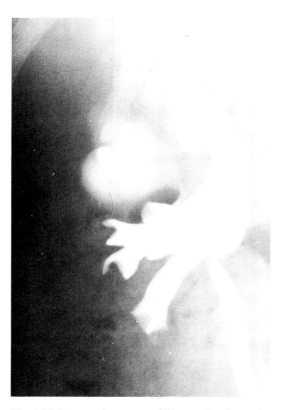

Fig. 8.39 Retrograde urogram filling a caliceal cyst that was the cause of repeated attacks of loin pain and fever.

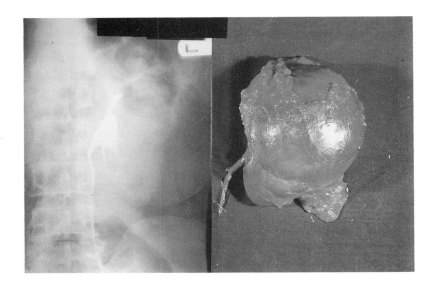

Fig. 8.41 Typical renal cyst in IVU (left) and specimen (right).

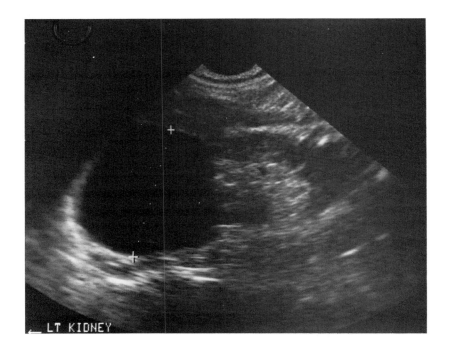

Fig. 8.42 Ultrasound appearance of a renal cyst (courtesy of Dr W. Hately).

Parapelvic cysts

These are simple cysts occurring near the hilum of the kidney, where they may compress adjacent calices against branches of the renal artery. Aspiration may be difficult and it may be safer to approach them through the renal sinus where a small window can be excised from their wall. It is not necessary to remove the entire cyst (Figs 8.44 & 8.45).

Medullary cystic disease

This is a very rare condition detected in young people with severe anaemia, salt wasting and uraemia [18]. It is probably inherited through a sex-linked dominant gene [19,20]. By the time the patient comes to autopsy the kidney is shrunken, and a cut section shows a remarkable group of cysts located just at the corticomedullary border (Fig. 8.46). It is sometimes confused with juvenile nephronophthisis [21].

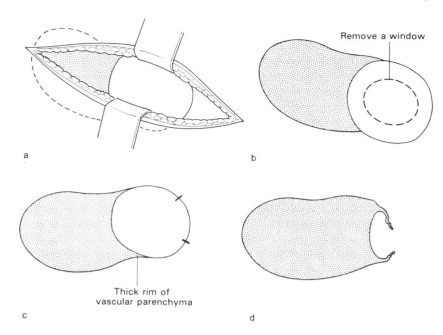

Fig. 8.43 (a–d) Treatment of a renal cyst. A small window is removed from the cyst wall, and there is no need to remove the rest of its wall.

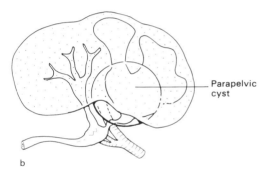

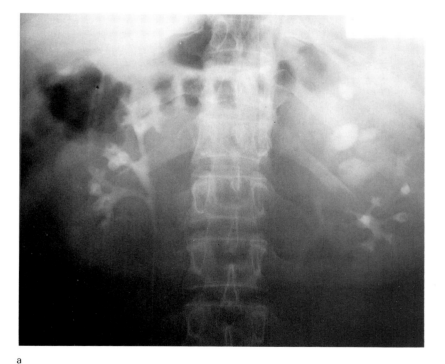

Fig. 8.44 (a) When a parapelvic cyst is obstructing a calix; it is approached though the renal sinus (b).

Medullary sponge kidney

Although this may be congenital, and there are reports of some families in which the condition has occurred in several members, along with Wilms' tumours, aniridia and unilateral hemi-hypertrophy, medullary sponge kidney is usually not a familial or congenital disorder, and is detected only in adolescence or early adult life [22,23] (Fig. 8.47).

The collecting tubules of the kidney are grossly dilated. The condition may affect only one papilla, a group of papillae, the entire kidney or both kidneys. Its cause is unknown. The author

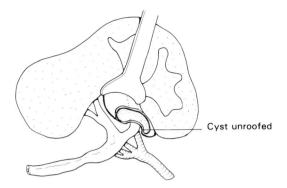

Fig. 8.45 It is only necessary to remove a small window from the wall of the parapelvic cyst.

Fig. 8.46 (*right*) Medullary cystic disease.

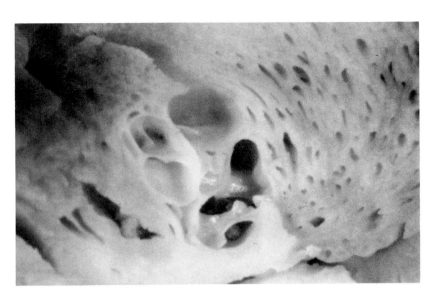

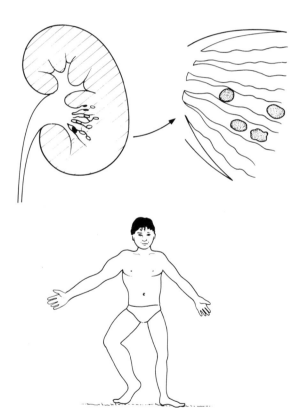

Fig. 8.47 Medullary sponge kidney.

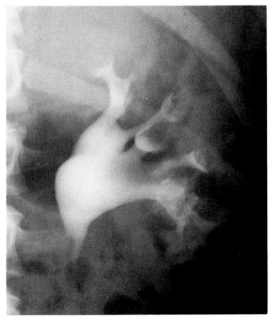

Fig. 8.48 Early medullary sponge kidney affecting only a few calices.

has followed one adolescent male from the age of 15 when a urogram (performed after a trivial injury had produced haematuria) showed a slight dilatation of the tubules of an adjacent group of calices in the lower pole (Fig. 8.48). Over the succeeding 20 years the patient developed a full-blown segmental form of medullary sponge kidney in the lower pole of one kidney which became complicated by stones and infection and eventually required a partial nephrectomy.

In more severe forms the entire kidney is enlarged, every collecting tubule converted into a long sac full of infected stones (Fig. 8.49). Urinary infection is continual and renal function progressively deteriorates. The symptoms arise from pain in the kidney, the repeated passage of calculi and infection.

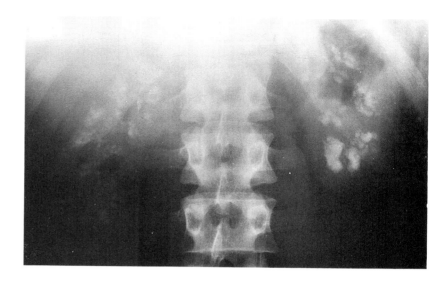

Fig. 8.49 Full-blown medullary sponge kidney with multiple stones in dilated collecting tubules.

If the disease is confined to one or two pyramids of the kidney they can be removed by partial nephrectomy. If stones are the predominant problem, they can be fragmented by extracorporeal shockware lithotripsy (ESWL), with antibiotics to control the concurrent infection. In the more severe cases the prognosis is very poor, and the unfortunate patients require continual treatment with antibiotics, and may eventually come to dialysis and transplantation.

In the early stages, the speckled calcification in these kidneys is easily confused with the nephrocalcinosis of renal tubular acidosis, a confusion made worse because, as a medullary sponge kidney gets worse, so renal tubular function deteriorates and leads to acidosis [23,24].

Acquired cystic disease in dialysis patients

Since more patients are being treated for long periods by dialysis a new entity has come to light in which multicystic changes, closely resembling those of the autosomal dominant adult disease, appear in one or both kidneys, and are eventually followed by multifocal carcinoma [25].

Cysts in von Hippel—Lindau disease

This is another genetically linked condition in which multiple renal cysts and cancers occur with increasing frequency as the patient lives longer [26].

References

1 Beck F, Moffat DB, Davies DP (1985) *Human Embryology*, 2nd edn, pp. 256—76. Oxford: Blackwell Scientific Publications.

2 Graves FT (1971) *The Arterial Anatomy of the Kidney: the Basis of Surgical Technique*. Bristol: John Wright.

3 Milovic IS, Oluic DI (1988) Thoracic renal ectopia. *Br J Urol* 62: 183.

4 Anderson JC, Hynes W (1949) Retrocaval ureter: case diagnosed preoperatively and treated successfully by plastic operation. *Br J Urol* 21: 209.

5 Torrey TW (1971) The early development of the human nephron. *Contrib Embryol* 239: 177.

6 Noe HN, Marshall JR, Edwards OP (1989) Nodular renal blastema in the multicystic kidney. *J Urol* 142: 486.

7 Thijssen AM, Carpenter B, Jimenez C, Schillinger J (1989) Multilocular cyst (multilocular cystic nephroma) of the kidney: a report of two cases with an unusual mode of presentation. *J Urol* 142: 346.

8 Quinn CM, Kelly DG, Cahalane SF (1988) Renal dysplasia — a clinicopathological review. *Br J Urol* 61: 399.

9 Tresidder GC, Blandy JP, Murray RS (1970) Pyelopelvic and ureterouretenic reflux. *Br J Urol* 42: 728.

10 Osathanondh V, Potter EL (1964) Pathogenesis of polycystic kidneys. Type 1 due to hyperplasia of interstitial portions of collecting tubules. *Arch Pathol* 77: 466.

11 Anderson GA, Degroot D, Lawson RK (1993) Polycystic renal disease. *Urology* 42: 358.

12 Gabow PA (1993) Medical progress: autosomal dominant polycystic kidney disease. *New Engl J Med* 329: 332.

13 Livera LN, Brookfield DSK, Egginton JA, Hawnaur JM (1989) Antenatal ultrasonography to detect fetal renal abnormalities: a prospective screening programme. *Br Med J* 298: 1421.

14 Wacksman J, Phipps L (1993) Report of the multicystic kidney registry: preliminary findings. *J Urol* 150: 1870.

15 Shokeir MHK (1978) Expression of 'adult' polycystic renal disease in the fetus and newborn. *Clin Gen* 14: 61.

16 Saggar-Malik AK, Jeffery S, Patton MA (1994) Autosomal dominant polycystic kidney disease. *Br Med J* 308: 1183.

17 Williams GB, Blandy JP, Tresidder GC (1969) Communicating cysts and diverticula of the renal pelvis. *Br J Urol* 41: 163.

18 Strauss MB (1962) Clinical and pathologic aspects of cystic disease of the renal medulla. An analysis of eighteen cases. *Ann Intern Med* 57: 373.

19 Smith CH, Graham JB (1945) Congenital medullary cysts with severe refractory anemia. *Am J Dis Child* 69: 369.

20 Goldman SH, Walker SR, Merigan TC, Gardner KD, Bull JMC (1966) Hereditary occurrence of cystic disease of the renal medulla. *New Engl J Med* 274: 984.

21 Spence HM, Singleton R (1971) What is sponge kidney disease and where does it fit in the spectrum of cystic disorders? *Trans Am Assoc Genitourin Surg* 63: 37.

22 Abeshouse BS, Abeshouse GA (1960) Sponge kidney: a review of the literature and a report of five cases. *J Urol* 84: 252.

23 Felts JH, Headley RN, Whitley JE, Yount EH (1964) Medullary sponge kidneys: clinical appraisal. *J Am Med Assoc* 188: 233.

24 Osther PJ, Hansen AB, Rohl HF (1988) Renal acidification defects in medullary sponge kidney. *Br J Urol* 61: 392.

25 Sasagawa I, Terasawa Y, Imai K, Sekino H, Takahashi H (1992) Acquired cystic disease of the kidney and renal carcinoma in haemodialysis patients: ultrasonographic evaluation. *Br J Urol* 70: 236.

26 Choyke P, Weiss G, Walther M *et al.* (1991) Natural history of von Hippel Lindau associated renal lesions: observations on serial computed tomography. *J Urol* 145: 560.

Chapter 9: Idiopathic hydronephrosis

Aetiology

Idiopathic hydronephrosis may occur at any age, and is today being detected *in utero* by ultrasound with increasing frequency. Other cases can develop at any subsequent age, and one may follow a suspicious kidney with serial examinations year by year, and then within a few months see a full-blown hydronephrosis develop for no apparent reason. The cause remains an enigma.

Pathology

The single underlying feature of idiopathic hydronephrosis is a ring of collagen in the ureteric muscle at the junction of the pelvis and ureter. Very rarely, the ring is a long cylinder extending down the ureter for 4–5 cm, but this is exceptional (Fig. 9.1). The smooth muscle of the renal pelvis above the site of obstruction is thickened, infiltrated and largely replaced with collagen [1]. The lumen of the renal pelvis is more or less distended, and the muscular wall hypertrophied. When there is a large gap between the lowermost segmental arteries the dilated renal pelvis bulges forwards between them, carrying the narrow zone outside the window and giving the appearance that the lower pole vessels are causing the obstruction (Fig. 9.2).

Peristaltic waves starting off in the calices fail to propagate smoothly down the ureter past the ring of collagen, and as a result there is an obstruction to the flow of urine. Murnaghan [2] considered that there was a discontinuity in the helical muscle fibres at this pelviureteric junction, but Notley [3] could not confirm this, finding only an increase in the amount of collagen amongst the muscular cells, and in the surrounding lamina propria — which (he considered)

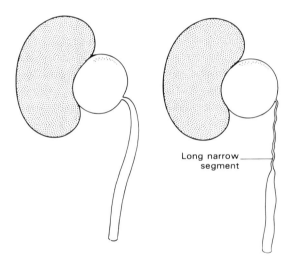

Long narrow segment

Fig. 9.1 Usually the obstructing segment is only a few millimetres long; occasionally it may extend over 4–5 cm.

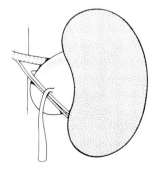

Fig. 9.2 As the dilated renal pelvis bulges out between the two lower anterior segmental arteries it carries the obstructing segment outside, giving the misleading impression that it is the lower pole artery which is causing the obstruction. (a) View from behind, and (b) view from the front.

Seen from behind the lower polar vessels appear to be causing the PUJ obstruction

Lower polar segmental artery and vein

a   b

might act as a rigid belt around the junction, preventing expansion.

In the urogram when there is a hydronephrosis it seems as if the ureter is attached high up along the convex border of the dilated renal pelvis (Fig. 9.3). In the literature there are many references to the 'high entry' of the ureter, or the 'squared-off' renal pelvis, but it is more probable that this is the result rather than the cause of the dilatation of the pelvis.

Effects of obstruction on the kidney

In time obstruction leads to atrophy of the renal parenchyma. The principal effect of this atrophy is borne by the papillae, relatively more tubules being destroyed than glomeruli. Because there are fewer tubules to render the urine concentrated the hydronephrotic kidney makes a larger volume of dilute urine and the effect of any obstruction is exaggerated.

Ultimately, entire nephrons are lost and there is a deterioration in the creatinine clearance from the obstructed kidney, but for a considerable time the obstructed kidney or idiopathic hydronephrosis remains a useful dialyser, and even when very thin, is still capable of sustaining life.

If infection supervenes at any time, then the devastating effect of inflammatory scarring — reflux nephropathy — are added to the slow atrophy caused by obstruction. This means that the presence of infection lends a measure of urgency to the need to relieve the obstruction.

Clinical features

Antenatal detection by ultrasound

Many hydronephrotic kidneys are today detected *in utero*, especially in the last 3 months of pregnancy when the fetus passes a relatively large volume of dilute urine. The hazard of precipitating premature labour rules out intervention, and it is now clear that a large number of these kidneys will recover spontaneously. Hence, the accepted practice is to follow the child by serial diethylenetriamine penta-acetic acid (DTPA) measurements, beginning at 1 month. If the renal function is satisfactory, surgery is deferred. A small number of kidneys will deteriorate over the course of the next year or two, but in the end only about 15% will require pyeloplasty [4–6].

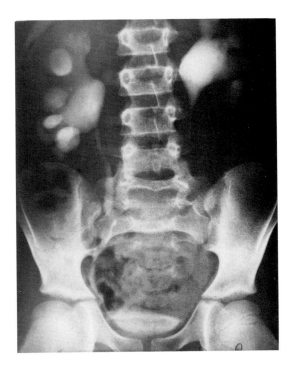

Fig. 9.3 Urogram showing a 'squared-off' renal pelvis on the right side.

Hydronephrosis detected in early infancy

Similar principles are applied to the hydronephroses which are discovered during early childhood. A mass is often noticed by chance when the mother or midwife is bathing the baby. Ultrasound quickly reveals a large urine-filled swelling, with more or less remaining renal parenchyma. Infants tend to secrete a larger volume of more dilute urine in the first few weeks of life, so that some of these patients, discovered very early on, recover spontaneously and will never need any operative intervention. On the other hand, if the renal function is already seriously impaired, operation should not be delayed. There is always time to allow a little delay for more information about the renal function.

Symptoms in adults

There are five easily recognizable syndromes.

Pain with diuresis. Young people, usually men, boasting of their prowess at drinking beer, give a characteristic history of pain in the loin, followed by vomiting, after drinking several pints of beer. It is all too easy to jump to the diagnosis of a duodenal ulcer. The diagnosis is easily made by means of an ultrasound or an IVU.

Loin pain and fever may be caused by an infection in the hydronephrotic sac. Curiously, this is often almost silent, even though the urine in the kidney may look like pea soup. Occasionally, the pyonephrosis makes the patient desperately ill with septicaemia, and its relief by percutaneous nephrostomy is an emergency.

A mass. Many patients notice a lump in the loin, even though it may not be clinically palpable. The patient who feels a lump in the loin is often right, and deserves an ultrasound scan.

Gastrointestinal symptoms. In later life, the patient may not associate the consumption of fluid with the onset of pain. Commonly, a hydronephrosis is detected by chance in the course of investigating other abdominal pains. If the hydronephrosis is on the right side, distension of tissues behind the duodenum may give rise to dyspepsia closely resembling the pain of a peptic ulcer, and patients have often undergone prolonged treatment for a non-existent duodenal ulcer before their hydronephrosis is discovered.

Similarly, a left-sided hydronephrosis may cause disturbance of bowel function. Many of these unfortunate patients are labelled as having colonic dysfunction, or are even dismissed as valetudinarians, especially when they get relief by inexplicable manoeuvres such as lying face down or bending over the side of the bed.

Hypertension. The routine investigation of a young person with hypertension sometimes reveals hydronephrosis. The dilated cortical tissue is secreting renin.

Physical signs

It is seldom possible to feel a large hydronephrosis except in a thin person and absence of any physical signs is the norm. Hypertension is an important feature.

Investigations

Ultrasound

Most hydronephroses are detected by ultrasound scan (Fig. 9.4). There can be a mistake here, for it is usual to overhydrate a patient before performing the ultrasound, and the physiological dilatation of the upper tract may be misdiagnosed as hydronephrosis.

Excretion urography

The IVU shows the characteristic features of the dilated renal pelvis (Fig. 9.5). The ureter is seldom shown and for this reason a retrograde ureterogram (Fig. 9.6) is a wise precaution immediately before proceeding to pyeloplasty, to ensure that the ureter is not one of the rare examples with a long narrow segment at its upper end.

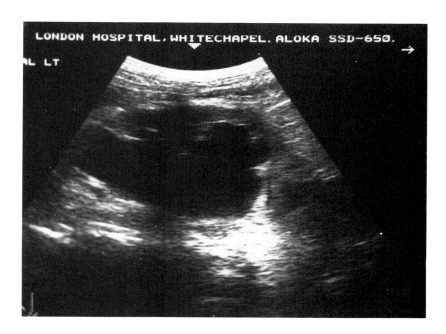

Fig. 9.4 Typical ultrasound scan showing hydronephrosis (courtesy of Dr W. Hately).

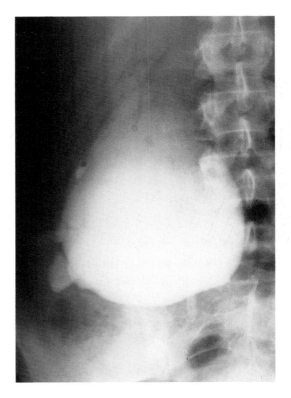

Fig. 9.5 Typical IVU appearance of hydronephrosis.

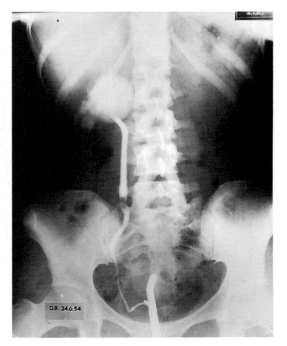

Fig. 9.6 Retrograde urogram in idiopathic hydronephrosis.

Diuresis urography

In patients who have been dehydrated before the IVU (which is usual) there may be no dilatation of the renal pelvis because there is only a low flow of urine. In these cases, the patient may be given a litre of water to drink, or intravenous frusemide to provoke a diuresis (Fig. 9.7). The same information is provided with more accuracy by means of diuresis renography.

Diuresis renography

DTPA is handled by the kidney by filtration, like inulin and contrast medium: it is filtered by the glomeruli but not absorbed or excreted in the tubules. It is readily labelled by ^{99m}technetium (^{99m}Tc) which emits gamma radiation. About 15 min after an intravenous injection of ^{99m}Tc–DTPA a dose of frusemide is given (Fig. 9.8). Normally the isotope is filtered, concentrated in the tubules, accumulates briefly in the pelvis and is then transported down the ureter. In obstruction, the isotope continues to accumulate.

The height of the peak of the DTPA renogram is a function of the blood flow to the kidney, and gives a useful notion of whether the remaining kidney tissue is worth trying to preserve. But a better image of the remaining tubular mass is obtained by an isotope-labelled dimercaptosuccinic acid (DMSA) scan using ^{99m}Tc–DMSA (Fig. 9.9).

Caution is needed when interpreting the diuresis renogram when the creatinine clearance is impaired for frusemide may then produce very little diuresis. If the frusemide is given 15 min before the isotope, it will show the same accumulation and failure of washout and may clarify otherwise equivocal results [7].

Deconvolution analysis

Using a computer it is possible to untangle (deconvolute) the data received in the gamma camera and compute the rate at which the isotope passes through the cortex independently of the rate at which it passes into and out of the renal pelvis [8]. The method relies on the accuracy with which the cortex and collecting system are mapped out, and is not without its critics.

In all these renographic tests, infection may give false results, since oedema of the kidney may reduce its blood flow. Hence, if the kidney is

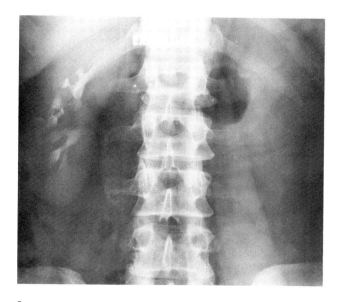

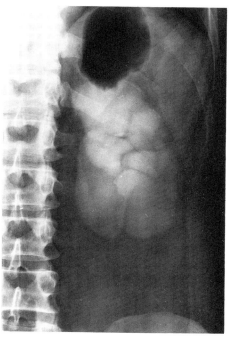

b

Fig. 9.7 (a) IVU at 20 min: no apparent 'function' on left. (b) A late film reveals the hydronephrosis.

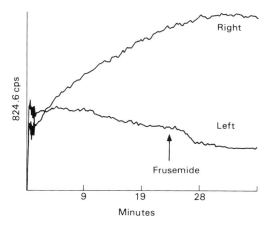

Fig. 9.8 A ^{99m}Tc–DTPA renogram followed by frusemide shows accumulation of isotope in the obstructed renal pelvis (courtesy of Dr Neil Garvie).

infected the renograms should be repeated after a period of drainage and antibiotics.

The Whitaker test

An objective method of detecting obstruction is to measure the pressure inside the renal pelvis during diuresis (see p. 62). Pressure flow studies were first performed at operation in children with hydronephrosis by Johnston [9] and were applied using percutaneous cannulae

by Whitaker first in children and then in adults [10,11]. It is rarely necessary, thanks to modern radioisotope techniques. It carries a slight risk of introducing infection into the closed obstructed system.

In practice, there are some cases where it is obvious that the kidney is reduced to nothing more than a thin bag of scarred tissue which ought to be removed, and others where there is a substantial thickness of renal tissue worth saving. Occasionally, the decision should be deferred until examination of the thickness of the renal tissue at the time of operation.

Complications of hydronephrosis

Infection

After the progressive diminution of renal function, infection is the most important complication. In the presence of obstruction, urine in the renal pelvis is leading freely into the renal lymphatics, and if the urine is infected, organisms readily enter the bloodstream. Septicaemia is an ever present risk. The curious thing is how often patients seem to remain well in spite of having a kidney full of purulent urine. The author has encountered two patients whose kidneys, when drained, yielded more than 4 l of pus.

When pyonephrosis is encountered, the first

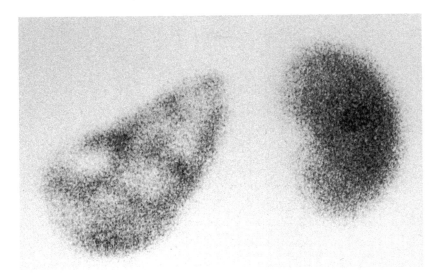

Fig. 9.9 A ^{99m}Tc−DMSA renogram gives an image of the remaining tubular mass in hydronephrosis (courtesy of Dr Neil Garvie).

step should be to drain it by means of a percutaneous nephrostomy. For the first few days, thick pus will drain away but will soon be followed by the production of a useful quantity of urine. The creatinine concentration in this urine should be measured from time to time until it becomes stable before making a decision as to whether to try to save the kidney or perform a nephrectomy.

Stones

Stones readily form in the pool of stagnant urine in hydronephrosis (Fig. 9.10). They are multiple and rounded like pebbles from the seashore in contrast to those stones which arise within the kidney, and give rise to secondary obstruction and hydronephrosis. The latter are not smooth and they retain the shape of the renal pelvis and its calices. When it is not easy to be sure whether the obstruction or the stone came first, a version of the Whitaker test may be used at operation or after percutaneous nephrolithotomy to see if there is an idiopathic obstruction at the pelviureteric junction.

Trauma

It is easier to burst a balloon when it is blown up, and for the same reason, a distended hydronephrosis is apt to be ruptured by external injury. The urogram performed as an emergency soon

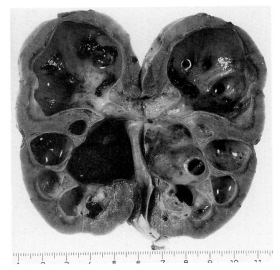

Fig. 9.10 Stones which form inside a hydronephrosis are typically smooth like the pebbles on the seashore.

after the patient is admitted with suspected closed renal injury may show the unexpected coexistence of a hydronephrosis and extravasation of urine, but more often the renal function is too poor to display the anatomy of the kidney. A computerized tomography (CT) scan will show the thinned out parenchyma. This sometimes raises a medicolegal question — did the injury cause the hydronephrosis? This may be easy to answer if the renal parenchyma is already severely atrophied at the time of injury. In other cases, it is impossible to be sure that the injury was not responsible for the obstruction.

Hypertension

Hypertension associated with a hydronephrosis may resolve with cure of the obstruction. In former days the lower pole artery used to be divided because it was believed to be causing the obstruction, and in these cases hypertension was a common sequel to the infarction of the lower pole.

Treatment

Pyeloplasty

There are many variations on the themes of the Anderson–Hynes dismembered pyeloplasty and the Culp–Scardino flap, but they have one principle in common — the use of a wide, well-vascularized flap of renal pelvis to enlarge the narrow part of the ureter. Essential to success is absence of any tension and free drainage.

The main difference between the various methods is whether or not the pelvis is detached from the ureter, but good results are provided by either method and the choice of technique should be determined by what is found when the kidney is explored.

Preliminary ureterography

In many cases, the ureter downstream of the pelviureteric junction will not have been shown in the preliminary urogram. The nightmare situation of embarking on an Anderson–Hynes pyeloplasty when there is a long narrow segment of ureter can be avoided by making it a rule always to perform a ureterogram immediately prior to the operation. If the retrograde is performed several days beforehand there is an unacceptable risk of introducing infection into the obstructed system.

Operative approach

The kidney may be approached from the loin using the standard 12th rib-tip incision, but in children and most slim young people the anterior approach of Anderson and Hynes has many advantages (Fig. 9.11). The colon is reflected medially off the kidney and the dilated renal pelvis presents itself into the wound. During

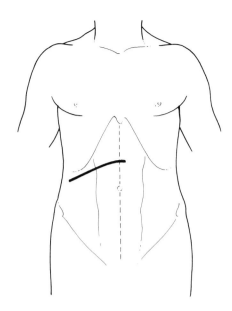

Fig. 9.11 Extraperitoneal approach to the renal pelvis through an anterior incision.

this approach the peritoneum may be opened without risk and in infants a transperitoneal abdominal approach allows both kidneys to be dealt with at the same sitting.

For well-muscled young males with a relatively small hydronephrosis, the loin approach may be easier.

Once the renal pelvis has been exposed, it is carefully freed from all its confusing coverings of connective tissue. When these have been swept aside, the relationship of the lower pole vessels if these are present becomes clear, and they are lifted up on a silicone sling (Fig. 9.12).

If the lower pole vessels are in the way, a dismembered pyeloplasty will be performed, and this can be modified if there is a long narrow upper segment of ureter [12,13] (Fig. 9.13).

It helps to fill the renal pelvis with 30–40 ml of saline with a syringe before marking out the flap with fine stay-sutures (Fig. 9.14). Unless this is performed while the pelvis is distended, it is easy to mark it wrongly. Cut through the ureter near the pelviureteric junction, and thread it behind the lower pole vessels, slit up and anastomose it to the loosely hanging flap of renal pelvis which has been previously marked out (Fig. 9.15).

If there is a long narrow segment of ureter, the flap can be made longer by using Culp's manoeuvre, carrying the flap in a spiral fashion round the pelvis [13] (Fig. 9.16). If there is no

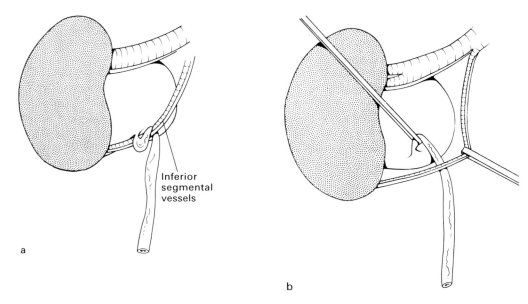

Fig. 9.12 (a & b) A sling is placed around the lower pole segmental vessels.

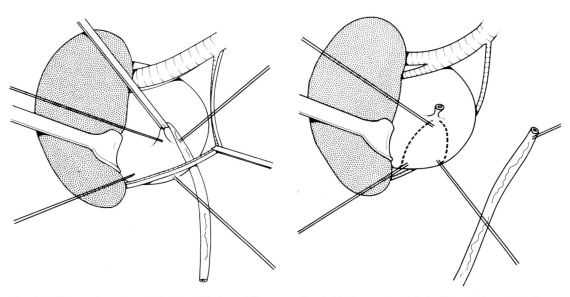

Fig. 9.13 Dismembered pyeloplasty. A U-shaped flap is formed from the redundant renal pelvis.

Fig. 9.14 The renal pelvis is distended, and the flap marked out with stay sutures.

lower pole vessel, there is no need to detach the ureter and either a simple flap or the Culp spiral modification can be adapted. Using either method, the anastomosis is made in a long ellipse to prevent subsequent contraction, and there must be no tension.

To splint or not to splint

The author always uses the combined splint-cum-nephrostomy tube of Cummings, and has

never had occasion to regret it. Others claim equally good results with a double-J splint, and there are some who feel strongly that no splint should be used. There is no hard evidence either way.

It is important to use only absorbable suture material for the anastomosis, but whether interrupted or continuous sutures are used is of little consequence. The author prefers to use continuous sutures of 4-0 chromic catgut, and follows Anderson's original advice to avoid

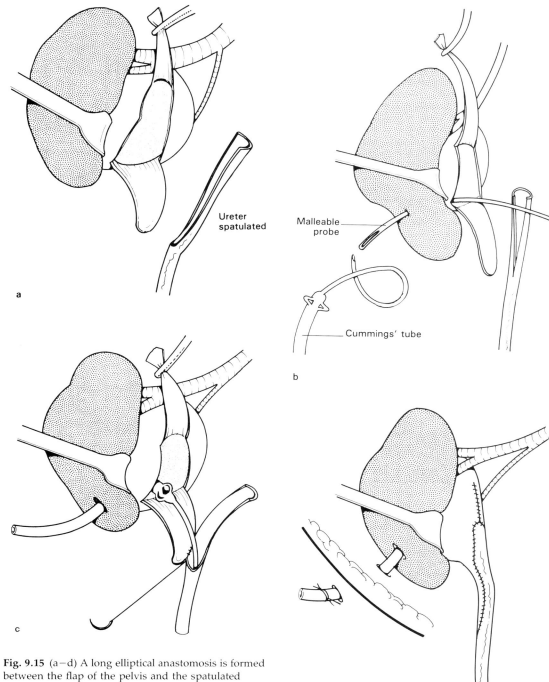

Ureter
spatulated

a

Malleable
probe

Cummings' tube

b

c

d

Fig. 9.15 (a–d) A long elliptical anastomosis is formed between the flap of the pelvis and the spatulated ureter.

having a knot at the apex of the U-shaped flap [12].

It is difficult to give firm advice about the use of antibiotics in this kind of conservative surgery. If there is an identified pathogenic organism in the urine — other than the expected commensals which accompany the presence of any tube in the urinary tract — then it is prudent to cover the operation with intravenous antibiotics directed against bacteraemia. However, during the postoperative period it is probably wiser to refrain from antibiotics while there is adequate drainage.

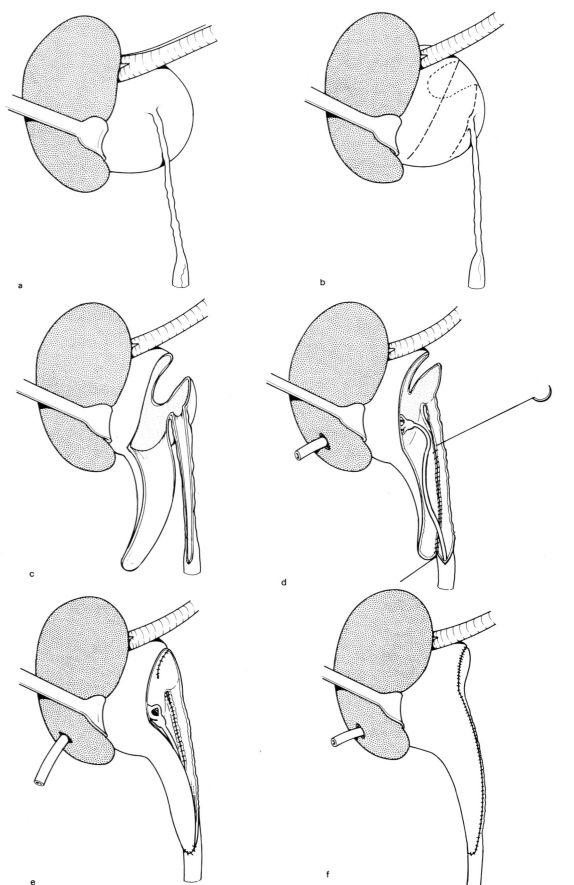

Fig. 9.16 (a–f) When there is a long narrow segment of ureter, Culp's spiral flap of renal pelvis is used.

Results

Few large long-term follow-up studies have been published of conservative pyeloplasty operations in adults [14]. Certain long-term complications are to be expected, notably recurrent pain and infection, hypertension and restenosis.

Stones have been seen to form on the suture material used to sew the ureter to the renal pelvis: they are almost inevitable if non-absorbable suture has been used for the anastomosis, but they can occur on absorbable sutures as well.

Hypertension is an important late sequel of even a successful pyeloplasty, and it is wise for the patient to be closely followed by the general practitioner.

In a few patients, despite an apparently successful operation — as judged by a free run-off down the anastomosis and no hold-up of contrast or isotope in the renal pelvis — the patient continues to experience recurrent pain in the loin, sometimes accompanied by verified infection in the urine. To some extent this kind of result, which is fortunately rare, represents a failure of selection of candidates for a conservative operation: in retrospect it is easy to say that it would have been better to have advised a nephrectomy.

In the majority, the outcome is excellent in terms of the absence of symptoms, infection, stones and deterioration of renal function, but when assessed by the appearance of the kidney in a urogram, the patient and the surgeon need to be warned that the kidney often continues to look disappointingly dilated (Fig. 9.17). This does not mean that it is obstructed — an isotope renogram with frusemide will check this — but it does mean that once there has been a thinning of the renal parenchyma and a deterioration in the muscular capacity of the renal pelvis, then the pyelographic appearances are unlikely to return to normal. This need not matter: the important point is that the obstruction has been permanently overcome and things will not deteriorate any further.

Secondary pelviureteric obstruction

Scarring in and around the pelviureteric junction occurs after surgery for renal calculi and after treatment for tuberculosis and other infections. The tissues do not lend themselves so easily to pyeloplasty and restenosis is a notorious complication. Fortunately, there are promising new alternatives.

Fig. 9.17 Urograms before and after successful pyeloplasty. Often the renal pelvis remains somewhat dilated: this does not necessarily signify obstruction.

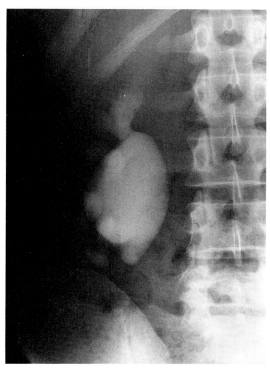

a

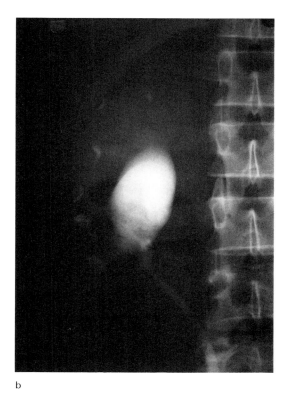

b

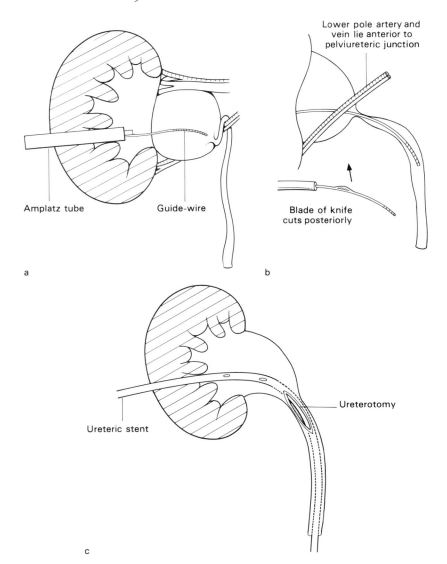

Lower pole artery and
vein lie anterior to
pelviureteric junction

Amplatz tube

Guide-wire

Blade of knife
cuts posteriorly

a

b

Ureteric stent

Ureterotomy

c

Fig. 9.18 (a—c) Percutaneous pyeloplasty: the narrow segment is incised under vision and the ureter left intubated for 6—8 weeks.

Percutaneous pyelolysis

An Amplatz tube is easily introduced into the dilated kidney of a hydronephrosis. Over a guide-wire a knife blade is slipped down the pelvis until the stenosis is encountered and divided under direct vision, taking care to direct the blade posteriorly so as not to cause haemorrhage from a lower pole segmental vessel. A double-J or similar stent is passed over the guide-wire (Fig. 9.18). The principle of this operation is a very old one: it was introduced by Davis as an intubated ureterotomy [15]. Davis pointed out that it was necessary to leave the stent in for at least 6 weeks, to give time for all the new collagen to finish its contraction [15].

Good results have been reported both in primary and secondary obstruction [16—18] with up to an 8-year follow-up. Some complications have been very serious — including complete loss of the ureter and arteriovenous fistula [19,20].

Balloon pyeloplasty

A similar principle uses an angioplasty balloon advanced up the ureter from below [21]. The way past the stricture is negotiated with a guide-wire, over which a balloon is passed and distended, and then replaced with a double-J stent (Fig. 9.19). Encouraging early results have been reported: it is too early to know the long-term results, but it seems that nothing is lost by making this very non-invasive attempt.

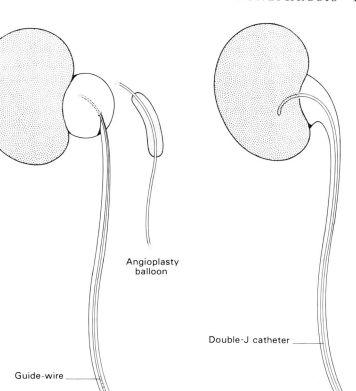

Angioplasty
balloon

Double-J catheter

Guide-wire

Fig. 9.19 Balloon pyeloplasty. An angioplasty balloon
is passed retrogradely over a guide-wire. After dilating
the stenosed segment a double-J catheter is left *in situ*.

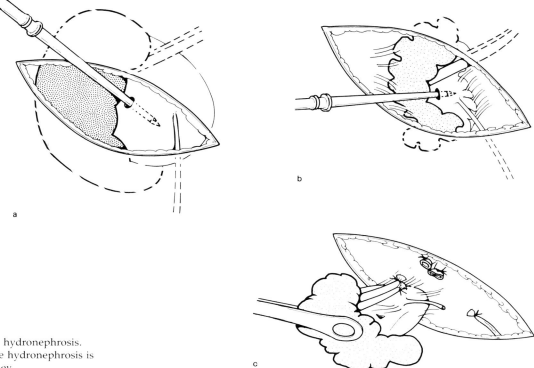

a

b

c

Fig. 9.20 (a–c) Nephrectomy for hydronephrosis.
Through a very small incision the hydronephrosis is
first emptied to collapse the kidney.

Nephrectomy in hydronephrosis

When the preoperative investigations show that the kidney has minimal function, or when at operation it is clear that the cortex is but a paper-thin shell, nephrectomy is the correct operation.

The operation can be made very easy if the distended kidney is first emptied out by a trocar and cannula. The huge swelling deflates like a balloon, leaving a thin crumpled bag of fibrous tissue which may be drawn up into a relatively small wound and removed (Fig. 9.20). There is no point in trying to remove a hydronephrosis intact.

References

1 Gosling JA, Dixon JS (1982) The structure of the normal and hydronephrotic upper urinary tract, in: O'Reilly PH, Gosling JA (eds) *Idiopathic Hydronephrosis*. Berlin: Springer.
2 Murnaghan GF (1958) Mechanism of congenital hydronephrosis with reference to factors influencing surgical treatment. *Ann Roy Coll Surg Engl* 23: 25.
3 Notley RG (1971) The structural basis for normal and abnormal ureteric motility. *Ann Roy Coll Surg Engl* 49: 248.
4 Koff SA, Campbell KD (1994) The non-operative management of unilateral neonatal hydronephrosis: natural history of poorly functioning kidneys. *J Urol* 152: 593.
5 Liu HYA, Dhillon HK, Yeung CK, Diamond DA, Duffy PG, Ransley PG (1994) Clinical outcome and management of prenatally diagnosed primary megaureters. *J Urol* 152: 614.
6 Koff SA, Peller PA, Young DC, Pollifrone DL (1994) The assessment of obstruction in the newborn with unilateral hydronephrosis by measuring the size of the opposite kidney. *J Urol* 152: 596.
7 English PJ, Testa JH, Shields RA *et al.* (1987) Modified method of diuresis renography for the assessment of equivocal pelviureteric junction obstruction. *Br J Urol* 59: 10.
8 Whitfield HN, Britton KE, Hendry WF *et al.* (1978) Frusemide intravenous urography in the diagnosis of pelviureteric junction obstruction. *Br J Urol* 51: 445.
9 Johnston HB (1969) The pathogenesis of hydronephrosis in children. *Br J Urol* 41: 724.
10 Whitaker RH, Buxton Thomas MS (1984) A comparison of pressure flow studies and renography in equivocal upper urinary tract obstruction. *J Urol* 131: 446.
11 Whitaker RH (1976) Equivocal pelvi-ureteric obstruction. *Br J Urol* 47: 771.
12 Anderson JC, Hynes W (1949) Retrocaval ureter: case diagnosed preoperatively and treated successfully by plastic operation. *Br J Urol* 21: 209.
13 Culp OS, DeWeerd JH (1951) A pelvic flap operation for certain types of ureteropelvic obstruction: preliminary report. *Mayo Clin Proc* 26: 483.
14 Notley RG, Beaugie J McN (1973) Long term follow-up of the Anderson–Hynes pyeloplasty. *Br J Urol* 45: 464.
15 Davis DM (1943) Intubated ureterotomy: a new operation for ureteral and ureteropelvic stricture. *Surg Gynecol Obstet* 76: 513.
16 Gerber GS, Lyon ES (1994) Endopyelotomy: patient selection, results and complications. *Urology* 43: 2.
17 Kavoussi LR, Albala DM, Clayman R (1993) Outcome of secondary open surgical procedure in patients who failed primary endopyelotomy. *Br J Urol* 72: 157.
18 Motala JA, Badlani GH, Smith AD (1993) Results of 212 consecutive endopyelotomies: an 8 year follow up. *J Urol* 149: 453.
19 Malden ES, Picus D, Clayman RV (1992) Arteriovenous fistula complicating endopyelotomy. *J Urol* 148: 1520–3.
20 Sutherland RS, Pfister RR, Koyle MA (1992) Endopyelotomy associated ureteral necrosis: complete necrosis using Boari flap. *J Urol* 148: 1490.
21 McLinton S, Steyn JH, Hussey JK (1993) Retrograde balloon dilatation for pelviureteric junction obstruction. *Br J Urol* 71: 152.

Chapter 10: Kidney and ureter — trauma

Closed trauma

Aetiology

Closed injury to the kidney occurs in sport and road traffic accidents [1–5]. Most injuries occur in otherwise healthy young men. The mechanism is a blow to the loin compressing the kidney between the 12th rib and the lumbar vertebrae (Fig. 10.1). A hydronephrotic kidney may be especially vulnerable, just as a distended balloon is more apt to burst than one which is half empty.

Pathology

Trauma may split the cortex, tear the collecting system, and open renal arteries and veins of different size. The consequence is more or less loss of blood, and more or less extravasation of urine (Fig. 10.2). In the most minor injuries the parenchyma is split, there is microscopic haematuria, minimal loss of blood and no shock develops. These are sometimes referred to as renal 'contusions' and their prognosis is so good that some authorities do not consider it necessary to investigate them further [6].

Gerota's fascia forms a firm thin envelope around the kidney. Blood leaking out of a damaged kidney builds up pressure and in most cases will stop bleeding by tamponade. The amount of blood loss in these cases is variable

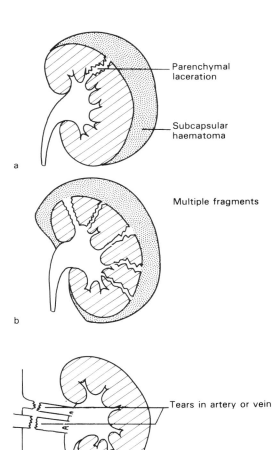

Fig. 10.2 Varying degrees of renal injury. (a) In most cases there are small tears in the renal parenchyma and the perirenal haematoma is contained within the envelope of Gerota's fascia. (b) In more severe injuries the kidney is ruptured into many smaller fragments, but bleeding is self-controlled by tamponade within Gerota's fascia. (c) In very severe injuries the renal pedicle is severed.

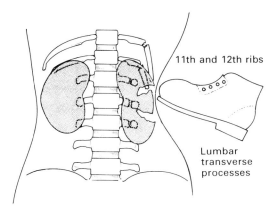

Fig. 10.1 Closed renal injury: the kidney is compressed between the 12th rib and the lumbar transverse processes. The lower ribs and the tips of the transverse processes are frequently fractured.

and unpredictable, and these patients can be difficult to manage [1,2].

In very severe injuries — usually resulting from massive deceleration — the renal artery and vein are torn across. Loss of blood is immediate and immense. The kidney is rendered instantly anoxic. It remains *in situ* at body temperature. This is an exceedingly rare accident. While it may seem almost impossible to make arrangements to make the diagnosis and get the patient to the operating room in time to mend the torn renal vessels, nevertheless sufficient numbers have been successfully diagnosed and the vascular injuries repaired to make the effort worthwhile.

Clinical features

Usually a fit young sportsman walks into the accident department because he has noticed blood in the urine. Earlier in the day he has been playing football, and someone kicked him in the loin. He feels well. He looks well. Blood is either detected in the urine by dipstick or is obvious to the naked eye [7]. For the doctor who sees him it is all too easy to dismiss the matter: in fact this is a very dangerous trap. He must be admitted and observed very carefully because he may be dead within 24 h.

The other method of presentation is part of the pattern of multiple trauma. The accident victim has obviously sustained many injuries [4,6]. That the kidneys might have been damaged can only be surmised because the loins are bruised or blood is found in the urine.

Investigation

When the patient is first seen it is quite imposs-ible to know how badly a kidney has been damaged. More important, it is impossible to know if the patient has a kidney on the other side. The first duty of any doctor confronting a patient with traumatic haematuria is to make sure there is a kidney on the other side.

The classical investigation is an IVU. This may show distortion of the renal outline on one side, with extravasation of contrast medium (Fig. 10.3) or it may show no secretion at all. A computerized tomography (CT) scan gives much better infor-mation, showing the full extent of the laceration of the renal parenchyma with a collection of blood outside the kidney, confined within Gerota's fascia (Fig. 10.4). Angiography is rarely indicated, but gives a more accurate and com-

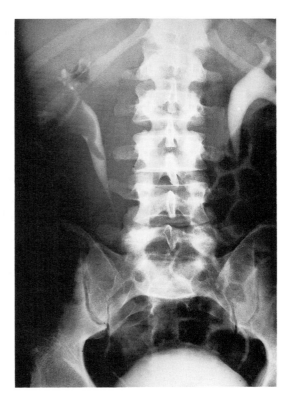

Fig. 10.3 IVU in closed renal injury of the right kidney: the pyelogram is distorted and there is a clot in the renal pelvis. There was no intervention and recovery was complete (courtesy of Dr Otto Chan).

plete diagnosis than either of the other methods [8]. If no secretion of contrast is seen at all, then a renal arteriogram may show damage to the renal artery (Fig. 10.5) and the question immediately arises whether or not to make an attempt to repair the damage (see below).

Management

In most cases, so long as it is certain that a kidney is present on the other side, it is safe to manage these patients by careful surveillance. This means regular measurements of pulse rate, blood pressure and abdominal girth, and examining each specimen of urine to confirm that the bleeding is reducing. The danger is that a small laceration in such a damaged kidney may bleed again, with a sudden deterioration in the patient's blood pressure, calling for immediate exploration, and for this reason it is usual to keep the patient under observation for at least 48 h.

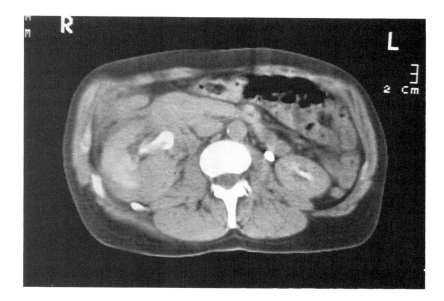

Fig. 10.4 A CT scan in closed renal injury of the right kidney. Note the fragmented renal parenchyma and the large perirenal haematoma. There was no intervention and recovery was complete (courtesy of Dr W. Hately).

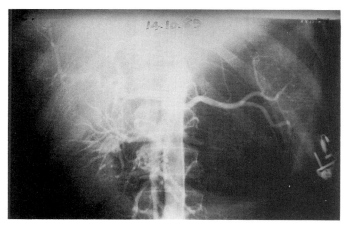

a

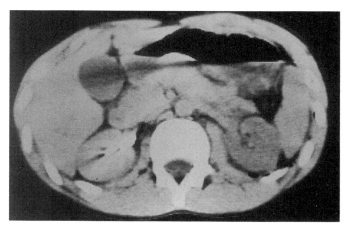

b

Fig. 10.5 Closed injury of the left kidney with a complete avulsion of the renal pedicle. (a) Angiogram shows a short stump of left renal artery. (b) Dynamic CT scan in the same case: no contrast in the left kidney but surprisingly small haematoma (courtesy of Dr Otto Chan).

Continuing haemorrhage

Patients who are obviously showing evidence of internal bleeding, but are in a stable state, should have a renal angiogram performed, at which time it may be possible to identify bleeding coming from a small branch and plug it with gelfoam or a small Gianturco coil [9] (Fig. 10.6).

In those who are obviously losing much blood, this angiographic approach makes it possible to block the renal artery with an angioplasty balloon, stemming the loss of blood, and giving time to bring the patient to the operating room to repair the damage [10]. The appropriate exper-

tise and adequate facilities may not be available and it may be safer to remove the patient to the operating room at once. One must remember that there can be tremendous bleeding not merely from the aorta but also from the inferior vena cava [11].

Through a long midline incision the aorta is secured at once, if possible before the perirenal haematoma is disturbed (Fig. 10.7). Once the renal artery has been found and taped, the haematoma can be evacuated, and the lacerations examined at leisure to see if it is possible to close the bleeding vessels, evacuate the thrombus, repair the injured vessels [12,13] and conserve as

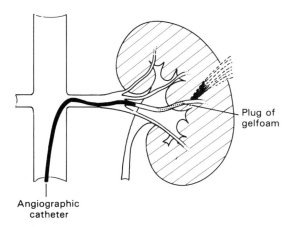

Fig. 10.6 Angiography may reveal a bleeding arterial branch which can be plugged with gelfoam or a Gianturco coil.

much of the parenchyma as possible. Wrapping the kidney in net made of collagen or some other synthetic suture material has been found to be useful [14]. Clearly nephrectomy will be necessary if the kidney is irrecoverable.

Complications

Secondary haemorrhage. There is a small but very real danger of delayed haemorrhage in patients who have a major laceration of the kidney. For this reason such patients are watched in hospital for at least 10 days.

Late hypertension. Hypertension may occur from one of two causes: (a) damage to the renal artery may be followed by stenosis; if this occurs it may be corrected by excision of the narrow segment and reanastomosis of the renal artery, or by bypass grafting; or (b) the kidney may become encased in fibrous tissue resulting from the perirenal haematoma, giving rise to the type of hypertension that can be produced in experimental animals by wrapping the kidney in cellophane [15].

Pseudocyst and urinoma. Although these are very uncommon, it is most important to recognize them, because they are so dangerous (Fig. 10.8). A collection of extravasated urine becomes

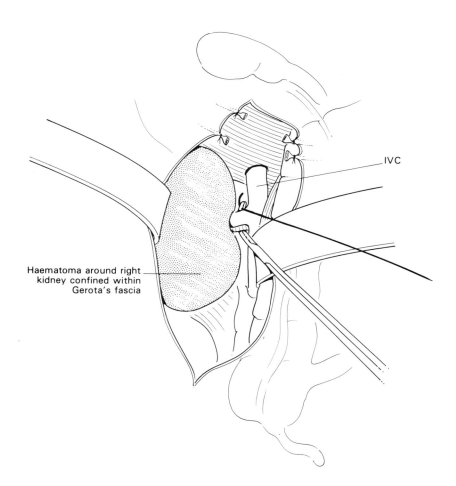

Fig. 10.7 Exploration for renal injury. The colon is reflected. The renal pedicle is secured as soon as possible without opening Gerota's fascia. IVC, inferior vena cava.

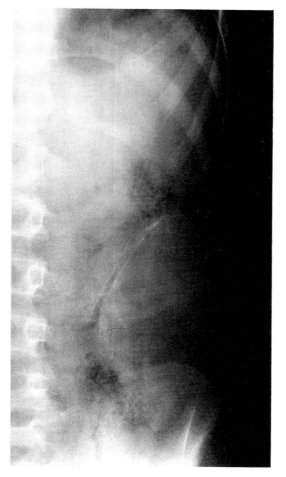

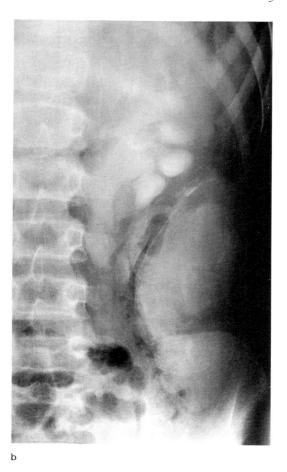

Fig. 10.8 Perirenal pseudocyst: (a) a plain radiograph showing the calcified wall of the pseudocyst, and (b) a delayed film of IVU showing contrast in the pseudocyst.

walled-off by fibrous tissue, but remains in communication with the renal pelvis [16,17]. The wall of the cavity becomes eventually more or less lined with urothelium, and in turn this leads to calcification and heterotopic bone formation, so that in time the urinoma takes on the appearance of an eggshell. The contents of the urinoma often become infected, but even if they do not, the absorption of urine from the granulation tissue lining the cavity leads to hyperchloraemic acidosis. Merely draining the cavity is seldom sufficient, and it is usually necessary to dissect out the lining of the cavity and repair the defect in the renal pelvis — a difficult and time-consuming operation.

Hydronephrosis. The haematoma around the lacerated kidney may compress the ureter and lead to hydronephrosis, but it is rarely possible to be sure that a hydronephrosis was not present before the injury.

Closed injury of the ureter

This is a very uncommon injury, which may be seen in major deceleration accidents. There may be extravasation of urine behind the peritoneum which leads to fat necrosis and sloughing of a considerable length of the ureter [18].

The clinical features that raise a question of the diagnosis are vomiting, ileus and distension of the bowel, as if there had been trauma to the bowel or pancreas. Even at laparotomy the diagnosis may be difficult to make in view of the extensive retroperitoneal haemorrhage and necrosis and it is only when urine issues from the drain afterwards that the diagnosis is considered.

Primary repair of the injury is seldom an option and instead percutaneous nephrostomy is performed to allow time for the inflammation to resolve before considering how to repair the damage.

Penetrating injuries of the kidney

These may be found in the course of exploration of a stab or gun-shot wound. It is usual to find that the bleeding has stopped by the time the kidney is inspected, but if it is continuing then the renal artery should be secured and occluded, and an attempt made to find and oversew the cut arterial branches using fine catgut sutures [4—6].

Experience in Vietnam taught that a nephrectomy was the safest course in high velocity missile injuries if the kidney appears to be injured, since the shock effect on the kidney would almost always lead to necrosis and massive secondary haemorrhage [19].

Arteriovenous fistula

One important complication of penetrating injuries of the renal parenchyma (and indeed of renal biopsy) is an arteriovenous fistula. It may lead to hypertension. There may be an audible bruit over the kidney. An angiogram will show the fistula and, unless the kidney has been totally destroyed (which occurs in the giant fistulae), it is usually possible to find and excise the fistula having first occluded the main renal artery (see p. 195).

Open and penetrating injuries of the ureter

The ureter may be injured by a knife or bullet, but it is rare for the damage to be noticed at the time of abdominal exploration [18,19]. More often, a leakage of urine from the wound drain brings the diagnosis to light and, as with closed injuries, a preliminary percutaneous nephrostomy will allow the kidney on the damaged side to be drained, and buy time for repair of the lesion to be planned and carried out when the patient has recovered from other major injuries.

How the ureter is repaired will depend on the site of the injury. In rare instances it may be possible to find the ends of the ureter, spatulate them and sew them together over a suitable splinting catheter. More often, it will be necess-ary to bridge the gap by means of a Boari flap or the interposition of a loop of ileum (see below).

Iatrogenic injuries to the ureter

The ureter is commonly injured during pelvic surgery when it is caught up by a ligature on the superior vesical and uterine vessels, crushed in a clamp or divided by accident. Ureters have been divided during laparoscopic sterilization in mistake for the fallopian tube and at appendicectomy when they are mistaken for a retrocaecal appendix. It is also quite easy for the ureter to be injured in the course of surgery for aortic aneurysms, particularly those with much surrounding fibrosis [20].

Today the ureter is most often injured at ureteroscopy or endopyelotomy [21,22].

Clinical features

If the ureter has been injured it is often obstructed, and patients complain of pain in the back, accompanied by fever and rigors when the urine is infected.

More often, the first symptom is a leak of urine from the vagina or the perineal part of an abdominoperineal excision of the rectum often after a delay of 5 days or more.

Investigations

Early diagnosis demands a willingness to consider the possibility that the ureter may have been injured after any pelvic operation, and a determination to get the appropriate investigations done without delay. When there is pain in the loin an ultrasound scan will usually reveal a dilated ureter and renal pelvis, and it may be helpful to confirm the suspicion by means of an excretion urogram (Fig. 10.9).

When fluid appears in the vagina it is quite understandable for the doctor to hope that it is not urine but merely lymph: this should never be an excuse not to make certain by sending a small quantity of the fluid to the laboratory where its content of creatinine or urea can be compared with that in the patient's plasma. No body fluid other than urine can possibly have a greater concentration of creatinine or urea than plasma.

If the IVU has not already been performed, it should be done now. It will usually show dilatation on the injured side, and it may, but not always, show a leakage of contrast medium into the vagina.

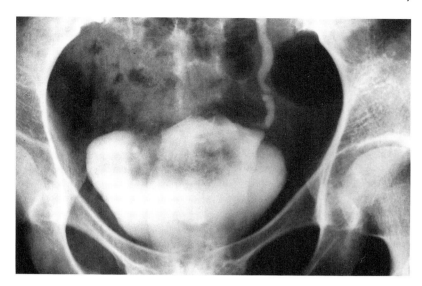

Fig. 10.9 IVU in iatrogenic injury of the ureter at hysterectomy. Contrast has leaked into the vagina to outline it.

Management

If the ureter is obstructed and especially when the patient is unwell because of infection, a percutaneous nephrostomy tube should be placed in the kidney to decompress it and allow infection to be brought under control with anti-biotics. Experience shows that the sooner these injuries are repaired the better, in spite of the widely accepted teaching in favour of delay [23,24].

Endoscopy

In all these patients it is necessary to confirm the diagnosis by retrograde urography (Fig. 10.10). It should be done not only on the side which is known to be injured, but on the other side as well, since it is not uncommon for both to have been damaged. It is easy to carry out a repair of both ureters there and then.

At this cystoscopy, a careful search is made for a vesicovaginal fistula since these may well accompany injury to the ureter [24], and again, the repair of both lesions may be carried out simultaneously.

Intubation

At the time of performing the retrograde uretero-gram, an attempt may be made to pass a guide-wire up the ureter from below, or, if there is a percutaneous nephrostomy in position, from above (Fig. 10.11). If the guide-wire can be wriggled past the site of the obstruction, a

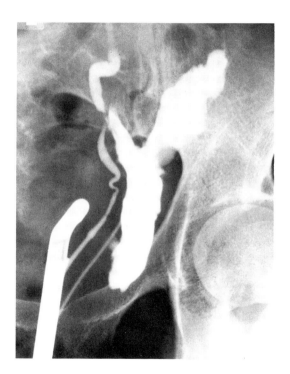

Fig. 10.10 Retrograde ureterogram showing contrast leaking out from the ureter (courtesy of Mr JC Smith).

double-J tube may be passed over it and left *in situ* for 4–6 weeks by which time the injured ureter may be found to heal completely without any stricture [25].

Operative repair

There are four alternative methods of repairing an injured ureter: the Boari–Ockerblad flap, the

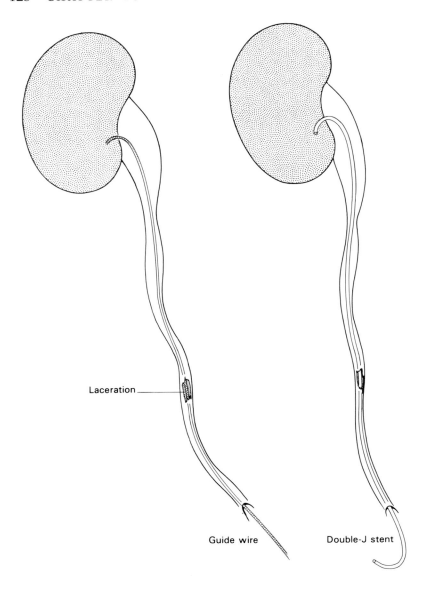

Laceration

Guide wire

Double-J stent

Fig. 10.11 If a guide-wire can be made to pass the site of the injury a double-J stent may be passed over it.

psoas hitch, transureteroureteric anastomosis and, for high injuries, an ileal loop.

The Boari—Ockerblad flap. This is the preferred and most reliable method [23,24,26]. The original incision is reopened unless the hysterectomy has been performed by the vaginal route, in which case a vertical midline incision gives marginally easier access than a Pfannenstiel incision especially in a fat person.

The injured ureter is followed down to the site of injury where it is seldom possible to see exactly how it has been injured — sometimes a distinct ligature can be found but usually the site of injury is concealed in scar tissue and oedema (Fig. 10.12). The ureter is divided at the site of

blockage. It always retracts cranially for several centimetres leaving a gap larger than first antici-pated (Fig. 10.13). The bladder is now filled, and a widely based flap is marked out with stay-sutures before the wall of the bladder is incised (Fig. 10.14). Careful haemostasis is obtained by suture ligature rather than diathermy. The opposite ureter is marked and protected by passing a catheter into it.

A long submucosal tunnel is made in the Boari flap, and the ureter is drawn down this into the bladder. The end of the ureter is spatulated, everted and sewn to the Boari—Ockerblad flap with interrupted fine absorbable sutures (Fig. 10.15). The flap is intubated, using a polyethylene tube led through the skin or a double-J tube. The

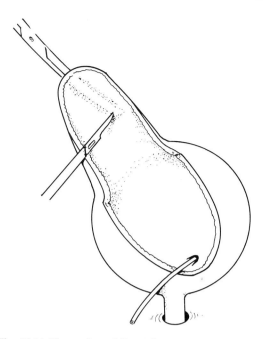

Fig. 10.14 The ∩-shaped Boari flap is raised and a submucosal tunnel formed with scissors.

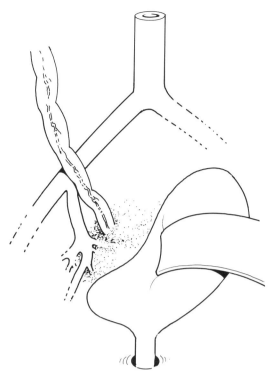

Fig. 10.12 The ureter is followed down to the site of the injury.

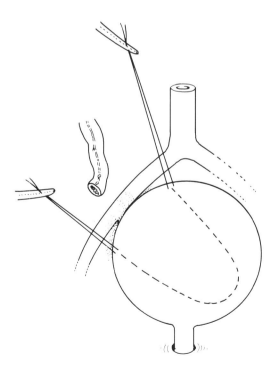

Fig. 10.13 The ureter is divided above the site of the injury: it always retracts. The bladder is filled and the ∩-shaped Boari flap marked out with stay-sutures.

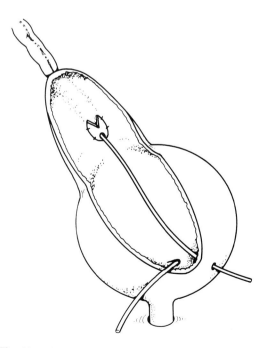

Fig. 10.15 The ureter is drawn through the submucosal tunnel, spatulated and sutured to the mucosa of the bladder over a suitable splinting catheter.

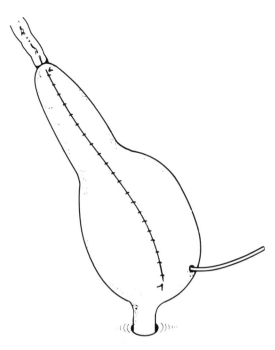

Fig. 10.16 The Boari flap is closed.

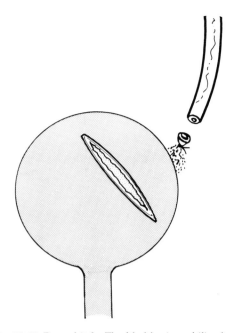

Fig. 10.18 Psoas hitch. The bladder is mobilized and incised at right angles to the line of the ureter.

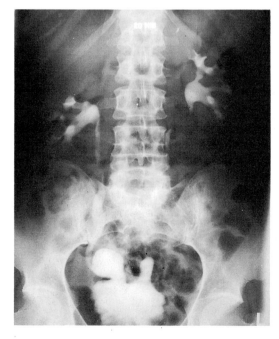

Fig. 10.17 IVU after bilateral Boari implantation. Usually it is not possible to see where the Boari flap has been made.

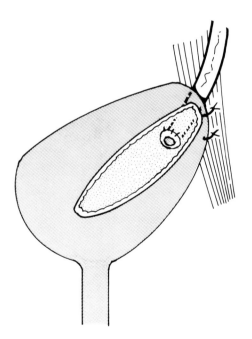

Fig. 10.19 The bladder is sutured to the tendon of psoas minor, when present, and the ureter is implanted through a long antireflux tunnel.

flap is closed in the line of the opening in the bladder using two layers of fine absorbable suture (e.g. 4-0 catgut or 5-0 Vicryl). It is sometimes helpful to attach the flap to adjacent fibrous tissue to make sure it lies correctly and that there is no tension at all on the anastomosis (Fig. 10.16).

The bladder is drained with a suitable catheter and the wound closed with absorbable sutures with a drain to the retropubic space.

Follow-up should include an intravenous pyelogram (IVP) at 3 months by which time it is usually very difficult to identify which ureter is the normal one and which had to be reimplanted (Fig. 10.17).

The psoas hitch. This is an alternative method [27]. Having found the injured ureter and divided it at the site of injury, the bladder is mobilized by dividing the superior vesical vessels on the opposite side. The bladder is then incised at right angles to the line of the ureter (Fig. 10.18), drawn up and attached with two or three stout sutures of absorbable material to the tendon of

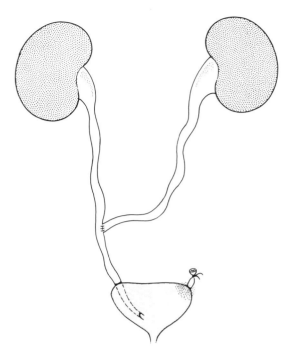

Fig. 10.20 The principle of ureteroureterostomy.

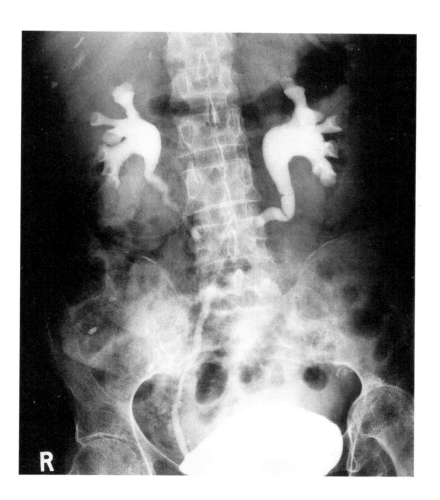

Fig. 10.21 Urogram after successful ureteroureterostomy (courtesy of Mr JC Smith).

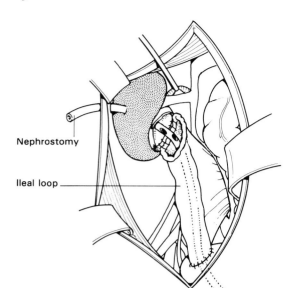

Fig. 10.22 A long gap in the ureter may be bridged with an ileal conduit.

psoas minor (when present) or to some adjacent strong fibrous tissue in those patients without this tendon. The implantation of the ureter is performed using an antireflux tunnel (Fig. 10.19).

Transureteroureteric anastomosis. The injured ureter is led behind the mesosigmoid to the good side, and there spatulated and anastomosed end-to-side onto the good ureter using very fine absorbable sutures [28] (Figs 10.20 & 10.21).

Of these three methods the Boari—Ockerblad technique is the most reliable and versatile [29,30]. It can even be brought right up to the kidney in some cases [22]. There is a temptation with the psoas hitch to allow a little tension on the anastomosis, and with transureteroureteric anastomosis there is a risk that the good ureter will be damaged [27].

The ileal loop. For very high injuries of the ureter where it is not possible to effect an end-to-end anastomosis it is usually safer to make an ileal conduit in the usual way, and anastomose one end to the ureter and the other to the bladder (Fig. 10.22).

References

1 Barnes DR (1973) The diagnosis and management of acute renal injuries. *South Afr J Surg* 11: 233.

2 McAndrew JD, Corriere JN (1994) Radiographic evaluation of renal trauma: evaluation of 1103 patients. *Br J Urol* 73: 352.

3 Cockett ATK, Frank IN, Davis RS, Linke CA (1975) Recent advances in the diagnosis and management of blunt renal trauma *J Urol* 113: 750.

4 Levy JB, Baskin LS, Ewalt DH *et al.* (1993) Nonoperative management of blunt pediatric major renal trauma. *Urology* 42: 417.

5 Spain DA, Berger Y, Boyarsky AH, Flancbaum LF (1993) Nonoperative management of bilateral shattered kidneys from blunt trauma. *Urology* 41: 579.

6 Mee SL, McAninch JW, Robinson AL, Auerback PS, Carroll PR (1989) Radiographic assessment of renal trauma: a 10 year prospective study of patient selection. *J Urol* 141: 1095.

7 Chandhoke PS, McAninch JW (1988) Detection and significance of microscopic hematuria in patients with blunt renal trauma. *J Urol* 140: 16.

8 Leppaniemi AK, Haapiainen RK, Lehtonen TA (1989) Diagnosis and treatment of patients with renal trauma. *Br J Urol* 64: 13.

9 Eastham JA, Wilson TG, Larsen DW, Ahlering TE (1992) Angiographic embolization of renal stab wounds. *J Urol* 148: 268.

10 Cass AS (1993) Preliminary vascular control before renal exploration for trauma. *Br J Urol* 71: 493.

11 Smith SRG (1988) Traumatic retroperitoneal venous haemorrhage. *Br J Surg* 75: 632.

12 Fay R, Brosman S, Lindstrom R, Cohen A (1974) Renal artery thrombosis: successful revascularization by autotransplantation. *J Urol* 111: 572.

13 Skinner DG (1973) Traumatic renal artery thrombosis: a successful thrombectomy and revascularisation. *Ann Surg* 177: 264.

14 Schoenenberger A, Mattler D, Roesler H *et al.* (1985) Surgical repair of the kidney after blunt lesions of intermediate degrees using a Vicryl mesh: an experimental study. *J Urol* 134: 804.

15 Page IH (1939) The production of persistent arterial hypertension by cellophane and perinephritis. *J Am Med Assoc* 113: 2046.

16 Arnold EP (1972) Pararenal pseudocyst. *Br J Urol* 44: 40.

17 Furtschegger A, Egender G, Jakse G (1988) The value of sonography in the diagnosis and follow-up of patients with blunt renal trauma. *Br J Urol* 62: 110.

18 Eastham JA, Wilson TG, Ahlering TE (1993) Urological evaluation and management of renal-proximity stab wounds. *J Urol* 150: 1771.

19 Brandes SB, Chelsky MJ, Buckman RF, Hanno PM (1994) Ureteral injuries from penetrating trauma. *J Trauma* 36: 766.

20 Spirnak JP, Persky L, Resnick MI (1985) The management of civilian ureteral gunshot wounds: a review of eight patients. *J Urol* 134: 733.

21 Bergqvist D, Takolander R (1982) Ureteral obstruction as a complication in aorto-iliac reconstructive surgery. *Scand J Urol Nephrol* 17: 391.

22 Chang R, Marshall FF (1987) Management of ureteroscopic injuries. *J Urol* 137: 1132.

23 Badenoch DF, Tiptaft RC, Thakar DR, Fowler CG, Blandy JP (1987) Early repair of accidental injury to the ureter or bladder following gynaecological surgery. *Br J Urol* 59: 516.

24 Blandy JP, Badenoch DF, Fowler CG, Jenkins BJ, Thomas NWM (1991) Early repair of iatrogenic injury to the ureter or bladder following gynecological surgery. *J Urol* 146: 761.

25 Selzman AA, Spirnak JP, Kursh ED (1995) The changing management of ureterovaginal fistulas. *J Urol* 153: 626

26 Cukier J (1966) L'operation de Boari: a propos de 63 observations. *Acta Urol Belg* 34: 15.

27 Ehrlich RM, Skinner DG (1975) Complications of transureteroureterostomy. *J Urol* 113: 467.

28 Smith IB, Smith JC (1975) Transureteroureterostomy: British experience. *Br J Urol* 47: 519.

29 Bowsher WG, Shah PJR, Costello AJ, Tiptaft RC, Paris AMI, Blandy JP (1982) A critical appraisal of the Boari flap. *Br J Urol* 54: 682.

30 Motiwala HG, Shah SA, Patel SM (1990) Ureteric substitution with Boari bladder flap. *Br J Urol* 66: 369.

Chapter 11: Kidney and ureter — inflammation

Glomerulonephritis

The various types of glomerulonephritis are diseases whose distinctive feature is damage to the glomerulus caused by an immune mechanism [1−3]. They are usually the concern of the nephrologist but the urological surgeon can hardly ignore a group of conditions which are responsible for 30−50% of end-stage renal failure needing dialysis or transplantation. Glomerulonephritis may present with haematuria, and may unexpectedly complicate some of the treatments the urologist is likely to use. The following is a very simplified account of what is in fact a very complex subject [1−4].

Mechanisms

Most antigen−antibody reactions result in the formation of insoluble immune complexes which are then disposed of by the reticuloendothelial system. If smaller soluble immune complexes are formed they may reach the kidney in the bloodstream and be deposited in the glomerulus. There is some question whether it is the nature of the antigen which determines the formation of soluble complexes, or a deficiency of the immune system itself. An alternative mechanism seems to involve trapping of the soluble antigen in the glomerulus with formation of immune complexes *in situ*.

Although the list of known antigens which may cause glomerulonephritis is a long one, in practice in most cases the cause is never known. Known antigens range from simple chemicals such as tridione, penicillamine and butazolidine, to complex antigens associated with viruses (mumps, measles, etc.), parasites (*Plasmodium malariae, Schistosoma*) and bacteria (Lancefield group A beta haemolytic streptococcus, staphylococcus, *Treponema pallidum*). In systemic lupus erythematosus the antigen is the patient's own DNA, and some cases of glomerulonephritis are caused by tumour antigens [1]. One of the most unusual is antiglomerular basement membrane (anti-GBM) antibody which reacts with an antigen in the GBM itself. Since this antigen is similar to that in the basement membrane of the alveoli of the lung, glomerulonephritis occurs together with haemorrhage in the lung — Goodpasture's syndrome.

Secondary damage to the glomerulus

Whether the primary event is deposition of complexes, or the reaction of anti-GBM antibody, a number of secondary events are triggered by the immune process. Complement fixation may be followed by the release of kinins which attract platelets and leucocytes, lead to the deposition of fibrin, and cause increased permeability of the glomerular capillary. The extent of this secondary damage is very variable, and is the basis for the classification of these diseases.

Classification

The working classification of glomerulonephritis has to take into account not only the severity of the damage as found by renal biopsy but also the clinical picture. These cover a wide range of manifestations and the resulting classification is very complex: the following is a simplification.

Minimal change glomerulonephritis

Here the glomeruli are normal under the light microscope, but electron microscopy shows fusion of the foot-processes of the epithelial cells (Fig. 11.1). Some argue that this is not a true glomerulonephritis at all, pointing out that these changes occur in conditions not associated with proteinuria. Rare in adults, minimal change glomerulonephritis is usually seen in children aged 2−4 years.

The clinical picture which accompanies these electron microscopic changes is the result of loss of albumen and cholesterol. The leak of albumen lowers the plasma oncotic pressure and leads to widespread oedema. Cholesterol is also leaked

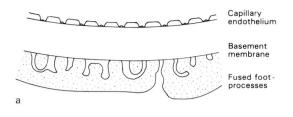

Capillary
endothelium

Basement
membrane

Fused foot-
processes

a

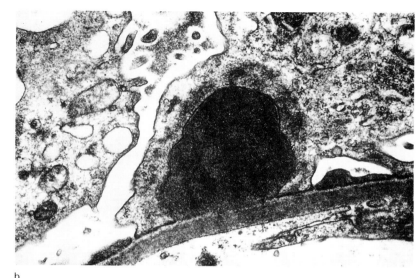

b

Fig. 11.1 (a) Diagram and (b) electrophotomicrograph of minimal change glomerulonephritis, in which the epithelial foot-processes are fused together (courtesy of Dr Suhail Baithun).

but reabsorbed to streak the oedematous kidneys with lipid. This is the nephrotic syndrome.

Although neither immune complexes nor anti-GBM antibody can be detected, an immune pathogenesis is suggested by its response to steroids and immunosuppressive drugs, and its predilection for families with a high incidence of asthma and eczema (immunological atopy). The proteinuria may be due to a factor produced by lymphocytes which increases glomerular permeability to protein, but the condition remains something of a mystery.

Membranous glomerulonephritis

Here the basement membrane is thickened by deposited immune complexes (Fig. 11.2). The antigen involved is usually unknown, but this type of glomerulonephritis is seen in systemic lupus erythematosus (host DNA), bowel and lung cancer, and penicillamine therapy. There is a strong association with the histocompatibility antigen human leucocyte antigen (HLA)-DR3, and a relative immune deficiency has been suggested as the underlying cause. It is mainly seen in adult males who present with proteinuria or the nephrotic syndrome. About 70% progress to end-stage renal failure, the remainder remit spontaneously.

Proliferative glomerulonephritis

Here the immune complexes have fixed complement and the basement membrane is more severely damaged by the secondary effects of inflammation. Red and white cells escape into Bowman's capsule, and mesangial and endothelial cells proliferate causing the glomerulus to bulge into the opening of the proximal tubule. Immunofluorescent stains show granular deposits of immune complexes and anti-GBM disease.

There are many variations on this theme: the histological changes may be patchy or diffuse, and they may affect mainly the mesangium or mainly the glomerulus (Figs 11.3 & 11.4). These different patterns serve to predict differences in clinical behaviour and response to treatment: the accumulation of 'crescents' of macrophages and epithelial cells in Bowman's space has a particularly bad significance.

With the more severe damage caused by the inflammation which follows fixation of complement there is massive haematuria with red cell casts in the urine, hypertension and oliguria. This is the nephritic syndrome. It is usually of rapid onset and is often associated with streptococcal infection. If only the mesangium and glomerulus is affected, the outlook is better than if Bowman's capsule is blocked by 'crescents' (Fig. 11.5).

End-stage renal failure

Here the glomeruli are replaced by functionless 'ghosts' and the tubules are more or less encased in fibrous tissue and distended with a pale eosinophilic substance (Fig. 11.6). At this stage it is seldom possible to know how the process began. These comprise about 15% of patients

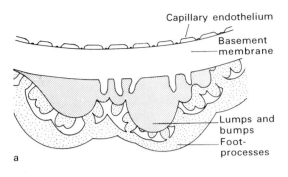

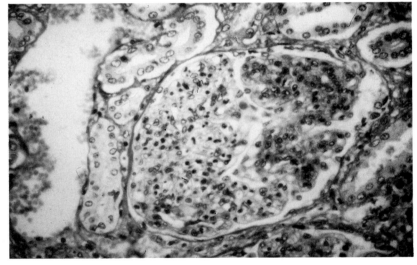

b

Fig. 11.2 (a) Diagram and (b) electrophotomicrograph of membranous glomerulonephritis. Lumps and bumps of soluble complex are trapped between the basement membrane and the foot-processes of the epithelial cells of Bowman's capsule (courtesy of Dr Suhail Baithun).

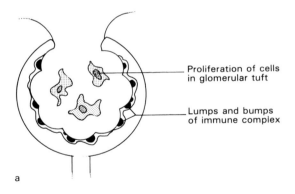

Fig. 11.3 (a) Diagram and (b) electrophotomicrograph of endocapillary proliferative glomerulonephritis. As well as the lumps and bumps of soluble complexes there is a proliferation of cells in the glomerular tuft (courtesy of Dr Suhail Baithun).

b

who need renal replacement by dialysis or transplantation.

Clinical syndromes

Within the spectrum of glomerulonephritis there are many different clinical entities. Surgeons should be aware of four of the more important ones.

Goodpasture's syndrome usually starts with a lung infection. Antibodies against alveolar membrane attack the immunologically similar basement membrane of the kidney, usually leading to a severe and irreversible attack of the nephritic syndrome.

Henoch—Schoenlein nephritis. The systemic immune response affects blood vessels of the skin,

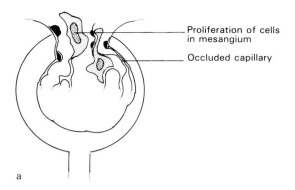

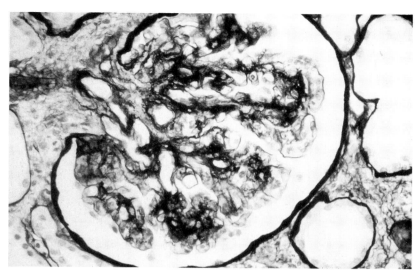

Fig. 11.4 (a) Diagram and (b) electrophotomicrograph of mesangial proliferative glomerulonephritis. The proliferation of cells in the mesangium may block the capillaries (courtesy of Dr Suhail Baithun).

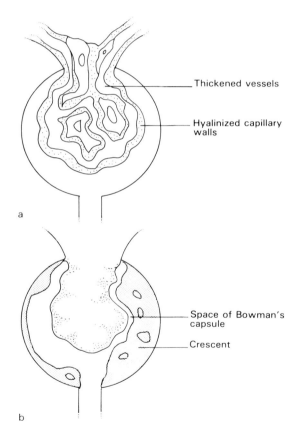

Fig. 11.5 (a & b) Diagrams of extracapillary proliferative glomerulonephritis. There is sclerosis of the vessels and Bowman's capsule is choked with cells that accumulate to form 'crescents'.

bowel and joints as well as the kidney. There is purpura, pain in the joints and abdomen and the nephritic syndrome.

Polyarteritis nodosa is characterized by a widespread immune process which produces fibrinoid necrosis in the walls of arteries and arterioles throughout the body. In the kidney, the arcuate arteries are affected as well as the arterioles leading to the glomeruli. Cells accumulate in Bowman's capsule.

Alport's syndrome is inherited as an autosomal dominant and appears in pre-pubertal boys. They have a change in the basement membrane, beginning as minimal change, and leading on to proliferative glomerulonephritis with crescent formation. The outlook for renal function is very poor.

Deposition of matrix in the kidney

Surgeons should be aware of three important conditions in which pathological matrix material is laid down in the renal parenchyma, progressively blocking and eventually replacing the glomerular vessels and the tubules.

Diabetic nephropathy. An eosinophilic material appears in many tissues of the body in diabetes mellitus. In the mesangium and glomerulus it causes thickening of the walls of arterioles and basement membrane (Fig. 11.7). By the time the kidney is severely affected there is invariably evidence of other complications of diabetes

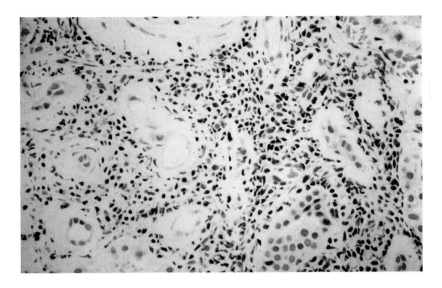

Fig. 11.6 Photomicrograph showing end-stage renal failure. The glomeruli are mere pale ghosts and the functionless tubules are blocked with eosinophilic hyaline material (courtesy of Dr Suhail Baithun).

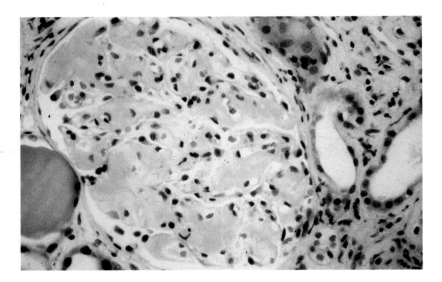

Fig. 11.7 Diabetic nephropathy. The mesangium and glomerulus are thickened by eosinophilic matrix (courtesy of Dr Suhail Baithun).

and more or less severe arterial calcification is common. Diabetic nephropathy is diagnosed by slowly progressive proteinuria, hypertension and renal failure. It is an increasingly common indication for dialysis and transplantation and one where the simultaneous transplantation of kidneys and pancreas offers the brightest prospect for the future [5].

Amyloid. Although its name implies 'like starch' amyloid is in fact an insoluble protein which is deposited throughout the body outside cells. It stains with Congo red, and shines green in polarized light. It occurs in a familial form as familial Mediterranean fever, and with chronic sepsis such as osteomyelitis and persistent urinary infection, notably in paraplegics.

In the kidney the amyloid infiltrates the mesangium and glomerular tuft, and may fill Bowman's space, but can be detected in most other tissues (Fig. 11.8). The result of the renal infiltration is the nephrotic syndrome. The kidneys are usually large and pale, but sometimes they become irregularly scarred and contracted. Slowly deteriorating renal function may at any time be suddenly worsened by renal vein thrombosis [6].

Myelomatosis. In multiple myeloma there is a similar deposit of light chain immunoglobulins which are produced by the tumour. These light chains appear in the urine as a protein which coagulates when warmed to 50°C and dissolves again when heated further — the Bence-Jones

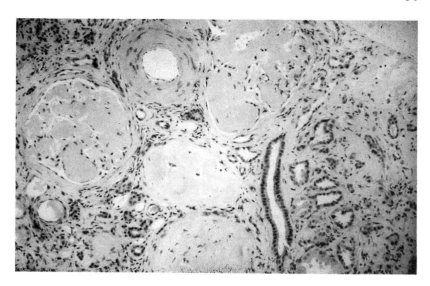

Fig. 11.8 Amyloid. A protein matrix infiltrates all the tissues of the kidney, including the glomerular tuft (courtesy of Dr Suhail Baithun).

protein. The renal changes may be reversed by intensive treatment with chemotherapy and dialysis [7].

Interstitial nephritis — acute

Aetiology

There are many known causes of non-infective inflammatory scarring of the kidney, e.g. drugs, heavy metals, antibiotics, non-steroidal anti-inflammatory drugs and analgesics [8]. Infection is one important cause especially in children with reflux, and in adults with a combination of infection and obstruction. In addition, there are probably many other causes remaining to be discovered.

Most of the agents which cause acute interstitial nephritis can also cause its chronic form.

Infection

It is difficult to produce renal infection in experimental animals unless the kidney has been injured in some way and pyelonephritis is often secondary to previous interstitial scarring of the kidney from some other cause.

Route of infection

Bacteria may find their way to the kidney through the bloodstream or up the urinary tract [9]. Blood-borne infection leads to diffuse inflammation in the kidney, which may progress to multiple abscesses throughout the renal parenchyma — a common autopsy finding in patients in whom infection has been a terminal feature.

Urine-borne infection has a characteristic pattern which follows the injection of infected urine up the collecting tubules: wedge-shaped areas of inflammation fan out from the calices into the cortex (Fig. 11.9): the reaction is most intense in the pyramids and papillae [8–10]. The oedema of inflammation impairs blood flow in the smaller arteries as shown by diminished uptake of radioactive isotopes and impairment of excretion of contrast medium [11] (Figs 11.10, 11.11).

Result of infection

As elsewhere in the body, acute inflammation in the kidney may have three possible outcomes: resolution, suppuration or scarring. Resolution is the usual result, leaving no visible or histological trace [8]. Suppuration in the renal pelvis and calices may occur, e.g. around a nephrostomy, and usually heals with an insignificant scar. Suppuration from blood-borne infection may rarely lead to a cortical abscess [10] (see p. 142).

The segmental inflammation which follows reflux or the combination of obstruction and infection, causes typical deep pitted scars [8–10] (see p. 148).

Clinical features

Acute pyelonephritis is very common and often preceded by lower urinary tract infection, with frequency and pain on voiding. The first symptom may be loin pain and pyrexia.

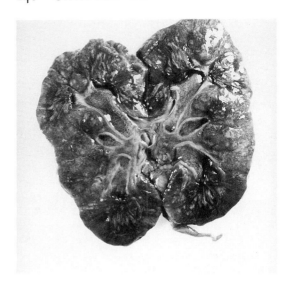

Fig. 11.9 Cross-section through a kidney with acute ascending pyelonephritis (courtesy of Dr E.A. Courtauld).

Investigations

An IVU at this stage will show the renal shadow to be enlarged and its outline hazy from oedema (Fig. 11.10). Excretion of contrast may be delayed, impaired or even completely absent. When the calices can be made out they may be narrowed and elongated because of the renal oedema.

The ^{99m}Tc−DMSA renogram shows that these changes are frequently patchy — some segments of the kidney may be silent, while others take up the isotope or excrete the contrast medium normally (Fig. 11.11). Occasionally, in severe infection, the kidney may seem to be completely non-functioning [11,12].

Urine examination

Microscopy of the urine will show leucocytes, and culture will reveal the causative organism. Very occasionally, it may be helpful to obtain urine from each kidney by ureteric catheterization in order to localize the infection.

Treatment

The first line of treatment is by antibiotics, selected according to the probable or known bacterial sensitivity of the organism in the urine.

In children, or in adults with repeated or severe attacks, an underlying mechanical cause must be excluded. In children this requires ultrasound and if necessary cystography to exclude reflux [13] (see p. 146).

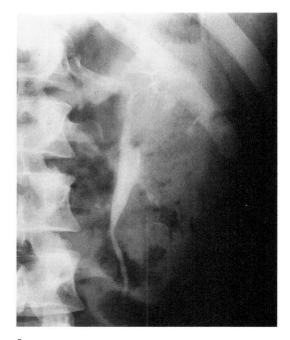

a

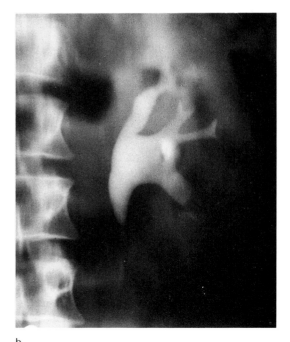

b

Fig. 11.10 (a) IVU during episode of acute pyelonephritis showing swollen parenchyma and spidery calices. (b) 8 weeks later: complete recovery after antibiotic therapy.

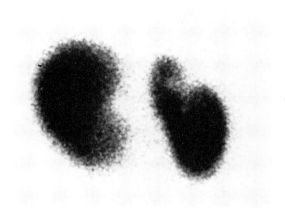

Fig. 11.11 DMSA renogram during an episode of acute pyelonephritis showing no perfusion in segments of the kidney (courtesy of Dr Neil Garvie).

In adults, a plain radiograph with ultrasound or IVU are needed to rule out the underlying mechanical causes of infection: calculus, obstruction, a pocket of undrained urine (e.g. in a diverticulum) or residual urine in the bladder.

Complications

Bacteraemia

Bacteraemia is the most serious of all the complications of urinary infection. Microorganisms from the urine leak through the urothelium and collecting tubules into the bloodstream. These are usually Gram-negative bacilli whose cell wall contains a lipopolysaccharide endotoxin which reacts with leucocytes to liberate a protein cachexin or 'tumour necrosis factor' which has four actions: (a) it stimulates the hypothalamus to cause pyrexia; (b) it releases histamine to cause vasodilatation and venous pooling; (c) it increases capillary permeability; and (d) it may impair the function of the myocardium [14−16].

There is an initial 'warm phase' when the patient may have fever, with rigors, bounding pulse and flushed face and limbs. Within about 30 min this is succeeded by the 'cold phase' with peripheral vasoconstriction and hypotension — septicaemic shock. During this phase there is reduced tissue perfusion leading to lactic acidosis which may be followed by pulmonary hypertension from plugging of the capillary bed in the lungs [17−19].

Every urological surgeon should be aware of this important and dangerous complication which strikes when least expected.

Whenever septicaemia is suspected, blood must be sent at once for culture. Keep the needle in the vein and inject specific anti-endotoxin serum, followed by a large dose of the most appropriate combination of antibiotics, guided if necessary by a call to the hospital laboratory for up-to-date advice. Transfer the patient to the intensive care unit where the cardiac output and the pressure in the right atrium can be monitored with a Swan−Ganz catheter to measure wedge pressure in the pulmonary artery, and monitor the rate at which saline is infused to fill up the intravascular space. Several litres of fluid may be needed.

If adequate fluid replacement fails to reverse hypotension, a low dose of dopamine is given to increase the flow through the renal and mesenteric arteries. Steroids are no longer used.

The patient usually begins to recover within 30−60 min. As the extracellular fluid begins to shift back into the blood compartment, and the peripheral vessels regain their tone, there is a danger of overloading the heart. Spontaneous diuresis usually takes care of the surplus fluid, but a diuretic may be needed.

Septicaemia is most often seen when there is a pocket of pus or infected urine under pressure: this must always be checked, e.g. with an ultrasound scan. Pus must be drained and obstruction to any part of the urinary tract must be relieved at once.

Disseminated intravascular coagulation (DIC)

If shock cannot be corrected in time the patient may enter a more serious phase. Bacterial endotoxin may activate the clotting cascade directly or through damage to endothelial cells. There is widespread coagulation within vessels including those of the kidney. The clotting factors are used up, and haemorrhage may be difficult to control. It may be helped by giving fresh frozen plasma or platelets.

About 20% of cases of bacteraemia are complicated by the adult respiratory distress syndrome. The alveolar membranes are thickened and the pulmonary capillaries blocked with cell debris preventing the effective exchange of respiratory gases. There is a 'white-out' on the chest X-ray. It carries a 90% mortality [14,19,20].

Osteomyelitis

Most patients survive an episode of bacteraemia but blood-borne organisms may settle in the skeleton. One site which is often missed is the junction of the vertebra and the intervertebral disc where an abscess may develop (Fig. 11.12). At first this is symptomless but later on there is persistent backache. There will not be any radiological changes for several weeks but a bone scan may detect the lesion.

Pyonephrosis

This is a combination of infection and obstruction. Its clinical features are those of an acute infection in the kidney, with pain and tenderness in the loin and high fever.

The most helpful investigation is an ultrasound scan. No time should be lost to decompress the kidney by percutaneous nephrostomy or ureteric catheterization. If neither is possible an open nephrostomy may be life-saving, but it is not a minor procedure.

Open nephrostomy

The kidney is exposed through a loin incision. The renal pelvis should be identified, which may be difficult when the tissues are inflamed: open it between stay-sutures (Fig. 11.13) and after aspirating the pus, pass a forceps from inside the pelvis through the parenchyma to draw in a catheter. Attempts to enter the pelvis blindly

from outside will often place the catheter in the renal sinus, not the lumen of the pelvis.

Nephrectomy for pyonephrosis

Today this is never an emergency operation, and is always difficult because a thick shell of fibrous inflammatory tissue surrounds the kidney and makes it difficult to identify the vessels in the pedicle. In such cases the technique of 'subcapsular nephrectomy' is useful.

Subcapsular nephrectomy

Approach the kidney through a loin incision, incise the capsule down to the kidney, and peel it off the renal parenchyma until the hilum is reached (Fig. 11.14). The peeled-back capsule is a thick layer which must be deliberately incised. Using a fully curved forceps pass a stout catgut ligature around the entire pedicle and tie it *en masse*. Then cut through the hilum bit by bit about 2 cm away from the encircling ligature, and suture ligate each vessel as you come across it with absorbable material.

Cortical abscess and carbuncle

Suppuration in the cortex usually follows bloodborne infection, especially in association with

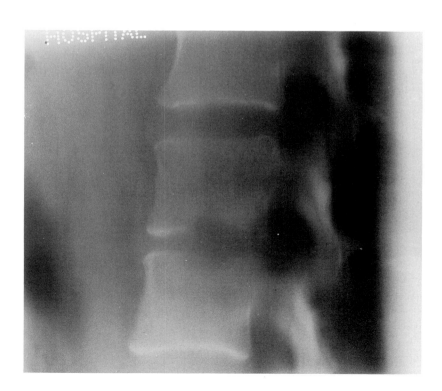

Fig. 11.12 Osteomyelitis of the vertebra.

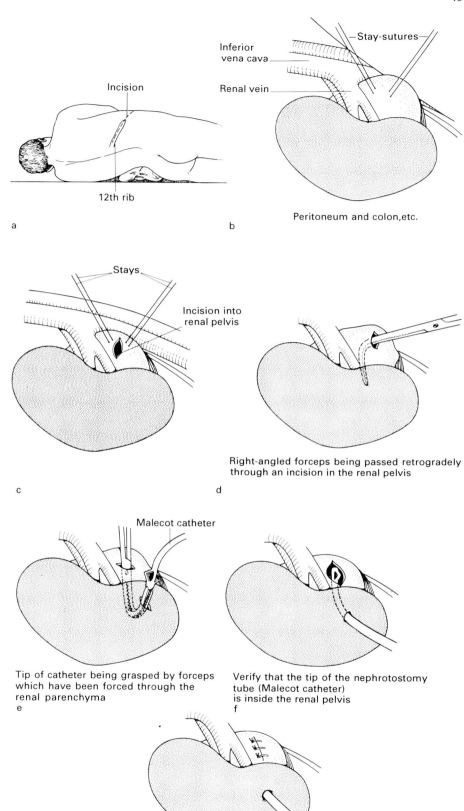

a

12th rib

Incision

b

Inferior vena cava

Renal vein

Stay-sutures

Peritoneum and colon,etc.

c

Stays

Incision into renal pelvis

d

Right-angled forceps being passed retrogradely through an incision in the renal pelvis

e

Malecot catheter

Tip of catheter being grasped by forceps which have been forced through the renal parenchyma

f

Verify that the tip of the nephrotostomy tube (Malecot catheter) is inside the renal pelvis

g   Close the incision in the renal pelvis with catgut

Fig. 11.13 Open nephrostomy (a) through a 12th rib-tip incision; (b) the renal pelvis is opened between stay-sutures; (c) and a forceps is passed from within (d) through the parenchyma to introduce the drainage tube from the outside (e–g).

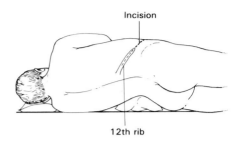

Incision

12th rib

a

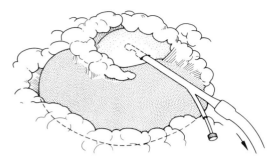

Emptying the pyonephrosis with an aspirating cannula
before attempting to dissect it
This reduces its bulk and makes dissection easier
b   and safer

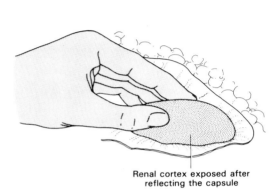

Renal cortex exposed after
reflecting the capsule

Reflecting the renal capsule off the parenchyma by
c finger dissection

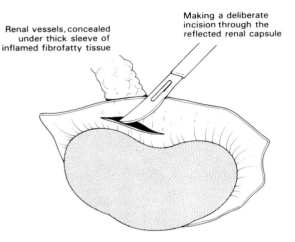

Renal vessels, concealed
under thick sleeve of
inflamed fibrofatty tissue

Making a deliberate
incision through the
reflected renal capsule

d

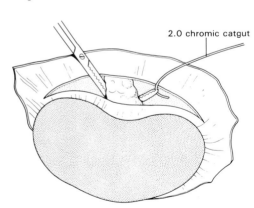

2.0 chromic catgut

The fully curved O'Shaughnessy or Mixter forceps
go right round entire renal vascular pedicle, to
e encircle both artery and vein

Incision into edge
of renal hilum

This surplus renal capsule
is removed

Catgut ligature in continuity around both renal
f artery and vein

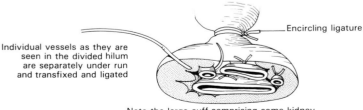

Individual vessels as they are
seen in the divided hilum
are separately under run
and transfixed and ligated

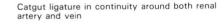

Encircling ligature

Note the large cuff comprising some kidney
parenchyma as well as part of the renal
g pelvis and structures of the hilum

Fig. 11.14 Subcapsular
nephrectomy. (a) The
kidney is approached
through a 12th rib
bed and (b) the
pyonephrosis is
aspirated. (c) The
capsule is peeled off the
kidney until the hilum is
reached where (d) the
capsule is incised to
reveal the vessels which
are first ligated *en masse*
(e), before cutting
through the hilum
piecemeal, suture
ligating each vessel as it
is encountered (f & g).

diabetes, immunosuppression and in intravenous drug abusers [21—23].

Clinical picture

The patient is ill with fever and loin tenderness. It is rare to elicit a history of previous infection such as a cutaneous boil. The IVU shows a soft tissue mass in the kidney whose outline is indistinct from oedema. The ultrasound and computerized tomography (CT) images may be difficult to distinguish from a renal cell carcinoma (Fig. 11.15). Angiography may be inconclusive. The diagnosis therefore rests on clinical suspicion which must be confirmed by aspiration of the abscess under ultrasound or CT control. Pus is sent for culture.

Treatment

Antibiotics are given according to bacteriological sensitivity, and over the next few weeks one expects to see the kidney return to normal. It is rarely necessary to explore or drain a parenchymal abscess, even in a child [23—25].

Emphysematous pyelonephritis

This occurs in diabetics. There is simultaneous coagulative necrosis and gas formation, giving a characteristic radiological appearance in the plain film and the CT scan (Fig. 11.16). The condition is usually lethal unless nephrectomy is performed [25,26].

Perinephric abscess

Perinephric abscess may complicate a neglected cortical abscess or pyonephrosis. Pus in the perirenal fat finds its way to the skin in the lumbar triangle of Petit (Fig. 11.17). Occasionally, the abscess may burst into the pleural cavity, bronchial tree or adjacent intestine [27—29].

Chronic pyelonephritis and papillary necrosis

Chronic pyelonephritis

Reflux nephropathy

Reflux nephropathy in children requires a combination of two congenital anatomical defects:

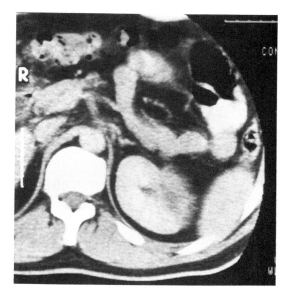

Fig. 11.15 CT scan of renal cortical abscess of left kidney — a 'renal carbuncle'.

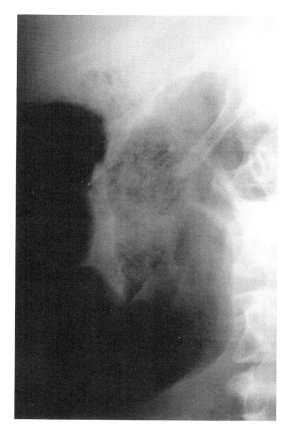

Fig. 11.16 Emphysematous pyelonephritis in a diabetic patient. Note the multiple gas shadows (courtesy of Dr Otto Chan).

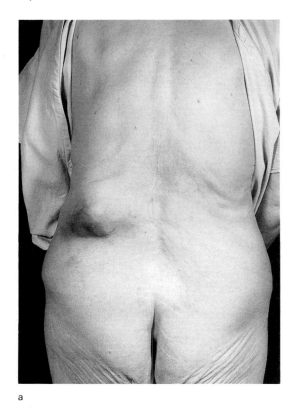

a

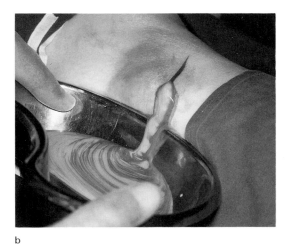

b

Fig. 11.17 (a) Clinical appearance of a perinephric abscess pointing in the lumbar triangle of Petit. (b) Incision and drainage of the same abscess.

one in the ureterovesical valve allowing urine to reflux up the ureter; the second in the renal papilla (Fig. 11.18) which permits infected urine to enter the renal parenchyma (Fig. 11.19) where inflammation is followed by a characteristic pitted scar in the renal cortex [30,31] (Figs 11.20 & 11.21).

Vesicoureteric reflux

The congenital defect in the ureterovesical valve is often associated with duplex ureters and ureterocele. Because the ureter from the lower half-kidney enters the bladder through a short tunnel its valve may be incompetent (see p. 55) (Fig. 11.22).

The ureter from the upper half-kidney often ends in a ureterocele which may cause obstruction, hence in duplex the lower half-kidney may be destroyed by reflux nephropathy and the upper half-kidney by hydronephrosis (Fig. 11.23). Defective vesicoureteric valves are also associated with outflow obstruction from urethral valves or dysfunctional voiding (Fig. 11.24).

Of children who present with urinary infection in the first few years of life 20–50% have reflux.

Of these one in three already have scars in the kidney which can be located by radiography or ^{99m}Tc–DMSA scanning. In later childhood these scars may secrete renin, and become an important cause of hypertension [32].

Since these scars have probably been present from infancy, the question has been whether surgical prevention of the reflux will prevent them getting any worse. This has been the subject of important controlled studies both national and international [33,34] whose results, while still strangely inconclusive, have been a remarkable vindication of this kind of scientific approach to a problem on which it was easy to take up an emotional stance [35]. A consensus has emerged along the following lines.

Investigations in children

Reflux is now often detected *in utero* by ultrasound scanning, but it is not related to the presence or absence of scarring. Scars do not always signify infection, and there may be infection in one kidney when the scarring is on the other side.

In children less than 6 months old, a micturating cystogram should be performed (Fig. 11.25):

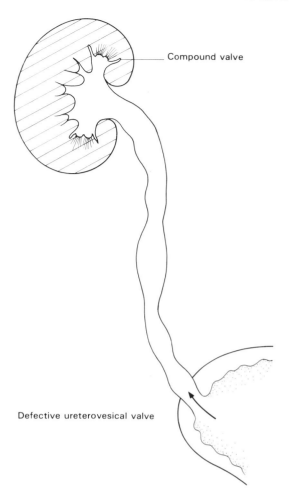

Compound valve

Defective ureterovesical valve

Fig. 11.18 If there is a defective ureterovesical valve as well as a compound papilla, urine is injected into the renal parenchyma.

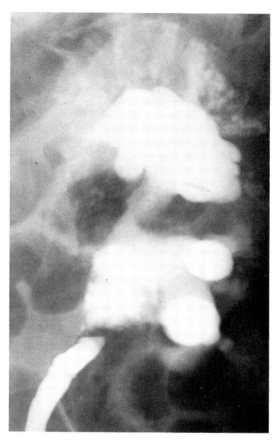

Fig. 11.19 Reflux of contrast medium into the renal parenchyma.

if reflux is present a ^{99m}Tc−DMSA scan is performed to show scarring (Fig. 11.26). Between 6 months and 4 years a plain radiograph is followed by an ultrasound scan, usually a micturating cystogram and a DMSA scan. After the age of 5, new scars are almost unknown and further investigations are needed only if a plain X-ray and ultrasound are abnormal. The technique of ultrasound scanning using agitated saline instead of contrast medium may replace cystography to detect reflux [36−39].

Reflux is classified into four grades by the International Reflux Study in Children (IRSC) [34] (Fig. 11.27). It is now generally accepted that grade I and II — the ureter and renal pelvis are not dilated — are of little consequence. The problem is what to do about grade III and IV where there is distension of the upper tract and the risk of intrarenal reflux.

The consensus seems to be that surgery is indicated when medical treatment fails to prevent recurrent episodes of infection. It does not prevent the formation of new scars: these are just as common in the surgical as in the medically treated group, but it does lessen the incidence of clinical infection.

Surgery is also indicated when the child cannot or will not take medication, or where supervision is difficult, for one of the lessons which emerges from these and other careful trials is the need for strict surveillance in both the non-operated and operated children. Non-operated patients must be kept on constant antimicrobial therapy (usually with nitrofurantoin or trimethoprim), but any breakthrough of infection must be promptly treated [33].

If surgical intervention is to be performed there are three methods in common use.

1 The Cohen technique [40]. The bladder is opened, the ureter is mobilized and brought to the other side through a long submucosal tunnel (Fig. 11.28).

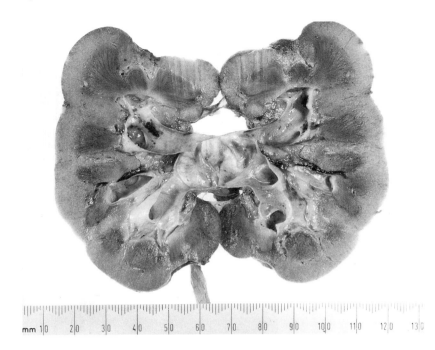

Fig. 11.20 Reflux nephropathy: characteristic scarring at the upper and lower poles of the kidney.

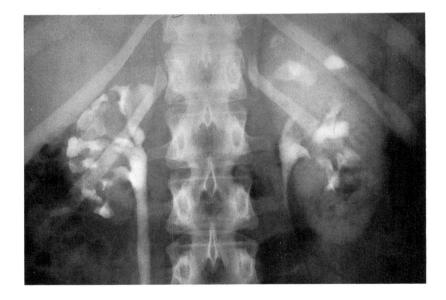

Fig. 11.21 IVU showing typical parenchymal scarring of the right kidney in a patient with uncorrected reflux.

2 The Leadbetter−Politano method [41] achieves the same objective but brings the ureter through a new tunnel under the bladder urothelium to its original position (Fig. 11.29).

3 The 'sting' (subtrigonal injection) procedure [42]. Through a cystoscope a small quantity of a paste made of collagen or silicone microspheres is injected under the ureteric orifice to produce a small mound, which changes the shape of the ureteric orifice into a crescent (Fig. 11.30). (Teflon paste was formerly used but has been shown to spread into the brain, see p. 23.)

The results of all these surgical manoeuvres are similar in expert hands. Reflux is prevented in more than 90% of cases in the older child. They are less successful in the neonate and when the ureter is grossly dilated. The calibre of the ureter may be reduced by tailoring it over a suitable catheter [43]. This is the field of the specialist paediatric urologist.

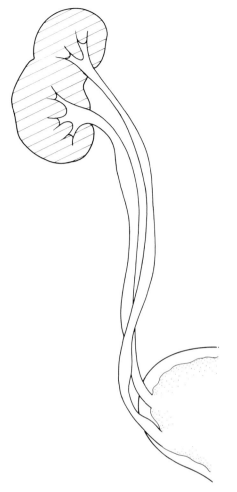

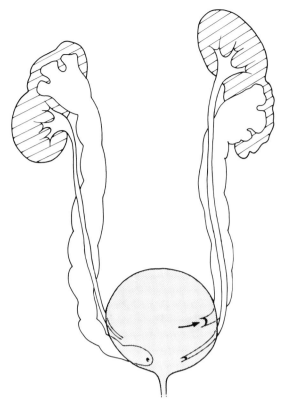

Fig. 11.23 In duplex there may be reflux up the ureter into the lower half-kidney, while the ureter from the upper half-kidney may be obstructed by a ureterocele: all four ureters may be so affected.

Fig. 11.22 In duplex, the ureter draining the lower half-kidney has a short intramural tunnel which does not prevent reflux.

Reflux nephropathy in adults

Parenchymal scarring in adults occurs when there is a combination of obstruction and infection, e.g. above a calculus. More often, when adults are seen with severely scarred kidneys, there is a history of recurrent urinary infection dating from infancy. Pregnancy is a particular hazard in these women: it may precipitate renal failure in a patient who is otherwise deteriorating slowly [44].

Correction of the reflux in adults seldom puts an end to the continuing symptoms of infection and loin pain on micturition, nor does it seem to halt the progressive deterioration in renal function. The changes in the scarred kidney continue, probably from an autoimmune inflammatory process which is now affecting the glomeruli as

well, enabling protein to escape into the filtrate [45].

Papillary necrosis

A second pathological process plays a part not only in severe acute infection, but also chronic scarring from many causes other than infection. This is papillary necrosis. The arterial supply to the renal papilla comes partly from the vasa recta, and partly from arteries at the fornix of the calix (see p. 49). Either vessel may become occluded when the papilla becomes oedematous or injected with urine, and the papilla becomes ischaemic (Fig. 11.31). A line of demarcation forms and the dead papilla may pass down the ureter to cause obstruction, or remain in the renal pelvis, to act as the nucleus for stone formation (Figs 11.32 & 11.33). The presence of the ischaemic papilla exacerbates existing inflammation and obstructive changes in the collecting tubules in the medullary rays.

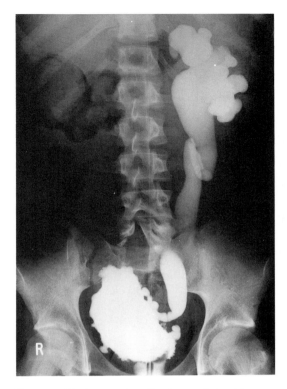

Fig. 11.24 Vesicoureteric reflux in an adult with a neuropathic bladder from spina bifida.

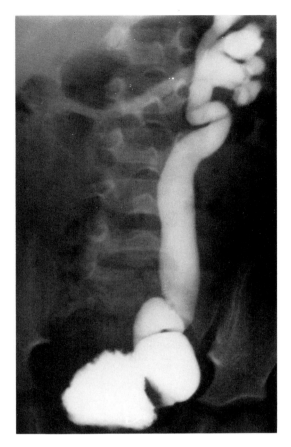

Fig. 11.25 Gross vesicoureteric reflux in a neonate.

Non-infective causes of scarring and papillary necrosis

A number of conditions may give rise to surgical complications, all with certain features in common with those of reflux nephropathy. Marsh in his valuable review calls them 'toxic nephropathies' [46].

Analgesic abuse

It has been estimated that in Britain 12% of end-stage renal failure is caused by analgesic abuse: this figure rises to 17.5% in Switzerland and 30% in Australia [47,48]. Phenacitin is the principal component of the analgesic mixtures which cause analgesic nephropathy, but other substances under suspicion include aspirin, codeine and paracetamol [49,50]. The scarring is similar to that caused by reflux nephropathy and it is also often complicated by papillary necrosis. There is sterile pyuria, proteinuria and progressive renal failure. The deterioration of renal function may be halted if the patient stops taking analgesics.

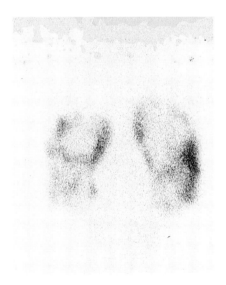

Fig. 11.26 DMSA scan in a baby with reflux nephropathy showing characteristic segmental defects in perfusion (courtesy of Mr R.H. Whitaker).

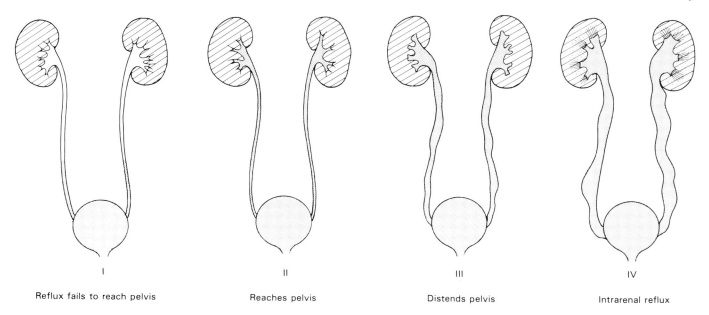

I	II	III	IV
Reflux fails to reach pelvis	Reaches pelvis	Distends pelvis	Intrarenal reflux

Fig. 11.27 The four grades of reflux.

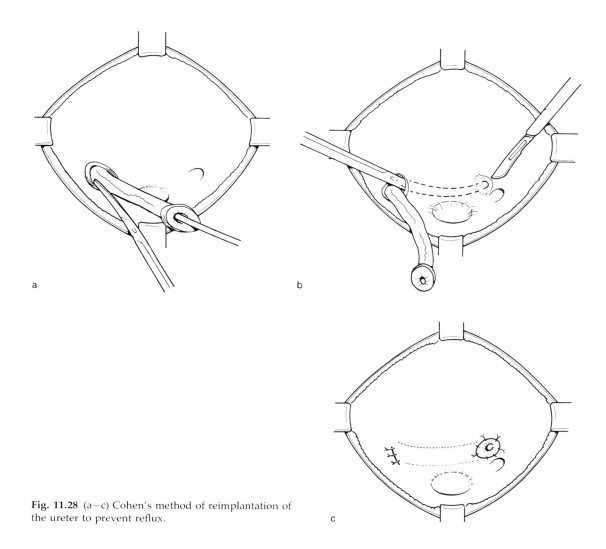

Fig. 11.28 (a–c) Cohen's method of reimplantation of the ureter to prevent reflux.

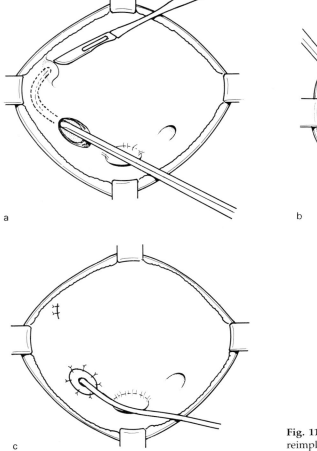

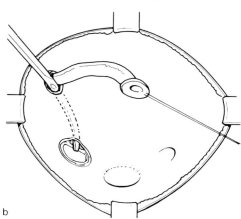

Fig. 11.29 (a–c) The Leadbetter–Politano method of reimplantation of the ureter to prevent reflux.

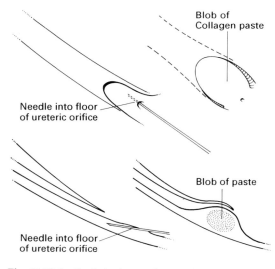

Fig. 11.30 In the 'sting' procedure, a small blob of collagen paste or similar compound is injected under the ureteric orifice.

Balkan nephropathy

Balkan nephropathy is thought to be caused by a mycotoxin produced by a fungus attacking grain stored in damp barns in Balkan countries. As with analgesic nephropathy, the scarring may be in the renal parenchyma, and may be complicated by papillary necrosis [51].

Both analgesic nephropathy and Balkan nephropathy predispose to transitional cell carcinoma in the renal pelvis and ureter which is frequently multicentric.

Sickle cell disease

Microinfarction in the homozygous patient with Sickle cell anaemia leads to papillary necrosis and scarring: in the heterozygote with sickle cell trait painless haematuria is common and loss of tubular concentrating function is the rule [52].

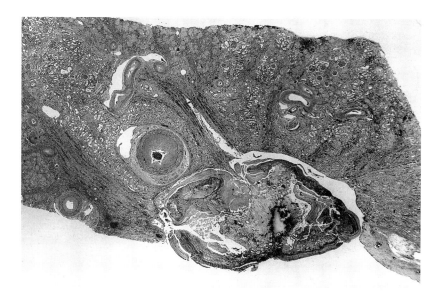

Fig. 11.31 Photomicrograph of necrosis of renal papilla (courtesy of Dr E.A. Courtauld).

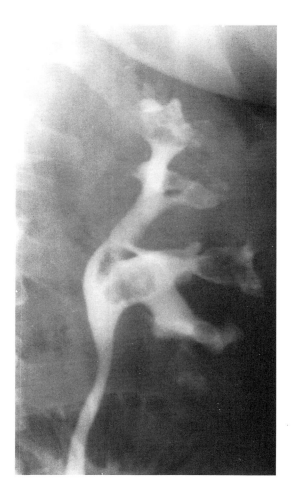

Fig. 11.32 IVU showing necrosis of most of the renal papillae: from a patient with diabetes and severe urinary tract infection.

Chronic surgical infections

Tuberculosis

Tuberculosis has become progressively less common in the last 40 years, so that today for most urologists it is a comparative rarity. However, with the recent acquired immune deficiency syndrome (AIDS) epidemic we may expect to see more tuberculosis in immune suppressed patients [53–55].

Pathology

Tubercle bacilli reach the urinary tract via the bloodstream from a primary focus in the lung, or bowel. There can also be tertiary spread from a lesion in the bone.

The bloodstream brings the mycobacteria to the kidney where they form multiple minute abscesses in the parenchyma (Fig. 11.34) which later invade the tubule, erode into a calix, spread to other calices and the pelvis, and finally progress down the ureter into the bladder. With the chronic infection there is healing by fibrosis. The fibrous tissue contracts, leading to obstruction of one or more calices. Similar obstruction may occur in the ureter [56] (Fig. 11.35).

The earliest lesions cannot be detected in the kidney until a small tuberculous abscess ruptures into the calix, giving rise to irritative symptoms and pyuria (Fig. 11.36). Untreated, these abscesses enlarge, coalesce and calcify until the

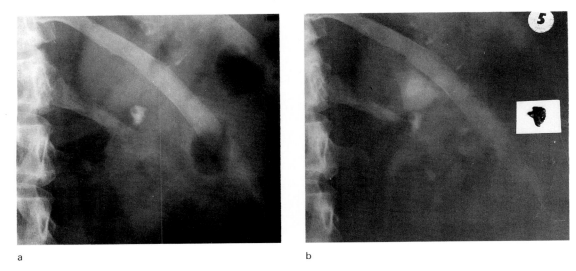

Fig. 11.33 (a) The dead papilla may calcify, forming a stone with a 'soft centre' (b), which may block a calix.

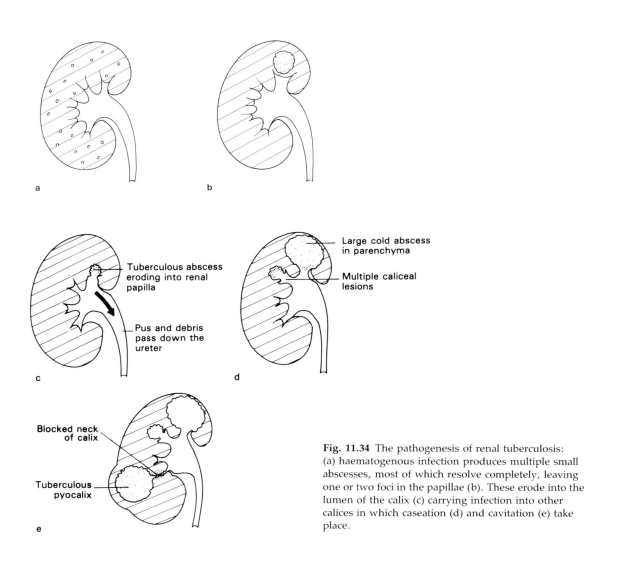

Fig. 11.34 The pathogenesis of renal tuberculosis: (a) haematogenous infection produces multiple small abscesses, most of which resolve completely, leaving one or two foci in the papillae (b). These erode into the lumen of the calix (c) carrying infection into other calices in which caseation (d) and cavitation (e) take place.

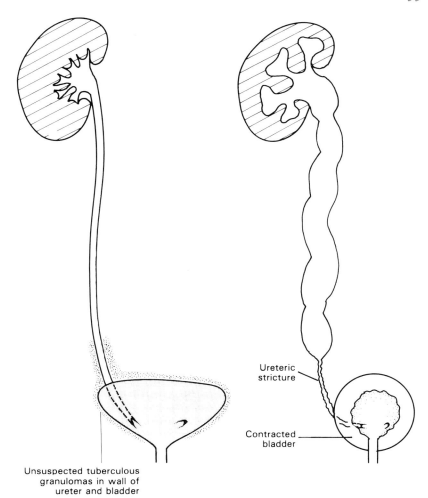

Fig. 11.35 Healing of tuberculosis in the ureter leads to a stricture.

Unsuspected tuberculous granulomas in wall of ureter and bladder

Ureteric stricture

Contracted bladder

entire kidney may be converted into a calcified mass — the so-called cement kidney (Fig. 11.37).

As the mycobacteria spread down the ureter they cause patches of granuloma in its wall and, on reaching the bladder, similar granulomas form in the vicinity of the ureteric orifice. Sometimes these are so oedematous that they resemble a papillary tumour. Later in the disease there is ulceration which may become confluent throughout the bladder.

The prostate and epididymis may be involved in the spread of the disease. In the epididymis, some of the infection may be haematogenous rather than via the lumen of the vas (see pp. 562).

Clinical features

It has always been a paradox that patients with tuberculosis should have so few symptoms even when the disease is quite far advanced. This is still true today, although most cases of tuberculosis are detected when sterile pyuria is found in the course of investigation for cystitis or prostatism [57,58].

Investigations

In all cases of sterile pyuria one should exclude cancer and tuberculosis. The mycobacteria are discovered by Ziehl–Neelsen or auramine staining of the urinary deposit. Because sperm also stains with this method, the finding of acid-fast material in the urine must be confirmed by culture on Loewenstein–Jensen medium. Using Bactec equipment a positive result can be provided within 1–2 weeks. It is no longer acceptable to confirm the diagnosis by inoculation of a guinea-pig because of the risk of accidental infection of laboratory staff [58].

An intravenous pyelogram (IVP) at an early stage will show a fuzzy, ill-defined cavity in one

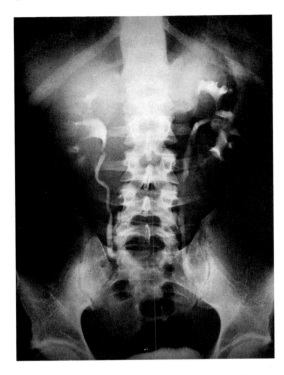

Fig. 11.36 Early tuberculosis: ulceration of papillae on the right side producing the typical 'fuzzy' appearance of the calices in the IVU (courtesy of Mr J.G. Gow).

or more calices, with perhaps a fleck of adjacent calcification. Later in the disease there will be more obvious areas of ulceration opening into the calices with larger areas of calcification [59] (Fig. 11.38). It is only in the late cases that massive calcification is seen (Figs 11.39 & 11.40).

The diagnosis may be expedited by passing a ureteric catheter into the suspect kidney and aspirating urine for culture and microscopy. Similarly, a biopsy from a suspicious lesion in the bladder may show the characteristic caseating lesions and the presence of acid-fast bacilli.

During the course of the preliminary work-up of the patient a chest radiograph is taken, sputum examined and liver function tests ordered.

Treatment

Treatment regimes are under continual review, but at the time of writing the usual one consists of combination chemotherapy using rifampicin 450 mg, isonicotinic acid hydrazide (INAH) 300 mg and ethambutol 800 mg daily for 3 months after which the ethambutol is discontinued and the other two agents maintained in the same dose for a further 6 months. Few urologists are

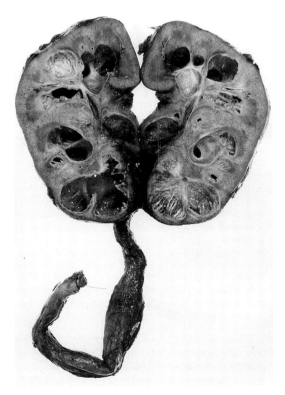

a

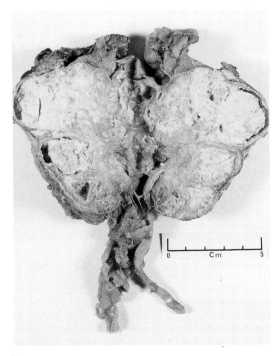

b

Fig. 11.37 (a) Multiple ulcerocavernous changes in tuberculosis. (b) The end stage — the 'cement' kidney.

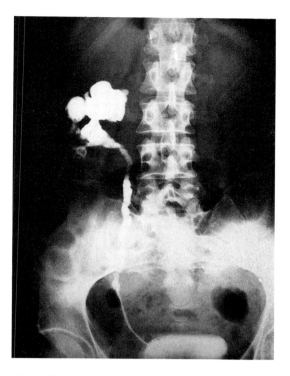

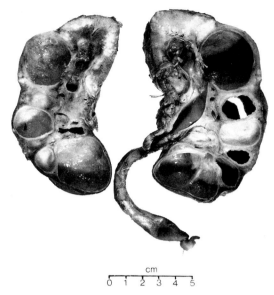

Fig. 11.39 Complete destruction of renal tissue following the spread of tuberculosis.

Fig. 11.38 Retrograde urogram showing advanced ulcerocavernous changes in the right kidney with granuloma and stricture formation in the right ureter (courtesy of Mr J.G. Gow).

likely to have much experience with treating tuberculosis and would be well advised to seek the help of a chest physician who will be familiar with the toxic side effects of the drugs that are used [60]. It is important to notify the case to the public health authorities.

In the West there has been a move towards shorter regimes of treatment: at the same time the pattern of tuberculosis overseas has changed, with the emergence of strains resistant to the first-line drugs. With the growing epidemic of tuberculosis secondary to AIDS we must expect dramatic changes in this picture in the next decade.

Surveillance

During this first few months of treatment the urinary tract is kept under very close surveillance, by ultrasound scanning supplemented where appropriate by IVU, because unnoticed tuberculous lesions heal very quickly and obstruction may develop silently in the ureter and lead to loss of a kidney.

A stricture at the upper end of the ureter will require a pyeloplasty or ureterocalicostomy (Fig. 11.41). At the lower end it may be necessary to reimplant the ureter by means of a Boari flap (Fig. 11.42). Obstruction in the middle third of the ureter is more difficult to deal with: on the right side the appendix may lend itself as an ideal substitute for the stenosed segment (Fig. 11.43) but on the left side it may be necessary to bridge the gap with ileum or colon (Fig. 11.44).

In the bladder, the healing process may shrink the bladder so much that it needs to be enlarged by enterocystoplasty to restore its reservoir function. The traditional solution has been to use the caecum, but this may generate high pressures and threaten the upper tract, and many surgeons now prefer a de-tubularized segment of bowel, even if the patient has to catheterize to empty it (see p. 326).

Tuberculosis of the prostate

In the prostate, tuberculosis leads to a characteristic hollowing out of the prostate (Fig. 11.45). This rare condition may be complicated by a cold abscess which points in the perineum and may rupture into the rectum. With combination chemotherapy even these fistulae can be expected to heal without surgical intervention so long as any stone that forms in the tract is removed.

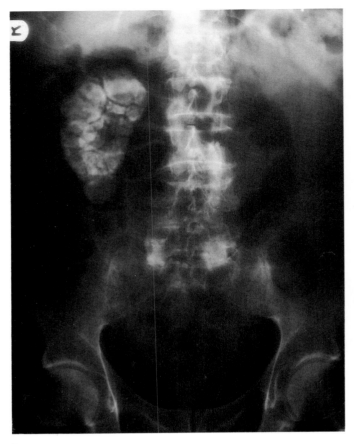
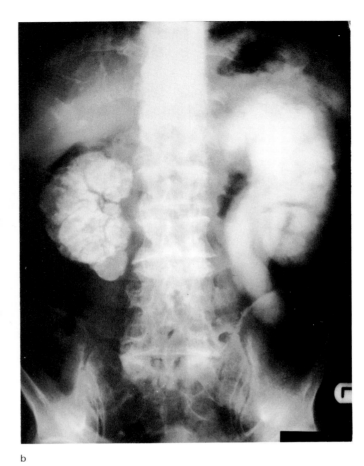

a   b

Fig. 11.40 (a) Plain X-ray showing massive calcification of the right kidney. (b) IVU showing obstruction of the left ureter.

Nephrectomy

Patients may present with a kidney that is completely destroyed, or it may have shrunk into a useless and contracted lump of scar tissue within a few weeks of chemotherapy. For such patients nephrectomy is the only appropriate treatment. This operation should be approached with considerable caution because dense adhesions can make what one expects to be a simple operation unusually difficult.

Nephrectomy for tuberculosis

Make a generous incision for safety. Open the peritoneum to make sure the bowel is safely reflected off the kidney. Always ligate the renal artery and vein with absorbable sutures in view of the risk of a chronic sinus if non-absorbable material is used.

In former times it was always necessary to remove the ureter to avoid the risk of late relapse. This is no longer necessary: in Gow's series of 265 nephrectomies not one developed relapse in the stump [59].

Cavernotomy

Previously, large tuberculous abscesses were sometimes seen which, after a course of anti-tuberculous treatment, were unroofed at a formal operation. Today, the need for this is almost unknown: it may occasionally be appropriate to aspirate the contents (if they are not too stiff).

Partial nephrectomy

Similarly, partial nephrectomy is no longer indicated. Either the kidney is sterilized with treatment and can be left alone, or it is so distorted by scarring that it is not worth saving.

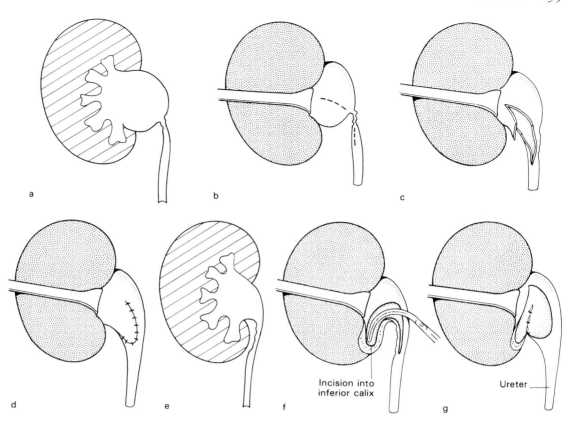

Fig. 11.41 A tuberculous stricture of the upper end of the ureter may be relieved by pyeloplasty (a—d) or by uretero-calicostomy (e—g).

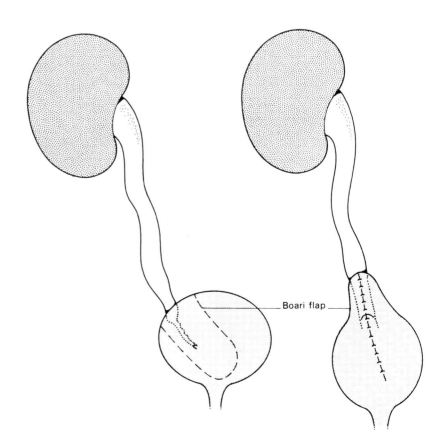

Fig. 11.42 A tuberculous stricture of the lower end of the ureter may be relieved by reimplanting the ureter into the bladder with a Boari flap, so long as the bladder is not too contracted; when the bladder is contracted it may be necessary to add on a piece of bowel.

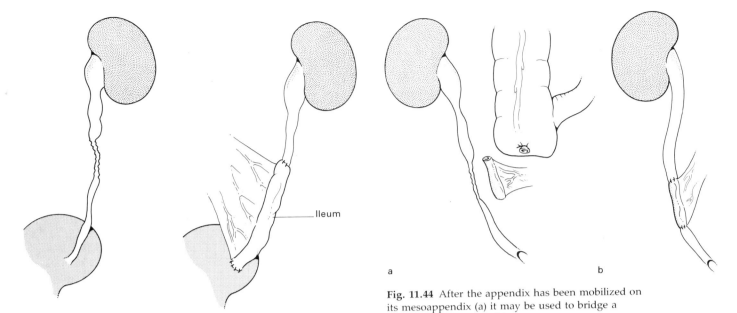

Fig. 11.44 After the appendix has been mobilized on its mesoappendix (a) it may be used to bridge a stricture in the ureter (b).

Fig. 11.43 A long length of stenosed ureter may be replaced with ileum.

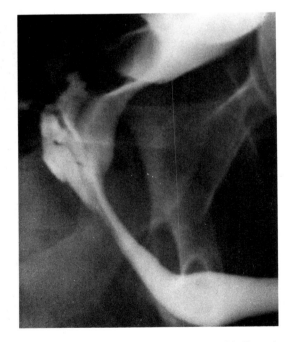

Fig. 11.45 Urethrogram showing the typical hollowed-out appearance caused by tuberculosis of the prostate with, in this case, a fistula tract which led back into the rectum.

Brucellosis

Brucella abortus is uncommon in Britain, but a major cause of disease overseas. How many people, and how many cattle, are infected in Britain is a matter for speculation [61]. Up to 30% of dairy workers and 90% of veterinary surgeons have antibodies to *Brucella* and a decade ago at least 30% of dairy herds were infected. Remarkably few of those presumably infected know anything about it: there are only about 600 new cases per annum in Britain.

Overseas it is a much more important problem [62]. *Brucella* may attack any organ in the body. It shares the complex immunology of tuberculosis and causes caseating lesions which lead to calcification and scarring in the organs it affects [63–65]. For the working urologist the important thing to remember is that it can produce odd calcifying granulomatous changes in the kidney, it can be diagnosed by immunological tests and responds to protracted treatment with tetracyclines.

Hydatid disease

Three species of the canine tape worm *Echinococcus granulosus* cause human disease [66,67].
1 Sylvatic *Echinococcus granulosus*, which has its life cycle between moose, deer and wolf or dog. It usually forms a self-limited unilocular cyst.
2 The more common pastoral *Echinococcus granulosus* is shared between sheep, pigs, cattle, horses and the domestic dog. This forms a rapidly expanding unilocular cyst.
3 *Echinococcus multilocularis* which is indigenous

to Europe, and is extremely dangerous, behaves like a cancer and is almost uniformly fatal. Its life cycle involves the lemming or field vole but it is quite possible that rats will do just as well [68].

The adult tape worm lives in the intestine of a canine (e.g. dog, wolf, fox or coyote, dingo or jackal) whose dried faeces containing the ova, scattered on grass, are eaten by grazing animals. Humans pick it up by fondling infested dogs and forgetting to wash their hands before eating (Fig. 11.46).

In humans, the ova hatch out, invade the bowel and form cysts in the viscera, most often the liver, but also the kidney and occasionally the lung [68,69].

Investigations

The cysts are multilocular and their walls almost always calcified (Fig. 11.47). The fluid within the cysts contains echoes from the many scolices present in the fluid (Fig. 11.48). The differential diagnosis lies between multicystic disease and renal cell cancer with cystic degeneration (Fig. 11.49). CT scanning will show the characteristic calcification which outlines the wall of the cysts in 50% of cases, but is more often stippled [70,71].

Aspiration of the contents of the cyst reveals multiple hooklets which are acid-fast, like tubercle bacilli [72,73] (Fig. 11.50).

An allergic wheal is produced if fluid from a cyst is injected under the skin — the Casoni test. This is unreliable, and has largely been replaced by serological tests, recently supplemented by an immunoassay for a specific circulating antigen [67]. False positive hydatid serological tests have been reported in patients with cancer of various organs (including the kidney), but it seems that these will usually be in a very low titre [74].

Skin tests and serum haemagglutinin titres are positive in about 90% of cases except in the sylvatic type when they are negative [67]. The complement fixation test was positive in 24 out of 30 cases and the enzyme-linked immuno-sorbent assay (ELISA) was positive in nine out of 11 [74].

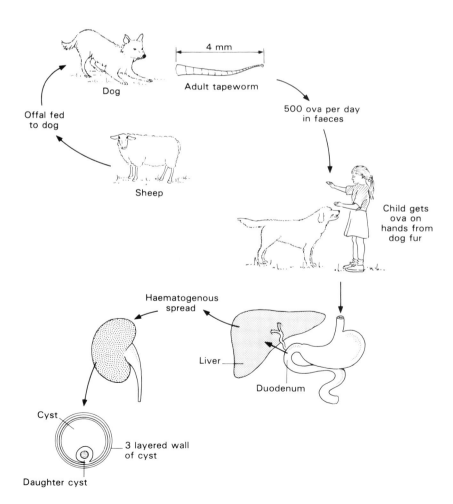

Fig. 11.46 The life cycle of *Echinococcus granulosus*.

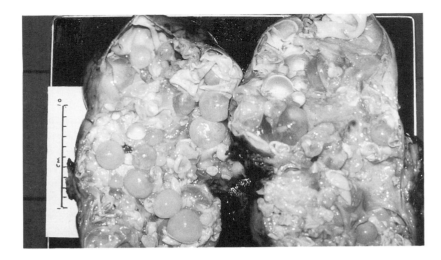

Fig. 11.47 Multiple hydatid cysts in a human kidney (courtesy of Mr G. Ravi).

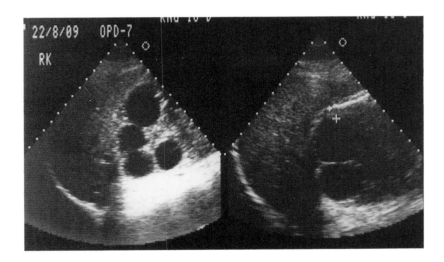

Fig. 11.48 Ultrasound showing partially calcified multiple cysts of hydatid cysts of the kidney (courtesy of Mr G. Ravi).

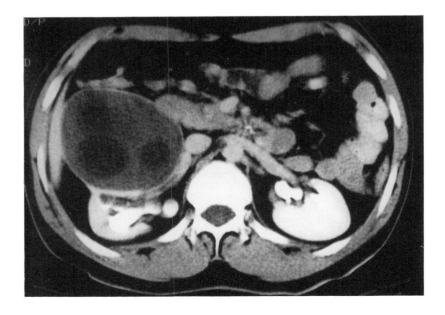

Fig. 11.49 CT scan showing multiple hydatid cysts of the right kidney (courtesy of Mr G. Ravi).

Treatment

Until recently there has been no medical treatment for hydatid disease. However, in the last decade a new family of drugs (e.g. albendazole) has given encouraging results [75–78].

It is seldom possible to save the kidney. It is important to make sure that the contents of the cysts are not spilled into the wound, otherwise each one will generate more cysts with a result equally disastrous and fatal as a massive local recurrence of cancer [75].

To prevent spillage, the cysts are approached through an appropriate loin incision, and the wound is protected with towels soaked in 1% formalin or hypertonic saline. The more obvious cysts are aspirated, then filled with hypertonic saline to kill the minute tape worms inside, and aspirated again. Finally, when there is no danger of the cysts bursting during removal, the kidney is removed *en bloc*, with as much care as in removing a cancer [70].

Chyluria and filariasis

In the Far East, chyluria is by no means uncommon. The patient presents with thick urine resembling anchovy sauce but usually without any other symptoms. Rarely, it is a cause of haematuria [79]. The only serious consequence may be the urinary loss of protein which occasionally leads to significant protein deficiency and loss of weight.

Investigations show a communication between the renal lymphatics and its collecting system [80] (Figs 11.51 & 11.52). The condition is traditionally attributed to the microscopic round worm *Wuchereria bancroftii* but it is rarely possible to confirm this diagnosis. Some cases have been seen of congenital origin [81], and there may well be some alternative cause for the phenomenon.

Wuchereria bancroftii lives in the lymphatics where it sets up an inflammatory response. The tiny worms creep at night into the peripheral blood where they are sucked up by feeding mosquitoes, and injected into the next victim (Fig. 11.53).

Investigations

A lymphogram will demonstrate communications between the kidney and lymphatics, but those with most experience of this condition make a therapeutic trial of an instillation of silver

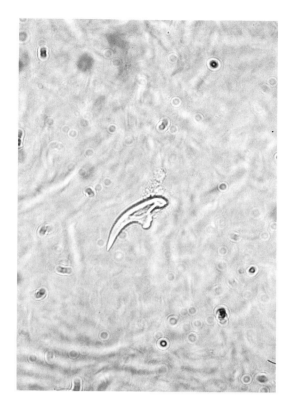

Fig. 11.50 Typical hooklet aspirated from a hydatid cyst. These stain acid-fast (courtesy of Professor J.D. Williams).

nitrate which stops the leak of lymph in about 80% of cases after two or three instillations [82,83].

Treatment

In most cases no treatment is needed [82]. Instillations of silver nitrate are simple and effective [83]. If the patient is obviously losing protein, the kidney is explored and stripped of all its surrounding tissue. A preliminary lymphogram using contrast stained with a blue dye may make the dissection more exact [80]. Every lymphatic trunk that is encountered must be meticulously ligated.

Actinomycosis

Actinomycosis is one of the rarest granulomas to occur in the urinary tract and is unlikely to be diagnosed without histological evidence [84].

Xanthogranuloma

This is a very important and by no means rare

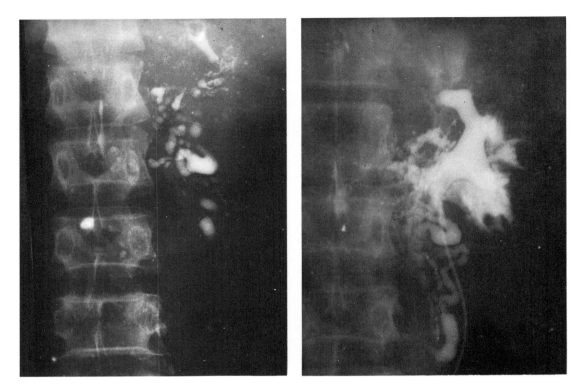

Fig. 11.51 Combined lymphangiogram (left) and retrograde urogram (right) in a patient with chyluria (courtesy of Professor Mya Thaung).

Fig. 11.53 The life cycle of *Wuchereria bancroftii*.

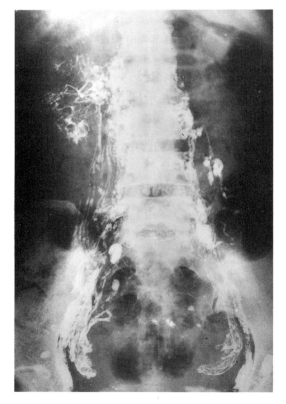

Fig. 11.52 Lymphangiogram in chyluria (courtesy of Mr Henry Yu).

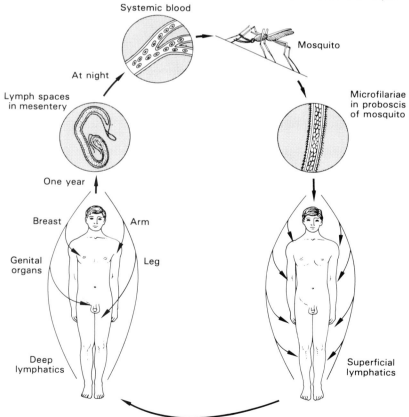

condition. It causes a mass in the kidney which has many of the features of an invasive clear cell carcinoma.

Pathology

Xanthogranuloma is usually associated with an infected calculus and *Proteus*. A variation on the theme of chronic pyelonephritis is set up in which huge macrophages, stuffed with lipid (resembling the clear cells of a renal carcinoma) infiltrate not only the renal pelvis and renal parenchyma, but also the surrounding tissues.

Macroscopically, there is a hard yellow mass, adherent to the surrounding tissues, often the intestine into which it may form a fistula. It can be a nightmare to the surgeon who, in trying to remove the mass thinks at first glance it is inoperable and despairs that he has cut through tumour [85–87] (Fig. 11.54).

Unfortunately, a frozen section may be misinterpreted because the lipid-laden macrophages of xanthogranuloma closely resemble the lipid-laden cells of renal cell cancer.

Clinical features

There is usually a stone. After a long time when the disease may be silent, the patient usually presents when very ill with a raised sedimentation rate and gross pyuria. Diabetes may coexist. It was formerly remarked that the condition was never bilateral but this has not proved to be true, and in one case bilateral nephrectomy was the only possible treatment.

Treatment

Antibiotics are useless. The only possible treatment is to resect the majority of the mass but this is by no means easy. A wide anterior approach is made, first reflecting the bowel, and then the entire mass is removed as completely as possible.

In its more severe forms, if nephrectomy is not performed the patient goes steadily downhill, but once removed, it does not recur [86,87].

Malacoplakia

This is a similar granuloma, but seldom associated with a stone. In the bladder it causes soft brown plaques to appear on the urothelium — hence its name. In the kidney, testis and prostate it can cause a destructive granuloma which riddles the tissue with innumerable abscesses. Histo-

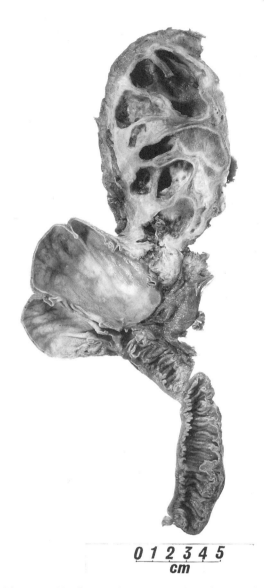

Fig. 11.54 Xanthogranulomatous pyelonephritis with a fistula between the right kidney and the ascending colon.

logically, the typical feature is the presence of Michaelis—Gutman bodies which are tiny, spherical and calcified. Like xanthogranuloma, malakoplakia erodes into adjacent bodies, and forms fistulae [88–90].

Clinical picture

There is fever, loss of weight, pain in the loin and investigations show a mass which is indistinguishable from xanthogranuloma, or indeed from cancer. The CT and angiographic images may be inconclusive. Only the evidence of urinary infection and fever make one suspicious that the condition may be benign. Untreated, these cases go downhill and die [89]. The mass must be excised completely [90].

Fungal infections of the kidney

Fungal infections occur when the normal bacterial flora are killed off by broad spectrum antibiotics, and the normal immune defences are depressed. They have been a major problem in renal transplantation and are increasingly seen in patients with AIDS. Many different fungi have been incriminated: *Cryptococcus* [91], *Nocardia* [92], *Aspergillosis* [93], *Torulopsis* [94] and most common of all *Candida*. Masses of *Candida* hyphae line the ureter or bladder, occlude a catheter and even give rise to a kind of bezoar [95].

Retroperitoneal fibrosis and other rare conditions

A number of strange conditions affect the retroperitoneal tissue and result in obstruction to the ureter. It is not at all clear whether these are all the same entity, or the final common pathway for a number of causes.

Retroperitoneal fibrosis

Retroperitoneal fibrosis was first described by Ormond in 1948 who reviewed his experience in 1960 [96,97]. In his case, a firm white plaque of fibrous tissue compressed both ureters and led to hydronephrosis. There is little doubt that in 1948 this was a new entity: the author made a search of the autopsy records of the London Hospital since 1907 and failed to discover any comparable condition prior to 1956. Since then many cases have been seen [98] including some 20 from the London Hospital, suggesting that some new pathological process may be at work.

Aetiology

The cause remains unknown. There have been many theories. Many drugs have been implicated, e.g. ergot derivatives, methysergide [99] and bromocriptine [100–103] and analgesics, the latter of which may also cause a different type of obstruction within the lumen of the ureter (see

p. 170) [104–107]. Cases have been reported after a wide variety of beta-blockers — sotalol, atenolol, oxyprenalol and metoprolol [108–110]. The reaction around the ureter seems different from the sclerosing peritonitis seen in patients taking Practolol where there is a diffuse fibrous involvement of the mesentery and peritoneum rather than the retroperitoneal tissues [111–113].

A second large group of cases are associated with aortic disease. Sometimes localized fibrosis has followed aortic reconstruction [114], more often the fibrosis has been part of the peri-aortic reaction before the operation began [115–118] (Fig. 11.55). Occasionally the peri-aortic fibrosis has caused obstruction followed by extravasation and a urinoma [117]. These have been comprehensively reviewed [118], and it seems clear that this is a distinct group. In a number of cases the retroperitoneal fibrosis accompanies, or is succeeded by, a very similar fibrosis surrounding the vessels in the porta hepatis where it causes obstruction to the portal vein and bile ducts [119,120]. In other patients the identical fibrosis is seen in the mediastinum, and may cause obstruction to the superior vena cava.

In many reported cases there has been evidence of vasculitis prior to the discovery of the retroperitoneal fibrosis: in one case this appears to have led to avascular necrosis of the femoral head [121].

An attempt has been made to offer a unifying

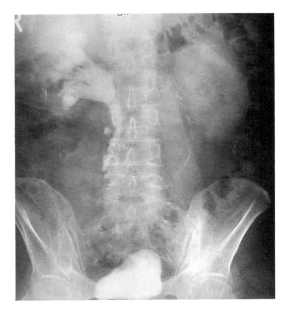

Fig. 11.55 Ureteric obstruction caused by an aortic aneurysm — note calcification in the wall of the aneurysm.

hypothesis, i.e. that the fibrosis is due to leakage of an insoluble ceroid from atheromatous plaques [122,123] but such an oversimple hypothesis fails to explain the bizarre clinical variety seen in this condition.

Pathology

Macroscopically, there is a hard white sheet of fibrous tissue in the retroperitoneal tissues. It is at its most dense just where the ureters are crossed by the gonadal vessels. The ureters are compressed and drawn medially. The aorta and vena cava may be completely concealed by the fibrous plaque (Fig. 11.56).

The extent of the plaque is very variable. It usually affects the middle third of the ureters, more on one side than on the other, but the author has seen instances where the fibrous tissue descends along the ureter as far as the bladder, and others where it reaches right up into the renal sinus. Sometimes the entire plaque is more or less acutely inflamed, vascular and oedematous, but as a rule it is uninflamed.

Histological examination of the fibrous tissue which is removed from around the aorta and vena cava shows scar tissue — collagen and fibrous tissue — together with a few lymphocytes and plasma cells. Except in cases where there is documented evidence of aortitis, examination of the fibrous tissue shows no evidence of extravasation of haemoglobin. Sometimes it is difficult to be sure that the fibrous tissue does not contain cancer cells and many sections must be examined before this, the more likely differential diagnosis, can be ruled out.

Arteritis in adjacent vessels is common [124], and this may be significant since in the long-term follow-up the principal cause of morbidity is vascular occlusive disease and hypertension. [125,126].

Clinical features

Patients present in many different ways. The most common picture is renal failure, hypertension and bilateral hydronephrosis. Others present with the complications of hypertension, e.g. retinopathy. A substantial number come into hospital with no specific complaint: they have lost weight, have backache and night-sweats. There is a markedly raised sedimentation rate and the clinical impression is of disseminated carcinoma. Patients are usually hypertensive.

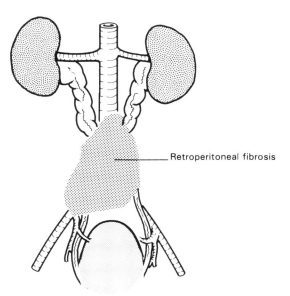

Retroperitoneal fibrosis

Fig. 11.56 Idiopathic retroperitoneal fibrosis: the ureters are compressed and drawn medially by a hard white sheet of fibrous tissue around the aorta and inferior vena cava.

Investigations

Urography shows a very typical appearance (Fig. 11.57). There is usually bilateral upper tract obstruction, and the ureters may be drawn towards the midline. Retrograde urography is diagnostic: catheters and contrast medium go easily up the ureters even though they are functionally obstructed (Fig. 11.58).

Under anaesthesia a mass may be palpable in the abdomen. CT scanning is inconclusive: it shows a flat plaque in the retroperitoneal area, but cannot distinguish a mass caused by idiopathic retroperitoneal fibrosis from one due to infiltration by carcinoma from a primary in the bowel, stomach or prostate.

Management

In the first instance the priority is to decompress the kidneys and this is easily performed by bilateral percutaneous nephrostomy. Since obstruction by retroperitoneal metastatic disease is more common than idiopathic fibrosis, a careful search is made for a primary cancer. Even then, the diagnosis may be in doubt.

Treatment

There are two alternative forms of treatment. The first is the most straightforward, to perform a

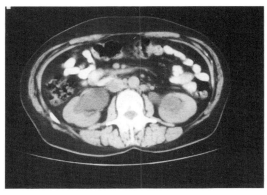

a

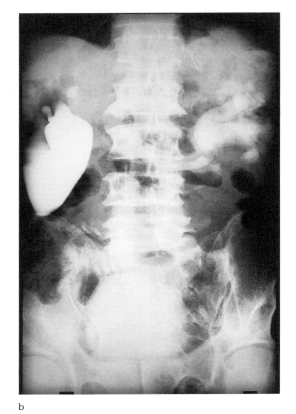

Fig. 11.57 (a) IVU and (b) CT scan in idiopathic retroperitoneal fibrosis (courtesy of Dr Otto Chan).

b

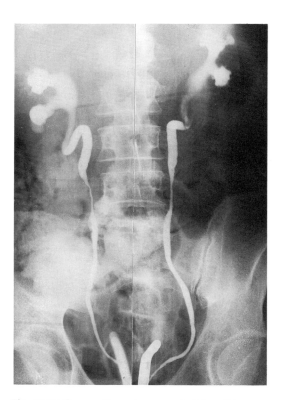

Fig. 11.58 Composite ureterogram in idiopathic retroperitoneal fibrosis. Typically the contrast goes easily along the obstructed ureters.

ureterolysis [127], but this is a considerable operation and many patients are unfit for such a procedure; the second is via medical agents.

Ureterolysis

Through a long transabdominal incision the colon is reflected off the ureter first on one side and then the other (Fig. 11.59). The plane of cleavage between the ureter and the surrounding sheath of fibrous tissue is dissected away, liberating the ureter [128] (Fig. 11.60). This is sometimes very difficult, since the fibrosis actually penetrates the muscular wall of the ureter and, when the lumen is breached, a nephrostomy is a mandatory precaution if one is not already in position. At this stage to prevent a return of the fibrosis it is safest to wrap each ureter in omentum (Fig. 11.61). Alternatives such as placing the ureter in the abdominal muscle or peritoneum have been followed by recurrence of the fibrosis [129].

Medical treatment

There have been many cases where immunosuppressive agents have been successfully used

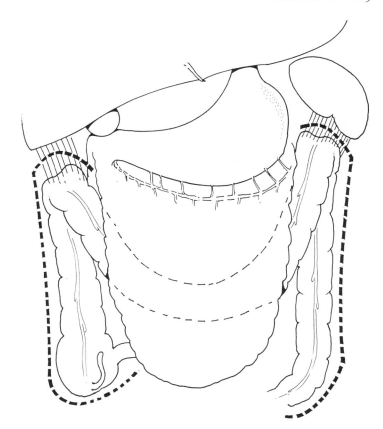

Fig. 11.59 The colon is mobilized on each side and reflected medially.

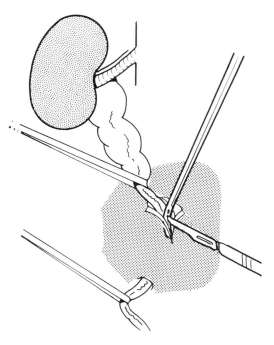

Fig. 11.60 The fibrous tissue is incised to release the ureter.

in the treatment of retroperitoneal fibrosis, usually with prednisolone alone but sometimes with added azathioprine [130]. If one can be certain that the diagnosis is not retroperitoneal cancer, steroids may be used, though in one of the author's cases they led to a pathological fracture of the vertebra and had to be discontinued.

Tamoxifen has been reported to cause the resolution of retroperitoneal fibrosis without the side effects of prednisolone [131].

Follow-up

Whether the ureters have been placed in the peritoneal cavity or wrapped in omentum, it is necessary to follow the patient carefully. Recurrence of the fibrosis is always a possibility, and so is a new manifestation of the fibrosis in the mediastinum or porta hepatis. Fortunately, a very useful index of return of active disease is provided by the sedimentation rate. This, and the blood pressure, should be monitored indefinitely in view of the long-term risk of

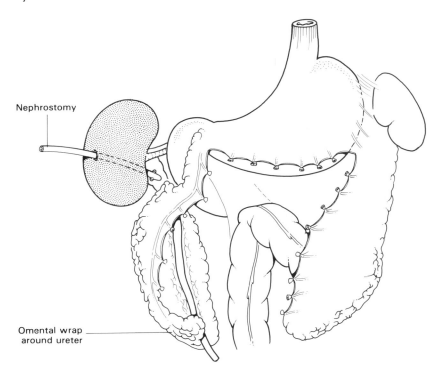

Nephrostomy

Omental wrap
around ureter

Fig. 11.61 After ureterolysis each ureter is wrapped in omentum.

atherosclerotic disease in one form or another [125,126].

Intraluminal obstruction of the ureter

First described by MacGregor *et al.* [104], very few cases have been reported [105,106]. The radiographic appearances resemble those of retroperitoneal fibrosis (Fig. 11.62) but the ureter, rather than being surrounded by fibrous tissue, is blocked by oedematous granuloma (Fig. 11.63). Bissada notes the association of this condition with arteritis [106,107].

Ureteric endometriosis

Endometriosis must always be included in the differential diagnosis of any unusual blockage of the ureter in a woman. Cyclical bleeding is seldom observed and the response to hormonal manipulation has been disappointing. Healing may be followed by obstructing fibrosis calling for reimplantation [132].

Primary amyloidosis of the ureter

The differential diagnosis of carcinoma of the ureter and retroperitoneal fibrosis should

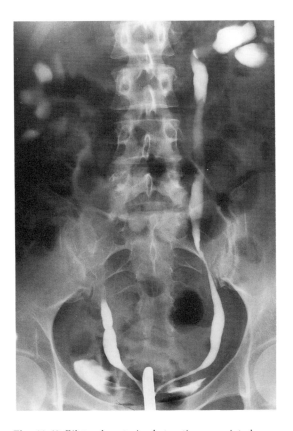

Fig. 11.62 Bilateral ureteric obstruction associated with analgesic abuse.

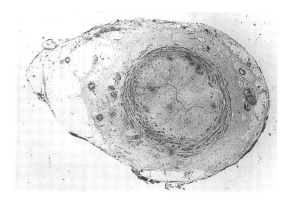

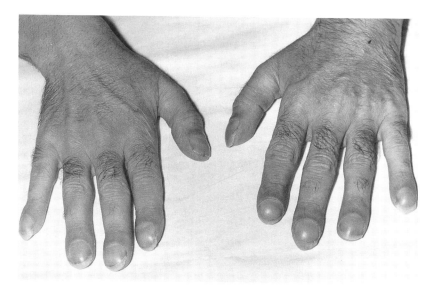

Fig. 11.63 (*above*) Cross-section through the site of the obstruction in the ureter in the same patient as Fig. 11.62 with analgesic abuse.

Fig. 11.64 (*right*) Clubbing in a patient with pelvic lipomatosis.

always include this rare entity. Few cases have been described, but they have presented with unilateral obstruction to the ureter of uncertain origin. Local resection and anastomosis has been successfully accomplished where the length of ureter has been short [133]. The important lesson of these cases is that frozen section can demonstrate the entity, and a nephroureterectomy can be avoided.

Pelvic lipomatosis

This is probably a completely unrelated disease. It occurs in males in their thirties, and is more common in those of African ancestry. It consists of a mass of firm fat, histologically normal, which surrounds and infiltrates the bladder, colon and ureters.

The presentation may be very variable and indeed the diagnosis is usually made by chance when investigating non-specific urinary symptoms such as frequency or dysuria [134,135].

Physical examination is seldom helpful. One patient had marked clubbing of the fingers (Fig. 11.64). One very helpful physical sign is revealed when sigmoidoscopy is attempted — the straight sigmoidoscope slips its whole length into the bowel as easily as a sword into a scabbard.

Investigations are pathognomonic. The IVP shows a startling deformity in the bladder which is lifted up out of the pelvis like a pear (Fig. 11.65). The ureters may be obstructed. CT scans show a thick layer of fat surrounding the pelvic organs [136] (Fig. 11.66). A biopsy is seldom necessary [137].

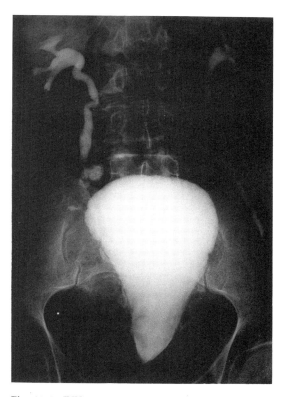

Fig. 11.65 IVU in pelvic lipomatosis (courtesy of Dr W. Hately).

The best way to treat this condition is disputed. It has been claimed that severe weight reduction may make the deposit of fat go away and that with a return of normal body weight the lipomatosis returns.

Surgical dissection of the fat from the bladder

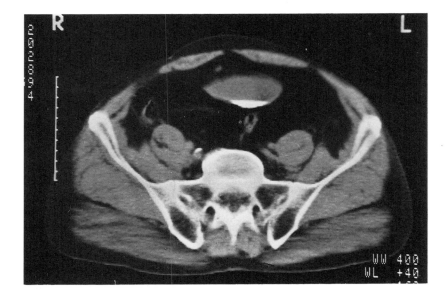

Fig. 11.66 CT scan in pelvic lipomatosis (courtesy of Dr Otto Chan).

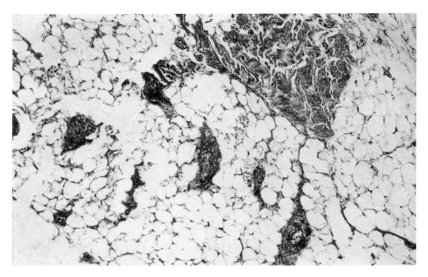

Fig. 11.67 Histology from pelvic lipomatosis: note that the muscle of the bladder is infiltrated with the fat.

and the ureters is fraught with difficulty. The fat is found to infiltrate both organs and there is no clean plane of cleavage (Fig. 11.67).

These patients need very careful follow-up. In the writer's small series death has followed from renal failure or hypertension within 5 years in every case.

Oedema around a calculus

A small ureteric calculus can cause a considerable oedematous inflammatory reaction in the wall of the ureter. Sometimes this can be so large as to resemble a tumour. When there is doubt, a CT scan will reveal the calculus which may be too small to be detected in a plain radiograph.

Tumours

Tumours of the ureter will cause intraluminal obstruction (see p. 203).

References

1 Williams DG, Peters DK (1987) Glomerulonephritis and renal manifestations of systemic disease, in: Weatherall DJ, Ledingham JGG, Warrell DA (eds) *Oxford Textbook of Medicine*, vol. 2, 2nd edn, pp. 18.36–56. Oxford: Oxford University Press.
2 Chapel HM, Haeney M (1984) *Essentials of Clinical Immunology*. Oxford: Blackwell Scientific Publications.
3 Mason PD, Pusey CD (1994) Glomerulonephritis: diagnosis and treatment. *Br Med J* 309: 1157.

4 Maxwell AP, Nelson WE, Hill EM (1988) Reversal of renal failure in nephritis associated with antibody to glomerular basement membrane. *Br Med J* 297: 627.

5 Watkins PJ (1982) ABC of diabetes: nephropathy. *Br Med J* 285: 627.

6 Marin JH, Brown AL, Daugherty GW (1962) Non-myelomatous amyloid disease of the kidney. *Proc Staff Meet Mayo Clin* 37: 567.

7 Rose PE, McGonigle R, Michael J, Boughton BJ (1987) Renal failure and the histopathological features of myeloma kidney reversed by intensive chemotherapy and peritoneal dialysis. *Br Med J* 294: 411.

8 Asscher AW (1987) Interstitial nephritis and urinary tract infection, in: Weatherall DJ, Ledingham JGG, Warrell DA (eds) *Oxford Textbook of Medicine*, 2nd edn, vol. 2, pp. 18.67–80. Oxford: Oxford University Press.

9 Childs S (1992) Current diagnosis and treatment of urinary tract infections. *Urology* 40: 295.

10 Bernstein J, Arant BS (1992) Morphological characteristics of segmental renal scarring in vesicoureteral reflux. *J Urol* 148: 1712.

11 Rushton HG, Majid M (1992) Dimercaptosuccinic acid renal scintigraphy for the evaluation of pyelonephritis and scarring: a review of experimental and clinical studies. *J Urol* 148: 1726.

12 Rosenberg AR, Rossleigh MA, Bass SHJ, Leighton DM, Farnsworth RH (1992) Evaluation of acute urinary tract infection in children by dimercaptosuccinic acid scintigraphy: prospective study. *J Urol* 148: 1746.

13 Lebowitz RL (1992) The detection and characterization of vesicoureteric reflux in the child. *J Urol* 148: 1640.

14 Edwards JD (1993) Management of septic shock. *Br Med J* 306: 1661.

15 Ledingham MMcA, McCartney AC, Ramsay G, Wright I (1988) Endotoxins as mediators. *Prog Clin Biol Res* 264: 125.

16 Lachman E, Pirsoe SB, Gaffin SL (1984) Anti-lipopolysaccharide immunotherapy in management of septic shock of obstetric and gynaecological origin. *Lancet* i: 981.

17 Schedel I, Drelchomsen U, Wentwig B *et al.* (1991) Treatment of Gram-negative septic shock with an immunoglobulin preparation: a prospective randomised clinical trial. *Crit Care Med* 19: 1104.

18 Ziegler EJ, Fisher CJ, Sprung CL *et al.* (1991) Treatment of Gram-negative bacteremia and septic shock with HA-1A human monoclonal antibody against endotoxin. *New Engl J Med* 324: 429.

19 Maier RY (1986) Multisystem organ failure. *Arch Surg* 121: 201.

20 Kaplan RL, Sahn SR, Petty TL (1989) Incidence and outcome of the respiratory distress syndrome in Gram-negative sepsis. *Arch Intern Med* 129: 867.

21 Rabinowitz JG, Kinkhabwala MN, Robinson T, Spyropoulos E, Becker JA (1972) Acute renal carbuncle. The roentgenographic classification of a medical enigma. *Am J Roentgenol* 116: 740.

22 Pedersen JF, Hancke S, Kristensen JK (1973) Renal carbuncle: antibiotic therapy govered by ultrasonically guided aspiration. *J Urol* 109: 777.

23 Whitfield JD, Noe HN (1989) Conservative management of renal carbuncles in children. *Urology* 34: 89.

24 Thomalla JV, Gleason P, Leapman SB, Filo RS (1993) Acute lobar nephronia of renal transplant allograft. *Urology* 41: 283.

25 Pontin AR, Barnes RD, Joffe J, Kahn D (1995) Emphysematous pyelonephritis in diabetic patients. *Br J Urol* 75: 71.

26 Nickas ME, Reese JH, Anderson RU (1994) Medical therapy alone for the treatment of gas forming intrarenal abscess. *J Urol* 151: 3998.

27 Salvatierra O, Bucklew WB, Morrow JW (1967) Perinephric abscess: a report of 71 cases. *J Urol* 98: 296.

28 Sherlock DJ, Holl-Allen RTJ (1984) Pyonephrosis necessitans: a report of two cases. *Br J Surg* 71: 644.

29 Gil-Salom M, Oron-Alpuente J, Ruiz del Castillo J, Chuan-Nuez P, Carretero-Gonzalez P (1989) Nephro-broncho-cutaneous fistula. *Br J Urol* 64: 652.

30 International Reflux Study Committee (1981) Medical versus surgical treatment of primary vesicoureteral reflux. *J Urol* 125: 277.

31 Blickman JG, Taylor GA, Lebowitz RL (1985) Voiding cystourethrography as the initial radiologic study in the child with urinary tract infection. *Radiology* 156: 659.

32 Smellie JM, Poulton A, Prescod NP (1994) Retrospective study of children with renal scarring associated with reflux and urinary infection. *Br Med J* 308: 1193.

33 Birmingham Reflux Study Group (1987) Prospective trial of operative versus non-operative treatment of severe vesicoureteric reflux in children: five years observation. *Br Med J* 295: 237.

34 International Workshop on Reflux and Pyelonephritis, New Orleans, 1991 (1992) Report. *J Urol* 148: 1639.

35 Allen TD, Arant BS, Roberts JA (1992) Commentary: vesicoureteral reflux — 1992. *J Urol* 148: 1758.

36 Whitaker RH, Sherwood T (1984) Another look at diagnostic pathways in children with urinary tract infection. *Br Med J* 288: 839.

37 Ozen HA, Whitaker RH (1987) Does the severity of presentation in children with vesicoureteric reflux relate to the severity of the disease or the need for operation? *Br J Urol* 60: 110.

38 Lebowitz RL (1992) The detection and characterization of vesicoureteric reflux in the child. *J Urol* 148: 1640.

39 Hanbury DC, Coulden RA, Farman P, Sherwood T (1990) Ultrasound cystography in the diagnosis of vesicoureteric reflux. *Br J Urol* 65: 250.

40 Cohen SJ (1975) Ureterozystoneostomie, eine neue antireflux technik. *Aktuelle Urol* 6: 1.

41 Politano VA, Leadbetter WF (1958) An operative technique for the correction of vesicoureteric reflux. *J Urol* 79: 932.

42 Aaronson IA (1995) Current status of the 'Sting' an American perspective. *Br J Urol* 75: 121.

43 Hendren WH (1969) Operative repair of megaureter in children. *J Urol* 101: 491.

44 Becker GJ, Ihle BU, Fairley KF, Bastos M, Kincaid-Smith P (1986) Effect of pregnancy on moderate

renal failure in reflux. *Br Med J* 292: 796.

45 Hanbury DC, Calvin J (1992) Proteinuria and enzymuria in vesicoureteric reflux. *Br J Urol* 70: 603.

46 Marsh FP (1987) Toxic nephropathies, in: Weatherall DJ, Ledingham JGG, Warrell DA (eds) *Oxford Textbook of Medicine*, vol. 2, 2nd edn, pp. 18.108–118. Oxford University Press, Oxford.

47 Akyol SM, Thompson M, Kerr DNS (1982) Renal function after prolonged consumption of aspirin. *Br Med J* 284: 631.

48 Editorial (1981) Analgesic nephropathy. *Br Med J* 282: 339.

49 Morlans M (1990) End stage renal disease and non-narcotic analgesics: a case control study. *Br J Clin Pharmacol* 30: 717.

50 Pommer W (1989) Regular analgesic intake and the risk of end stage renal failure. *Am J Nephrol* 9: 403.

51 Balkan Endemic Nephropathy (1991) Two international workshops. Belgrade Yugoslavia, 1989 and 1990. *Kidney Int Supp* 34: 1.

52 Akinkugbe OO (1967) Renal papillary necrosis in sickle-cell haemoglobinopathy. *Br Med J* 3: 283.

53 Editorial (1984) Tuberculosis in hospital doctors. *Br Med J* 289; 1327.

54 Watson JM, Gill ON (1990) HIV infection and tuberculosis. *Br Med J* 300: 63.

55 Editorial (1980) Tuberculosis in patients having dialysis. *Br Med J* 1: 349.

56 Medlar EM (1926) Cases of renal infection in pulmonary tuberculosis. *Am J Clin Path* 2: 401.

57 Lattimer JK, Wechsler H, Ehrlich RM (1969) Current treatment for renal tuberculosis. *J Urol* 102: 2.

58 Edwards D, Kirkpatrick CH (1986) The immunology of mycobacterial diseases. *Am Rev Respir Dis* 134: 1062.

59 Gow JG, Barbosa S (1984) Genitourinary tuberculosis. A study of 1117 cases over a period of 34 years. *Br J Urol* 56: 449.

60 Weinberg AC, Boyd SD (1988) Short course chemotherapy and role of surgery in adult and pediatric genitourinary tuberculosis. *Urology* 31: 95.

61 Henderson RJ (1973) Brucellosis: the situation in Britain. *Health Trends* 5: 10.

62 Ibrahim AIA, Awad R, Shetty SD, Saad M, Bilal NE (1988) Genitourinary complications of brucellosis. *Br J Urol* 61: 294.

63 Abernathy RS, Price WE, Spink WW (1955) Chronic brucella pyelonephritis simulating tuberculosis. *J Am Med Assoc* 1259: 1534.

64 Zinneman HH, Glenchur H, Hall WH (1961) Chronic renal brucellosis: a report of a case with studies of blocking antibodies and precipitins. *New Engl J Med* 265: 872.

65 Kelalis PP, Greene LF, Wee LA (1962) Brucellosis of the urogenital tract: a mimic of tuberculosis. *J Urol* 88: 347.

66 Gilles HM (1990) Parasitic infections, in: Chisholm GD, Fair WR (eds) *Scientific Foundations of Urology*, 3rd edn, pp. 152–6. Oxford: Heinemann.

67 Craig PS, Zehle E, Romig T (1986) Hydatid disease: research and control in Turkana. II. The role of immunological techniques for the diagnosis of hydatid disease. *Trans Roy Soc Trop Med Hyg* 80: 183.

68 Afsar H, Yagci F, Abyasti N, Meto S (1994) Hydatid disease of the kidney. *Br J Urol* 73: 17.

69 Haddad FS (1987) Primary retroperitoneal pelvic echinococcal cyst. *J Urol* 137: 1248.

70 Shetty SD, Al-Saigh A, Ibrahim AIA, Patil KP, Bhattachan CL (1992) Management of hydatid cysts of the urinary tract. *Br J Urol* 70: 258.

71 Karabekios S, Gouliamos A, Kalovidouris A, Vlahos L, Papavasiliou C, Sakkas J (1989) Features of computed tomography in hydatic cysts of the urinary tract. *Br J Urol* 64: 575.

72 Symmers WStC (1973) Acid-fast staining of hooklets of *Echinococcus granulosus*. *Lancet* i: 942.

73 Brundelet PJ (1973) Acid-fast staining of hooklets of *Taenia echinococcus*. *Lancet* i: 678.

74 Dar FK, Buhidma MA, Kidwai SA (1984) Hydatid false positive serological test results in malignancy. *Br Med J* 288: 1197.

75 Dawson JL, Stamatakis JD, Stringer MD, Williams R (1988) Surgical treatment of hepatic hydatid disease. *Br J Surg* 75: 946.

76 Yasawy MI, Al Karawi MA, El-Sheikh Mohamed AR (1990) Prospective study of effects of albendazole on hydatid disease. *Ann Saudi Med* 10: 105.

77 Taylor DH, Morris DL (1989) Combination chemotherapy is more effective in postspillage prophylaxis for hydatid disease than either albendazole or praziquantel alone. *Br J Surg* 76: 954.

78 Nahmias J, Goldsmith R, Soibelman M, El-On J (1994) Three to seven year follow-up after albendazole treatment of 68 patients with cystic echinococcosis (hydatid disease). *Ann Trop Med Parasit* 88: 295.

79 Edwards BD, Eastwood JB, Shearer RJ (1988) Chyluria as a cause of haematuria in patients from endemic areas. *Br J Urol* 62: 609.

80 Cahill K, Kaiser R (1964) Lymphangiography in Bancroftian filariasis. *Trans Roy Soc Trop Med Hyg* 58: 356.

81 Grieg JD, MacKenzie JR, Azmy AAF (1989) Congenital pyelolymphatic fistula in a child with chyluria. *Br J Urol* 63: 550.

82 Tan LB, Chiang CP, Huang CH, Chou YH, Wang CJ (1990) Experiences in treatment of chyluria in Taiwan. *J Urol* 144: 710.

83 Sabnis RB, Punekar SW, Desai RM, Bradoo AM, Bapat SD (1992) Instillation of silver nitrate in the treatment of chyluria. *Br J Urol* 70: 660.

84 Cvetkov MC, Elenkov C, Georgiev M, Topov U, Stefanova G (1995) Renal actinomycosis complicated by renoduodenal fistula and diabetes mellitus. *Br J Urol* 75: 104.

85 Elliott CB, Johnson HW, Balfour JA (1968) Xanthogranulomatous pyelonephritis and perirenal xanthogranuloma. *Br J Urol* 40: 548.

86 Husain I, Pingle A, Kazi T (1979) Bilateral diffuse xanthogranulomatous pyelonephritis. *Br J Urol* 51: 162.

87 Petronic V, Buturovic J, Isvaneski M (1989) Xanthogranulomatous pyelonephritis. *Br J Urol* 64: 336.

88 Gupta RK, Schuser RA, Christian WD (1972) Autopsy findings in a unique case of malacoplakia. *Arch Pathol* 93: 42.

89 Scullin DR, Hardy R (1972) Malacoplakia of the

urinary tract with spread to the abdominal wall. *J Urol* 107: 908.

90 Bowers JH, Cathey WJ (1971) Malakoplakia of the kidney with renal failure. *Am J Clin Pathol* 55: 765.

91 Salyer WR, Salyer DC (1973) Involvement of the kidney and prostate in cryptococcosis. *J Urol* 109: 695.

92 Presant CA, Wiernick PH, Serpick AA (1970) Disseminated extrapulmonary nocardiasis presenting as a renal abscess. *Arch Pathol* 89: 560.

93 Melchior J, Mebust WK, Walk WL (1972) Ureteral colic from a fungus ball: unusual presentation of systemic aspergillosis. *J Urol* 108: 698.

94 Khauli RB, Kalash S, Young JD (1983) Torulopsis glabrata perinephric abscess. *J Urol* 130: 968.

95 Schoenebeck J, Winblad B, Ansehn S (1972) Renal candidiasis complicating caecocystoplasty. *Scand J Urol Nephrol* 6: 129.

96 Ormond JK (1948) Bilateral ureteral obstruction due to envelopment and compression by one inflammatory process. *J Urol* 59: 1072.

97 Ormond JK (1960) Idiopathic retroperitoneal fibrosis. *J Am Med Assoc* 174: 1561.

98 Raper FP (1956) Idiopathic retroperitoneal fibrosis involving the ureters. *Br J Urol* 28: 436.

99 Graham JR (1964) Methysergide for prevention of headache: experience in 500 patients over 3 years. *New Engl J Med* 270: 67.

100 Bowler JV, Ormerod IE, Legg NJ (1986) Retroperitoneal fibrosis and bromocriptine. *Lancet* ii: 466.

101 Demonet JF, Rostin M, Dueymes JM *et al.* (1986) Retroperitoneal fibrosis and treatment of Parkinson's disease with high doses of bromocriptine. *Clin Neuropharmacol* 9: 200.

102 Murphy F, Pickard RS (1989) Bromocriptine-associated retroperitoneal fibrosis presenting with testicular retraction. *Br J Urol* 64: 318.

103 Herzog A, Minne H, Ziegler R (1989) Retroperitoneal fibrosis in a patient with macroprolactinoma treated with bromocriptine. *Br Med J* 298: 1315.

104 MacGregor GA, Jones NF, Barraclough MA, Wing AJ, Cranston WI (1973) Ureteric stricture with analgesic nephropathy. *Br Med J* 2: 271.

105 Lewis CT, Molland EA, Marshall VR, Tresidder CG, Blandy JP (1976) Analgesic abuse, ureteric obstruction and retroperitoneal fibrosis. *Br Med J* 2: 76.

106 Bissada NK, Finkbeiner AE (1978) Idiopathic segmental ureteritis. *Urology* 12: 64.

107 Bissada NK (1978) Personal communication to JPB.

108 Laakso M, Arvala I, Tervonen S, Sotarauta M (1982) Retroperitoneal fibrosis associated with sotalol. *Br Med J* 285: 1085.

109 Thompson J, Julian DG (1982) Retroperitoneal fibrosis associated with metoprolol. *Br Med J* 284: 83.

110 McCluskey DR, Donaldson RA, McGeown MG (1980) Oxyprenalol and retroperitoneal fibrosis. *Br Med J* 281: 1459.

111 Bedtzen K, Soborg M (1975) Sclerosing peritonitis and practolol. *Lancet* i: 629.

112 Brown P, Baddeley H, Read AE, Davies JD, McGarry J (1974) Sclerosing peritonitis, an unusual reaction to a beta-adrenergic-blocking drug (Practolol). *Lancet* ii: 1477.

113 Windsor WO, Kurrein F, Dyer NH (1975) Fibrinous peritonitis: a complication of Practolol therapy. *Br Med J* 1: 68.

114 Bergqvist D, Takolande R (1983) Ureteral obstruction as a complication in aorto-iliac reconstructive surgery. *Scand J Urol Nephrol* 17: 391.

115 Darke SG, Glass RE, Eadie DGA (1977) Abdominal aortic aneurysm: perianeurysmal fibrosis and ureteric obstruction and deviation. *Br J Surg* 64: 649.

116 Sethia B, Darke SG (1983) Abdominal aortic aneurysm with retroperitoneal fibrosis and ureteric entrapment. *Br J Surg* 70: 434.

117 Allison MC, McLean L, Robinson LQ, Torrance CJ (1985) Spontaneous urinoma due to retroperitoneal fibrosis and aortic aneurysm. *Br Med J* 291: 176.

118 Blasco FJ, Saladie JM (1991) Ureteral obstruction and ureteral fistulas after aortofemoral or aortoiliac bypass surgery. *J Urol* 145: 237.

119 Gellstrom HR, Perez-Stable EC (1966) Retroperitoneal fibrosis with disseminated vasculitis and intrahepatic sclerosing cholangiitis. *Am J Med* 40: 184.

120 Mosimann F, Mange B (1980) Portal hypertension as a complication of idiopathic retroperitoneal fibrosis. *Br J Surg* 67: 804.

121 Appell RA, Weiss RM (1976) Retroperitoneal fibrosis and avascular necrosis of the femoral head. *J Am Med Assoc* 236: 2886.

122 Bullock N (1988) Idiopathic retroperitoneal fibrosis (editorial). *Br Med J* 297: 240.

123 Mitchinson MJ (1986) Retroperitoneal fibrosis revisited. *Arch Pathol Lab Med* 110: 784.

124 Lepor H, Walsh PC (1979) Idiopathic retroperitoneal fibrosis. *J Urol* 122: 1.

125 Tiptaft RC, Costello AJ, Paris AMI, Blandy JP (1982) The long term follow up of idiopathic retroperitoneal fibrosis. *Br J Urol* 54: 620.

126 Mundy AR, Kinder CH, Flannery JF, Joyce ORL (1982) Hypertension and thromboembolism in idiopathic retroperitoneal fibrosis. *Br J Urol* 54: 625.

127 Tresidder GC, Blandy JP, Singh M (1972) Omental sleeve to prevent recurrent retroperitoneal fibrosis around the ureter. *Urol Int* 27: 144.

128 Heller JE, Teggatz J (1992) Idiopathic retroperitoneal fibrosis infiltrating ureteral wall. *Urology* 40: 277.

129 Cooksey G, Powell PH, Singh M, Yeates WK (1982) Idiopathic retroperitoneal fibrosis: a long term review after surgical treatment. *Br J Urol* 54: 628.

130 McDougall WS, MacDonell RC (1991) Treatment of idiopathic retroperitoneal fibrosis by immunosuppression. *J Urol* 145: 112.

131 Clark CP, Vanderpool D, Preskitt JT (1991) The response of retroperitoneal fibrosis to tamoxifen. *Surgery* 109: 502.

132 Pollack HM, Wills JS (1978) Radiographic features of ureteral endometriosis. *Am J Roentgenol* 131: 627.

133 Willen R, Willen H, Lindstedt E, Ekelund L (1983) Localized primary amyloidosis of the ureter. *Scand J Urol Nephrol* 17: 385.

134 Crane DB, Smith MJV (1977) Pelvic lipomatosis: 9

year follow up. *J Urol* 118: 547.

135 Susmano DE, Dolin EH (1979) Computed tomography in diagnosis of pelvic lipomatosis. *Urology* 13: 215.

136 Werbhoff LH, Korobkin M, Klein RS (1979) Pelvic lipomatosis: diagnosis using computed tomography. *J Urol* 122: 257.

137 Heyns CF (1991) Pelvic lipomatosis: a review of its diagnosis and management. *J Urol* 146: 267.

Chapter 12: Kidney and ureter — neoplasms

Embryoma of the kidney — Wilms' tumour

There are only about 500 new cases of Wilms' tumour every year in the USA. Males and females are equally affected and there appear to be no ethnic differences. Most cases appear within the first 4 years of life but it occurs very rarely in adults. The peak incidence is at 2 years [1,2].

There are two main types: one inherited, the other not. The inherited group has an autosomal dominant with varying penetrance and expressivity [3,4] and loss of genetic material on the short arm of chromosome 11 [5]. In this group multiple tumours occur in a single family tree — and are often bilateral. In the hereditary group the children of those who are cured by treatment have about a 40% chance of developing one — 10 times more than those in the non-hereditary group [4].

Other congenital anomalies are associated with Wilms' tumour: aniridia, hemihypertrophy, the Beckwith—Wiedemann syndrome and hypospadias [6,7]. Occasionally, small islands of Wilms' tumour ('tumourlets') are discovered in multicystic dysplastic kidneys [8].

Pathology

Macroscopic. The Wilms' tumour is typically large, soft and heterogeneous on cut section (Fig. 12.1). It is very vascular and easily ruptured at operation.

Histology. The mesenchyme of the metanephros from which a Wilms' tumour originates is multipotential, and within a Wilms' tumour there can be blastema, stromal and epithelial elements: these are classified as favourable or unfavour-

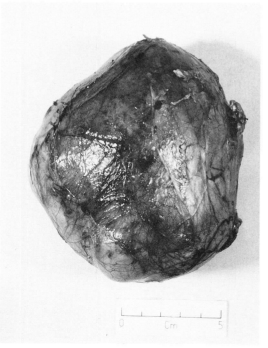

a

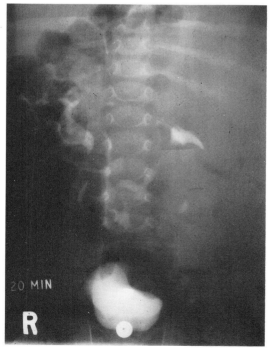

b

Fig. 12.1 (a) Macroscopic appearance of an embryoma of the kidney — Wilms' tumour. (b) IVU from the same patient.

able. The unfavourable are sheets of anaplastic tissue, clear cell sarcoma and malignant rhabdomyosarcoma (Figs 12.2 & 12.3). With modern combination chemotherapy and surgery the difference in survival is significant — 95% of those with favourable versus 50% of those with unfavourable features (Tables 12.1) [9—13].

Congenital mesoblastic nephroma. This tumour is usually noticed at birth or soon after and accounts for about one-third of tumours in children under 6 months. It forms a large lump of spindle cells resembling myoblasts or fibroblasts together with scattered primitive glomeruli (Fig. 12.4). It invades locally. The child usually does well as long as the mass is completely excised but these tumours are not to be regarded as benign [14].

Spread and staging

Wilms' tumour spreads by direct invasion, lymph node involvement and haematogenous metastasis. This underlies the system of staging [15]. The most important prognostic indicators are regional lymph node invasion, tumour spill at operation and tumour thrombus in the vena cava (Fig. 12.5).

Stage 1. Tumour limited to kidney; complete excision; capsule intact; no spill; no residual tumour beyond margins of resection.

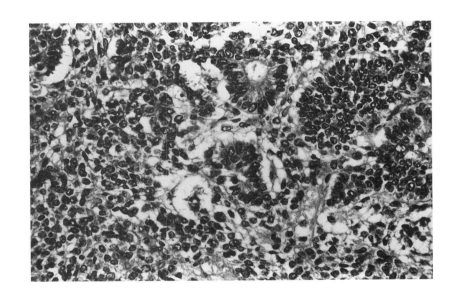

Fig. 12.2 Embryoma of the kidney (Wilms' tumour) — favourable histology (courtesy of Dr Suhail Baithun).

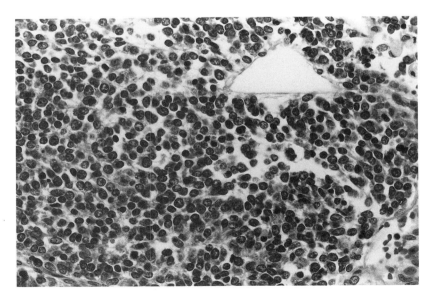

Fig. 12.3 Embryoma of the kidney (Wilms' tumour) — unfavourable histology (courtesy of Dr Suhail Baithun).

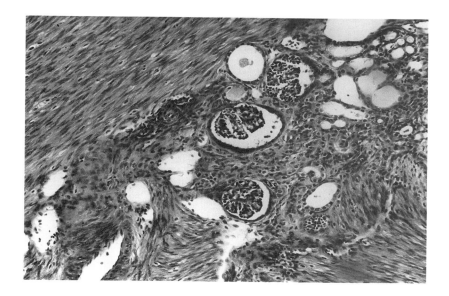

Fig. 12.4 Mesoblastic nephroma of the kidney (courtesy of Dr E.A. Courtauld).

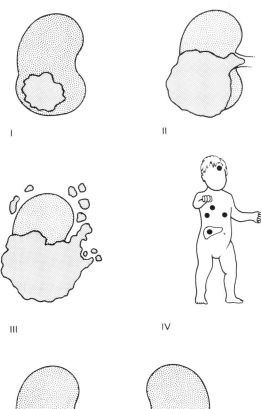

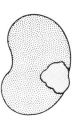

Fig. 12.5 Staging of embryoma of the kidney (see text for explanation of stages I–V).

Stage II. Tumour outside kidney, but completely excised; regional extension of tumour; vessel invasion; local spill or previous biopsy; no residual tumour beyond margins of resection.

Stage III. Residual tumour in abdomen; lymph node involvement; tumour spill; tumour extending beyond resection margins or incompletely removed.

Stage IV. Metastases in lung, liver, bone or brain.

Stage V. Bilateral renal involvement at time of diagnosis.

A joint study of 1439 patients showed 4-year survival rate as detailed in Table 12.1 [10].

Clinical features

Classically, a Wilms' tumour presents as a mass accidentally noted by the mother when bathing the child — 'a large lump in a wasted baby' (Fig. 12.6). Other presenting features include haematuria, abdominal pain and fever.

Table 12.1 A joint study of 1439 patients (data from [10]).

Stage	Histology	4-year survival (%)
I	Favourable	96.5
II	Favourable	92.2
III	Favourable	86.9
IV	Unfavourable	73.0

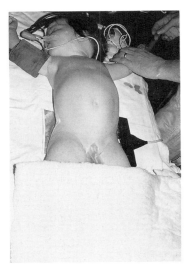

Fig. 12.6 Wilms' tumour — 'a large lump in a wasted baby'.

Investigations

Ultrasound scanning will reveal a large solid mass (Fig. 12.7) and may detect tumour in the vena cava or right atrium. A plain radiograph may help in distinguishing a Wilms' tumour from a neuroblastoma which is usually calcified. If an IVU has been done it will show the kidney distorted by the tumour rather than displaced (Fig. 12.8). A computerized tomography (CT) scan is necessary and justifies heavy sedation or a general anaesthetic since it gives additional information about spread to the liver and lungs, and detects tumour in the other kidney in about 5% of cases (Fig. 12.9). CT scanning has virtually replaced angiography except when partial nephrectomy is being contemplated for bilateral tumours.

Treatment

Wilms' tumours are so rare and the price for an error in management so high, that every child with a Wilms' tumour should be referred to a specialist centre engaged in multicentre trials where every protocol of treatment is continually audited [16].

Wilms' tumours are treated by a combination of radical surgery, chemotherapy and (rarely) radiotherapy. This combination is continually reviewed in the light of each cooperative trial. The key agents are actinomycin D and vincristine: doxorubicin and cyclophosphamide are used in some of the more advanced cases [17,18].

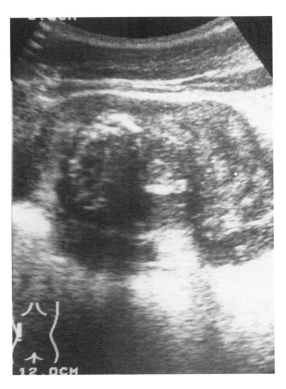

Fig. 12.7 Ultrasound scan of a Wilms' tumour (courtesy of Miss Leela Kapila).

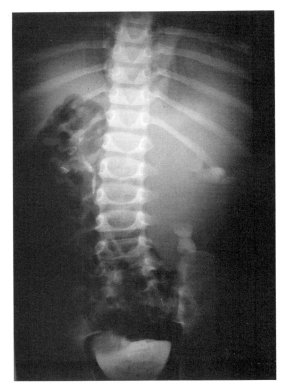

Fig. 12.8 IVU of a left-sided Wilms' tumour showing gross distortion of the calices (courtesy of Dr W. Hately).

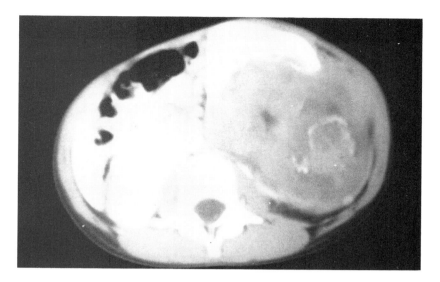

Fig. 12.9 CT scan of the same Wilms' tumour as in Fig. 12.7 (courtesy of Miss Leela Kapila).

Although these tumours are very radio-sensitive, but radiotherapy has only an adjuvant role [17] for residual pulmonary metastases and bilateral disease.

Recent audits of treatment regimes have shown that (a) short courses of chemotherapy are just as effective as long ones; (b) 6 months of actino-mycin D with vincristine is adequate for stage I disease (favourable); (c) there is no benefit from added radiation or doxorubicin in stage II (favourable); (d) 1000 cGy radiation is just as effective as 2000 cGy for stage III (favourable); and (e) in stage IV disease there is no advantage in adding cyclophosphamide.

Nephrectomy for Wilms' tumour

Through a long incision, extended if necessary into the chest, the bowel is reflected off each kidney so that both can be carefully inspected. These large soft tumours must be handled very gently to avoid tumour spill. It is worthwhile extending the resection when tumour has invaded the wall of the colon or duodenum. There is no advantage in performing a complete para-aortic or paracaval node dissection, but the nodes should be sampled for staging. Extension of tumour into the inferior vena cava is treated by taping the vena cava and contralateral renal vein before opening it to extract the thrombus. In doing this, extra care is necessary to verify the contralateral renal vein: the vena cava is often compressed to a thin ribbon, and it is all too easy to divide the contralateral renal vein in mistake for the one draining the tumour (Fig. 12.10).

Bilateral Wilms' tumours

CT scanning identifies tumour in the opposite kidney, nevertheless it should always be examined at operation. It is well worth trying to save the other kidney: 87% of patients with bilateral tumours survived for 2 years, which included 19 of 22 in whom residual disease was left behind [8].

If the contralateral tumour can be removed by

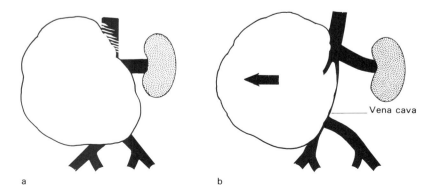

Fig. 12.10 (a & b) Nephrectomy for Wilms' tumour: the renal vein on the side of the tumour is often compressed, and it is all too easy to ligate the contralateral renal vein by mistake.

a   b

partial nephrectomy this should be performed. In many centres this is preceded by a preliminary course of chemotherapy. If partial nephrectomy is not feasible then biopsies should be taken from the tumour and local lymph nodes. Chemotherapy will be longer and more intensive.

In very advanced Wilms' tumours there is a place for second-look surgery after chemotherapy which may render inoperable disease operable.

Wilms' tumours in adults

These are exceedingly rare and by the time they are diagnosed they are usually advanced and show little response to chemotherapy. Nevertheless, a combination of surgery, chemotherapy and local radiotherapy is usually given [18−20]. Very rarely metastases from Wilms' tumours have been seen up to 15 years after apparently successful treatment of the primary [21].

Tumours of the renal parenchyma

Adenocarcinoma of the kidney

Epidemiology

The incidence of renal adenocarcinoma cancer varies from three per 100 000 in Bombay to seven per 100 000 in New York State [22]: it is low in Japan [23] and less common in England than in Scotland but in both it is increasing [24] (Fig. 12.11). It is most common in Scandinavians and North American whites, and least in Africans and Asians [25].

Adenocarcinoma of the kidney is about twice as common in men as in women. In England and Wales it accounts for 1.6% of cancer deaths in males. Its peak incidence is in the sixth and seventh decades and though rare under 20 it has been well described in children [26].

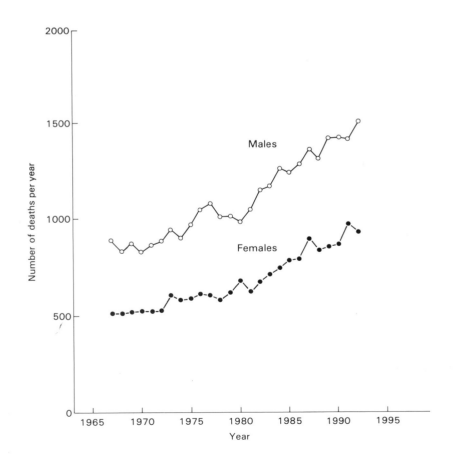

Fig. 12.11 Graph showing the steady increase in deaths from renal cell carcinoma in England and Wales (from Registrar General, Office of Population Census and Surveys).

Aetiology

In animals renal cancer can be caused by viruses, radiation and a variety of carcinogens [27–31]. In mice and rats there are strains with a high incidence and a dominant inheritance has been noted both in monkeys [32] and humans [33] where it is related to blood group A, colour blindness and certain human leucocyte antigen (HLA) factors [34]. It has been suggested that people with kidney cancer in the family should undergo a renal ultrasound scan every 2–3 years from the age of 30 [34].

In patients undergoing dialysis the increased risk of cancer justifies regular screening [35]. Certain occupations (e.g. fire-fighting and painting) may carry an increased hazard [36].

Some interesting cytogenetic differences have been reviewed in renal tumours [37]. Unilateral tumours have loss of genetic material from chromosome 3, bilateral tumours lack a sex chromosome and have extra material on chromosome 7 [38]. Since chromosome 3 encodes for acylpeptide hydrolase it is possible that this could become a useful tumour marker.

Pathology

Macroscopically, renal cell cancers are bright yellow masses with an apparent capsule, areas of haemorrhage, cyst formation and calcification (Fig. 12.12). They often invade the renal vein. Occasionally, a tumour forms a nodule in the wall of a benign renal cyst [39]. Multiple tumours are associated with von Hippel–Lindau disease in which there is a benign haemangioblastoma in the central nervous system associated with renal cysts and multiple renal cell carcinomas [40,41].

Microscopically, the most common cell type resembles the cells of the proximal renal tubule [30], having large clear cells containing glycogen and lipid (Fig. 12.13). About 10% show other cell types, with eosinophilic granular cells containing less glycogen and lipid, spindle cell elements resembling sarcoma (which carry a poor prognosis [42]) and areas of haemorrhage, necrosis and calcification. Papillary elements may cause confusion with transitional cell carcinoma (Fig. 12.14).

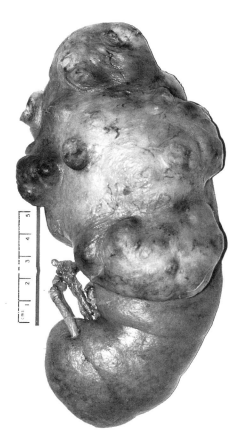

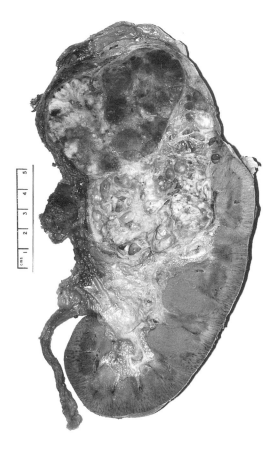

Fig. 12.12 (a & b) Macroscopic appearance of an adenocarcinoma of the kidney (courtesy of Mr Philip Clark).

a

b

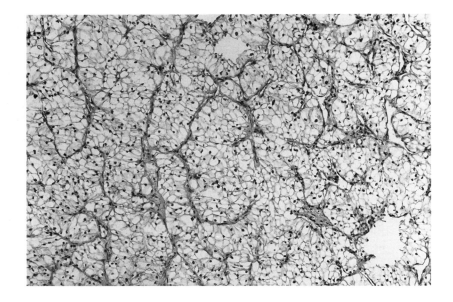

Fig. 12.13 Clear cell carcinoma of the kidney.

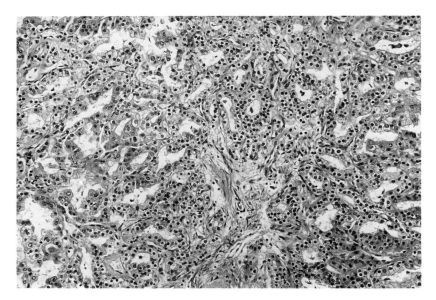

Fig. 12.14 Tubulopapillary pattern of adenocarcinoma of the kidney (courtesy of Dr EA Courtauld).

Oncocytoma

These are mahogany brown tumours made up of eosinophilic epithelial cells (Fig. 12.15). They have such a good prognosis after nephrectomy that it has been suggested that they are a distinct, benign entity. They have no abnormality on chromosome 3 [43]. Much effort has been made to detect them, and perhaps avoid nephrectomy. It was claimed that they had a characteristic 'cartwheel' pattern in the angiogram. Sadly, experience shows that they overlap with renal cell carcinoma, are quite capable of metastasizing and must be treated like any other cancer of the kidney [44–47].

Grade

Frequency of mitoses is used as the basis for grading renal adenocarcinoma [48], G1 being highly differentiated and G3 poorly or undifferentiated. DNA flow cytometry adds little to subjective evaluation of differentiation [49] failing to pick out small areas containing highly malignant cells, but perhaps DNA cytophotometry may be more accurate [50].

Stage

The Union Internationale Contre le Cancer (UICC) TNM system [48] recognizes the following

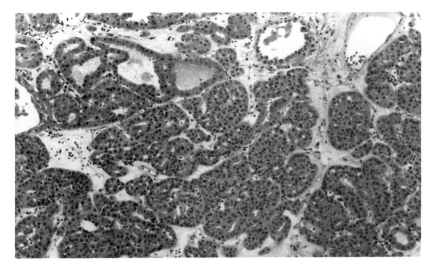

Fig. 12.15 Oncocytoma of the kidney — brightly eosinophilic cells (courtesy of Dr Jo Martin).

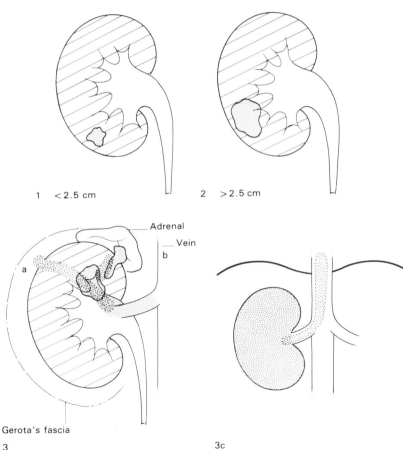

1 < 2.5 cm   2 > 2.5 cm

Adrenal
Vein
b
a

Gerota's fascia
3   3c

Fig. 12.16 UICC system of staging of adenocarcinoma of the kidney (see text for further details).

system of clinicopathological staging (Fig. 12.16):
- **T1** Tumour less than 2.5 cm diameter, limited to kidney.
- **T2** Tumour more than 2.5 cm diameter, limited to kidney.
- **T3** Into major veins, adrenal gland, perinephric tissue, but not beyond Gerota's fascia:
  T3a into fat;

T3b into veins or vena cava below diaphragm; **T3c** into vena cava above diaphragm.
- **N1** Single node less than 2 cm.
- **N2** Single node more than 2 cm and less than 5 cm.
- **N3** Nodes more than 5 cm.
- **M1** Distant metastases.

Prognostic features

Staging is the single most important prognostic factor [51]. Others include the size of the tumour, invasion of veins and the histological grade.

Size of tumour. Bell pointed out a generation ago [52] that tumours of less than 3 cm in diameter were generally benign, and those over 3 cm in diameter were malignant, although even in his experience of 62 tumours of less than 3 cm in diameter no less than three (4.8%) had metastasized. Small tumours were detected in 350 out of 16 294 (2.1%) autopsies in Sweden: 115 had been noted in life, but 24% of the unnoticed cancers had already metastasized, amongst which three out of 82 were less than 3 cm in diameter [53,54].

So long as the tumours are small and confined to the kidney at the time of nephrectomy, the prognosis is excellent [55,56] with a 70–80% 5-year survival while the overall 5-year survival for all cases without metastases is about 65% [57]. If tumours are detected when they are very small and treated by radical nephrectomy, the survival rate exceeds 95% [57,58].

Invasion of veins. Microscopic invasion of small veins in the kidney has surprisingly little effect on the prognosis but the prognosis is worse if there is tumour thrombus in the main renal vein [59].

Histology. Grade 3 tumours do worse than grade 1. There is also a difference in the prognosis according to the pattern of cell growth; in descending order: clear cell cancers, papillary patterns, granular cell tumours and worst of all those with a spindle cell element [42,59].

Clinical features

Classical symptoms

The cardinal symptoms of renal cell carcinoma are haematuria, pain and a mass in the loin. Haematuria occurs in only 60% of cases [58] and it is the other presenting features which make this such a challenging clinical entity [60,61].

Unusual symptoms

1 Often accompanied by loss of weight, night-sweats and a raised sedimentation rate, fever of unknown origin is a deceiving presentation caused by a pyrogen secreted by the cancer. Extracts of renal cell carcinoma cause fever when injected into laboratory animals [60].

2 Alterations in the blood picture are common. The usual one is erythrocytosis, i.e. a haemo-globin level over 15.5 g/dl. It differs from true polycythaemia in having no increase in platelets or splenomegaly. It is due to an increase in erythropoietin secreted by the tumour [60,61].

3 The converse, anaemia, is also common and caused not by loss of blood in the urine, but a marrow toxin secreted by the tumour [61]. Hypertension is often present, and is associated with elevated renin levels in the blood [61].

4 Hypercalcaemia (serum calcium over 10.5 mg/dl) is a common and dangerous clinical feature. Sometimes due to widespread bony met-astases, more often it is caused by production of parathyroid hormone by the tumour [61]. Hyper-calcaemia is more common the more advanced the disease but is not related to any specific cell type [62].

5 Stauffer [63] described a syndrome of hepato-splenomegaly with disordered liver function, without metastases. It was reversed by neph-rectomy. Like the return of erythrocytosis after nephrectomy, the return of Stauffer's syndrome may signify the development of metastases and carries a poor prognosis [63,64].

6 Some tumours secrete glucagon, which leads to enteropathy and diarrhoea [65].

7 Tumour proteins may cause glomerulonephritis by depositing immune complex on the basement membrane [66].

8 Amyloid may be deposited in many tissues including that of the contralateral kidney. It usually persists despite removal of the cancer [66].

9 Paraneoplastic motor neurone disease has been described in renal cell cancer [67].

Investigations

Intravenous urogram

The IVU is still the most common investigation for haematuria, and will usually provide all the information needed to make a diagnosis of cancer of the kidney: typically it shows a mass, sometimes with calcification here and there, which distorts the collecting system and the renal outline (Fig. 12.17).

Ultrasound

When the IVU does not show clearly whether the

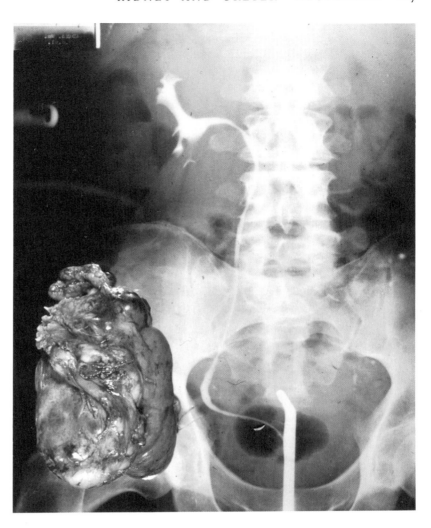

Fig. 12.17 Retrograde urogram of an adenocarcinoma of a kidney photographed with the specimen.

mass is solid or cystic, the ultrasound scan will distinguish between them. Cysts have a spherical outline with a complete absence of echoes within.

Difficulty arises when there are several cysts close together, or when haemorrhage into a cyst gives rise to echoes within it. If necessary fine needle aspiration of the contents of the cyst will settle the issue by excluding malignant cells. If contrast is introduced, the interior of the cyst can be shown to be smooth.

The ultrasound scan is particularly useful in showing tumour thrombus in the vena cava (Fig. 12.18).

CT scanning

CT scanning has greatly improved the precision of preoperative diagnosis. It will usually demonstrate tumour in the renal vein and vena cava, and detects small lung metastases which would otherwise be missed in a conventional radiograph (Figs 12.19 & 12.20).

Angiography

Today, angiography is rarely needed, all the information necessary to make a decision being provided by ultrasound and CT scans. However, angiography can be helpful in showing the arterial supply of the tumour if partial nephrectomy is contemplated (Fig. 12.21).

Embolization

Some years ago embolization of the renal artery with a balloon, gelfoam, chopped muscle or a Gianturco coil was used to facilitate the subsequent operation [68,69]. In practice, pain and fever are common following embolization and

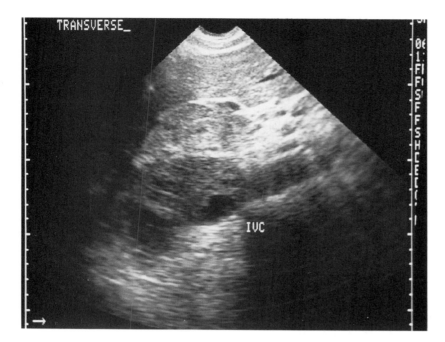

Fig. 12.18 Ultrasound showing tumour in the inferior vena cava (courtesy of Dr W. Hately).

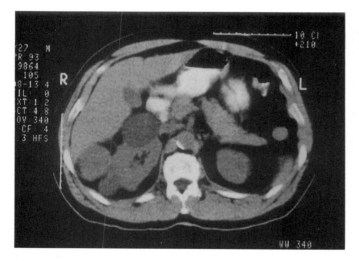

Fig. 12.19 CT scan showing the right kidney with both cysts and a tumour to show the difference. The cysts are echo free.

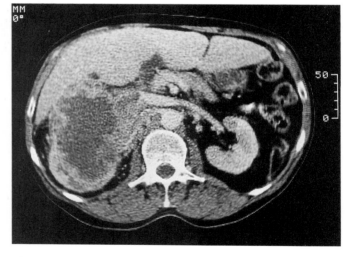

Fig. 12.20 CT scan showing on the right a Grawitz tumour invading the inferior vena cava (courtesy of Dr Otto Chan).

disasters have been reported when material used to block the renal artery found its way into a cerebral, spinal, coronary, retinal or superior mesenteric artery. At operation, the tumour was often found to have a rich blood supply from subcapsular vessels. The method is now generally given up for all but exceptional cases.

Magnetic resonance imaging (MRI)

MRI has the advantage over other forms of imaging in that it shows more clearly than any

other technique the exact extent of tumour thrombus in the vena cava [70] (Fig. 12.22).

Differential diagnosis

A solid mass in the kidney is rarely anything other than a renal cell carcinoma. Oncocytoma must be regarded as malignant until nephrectomy has been performed. A chronic abscess of the cortex is usually accompanied by more fever than a tumour, and the CT scan usually suggests an abscess rather than a cancer. The

and frozen section may be misleading (see p. 164).

Multiple cysts in the kidney may be impossible to distinguish from the cystic form of carcinoma, especially the so-called multilocular cystic adenoma (see p. 198). In practice, it is not possible to be certain of the benign nature of many of the other tumours until the nephrectomy specimen has been examined histologically (see p. 198).

Angiomyolipoma has a characteristic appearance in the CT scan (see p. 198).

A renal pseudotumour — the normal column of Bertin — is easy to recognize on the CT scan (see p. 197).

Larger sarcomas and haemangiosarcomas of the kidney will only be recognized after nephrectomy.

Treatment

The standard treatment of a cancer of the kidney is radical nephrectomy. The chief precaution before operation is to check that there is no evidence of tumour in the vena cava: this evidence is provided by the ultrasound, CT and MRI scans, but when in doubt superior and inferior cavography should be performed (Fig. 12.23).

Radical nephrectomy for cancer

The anterior approach. Through a generous midline or transverse incision the colon and duodenum are reflected medially. The renal artery is tied in continuity before ligating and dividing

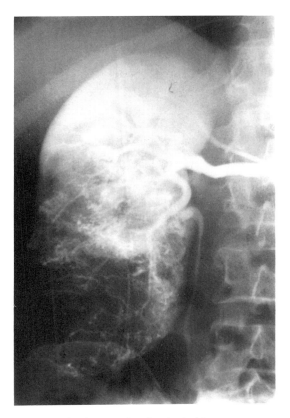

Fig. 12.21 Angiogram showing typical tumour circulation of an adenocarcinoma.

diagnosis is settled by aspiration of pus from the middle of the abscess.

Xanthogranuloma is nearly always accompanied by a calculus, but the diagnosis may remain in doubt even at the time of operation

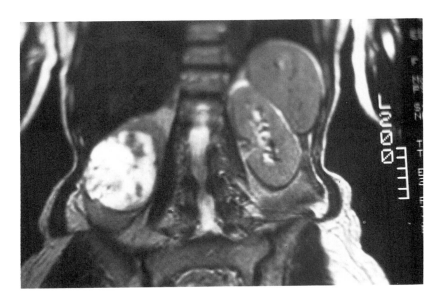

Fig. 12.22 MRI showing Grawitz adenocarcinoma of the right kidney.

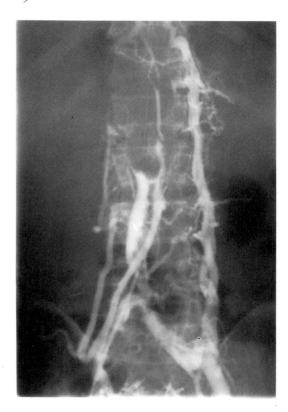

Fig. 12.23 Inferior cavogram showing tumour blocking the inferior vena cava.

the renal vein. Haemorrhage from small collateral vessels is diminished and the dissection becomes easier once the main artery to the kidney has been ligated (Fig. 12.24).

On the right side when there is a very large tumour the renal artery is found where it lies between the aorta and vena cava (Fig. 12.25). On the left side, the left renal artery may be located behind the duodenojejunal flexure. If necessary access may be improved by dividing the inferior mesenteric vein (Fig. 12.26).

In approaching the renal veins, it is well to watch out for large lumbar veins which can enter the renal vein just where it joins the vena cava, while on the left side, a double vein encircling the aorta is a common anatomical variant (Fig. 12.27).

Thoracoabdominal approach. For large tumours of the upper pole of either kidney a 10th rib thoraco-abdominal incision may give better access (Fig. 12.28). Many prefer the loin approach, with or without entering the thorax. Whatever the approach, once the vessels have been secured, the kidney and all its surrounding tissues within

the envelope of Gerota's fascia, including the adrenal gland are removed *en bloc* [71].

Tumour in the renal veins

The management of tumour in the renal vein depends on how far it has grown into the inferior vena cava. Often only a small finger of tumour thrombus protrudes into the vena cava from a cancer in the right kidney. On the right side, having ligated the right renal artery in continuity, the back of the vena cava is exposed by dividing the lumbar veins. The vena cava above and below the right renal vein, and the left renal vein, are all secured with Rummel tourniquets (Fig. 12.29). Only then is the cava opened, the tumour thrombus extracted and the vein sutured (Fig. 12.30).

If the thrombus is growing into the edge of the cava it is necessary to remove a cuff of cava along with the renal vein. If the whole thickness of the vena cava is invaded by tumour, it is safe to remove a segment of the vein, knowing that collateral venous circulation will prevent infarction of the opposite kidney (Fig. 12.31).

When tumour thrombus is discovered in the left renal vein it is essential to make a wide anterior approach in order to gain safe access to the vena cava and the large veins that drain into it (Fig. 12.32).

Tumour thrombus extending above the liver

If the CT, MRI and venograms have shown tumour thrombus extending above the liver, the cardiothoracic team should be involved in planning the operation. In principle, a long midline incision is made, first into the abdomen to confirm the preoperative findings and then it is carried up into the chest by splitting the sternum. The inferior vena cava is occluded where it enters the right atrium unless tumour thrombus has extended into the right atrium. The superior vena cava and ascending aorta are cannulated and the patient is put on a cardiopulmonary bypass. The limiting factor for this operation is hepatic ischaemia time and this can be prolonged by lowering the body core temperature [72–76].

This very major surgery calls for detailed planning in advance. Those who survive the operation have a 30% 5-year survival, determined more by the presence of perinephric spread or lymph node spread than the threat of cancer in the middle of the heart [73–76]. Enthusiasm for these big procedures does however need to be

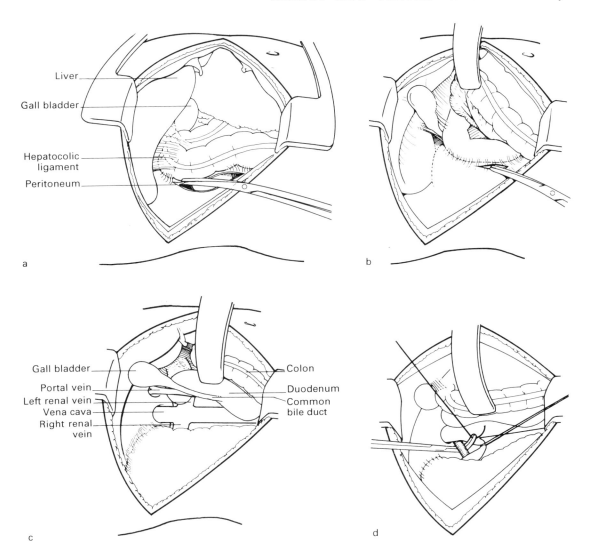

Fig. 12.24 (a) On the right side the colon and (b) duodenum are mobilized medially to reveal (c) the inferior vena cava and the right renal vessels. (d) The right renal artery is ligated in continuity.

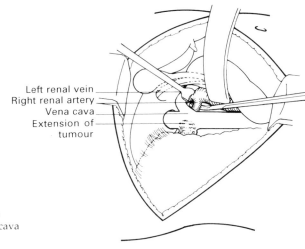

Fig. 12.25 The right renal artery may be ligated in continuity where it lies between the inferior vena cava and the aorta.

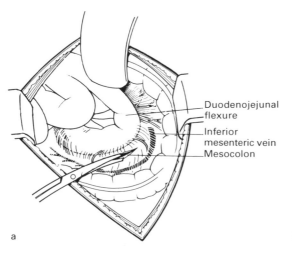

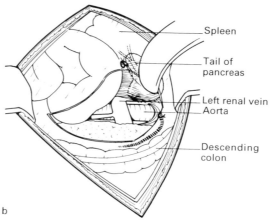

Duodenojejunal flexure

Inferior mesenteric vein

Mesocolon

Spleen

Tail of pancreas

Left renal vein

Aorta

Descending colon

a

b

Fig. 12.26 (a & b) With large tumours the left renal artery may be found by dividing the peritoneal reflexion over the lateral aspect of the duodenum, if necessary dividing the inferior mesenteric vein.

tempered with common sense: there is at least one long-term survivor whose bilateral renal cell cancers had tumour thrombus extending above the diaphragm which were not removed [77].

Partial nephrectomy

Small tumours at one or other pole of the kidney may be removed by partial nephrectomy with a good margin. Expose the kidney through a wide approach. Tape the renal artery and occlude it with a vascular clamp (Fig. 12.33). Remove the tumour with a good margin of healthy tissue (Fig. 12.34), confirming the clear margin with peroperative ultrasound [78] or frozen section. Before the renal artery is unclamped, every tiny vessel in the cut surface of the kidney is secured by meticulous suture ligature using fine absorbable suture material. Remove the clamp and catch up any remaining vessels.

For tumours in the middle third of the kidney a very similar procedure can be carried out, taking a wedge of parenchyma. When a pro-

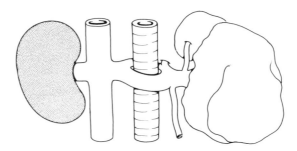

Fig. 12.27 A large lumbar vein often enters the back of the left renal vein, which may encircle the aorta.

longed dissection is anticipated, cool the kidney with sterile ice slush.

As a last resort the renal artery and vein can be cut across and the kidney perfused with transplant solution and the dissection performed with the help of the dissecting microscope [79]. There have been many proponents of this kind of 'bench surgery' but in practice there are few operations that cannot be done *in situ* [80].

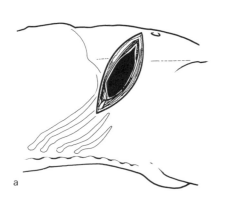

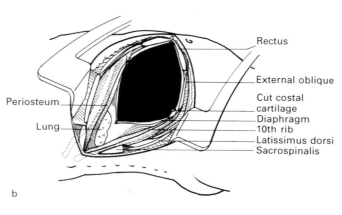

Rectus

External oblique

Cut costal cartilage

Diaphragm

10th rib

Latissimus dorsi

Sacrospinalis

Periosteum

Lung

a

b

Fig. 12.28 Tenth rib thoracoabdominal approach to the kidney. (a) The anterior part of the incision is made first, to make sure the tumour is operable; and (b) the incision is carried back along the 12th rib. If the periosteum is stripped off the upper border of the rib there is no need to resect it.

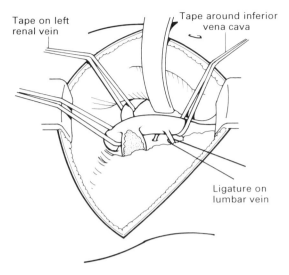

Fig. 12.29 When there is tumour in the right renal vein and vena cava, after ligating the right renal artery, the cava and left renal vein are secured with tapes.

Partial nephrectomy has often been performed for bilateral tumours. The operation has sometimes been simplified, the main mass of tumour being enucleated from its false capsule [81] but the histology of the edge of the capsule always shows that tumour has spread through into the healthy parenchyma, and there is no evidence that this operation has changed the natural history of this slow-growing disease [81,82] perhaps because the tumours are multicentric in about 10% of cases [83].

Adjuvant therapy

In discussing any treatment for renal cell cancer it is difficult to make allowances for the unpredictable natural history of this disease. Until recently, tumours were seldom detected until they were very large, often over 1 kg, and evidently present for many years. Others have

Fig. 12.30 (a) The vena cava is opened, (b) the tumour is extracted, and the cava is closed. (c) If the tumour thrombus is limited to the renal vein a Satinsky clamp may be applied to the inferior vena cava after (d) making sure the Rummel tapes are in readiness.

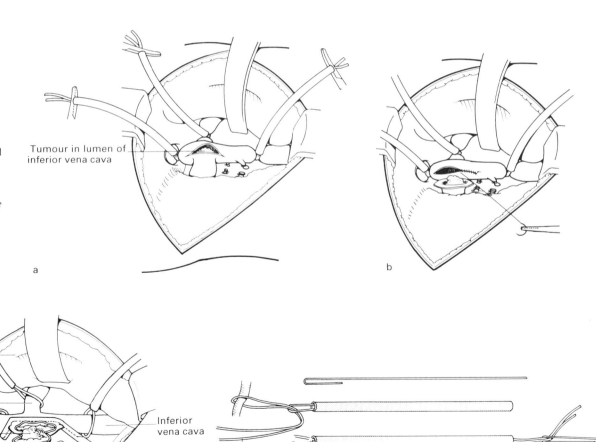

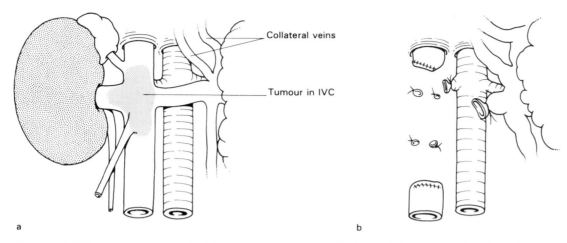

Fig. 12.31 (a) When tumour has blocked the inferior vena cava (IVC), there will be an adequate collateral circulation, and the entire segment of vena cava (b) may be removed.

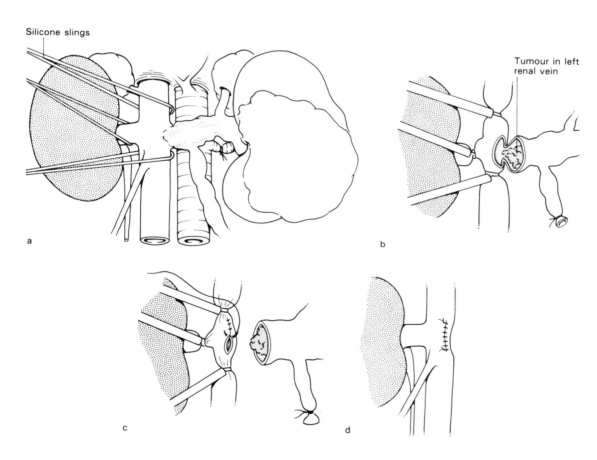

Fig. 12.32 When the vena cava is invaded by tumour from the left renal vein a wide anterior approach is used (a), the vena cava is (b) taped and opened, the tumour extracted and the cava closed (c & d).

been observed for as long as 35 years without metastasizing [84,85].

Adjuvant node dissection

One in five patients who were cancer free at 5 years, go on to die of metastases by the 10th year [86]. It is commonplace for patients to develop metastases many years after the original nephrectomy. Against this background it needs very prolonged prospective studies to show any meaningful benefit from any kind of adjuvant treatment. Hence, it is impossible to know whether removing lymph nodes *en bloc* with the

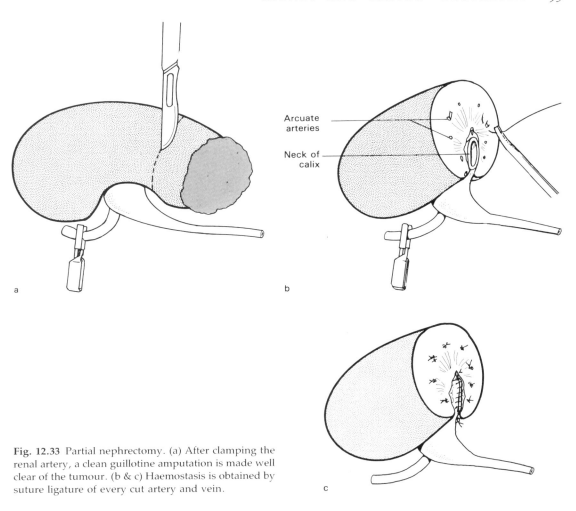

Fig. 12.33 Partial nephrectomy. (a) After clamping the renal artery, a clean guillotine amputation is made well clear of the tumour. (b & c) Haemostasis is obtained by suture ligature of every cut artery and vein.

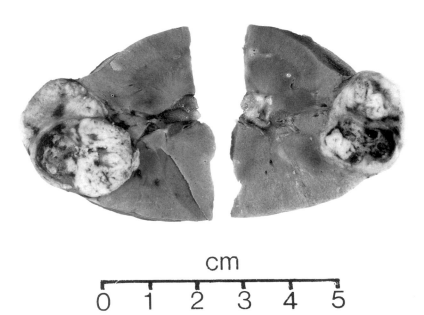

Fig. 12.34 A small tumour removed by partial nephrectomy.

nephrectomy makes any difference to survival though this is often advocated [87]. It is always helpful to sample the adjacent nodes in order to stage the tumour, especially if adjuvant therapy is being considered.

Adjuvant chemotherapy

Chemotherapy for metastatic renal cancer has been disappointing, giving at best a 15% partial response — a benefit which does not justify the toxicity and expense of the treatment [88].

Adjuvant radiotherapy

After initial enthusiasm for using radiotherapy either before or after nephrectomy more careful studies showed that radiation, if anything, actually made the outlook worse [89,90], a result which is nowadays interpreted in terms of the immunosuppressive effect of radiation.

Hormone therapy

There is an unexplained incidence of spontaneous regression of metastases [91] — up to 24% in some series. In a prospective surveillance study Oliver [27] documented a large number of patients who showed spontaneous regression as well as lack of progression.

Claims for any adjuvant therapy must therefore be viewed against this background. Medroxyprogesterone acetate (Provera), is still widely used, though controlled studies show that patients on Provera do if anything worse than controls [92,93].

Immunotherapy

Three agents have been investigated: bacille Calmette–Guérin (BCG), alpha interferon and interleukin-2 which increase host T cell activity, especially when the tumours are well differentiated. About 20% of patients may expect a measurable response, and about 5% a complete remission — not a spectacular advance but still twice the spontaneous regression rate observed on surveillance [94–99].

A suggestion that blood transfusion might worsen the outcome of surgery for renal cancer by producing immunosuppression, has not been confirmed [100,101].

Nephrectomy in presence of metastases

Many surgeons cling to the hope that removing the primary tumour may encourage the immune defences of the body to deal with residual metastases. The occasional remission after nephrectomy that most surgeons of experience can remember once or twice in their career supports this optimism but there is no proof that remission is more likely to follow operation than doing nothing.

There may be good reasons for removing the primary tumour, e.g. bleeding and pain, or when it is hoped to obtain some benefit by some new form of treatment, perhaps with interleukin-2 where there are sound theoretical reasons for reducing the tumour burden. But the surgeon must think twice before inflicting a painful, and perhaps dangerous, operation on a patient whose life expectancy is already limited. It is easy to make the patient worse [84,102].

Embolization and nephrectomy

There was a hope that preliminary embolization of a cancer might release antigenic material which would provoke an immunological response and result in the disappearance of metastases. It does not make the operation any easier (see p. 187). The desired effect on metastases has not been confirmed [103].

Screening and prevention

Ultrasound scanning now makes it possible to detect tumours less than 3 cm in diameter, and so it is already possible to find tumours at a stage when they are virtually all curable. Removal of these incidentally found tumours gives results which are much better than those of tumours detected in the usual way: up to 95% surviving for 5 years without disease [57,104]. This may explain the recent improvement in the survival of patients with kidney cancer [105,106]. Given the low background of occult renal tumours found at autopsy [54,55] there is a strong argument for screening for kidney cancer.

Renal pseudotumour — column of Bertin

This common variation of normal anatomy can still be a trap for the unwary (Fig. 12.35). A form of duplex kidney results in an extra large column of Bertin at the junction of the upper and lower

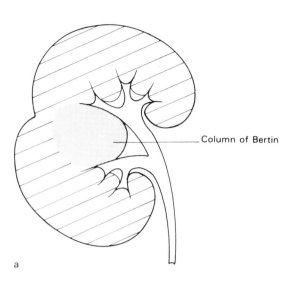

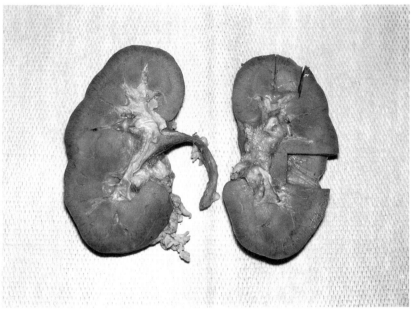

Fig. 12.35 (a & b) A large column of Bertin may mimic a renal cell cancer.

moieties. If the patient has had haematuria, the IVU will show a soft tissue 'mass' in this position. CT scanning will show that it shares the same density as the rest of renal parenchyma. If doubt remains, a biopsy will show normal renal tissue.

Adenoma

Adenomas are in fact small carcinomas of the kidney. Although those of less than 3 cm in diameter seldom metastasize they cannot be relied upon: in an autopsy series 4% of such small tumours had already metastasized [53,54]. New methods of screening are disclosing more and more of them and removal gives excellent survival figures [57].

Multilocular cystic adenoma

In the course of a routine investigation of haematuria the IVU may show a multicystic mass in the middle of the kidney. CT and angiography cannot distinguish it from cancer (Fig. 12.36). The only safe course is nephrectomy, although it is probably an innocent hamartomatous malformation [107].

A somewhat similar clinical problem is posed by the bilateral renal masses seen in von Hippel–Lindau disease, where there may be angiomatous cysts of the cerebellum, retina, pancreas and kidneys: here local resection of the mass is advised [108].

Angiomyolipoma

This unusual tumour of the kidney is often but not always associated with tuberous sclerosis [44,109–117]. It contains a large amount of fat which gives it a very typical radiographic (Fig. 12.37) and CT appearance (Fig. 12.38).

Macroscopically, these are very soft, friable and exceedingly vascular tumours which bleed at the lightest touch.

Histologically, they are mostly made up of benign fat, smooth muscle and blood vessels (Fig. 12.39). Malignant elements are present in about a quarter of them and may cause hypercalcaemia and lead to metastases.

Clinical features

Half of the patients with this tumour have features of tuberous sclerosis, an autosomal dominant disorder characterized by mental retardation, fits, adenoma sebaceum on the face, retinal phakomas, subependymal brain calcification, astrocytomas, and hamartomatous or cystic changes in the heart, lungs and kidneys. Half of the patients with tuberous sclerosis have kidney tumours, which may be multifocal and bilateral.

The other half of the angiomyolipomas occur in patients without tuberous sclerosis: many of these present with bizarre symptoms often resulting from bleeding into or around the tumour, e.g. loin pain, intestinal symptoms,

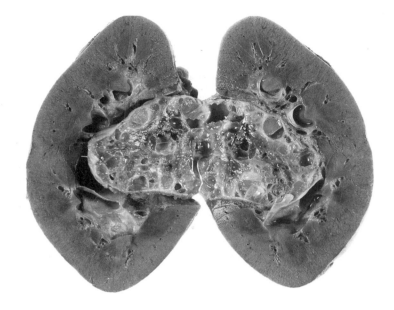

Fig. 12.36 Multilocular cystic adenoma. It is impossible to know that this is benign before nephrectomy.

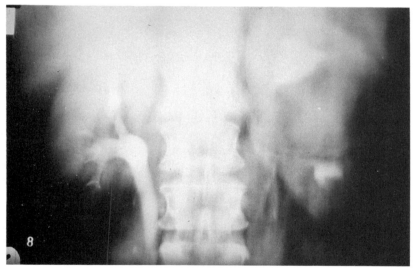

Fig. 12.37 IVU of angiomyolipoma associated with tuberous sclerosis (courtesy of Dr Otto Chan).

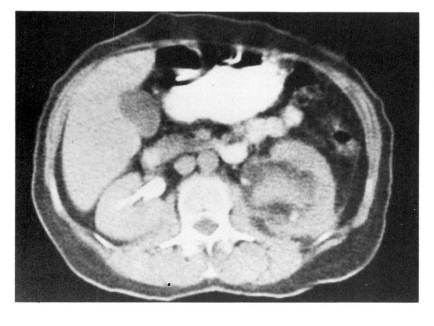

Fig. 12.38 CT scan of angiomyolipoma: note the large masses of fatty tissue (courtesy of Dr Otto Chan).

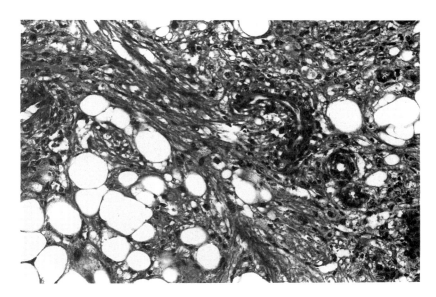

Fig. 12.39 Photomicrograph of angiomyolipoma. Note the masses of fatty tissue (courtesy of Dr Suhail Baithun).

meteorism or sudden collapse from severe massive retroperitoneal haemorrhage [108–117].

Diagnosis

The preoperative diagnosis may be suspected on the basis of the CT appearances, but it is never possible to be sure that the tumour is benign. However, the rather small chance of local or distant spread justifies partial nephrectomy whenever this is feasible. In doing this it is essential to find and tape the main renal artery early in the operation, before handling the tumour sets off daunting haemorrhage.

Bilateral nephrectomy for the large bulky tumours is justified, and may be followed by transplantation with very little risk of the immunosuppression precipitating metastases.

Haemangioma and haemangiosarcoma

A variety of benign tumours arising from the endothelium of arteries and veins, like the common hamartomas of the liver, are also seen in the kidney, but much less often [118].

Histologically, they consist of blood vessels of varying size interconnected by sinusoids. Rarely, they may form a mass of endothelial hyperplasia — 'Masson's tumour'. They may occur anywhere along the urinary tract and, very unusually, may be seen at the lower end of the ureter. They may be bilateral.

Clinical features

When they are small, angiomas of the kidney are notoriously difficult to diagnose. They give rise to episodes of haematuria, sometimes provoked by exercise. When the usual investigations are performed for haematuria nothing abnormal may be detected in the IVU, but a cloud of blood is seen to puff out of the ureter on cystoscopy. Occasionally, a tiny irregularity in a calix can be seen in the IVU, resembling papillary necrosis or early tuberculosis.

Ureteroscopy may confirm that bleeding is issuing from one calix, and occasionally it is possible to stop the haemorrhage by coagulation of the offending spot with the neodymium-yttrium aluminium garnet (YAG) laser.

Angiography during the bleeding phase may localize the source of the bleeding and allow it to be plugged there and then, or identify which part to remove by partial nephrectomy. Occasionally, the mere injection of hypertonic contrast medium in the course of the angiogram is enough to stop the bleeding.

The more rare large lesions cannot be distinguished from those with malignant sarcomatous change or a renal cell cancer with a large arteriovenous shunt, and there is no practical alternative to nephrectomy.

Juxtaglomerular tumour — reninoma

This rare variant on the theme of haemangiopericytoma is derived from the juxtaglomerular cells which secrete renin. Young patients with hypertension are found to have elevated blood levels of aldosterone and renin. Because they are so small, finding them can be difficult. The intravenous pyelogram (IVP) may look normal but there may be more renin in one renal vein than the other [119].

Macroscopically, they are single, usually less than 4 cm in diameter, and grey–yellow in colour. Histologically, they resemble haemangiopericytomas (Fig. 12.40). Immunofluorescence shows their cells are full of renin. Local excision cures the patient of hypertension and they are believed not to metastasize or recur.

Sarcoma of the kidney

Sarcomas may arise from any of the connective tissues of the kidney [44,110]. They present as masses in the kidney and have a poor prognosis. Histologically, the only way to tell them from the adult form of a Wilms' tumour is to show that they have no renal components.

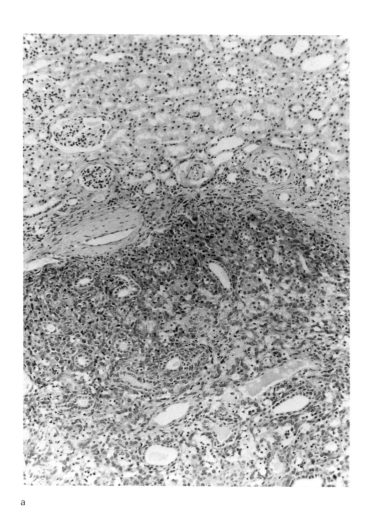

a

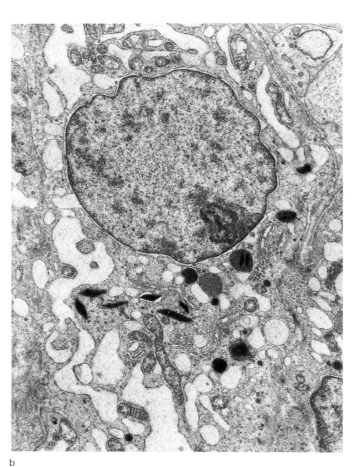

b

Fig. 12.40 (a) Light photomicrograph of a renin-secreting juxtaglomerular cell tumour, stained with an antiserum to human renin and an immunoperoxidase method. The dark staining tumour cells contain renin; the tubule component of the tumour does not contain renin. There is no stainable renin in the adjacent kidney due to suppression of renin synthesis by high circulating levels of angiotensin II. (b) Electron micrograph showing a renin-secreting cell in a juxtaglomerular cell tumour. The spaces consist of dilated rough endoplasmic reticulum indicating active synthesis and the renin storage granules including characteristic paracrystalline photogranules are seen. × 19 000 (courtesy of Dr G.B.M. Lindop and the Editor of *Histopathology*).

Carcinoma of the renal pelvis and ureter

Epidemiology

Except in the Balkans, urothelial cancers of the kidney and ureter are comparatively rare, occurring once for every 12 cases of cancer of the bladder and twice as often in men as in women, with a peak incidence around 45 years. They occur in about 3% of patients undergoing treatment for urothelial cancer of the bladder [120] (Fig. 12.41).

Aetiology

All the aetiological agents that cause cancer of the bladder also cause cancer in the urothelium of the renal pelvis and ureter, e.g. industrial aminophenols and smoking [120,121]. There is some evidence that certain families carry an autosomal dominant gene making them unusually prone to carcinoma of the renal pelvis and ureter as well as other malignancies [122]. Two causes deserve special attention: analgesic abuse and Balkan nephropathy.

Analgesic abuse

About a decade after a form of interstitial nephritis was recognized to be caused by overconsumption of analgesics containing phenacitin, phenazone and caffeine [123], an epidemic of cancers in the renal pelvis and ureter was identified in those who survived the nephropathy. In Australia and Germany, it was associated with 22% of renal pelvic tumours and 11% of tumours of the ureter [124–126].

Balkan nephropathy

Although several aetiological agents have been postulated as the cause of this condition, it seems likely that it is caused by a toxin secreted by a mould growing on maize stored in damp barns [127].

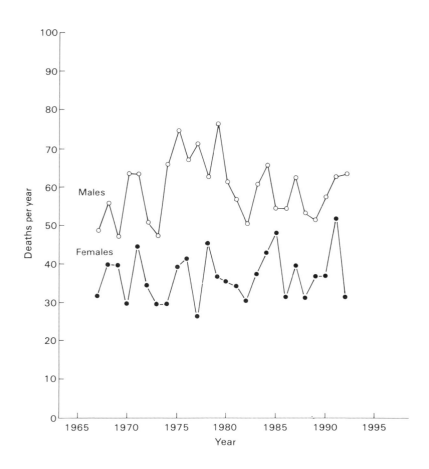

Fig. 12.41 Deaths from carcinoma of the renal pelvis and ureter for England and Wales (from Registrar General, Office of Population Census and Surveys). Note that the very small number remains more or less constant.

Metaplasia

Almost any type of chronic irritation may lead to metaplasia of the urothelium, either to squamous epithelium, as in stones and bilharziasis, or columnar epithelium as with chronic cystitis where it is preceded by follicular cystitis and the formation of von Brunn's nests.

Pathology

As in the bladder, the macroscopic appearances of these tumours varies with their degree of malignancy: the most well differentiated tend to be papillary, the more anaplastic ones more solid (Fig. 12.42).

The histological classification of urothelial cancers of the renal pelvis and ureter is identical to that of the urinary bladder. Most tumours are transitional cell carcinomas and three grades of malignancy are recognized [121,128,129]. (see p. 292). There is also the rare 'inverted papilloma' which is almost always benign, needing local excision. It may be bilateral [130,131].

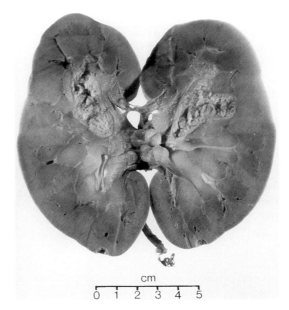

Fig. 12.42 Papillary transitional cell carcinoma of the renal pelvis.

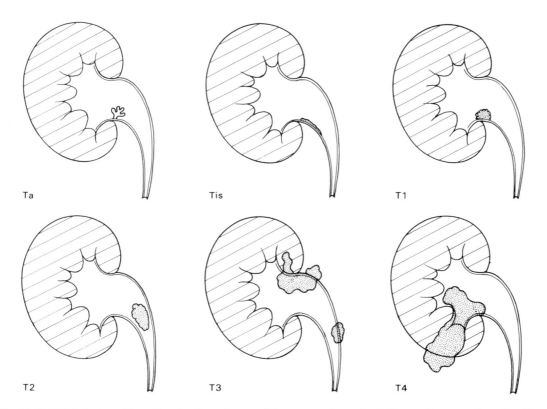

Fig. 12.43 TNM staging of transitional cell carcinoma of the upper urinary tract. Ta, papillary, non-invasive; Tis, carcinoma *in situ*; T1, not invading muscle; T2, invading muscle; T3, invading renal parenchyma or outside muscle; T4, invading outside kidney.

The staging of transitional cell cancers in the renal pelvis and ureter follows the principles that obtain in the bladder which can be applied to the kidney, except that the muscle of the renal pelvis is so thin that in practice it is difficult to draw a distinction between T2 and T3 (superficial and deep muscle invasion) [128−130] (Fig. 12.43). The UICC system [48] is described in Table 12.2.

Spread

Tumour spread is by direct invasion into the muscle of the renal pelvis and ureter, thence into the fat of the renal sinus, the parenchyma, regional lymph nodes and veins. Tumour may be implanted downstream in the ureter and bladder, but one cannot distinguish them from new foci of tumour.

Bilateral tumours may occur, and sooner or later a tumour in the upper tract is likely to be followed by urothelial tumours in the bladder [132,133].

Table 12.2 UICC TNM staging for cancer of the renal pelvis and ureter

Ta	Papillary, non-invasive tumour
Tis	Carcinoma *in situ*
T1	Invades subepithelial connective tissue
T2	Invades muscularis
T3	Invades (pelvis) into peripelvic fat or renal parenchyma; (ureter) into periureteric fat
T4	Invades adjacent organs, or through kidney into perinephric fat

Clinical features

Most of these patients are diagnosed when haematuria is investigated [132,134]. In cancer of the ureter obstruction may give rise to pain from hydronephrosis, which can be surprisingly acute, or the obstructed upper tract may become infected. There are seldom any physical signs.

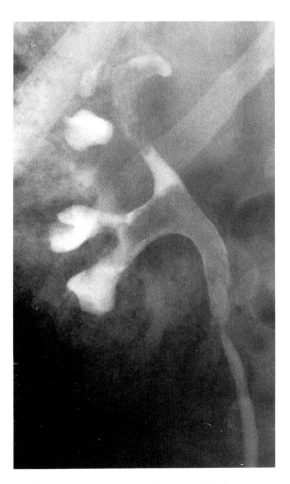

Fig. 12.44 IVU of carcinoma in the renal pelvis (courtesy of Dr W. Hately).

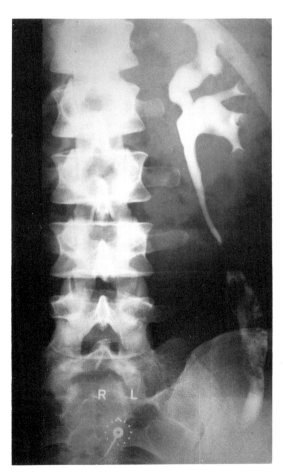

Fig. 12.45 IVU of carcinoma in the ureter (courtesy of Dr W. Hately).

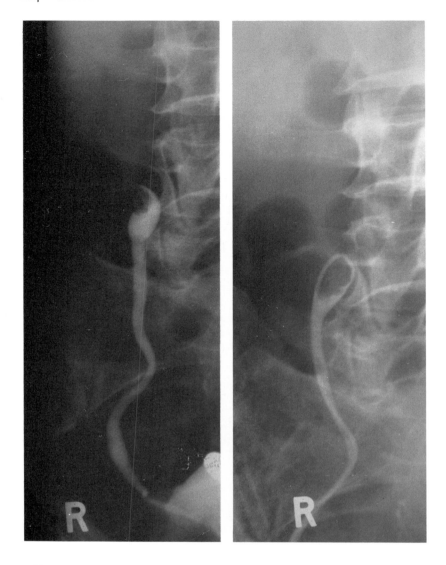

Fig. 12.46 Retrograde urogram of carcinoma in the ureter.

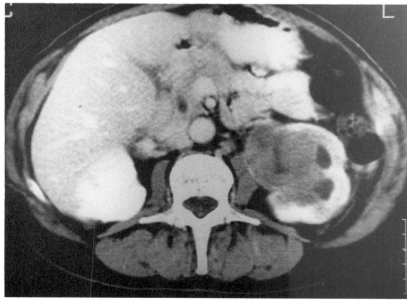

Fig. 12.47 CT scan image of a carcinoma occupying the left renal pelvis (courtesy of Dr W. Hately).

Investigations

The classical investigation has been the IVU, which reveals an irregularity or a filling defect in the renal collecting system (Fig. 12.44). In the ureter, there is a classic combination of a filling defect and dilatation of the ureter both up- and downstream (Fig. 12.45). When the definition is unclear a retrograde ureteropyelogram may be helpful (Fig. 12.46). CT and MRI scans will show the mass and help define how far it has spread (Figs 12.47). Ultrasound scanning is seldom helpful.

Ureteroscopy

It is often possible to see and obtain a biopsy from a tumour under direct vision with the ureteroscope.

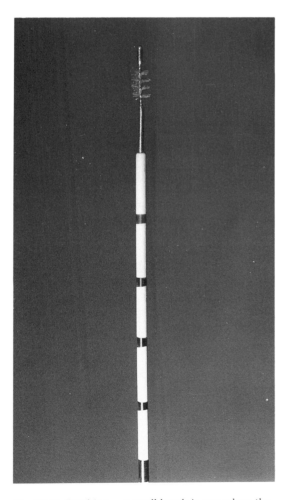

Fig. 12.48 Brushing — a small brush is passed up the ureter, and rubbed against the tumour. The brush is agitated by ultrasound and the deposit centrifuged and stained.

Cytology

If anaplastic cells are detected in the bladder urine it is likely that any tumour in the upper trace will be anaplastic, and to find only apparently normal transitional cells in the urine does not exclude a well-differentiated tumour.

Brushing

Passing a brush (Fig. 12.48) up a ureteric catheter may provide cells from the tumour which, when fixed and freed from the brush by ultrasound, will give a preparation almost as diagnostic as a histological one.

Treatment

Radical nephroureterectomy

The classical operation for carcinoma of the upper tract is nephroureterectomy. If the ureter is not removed then recurrences will occur in the stump in about 15% of cases [134–137].

There are several ways of performing this operation: a very long midline incision makes it possible to remove the ureter together with the cuff where it enters the bladder [134]. Less invasive is a technique which allows the kidney to be removed through an upper transverse incision and the lower third of the ureter and cuff of bladder to be removed through a Pfannenstiel incision [138] (Fig. 12.49).

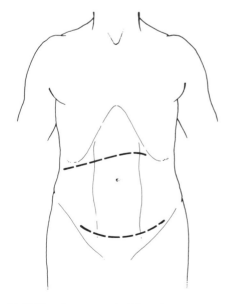

Fig. 12.49 Two transverse incisions for nephroureterectomy.

The excision of the cuff of bladder is most safely performed through the open bladder, with a ureteric catheter placed in the other ureter for safety (Fig. 12.50).

Most tumours arise in the upper part of the ureter and for these Semple's manoeuvre is least invasive [139]. With the patient in the cystoscopy position, the ureteric orifice and intramural ureter are deeply resected (Fig. 12.51) and careful haemostasis obtained with the resectoscope. Then, through a transverse incision, the kidney is mobilized and its pedicle divided. The ureter is followed down and, with a little traction, brought out into the wound (Fig. 12.52). Semple's manoeuvre [139] is not appropriate for a tumour in the lower third of the ureter, and it should not be used for ureters that are surrounded by fibrosis, e.g. in tuberculosis, when the common iliac artery can be injured.

It has been suggested that one should remove the kidney more radically, together with all its surrounding fat, Gerota's fascia and the regional lymph nodes. No controlled trials support this concept. What we do know is that in undifferentiated tumours the lymph nodes are often involved [140] and if they are, the patients do very badly [141] unless adjuvant treatment is given (see p. 209).

Conservative surgery

Experience with cancer of the bladder suggests that superficial well-differentiated tumours could be adequately treated by local excision or coagulation with diathermy or laser [142,143]. Before the introduction of the ureteroscope it was necessary to expose the kidney, open the pelvis and excise a localized tumour with a cuff of healthy renal pelvis (Fig. 12.53), and do the same with a localized tumour of the ureter (Figs 12.54 & 12.55). In a tumour of the lower end of the ureter local resection could be followed by reimplantation of the ureter with, if necessary, a Boari flap.

The ureteroscope makes it possible to see inside the renal pelvis, and apply diathermy coagulation or the neodymium-YAG laser beam to small tumours (Fig. 12.56). When the tumours cannot be seen with the ureteroscope, a percutaneous track allows a nephroscope to resect or coagulate them (Fig. 12.57). To prevent seeding of tumour along the nephroscope track local

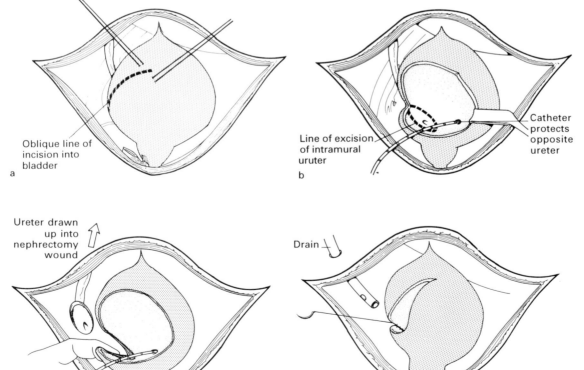

a   Oblique line of incision into bladder

b   Line of excision of intramural ureter   Catheter protects opposite ureter

c   Ureter drawn up into nephrectomy wound

d   Drain

Fig. 12.50 (a) The bladder is opened obliquely. (b) An ellipse of bladder is removed with the ureter, taking care to protect the other ureter with a catheter (c). The bladder is closed (d).

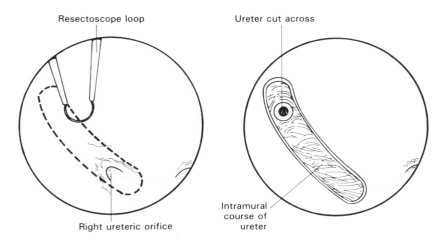

Fig. 12.51 Semple's manoeuvre. The ureter is resected down to fat with the resectoscope.

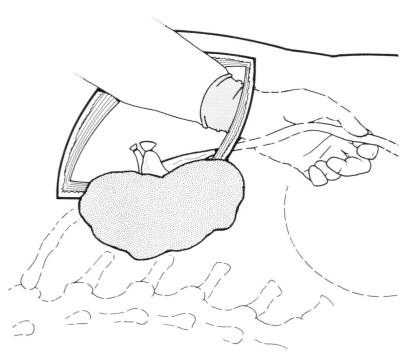

Fig. 12.52 After mobilizing the kidney, the ureter is followed down between finger and thumb until its lower end comes free.

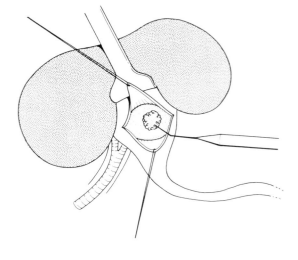

Fig. 12.53 Open removal of a papillary tumour of the renal pelvis.

irradiation by means of an iridium wire has been used [144,145]

Results

The results of treatment of urothelial cancer of the renal pelvis and ureter depend less on what treatment has been given than on the original grade and stage of the cancer. In the author's series, G1 urothelial tumours of the upper tract whether treated conservatively or by nephro-ureterectomy had an overall 97% 5-year survival [135] justifying an attempt to conserve the kidney when possible. On the other hand G3 tumours

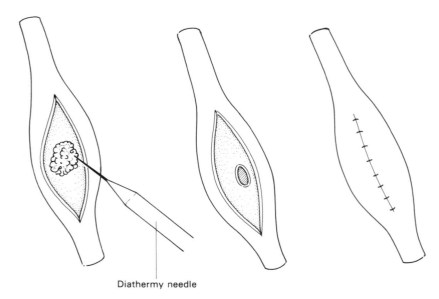

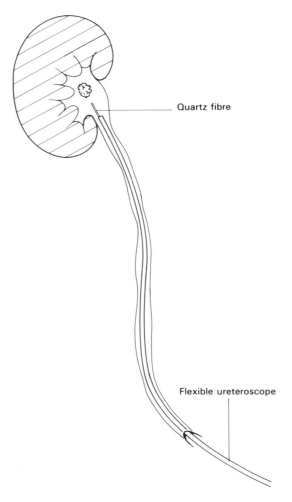

Diathermy needle

Fig. 12.54 Local excision of a small papillary tumour of the ureter. The ureter is incised, the tumour resected with diathermy, and the ureter closed.

Quartz fibre

Flexible ureteroscope

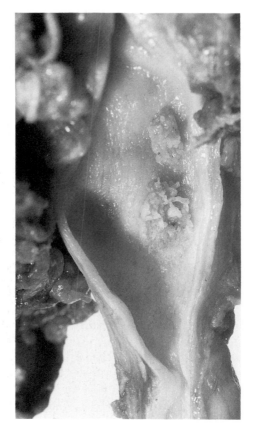

Fig. 12.55 Small papillary tumour of the ureter suitable for local excision.

Fig. 12.56 A small papillary tumour of the renal pelvis may be visible through a flexible ureteroscope: if so, it can be coagulated with a neodymium-YAG laser.

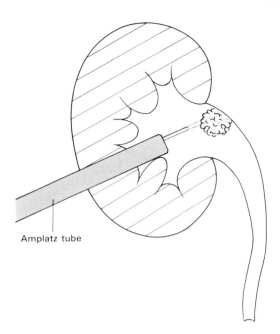

Fig. 12.57 Through an Amplatz tube introduced into the renal pelvis over a guide-wire, a small papillary tumour can be seen, biopsied and coagulated with a neodymium-YAG laser or diathermy.

had only a 40% overall survival [135], hence the need for adjuvant therapy [146].

Adjuvant radiotherapy

In many centres postoperative radiotherapy is given for those cases where the cancer is found to have invaded through the muscle of the pelvis or reached the lymph nodes. Since invasion is almost inevitable in patients with G3 cancer [135] it would be logical to give any adjuvant treatment before the operation when there is biopsy or cytological evidence that the tumour is other than well differentiated [147].

Because these cases are so uncommon, it has so far not been possible to set up a prospective trial to test this concept. The author has a patient with a biopsy-proven G3 invasive tumour, treated by preoperative radiotherapy, in which the nephroureterectomy specimen showed no tumour: he has survived 7 years without recurrence.

An equally strong argument can be made for giving combination chemotherapy to G3 cases before nephroureterectomy. Fair [148] has had at least one case in which invasive multifocal G3 cancer of the renal pelvis involving lymph nodes (proven by needle aspiration) responded to a combination of mitomycin, vinblastine and actinomycin C (MVAC) and at subsequent nephroureterectomy only a trace of carcinoma *in situ* could be found in the specimen.

Such anecdotes prove nothing, therefore trials are needed which combine the experience of many centres to test the hypothesis that G3 tumours need something more than surgery alone.

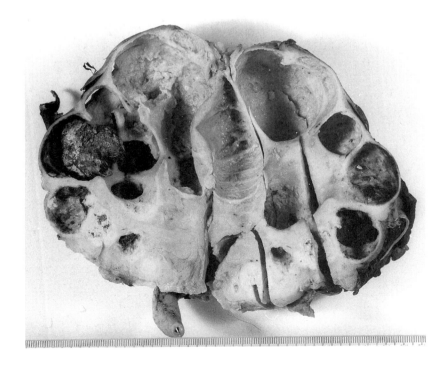

Fig. 12.58 Squamous cell carcinoma of the renal pelvis associated with a renal calculus.

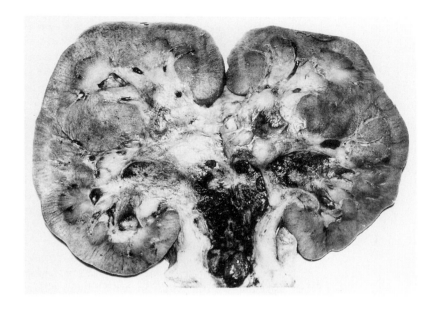

Fig. 12.59 Adenocarcinoma of the renal pelvis secondary to calculus.

Squamous carcinoma of the renal pelvis and ureter

About 10% of upper tract tumours are squamous cell cancers arising in metaplastic urothelium from long-standing irritation, usually from a calculus. They seldom gives rise to haematuria, and are diagnosed late, when invasion of adjacent organs gives rise to pain (Fig. 12.58).

Adenocarcinoma of the renal pelvis and ureter

Adenocarcinoma may arise in the renal pelvis after protracted upper urinary tract infection or *de novo*. It is very rare, is seldom diagnosed early and does badly [149] (Fig. 12.59).

References

1 Mesrobian H-GJ (1988) Wilms' tumor: past, present, future. *J Urol* 140: 231.

2 Young JL, Miller RW (1975) Incidence of malignant tumors in US children. *J Pediatr* 86: 254.

3 Breslow NE, Beckwith JB (1982) Epidemiological features of Wilms' tumor: results of the National Wilms' Tumor Study. *J Natl Cancer Inst* 68: 429.

4 Coppes MJ, Williams BRG (1994) The molecular genetics of Wilms' tumor. *Cancer Invest* 12: 57.

5 Weissman BE, Saxon PJ, Pasquale SR *et al.* (1987) Introduction of a normal human chromosome 11 into a Wilms' tumor cell line controls its tumorigenic expression. *Science* 236: 175.

6 Miller RV, Fraumeni JF, Manning MD (1964) Association of Wilms' tumor with aniridia, hemihypertrophy and other congenital malformations. *New Engl J Med* 270: 922.

7 Pendergrass TW (1976) Congenital anomalies in children with Wilms' tumor: a new survey. *Cancer* 37: 403.

8 Dimmick JE, Johnson HW, Coleman GU, Carter M (1989) Wilms tumorlet, nodular renal blastema and multicystic renal dysplasia. *J Urol* 142: 484.

9 Beckwith JB, Palmer NF (1978) Histopathology and prognosis of Wilms' tumor. Results from the first National Wilms' Tumor Study. *Cancer* 41: 1937.

10 D'Angio GJ, Breslow N, Beckwith JB *et al.* (1989) Treatment of Wilms' tumor: results of the third National Wilms' Tumor Study. *Cancer* 64: 349.

11 Bolande RP (1972) Congenital mesoblastic nephroma of infancy. *Perspect Pediatr Pathol* 1: 227.

12 Howell CG, Othersen HB, Kiviat NE (1982) Therapy and outcome in 51 children with mesoblastic nephroma: a report of the National Wilms' Cancer Study. *J Pediatr Surg* 17: 826.

13 Zuppan CW, Beckwith JB, Luckey DW (1988) Anaplasia in unilateral Wilms' tumor: a report from the National Wilms' Tumor Study Pathology Center. *Hum Pathol* 19: 1199.

14 Gormley TS, Skoog SJ, Jones RV, Maybee D (1989) Cellular congenital mesoblastic nephroma: what are the options. *J Urol* 142: 479.

15 Farewell VT, D'Angio GJ, Breslow N, Norkool P (1981) Retrospective validation of a new staging system for Wilms' tumor. *Cancer Clin Trials* 4: 167.

16 Pritchard J (1989) Overtreatment of children with Wilms' tumour outside paediatric oncology centres. *Br Med J* 299: 853.

17 Habib F, McLorie GA, McKenna PH, Khoury AE, Churchill BM (1993) Effectiveness of preoperative chemotherapy in the treatment of Wilms' tumor with vena caval and intracardiac extension. *J Urol* 150: 933.

18 Pritchard J, Imeson J, Barnes J *et al.* (1995) Results of the United Kingdom children's cancer study group first Wilms' tumor study. *J Clin Oncol* 13: 124.

19 Boilletot A, Tournade MF, Delemarre JF *et al.* (1985)

Wilms' tumor in adult patients: SIOP results in 15 patients, in: *Proceedings of the Third European Conference on Clinical Oncology*. Stockholm, p. 179.

20 Williams GB, Colbeck RA, Gowing NFC (1992) Adult Wilms' tumour: review of 14 patients. *Br J Urol* 70: 230.

21 Rao SP, Miller ST, Wrzolek M, Haller JP, Klotz D (1993) Skeletal muscle metastasis in a patient with Wilms' tumor and multiple late recurrences. *Cancer* 71: 1343.

22 Mellembaard A, Carstensen B, Norgaard N *et al.* (1993) Trends in the incidence of cancer of the kidney, pelvis, ureter and bladder in Denmark 1943–1988. *Scand J Urol Nephrol* 27: 327.

23 Skeet RG (1990) Epidemiology of urogenital tumours, in: Chisholm GD, Fair W (eds) *Scientific Foundations of Urology*, 3rd edn, pp. 427–32. Oxford: Heinemann.

24 Ritchie AWS, Kemp IW, Chisholm GD (1984) Is the incidence of renal carcinoma increasing? *Br J Urol* 56: 571.

25 Page HS, Asire JH (eds) (1985) *Cancer Rates and Risks*. NIH Publication No. 85, p. 691. Bethesda.

26 Futrell JW, Filston HC, Reid JD (1978) Rupture of a renal cell carcinoma in a child: five year tumor-free survival and literature review. *Cancer* 41: 1565.

27 Oliver RTD (1989) Medical management of renal cell carcinoma, in: Oliver RTD, Blandy JP, Hope-Stone HF (eds) *Urological and Genital Cancer*, pp. 180–91. Oxford: Blackwell Scientific Publications.

28 Murphy GP, Mirand EA, Johnson GS, Schmidt JD, Scott WW (1966) Renal tumors induced by a single dose of dimethylnitrosamine: morphologic, functional, enzymatic and hormonal characterization. *Invest Urol* 4: 39.

29 Skinner MS, Mizell M (1978) The effect of different temperatures on herpes virus induction and replication in Lucke explants. *Lab Invest* 26: 671.

30 Wallace AC, Nairn RC (1972) Renal tubular antigens in kidney tumors. *Cancer* 29: 977.

31 La Vecchia C (1990) Smoking and renal cell carcinoma. *Cancer Res* 50: 5231.

32 Ratcliffe HL (1940) Familial occurrence of renal carcinoma in rhesus monkey (*Macaca mulatta*). *Am J Pathol* 16: 619.

33 Reddy ER (1981) Bilateral renal cell carcinoma, unusual occurrence in three members of one family. *Br J Radiol* 54: 8.

34 Levinson AK, Johnson DE, Strong LC, Pathak S, Huff V, Saunders GF (1990) Familial renal cell carcinoma: hereditary or coincidental? *J Urol* 144: 849.

35 Terasawa Y, Suzuki Y, Morita M, Kato M, Suzuki K, Sekino H (1994) Ultrasonic diagnosis of renal cell carcinoma in hemodialysis patients. *J Urol* 152: 846.

36 Delahunt B, Bethwaite PB, Nacel JN (1995) Occupational risk for renal cell carcinoma: a case control study based on the New Zealand Cancer Registry. *Br J Urol* 75: 578.

37 Weaver DJ, Michalski K, Miles JH (1989) Cytogenetics of bilateral renal cell carcinoma. *J Urol* 142: 697.

38 Erlandsson R, Boldog F, Persson B *et al.* (1991) The gene from the short arm of chromosome 3 at D3F15S2 frequency deleted in renal cell carcinoma encodes acylpeptide hydrolase. *Oncogene* 6: 1293.

39 Weitzner S (1971) Clear cell carcinoma of the free wall of a simple renal cyst. *J Urol* 106: 515.

40 Greene LF, Rosenthal MH (1951) Multiple hypernephromas of the kidney in association with Lindau's disease. *New Engl J Med* 244: 633.

41 Maher ER (1993) The gene for von Hippel–Lindau disease. *Br Med J* 307: 279.

42 Fuhrman SA, Lasky LC, Limas C (1992) Prognostic significance of morphological parameters in renal cell carcinoma. *Am J Surg Pathol* 6: 655.

43 Meloni AM, Bridge J, Sandberg AA (1992) Reviews on chromosome studies in urological tumors. I. Renal tumors (review). *J Urol* 148: 253.

44 Dickersin CR, Colvin RB (1988) Pathology of renal tumors, in: Skinner DG, Lieskovsky G (eds) *Diagnosis and Management of Genitourinary Cancer*, pp. 118–49. Philadelphia: WB Saunders.

45 Van der Valt JD, Reid HA, Risdon RA, Shaw J (1983) Renal oncocytoma. A review of the literature and a report of an unusual multicentric case. *Virch Archiv* (A) 398: 2191.

46 Zhang G, Monda L, Wasserman FF, Fraley EE (1985) Bilateral renal oncocytoma: report of two cases and literature review. *J Urol* 133: 84.

47 Frydenberg M, Eckstein RP, Saalfield JAAH, Breslin FHD, Alexander JH, Roche J (1991) Renal oncocytomas — an Australian experience. *Br J Urol* 67: 352.

48 Union Internationale Contre le Cancer (UICC) (1992) *TNM Classification of Malignant Tumours*, 4th end, 2nd revision. Berlin: Springer.

49 Grignon DJ, Ayala AG, El-Naggar A *et al.* (1989) Renal cell carcinoma: a clinicopathologic and DNA flow cytometric analysis of 103 cases. *Cancer* 64: 2133.

50 Rauschmeier H, Hofstadter F, Jakse G (1984) Tumor grading: an important prognostic factor in renal cell carcinoma. *World J Urol* 2: 103.

51 Paulson DF (1984) Prognostic factors predicting treatment response. *World J Urol* 2: 99.

52 Bell ET (1959) *Renal Disease*, 2nd edn, p. 435. Philadelphia: Lea & Febiger.

53 Hellsten S, Berge T, Wehlin L (1981) Unrecognised renal cell carcinoma: clinical and pathological aspects. *Scand J Urol Nephrol* 15: 273.

54 Hellsten S, Berge T, Linell F (1983) Clinically unrecognised renal carcinoma: aspects of tumour morphology, lymphatic and haematogenous metastatic spread. *Br J Urol* 55: 166.

55 Guinan PD, Vogelzand NJ, Fremgen AM *et al.* (1995) Renal cell carcinoma: tumor size, stage and survival. *J Urol* 153: 901.

56 Gibbons RP, Montie JE, Correa RJ, Mason JT (1976) Manifestations of renal cell carcinoma. *Urology* 8: 201.

57 Erden I, Beduk Y, Karalezli G, Aytac S, Anafarta K, Safak M (1993) Characterisation of renal masses with colour flow Doppler ultrasonography. *Br J Urol* 71: 661.

58 Best BG (1987) Renal carcinoma: a ten year review 1971–80. *Br J Urol* 60: 100.

59 Tomera KM, Farrow BM, Liever MM (1983) Well differentiated (grade 1) clear cell renal carcinoma. *J Urol* 129: 933.

60 Samaan NA (1979) Paraneoplastic syndromes associated with renal carcinoma, in: Johnson DE, Samuels ML (eds) *Clinical Conference on Cancer — Cancer of the Genitourinary Tract*, pp. 73–8. New York: Raven Press.

61 Sufrin G, Mirand EA, Moore RH *et al.* (1977) Hormones in renal cancer. *J Urol* 117: 433.

62 Fahn H-J, Lee Y-H, Chen M-T, Huang J-K, Chen K-K, Chang LS (1991) The incidence and prognostic significance of humoral hypercalcemia in renal cell carcinoma. *J Urol* 145: 248.

63 Stauffer MH (1961) Nephrogenic hepatosplenomegaly. *Gastroenterology* 40: 694.

64 Walsh PN, Kissane JM (1968) Nonmetastatic hypernephroma with reversible hepatic dysfunction. *Arch Intern Med* 122: 214.

65 Gleeson MH, Bloom SR, Polak JM *et al.* (1970) An endocrine tumour in kidney affecting small bowel structure, motility and function. *Gut* 11: 1060.

66 Cronin RE, Kaehny WD, Miller PD *et al.* (1976) Renal cell carcinoma: unusual systemic manifestations. *Medicine* 55: 291.

67 Evans BK (1990) Paraneoplastic motor neuron disease and renal cell carcinoma: improvement after nephrectomy. *Neurology* 40: 960.

68 Kato T (1992) Embolization of the kidney, in: Waxman J, Williams G (eds) *Urological Oncology*, p. 216. London: Arnold.

69 Mebust WK, Weigel JW, Less KR, Cox GG, Lewel WR, Krishnan EC (1984) Renal cell carcinoma — angioinfarction. *J Urol* 131: 24.

70 Horan JJ, Robertson CN, Choyke PL *et al.* (1989) The detection of renal carcinoma extension into the renal vein and inferior vena cava: a prospective comparison of venacavography and magnetic resonance imaging. *J Urol* 142: 943.

71 Winter P, Miersch WD, Vogel J, Jaeger N (1990) On the necessity of adrenal extirpation combined with radical nephrectomy. *J Urol* 144: 842.

72 Skinner DG, Pfister RF, Colvin R (1972) Extension of renal cell carcinoma into the vena cava: the rationale for aggressive surgical management. *J Urol* 107: 711.

73 Marshall FF, Reitz BA, Diamond DA (1984) A new technique for management of renal cell carcinoma involving the right atrium: hypothermia and cardiac arrest. *J Urol* 131: 103.

74 Pritchett RT, Lieskovsky G, Skinner DG (1986) Extension of renal cell carcinoma into the vena cava: clinical review and surgical approach. *J Urol* 135: 460.

75 Reissigl A, Janetschek G, Eberle J *et al.* (1995) Renal cell carcinoma extending into the vena cava: surgical approach, technique and results. *Br J Urol* 75: 138.

76 Davits RJAM, Blom JHM, Schroder FH (1992) Surgical management of renal carcinoma with extensive involvement of the vena cava and right atrium. *Br J Urol* 70: 591.

77 Schorn A, Marberger M (1984) Long-term survival of untreated bilateral renal cell carcinoma with supradiaphragmatic vena caval thrombus. *J Urol* 131: 108.

78 Assimos DG, Boyce WH, Woodruff RD, Harrison LH, McCullough DL, Kroovand RL (1991) Intraoperative renal ultrasonography: a useful adjunct to partial nephrectomy. *J Urol* 146: 1218.

79 Marshall FF (1984) The *in situ* surgical management of renal cell carcinoma and transitional cell carcinoma of the kidney. *World J Urol* 2: 130

80 Novick AC, Streem S, Montie JE *et al.* (1989) Conservative surgery for renal cell carcinoma: a single-center experience with 100 patients. *J Urol* 141: 835.

81 Morgan WR, Zincke H (1990) Progression and survival after renal-conserving surgery for renal cell carcinoma: experience in 104 patients and extended follow-up. *J Urol* 144: 852.

82 Tochimoto M, Matsumoto T (1994) Histological evaluation of enucleation for renal cell carcinoma using radical nephrectomy specimens. *Jap J Urol* 85: 1097.

83 Cheng WS, Farrow GM, Zincke H (1991) The incidence of multicentricity in renal cell carcinoma. *J Urol* 146: 1221.

84 Ljunberg B, Duchek M, Hietala S-O, Roos G, Stenling R (1988) Renal cell carcinoma in a solitary kidney: late nephrectomy after 35 years and analysis of tumor deoxyribonucleic acid content. *J Urol* 139: 350.

85 Herr HW (1994) Partial nephrectomy for renal cell carcinoma with a normal opposite kidney. *Cancer* 73: 160.

86 Herrlinger A, Schrott KM, Sigel A, Giedl J (1984) Results of 381 transabdominal radical nephrectomies for renal cell carcinoma with partial and complete *en-bloc* lymph node dissection. *World J Urol* 2: 114.

87 Robson CJ (1982) The natural history of renal cell carcinoma. *Prog Clin Biol Res* 100: 447.

88 Cockburn AG, White R de V (1984) Chemotherapy of advanced renal adenocarcinoma. *World J Urol* 2: 136.

89 Peeling WB, Mantell BS, Shepheard BGF (1969) Post-operative irradiation in the treatment of renal cell carcinoma. *Br J Urol* 41: 23.

90 Finney R (1973) The value of radiotherapy in the treatment of hypernephroma: a clinical trial. *Br J Urol* 45: 259.

91 Freed SZ, Halperin JP, Gordon M (1977) Idiopathic regression of metastases from renal cell carcinoma. *J Urol* 118: 538.

92 van der Werf-Messing B, van Gilse HA (1971) Hormonal treatment of metastases of renal carcinoma. *Br J Cancer* 25: 423.

93 Pizzocaro G, Piva L, Salvioni R, Di Fronzo G, Ronchi E, Miodini P and the Lombardy Group (1986) Adjuvant medroxyprogesterone acetate and steroid hormone receptors in category Mo renal cell carcinoma. An interim report of a prospective randomised study. *J Urol* 135: 18.

94 Garnick MB, Reich SD, Maxwell B, Coval-Goldsmith S, Richie JP, Rudnick SA (1988) Phase I/II study of recombinant interferon gamma in advanced renal cell carcinoma. *J Urol* 139: 251.

95 Grups JW, Frohmuller HGW (1989) Cyclic interferon gamma treatment of patients with metastatic renal carcinoma. *Br J Urol* 64: 218.

96 Rosenthal MA, Cox K, Raghavan D *et al.* (1992) Phase II clinical trial of recombinant alpha-2 interferon for biopsy-proven metastatic or recurrent renal carcinoma. *Br J Urol* 69: 491.

97 Onishi T, Machida T, Masuda F et al. (1991) Assessment of tumour-infiltrating lymphocytes, regional lymph node lymphocytes and peripheral blood lymphocytes and their reaction to interferon gamma in patients with renal carcinoma. Br J Urol 67: 459.

98 Fossa SD, Raabe N, Moe B (1989) Recombinant interferon-alpha with or without vinblastine in metastatic renal carcinoma. Br J Urol 64: 468.

99 Schornagel JH, Verweij J, ten Bokkel Huinink WW et al. (1989) Phase II study of recombinant interferon alpha 2A and vinblastine in advanced renal cell carcinoma. J Urol 142: 253.

100 Manyonda IT, Shaw DE, Foulkes A, Osborn DE (1986) Renal cell carcinoma: blood transfusion and survival. Br Med J 293: 537.

101 Moffat LEF, Sunderland GT, Lamont D (1987) Blood transfusion and survival following nephrectomy for carcinoma of kidney. Br J Urol 60: 316.

102 Onishi T, Machida T, Masuda F et al. (1989) Nephrectomy in renal carcinoma with distant metastasis. Br J Urol 63: 600.

103 Kurth KH, Cinqualbre J, Oliver RTD, Schulman CC (1984) Embolization and subsequent nephrectomy in metastatic renal cell carcinoma. World J Urol 2: 122.

104 Ozen H, Colowick A, Freiha FS (1993) Incidentally discovered solid renal masses: what are they? Br J Urol 72: 274.

105 Nakano E, Iwasaki A, Seguchi I, Kikado Y, Sugao H, Koide T (1992) Incidentally diagnosed renal cell carcinoma. Eur Urol 21: 294.

106 Ueda T, Yasumasu T, Uozumi J, Naito S (1991) Comparison of clinical and pathological characteristics in incidentally detected and suspected renal carcinoma. Br J Urol 68: 470.

107 Thijseen AM, Carpenter B, Jimenez C, Schillinger J (1989) Multilocular cyst (multilocular cystic nephroma) of the kidney: a report of two cases with an unusual mode of presentation. J Urol 142: 346.

108 Frydenberg M, Malek RS, Zincke H (1993) Conservative renal surgery for renal cell carcinoma in von Hippel—Lindau's disease. J Urol 149: 461.

109 Steiner MS, Goldman SM, Fishman EK, Marshall FF (1993) The natural history of renal angiomyolipoma. J Urol 150: 1782.

110 Koike H, Muller SC, Hohenfellner R (1994) Management of renal angiomyolipoma: a report of 14 cases and review of the literature. Eur Urol 25: 183.

111 Blute ML, Malek RS, Segura JW (1988) Angiomyolipoma: clinical metamorphosis and concepts for management. J Urol 139: 20.

112 Kennelly MJ, Grossman HB, Cho KJ (1994) Outcome analysis of 42 cases of renal angiomyolipoma. J Urol 152: 1988.

113 Taylor RS, Joseph DB, Kohaut EC, Wilson ER, Bueschen AJ (1989) Renal angiomyolipoma associated with lymph node involvement and renal cell carcinoma in patients with tuberous sclerosis. J Urol 141: 930.

114 Person Y (1992) Renal transplantation in tuberous sclerosis. Br Med J 305: 313.

115 Webb DW, Osborne JP (1992) New research in tuberous sclerosis. Br Med J 304: 1647.

116 Lowe BA, Brewer J, Houghton DC, Jacobson E, Pitre T (1992) Malignant transformation of angiomyolipoma. J Urol 147: 1356.

117 Tong YC, Chieng PU, Tsai TC, Lin SC (1990) Renal angiomyolipoma: report of 24 cases. Br J Urol 66: 585.

118 Appell RA, Thistlethwaite JR (1977) Leiomyosarcoma of renal vein. Urology 9: 680.

119 Lindop GMB, Leckie BJ, Mimran A (1993) Renin-secreting tumors, in: Robertson JIS, Nicholls GM (eds) The Renin—Angiotensin System, pp. 54.1—54.12. London: Gower Medical Publishing.

120 Schwartz CB, Bekirov H, Melman A (1992) Urothelial tumors of upper tract following treatment of primary bladder transitional cell carcinoma. Urology 40: 509.

121 Benningtson JL, Beckwith JB (1975) Tumours of the kidney, renal pelvis and ureter, in: Atlas of Tumor Pathology, 12. Washington DC: Armed Forces Institute of Pathology.

122 Greenland JE, Weston PMT, Wallace DMA (1993) Familial transitional cell carcinoma and the Lynch syndrome II. Br J Urol 72: 177.

123 Pommer W (1989) Regular analgesic intake and the risk of end stage renal failure. Am J Nephrol 9: 403.

124 Johansson S, Angervall L, Bengtsson U et al. (1974) Uroepithelial tumors of the renal pelvis associated with abuse of phenacitin-containing analgesics. Cancer 33: 743.

125 Kench P (1977) Analgesic nephropathy complicated by development of transitional cell carcinoma of the renal pelvis and ureter. Med J Austral 2: 607.

126 Steffens J, Nagel R (1988) Tumours of the renal pelvis and ureter: observations in 170 patients. Br J Urol 61: 277.

127 Balkan Endemic Nephropathy (BEN) (1991) Two International Workshops, Belgrade, Yugoslavia. Kidney Int Suppl 34: 1.

128 Auld CD, Grigor KM, Fowler JW (1984) Histopathological review of transitional cell carcinoma of the upper urinary tract. Br J Urol 56: 485.

129 Booth CM, Cameron KM, Pugh RCB (1980) Urothelial carcinoma of the kidney and ureter. Br J Urol 52: 430.

130 Schultz RE, Boyle DE (1988) Inverted papilloma of renal pelvis associated with contralateral ureteral malignancy and bladder recurrence. J Urol 139: 111.

131 Page CM, Nelson JH, Drago JR (1991) Multifocal synchronous inverted papillomas involving the ureter. J Urol 145: 357.

132 Mazeman E (1976) Tumours of the upper urinary tract calyces, renal pelvis and ureter. Eur Urol 2: 120.

133 Anselmo G, Rissotti A, Felici E, Bassi E, Maccatrozzo L (1987) Multiple simultaneous bilateral urothelial tumours of the renal pelvis. Br J Urol 60: 312.

134 Mills C, Vaughan ED (1983) Carcinoma of the ureter: natural history, management and 5-year survival. J Urol 129: 275.

135 Mufti GR, Gove JRW, Badenoch DF et al. (1989) Transitional cell carcinoma of the renal pelvis and ureter. Br J Urol 63: 135.

136 Nielsen K, Ostri P (1988) Primary tumors of the renal pelvis: evaluation of clinical and pathological

features in a consecutive series of 10 years. *J Urol* 140: 19.

137 Woodhouse CRJ (1989) Conservative versus radical surgery for renal transitional cell carcinoma and adenocarcinoma, in: Oliver RTD, Blandy JP, Hope-Stone HF (eds) *Urological and Genital Cancer*, pp. 171−5. Oxford: Blackwell Scientific Publications.

138 Richie JP (1988) Carcinoma of the renal pelvis and ureter, in: Skinner DG, Lieskovsky G (eds) *Diagnosis and Management of Genitourinary Cancer*, pp. 323−36. Philadelphia: WB Saunders.

139 Abercrombie GF, Eardley I, Payne SR, Walmsley BH, Vinnicombe J (1988) Modified nephroureterectomy. Long term follow up with particular reference to subsequent bladder tumours. *Br J Urol* 61: 198.

140 McDonald JR, Priestley JT (1944) Carcinoma of the renal pelvis. *J Urol* 51: 245.

141 Grabstald H, Whitmore WF, Melamed MR (1971) Renal pelvic tumors. *J Am Med Assoc* 218: 845.

142 Wallace DMA, Wallace DM, Whitfield HN, Hendry WF, Wickham JEA (1981) The late results of conservative surgery for upper tract urothelial carcinomas. *Br J Urol* 53: 537.

143 Ziegelbaum M, Novick AC, Streem SB, Montie J E, Pontes JE, Straffon RA (1987) Conservative surgery for transitional cell carcinoma of the renal pelvis. *J Urol* 138: 1146.

144 Woodhouse CRJ, Kellett MJ, Bloom HJG (1986) Percutaneous renal surgery and local radiotherapy in the management of renal pelvic transitional cell carcinoma. *Br J Urol* 58: 245.

145 Huang A, Low RK, White R deV (1995) Nephrostomy tract tumor seeding following percutaneous manipulation of a ureteral carcinoma. *J Urol* 153: 1041.

146 Reitelman C, Sawczuk IS, Olsson CA, Puchner PJ, Benson MC (1987) Prognostic variables in patients with transitional cell carcinoma of the renal pelvis and proximal ureter. *J Urol* 138: 1144.

147 Babaian RJ, Johnson DE (1980) Primary carcinoma of the ureter. *J Urol* 123: 357.

148 Fair WR (1988) Personal communication to JPB.

149 Wan J, Ohl DA, Weatherbee L (1993) Primary mucinous adenocarcinoma of renal pelvis in solitary pelvic kidney. *Urology* 41: 292.

Chapter 13: Kidney and ureter — calculi

The history of surgery begins with the surgery of stones, and urologists can authenticate their claim to seniority by referring to Hippocrates who enjoined doctors to leave cutting for stone to those who had specialized in that art.

Epidemiology

The reported incidence of stones in the urinary tract varies widely, suggesting that there may be factors in the diet or water which favour stone formation — the so-called 'stone belts'. This concept must be viewed with caution: more stones are found the more they are looked for. In Europe, the steady increase in the incidence of urinary calculi was interrupted by World War I and II [1]. This was attributed to dietary changes, but it could equally reflect the availability of doctors. Today in Europe calculi are common: almost 20% of doctors get stones, surgeons more than anaesthetists, who in turn get more than general practitioners [2].

Aetiology

Background

In the formation of a urinary calculus, several of the following factors often occur.

Nucleation

Crystals form on nuclei, and for stones this can be a foreign body such as a non-absorbable suture, the fragment of a catheter, necrotic tissue, bacteria or another stone [3,4].

Precipitation

The common solutes which form calculi, calcium and oxalate, are present in normal urine in concentrations which exceed the normal solubility product [3,4] (Fig. 13.1). In some disorders a metabolic abnormality causes the urine to have an abnormal amount of the solute, but more

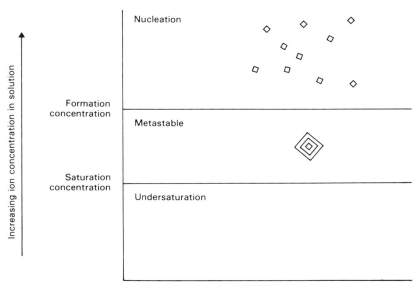

Fig. 13.1 Effects of increasing ion concentration in the urine.

often the absolute quantities are not greater, but the urine has become more concentrated, making precipitation inevitable, hence the importance of keeping the urine well diluted in any therapeutic regime, and the importance of heat, shortage of water, and endemic diarrhoeal diseases in the epidemiology of calculous disease [5].

Protective factors

There are proteins in urine which impart their electrical charge to the crystals which they coat and keep them in suspension by repelling each other [3,6]. Magnesium ions in the urine may play a part in this.

Other proteins have the contrary effect and stick the particles together: one of these is the Tamm−Horsfall protein secreted by renal tubules [7].

Urine pH

Some crystals (e.g. calcium phosphate) are more soluble in acid urine; others (e.g. uric acid and cystine) are more soluble in alkaline urine.

Matrix

It is not enough that crystals should precipitate in the urine: loose grains would be flushed out the next time the patient passed urine. Another factor is always present, the protein matrix, which glues particles together into a coherent mass [8]. Matrix forms from 2.5 to 60% of the dry weight of stones, even those in which supersaturation is the most obvious underlying factor, e.g. uric acid and cystine calculi.

Common forms of calculi

Against this background it is appropriate to consider some of the different types of stone.

Cystine

Cystinuria is the purest example of the simple supersaturation stone. A defect in the cellular transport of four amino acids, cystine, ornithine, arginine and lysine, is inherited as an autosomal dominant. Homozygous patients pass about 1 g cystine every 24 h, heterozygous patients about half this quantity. The homozygous cystinuric will almost inevitably form stones [9,10].

Uric acid

Uric acid is filtered in the glomeruli, reabsorbed in the proximal and secreted again in the distal tubule. It is more soluble in alkaline than in acid urine.

Some uric acid stone formers have a normal load of uric acid in the urine, but secrete a persistently acid urine. Others have an excessive load of uric acid, e.g. in gout, protein hypercatabolism after chemotherapy for cancer, or with thiazide diuretics. As a general rule, one must expect about a quarter of those with gout to have stones and about a quarter of those with uric acid stones to have gout.

Dehydration from heat or diarrhoeal disease is the main factor in causing uric acid stones in the tropics [5] where they are a common cause of obstructive anuria [11].

Xanthine stones

Patients given allopurinol to inhibit xanthine oxidase and prevent xanthine turning into uric acid may form calculi from the excess of xanthine in the urine.

Silicate stones

Excessive consumption of magnesium trisilicate for indigestion over a long period of time may result in silicate calculi forming in the urinary tract. These are usually radiolucent.

Calcium stones

The most common type of stone is made of calcium oxalate. Some patients with stones have an excessive quantity of calcium in their urine (hypercalciuria), others have an excess of oxalate. Excess of either will result in exceeding the solubility product of calcium oxalate [3,4].

Hypercalciuria

Hypercalciuria can be classified into three types: absorptive, resorptive and renal [12].

In absorptive hypercalciuria an excessive proportion of dietary calcium is absorbed, possibly from undue sensitivity of the bowel to vitamin D. If dietary calcium is restricted the urinary levels fall, rebounding when calcium is restored.

In resorptive hypercalciuria an excess of parathyroid hormone increases the resorption of calcium from bones as well as increased bone destruction. There is an elevated level of para-thyroid hormone and plasma calcium.

In renal hypercalciuria there is a 'renal leak' of calcium, of unknown cause, which results in a low plasma calcium. This may give rise to secondary hyperparathyroidism (see p. 66).

Hyperoxaluria

Most of the oxalate in the urine comes from metabolism but some comes from food, particularly citrus fruits, rhubarb, coffee, cola drinks, chocolate and tea. Hyperoxaluria is seen in three forms: genetic, toxic and intestinal [12].

Genetic hyperoxaluria. In this group of autosomal recessive disorders there are deficiencies of the enzymes glyoxalate carboligase or D-glycerate dehydrogenase which result in an excess of oxalate being formed and finding its way into the urine, which contains more than 100 mg a day. Oxalate crystals accumulate in the soft tissues of the body and multiple stones accumulate in the kidney and lead to renal failure. Renal transplantation alone is futile because more oxalate forms in the new kidney but may be successful if a liver transplant is put in at the same time to supply the missing enzymes.

Toxic hyperoxaluria. Ethylene glycol poisoning, overdose of ascorbic acid and some fluorocarbons cause deposits of oxalate.

Intestinal hyperoxaluria. Bile acids are absorbed in the distal ileum, to be re-excreted in the bile.

In malabsorption of many types, e.g. Crohn's disease, there is a failure in the reabsorption of these fatty acids, a lack of them in bile and a failure to absorb dietary fat which binds with the calcium that will normally have bound to oxalate, and an excess of oxalate is absorbed (Fig. 13.2). Cholestyramine and aluminium antacids may take up the surplus oxalate.

Infection stones

These stones occur in association with infection by urea-splitting organisms, notably *Proteus*, *Klebsiella* and *Pseudomonas* which make the urine alkaline. The stones are a mixture of magnesium ammonium phosphate, calcium phosphate and calcium carbonate ($MgNH_4PO_4$ and $Ca_{19}[PO_4]_6 CO_3$). It resembles the mineral struvite, a useful shorthand term. Struvite forms in the presence of infection or on a foreign body such as an unabsorbable suture or an indwelling catheter. Successive shells of struvite often form around a core of uric acid or cystine if the urinary tract becomes infected.

Renal tubular acidosis

These patients have a defect in the metabolism of the distal renal tubule which may be inherited as an autosomal dominant trait (see p. 61). There are low levels of plasma bicarbonate and potassium, and an inability to acidify the urine below pH 6. Multiple small stones form in the kidneys (nephrocalcinosis), the calculi sometimes being formed of pure calcium phosphate [13].

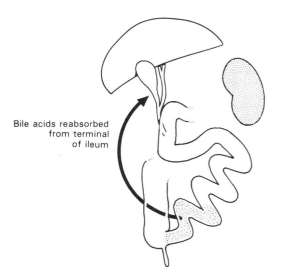

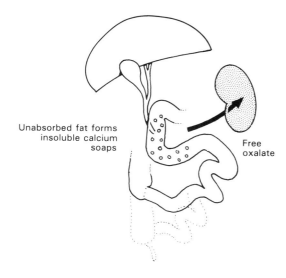

Bile acids reabsorbed from terminal of ileum

Unabsorbed fat forms insoluble calcium soaps

Free oxalate

Fig. 13.2 Hyperoxaluria from disease or loss of the terminal ileum.

Stone formation in a cavity

Wherever there is a large collection of stagnant urine, e.g. hydronephrosis, hydrocalicosis, chronic retention of urine in the bladder or a diverticulum, stones tend to form. These are usually a mixture of calcium oxalate and struvite, for secondary infection is common by the time the diagnosis is made. They are typically smooth and rounded like pebbles (Fig. 13.3).

Formation of calculi in the kidney

There are four mechanisms of formation of calculi in the kidney.

Concretions

Most stones that form in a papilla begin as multiple minute calcium oxalate stones [14] (Fig. 13.4). Later, an accumulation of these minute concretions forms a layer under the tip of the papilla — Randall's plaque. This subsequently separates into the lumen of the calix [15].

Papillary necrosis

A second mechanism for stone formation in the renal papilla is ischaemic necrosis seen with many of the conditions that cause interstitial nephritis (see p. 149). The dead papilla acts as a nucleus for secondary accumulation of calcium oxalate or struvite (see p. 153).

Medullary sponge kidney

In this condition (see p. 103) the renal collecting tubules become grossly dilated. Stones may form as a result of stasis, but there may also be an element of renal tubular acidosis. The condition may appear in one calix and gradually spread through the kidney (Fig. 13.5). Its cause is

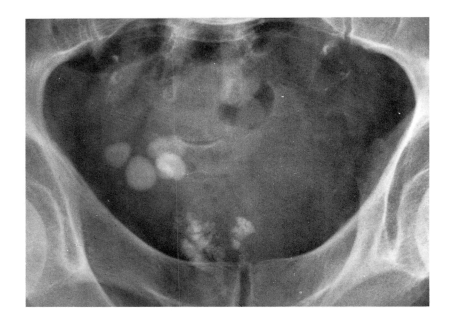

Fig. 13.3 Stones which form in stagnant urine are smooth and round as in this bladder with chronic retention.

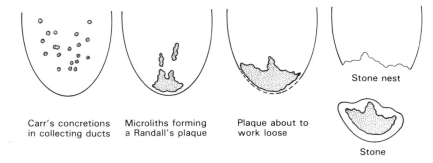

Carr's concretions in collecting ducts   Microliths forming a Randall's plaque   Plaque about to work loose   Stone nest   Stone

Fig. 13.4 Most calculi originate in the kidney as Carr's concretions in the collecting tubules, which accumulate to form Randall's plaques in the papillae, which finally work loose.

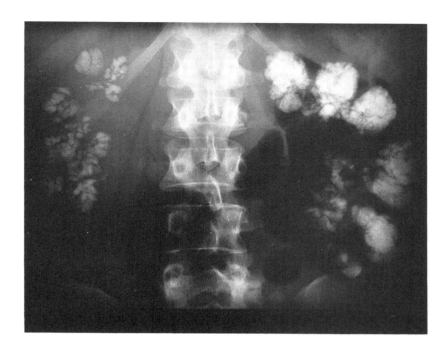

Fig. 13.5 Bilateral medullary sponge kidney showing multiple calculi in the dilated collecting tubules (courtesy of Dr Otto Chan).

unknown, but it is associated with unilateral hemihypertrophy and other congenital conditions such as aniridia [16].

Hydronephrosis and hydrocalix

A fourth type of stone is seen in a chronically dilated renal pelvis or calix: these stones are usually multiple and rounded and may be so numerous that they are called 'milk of calcium stones'.

Recumbency stones

In spinal injury and major trauma, stone formation was once a common complication. There were several contributing factors: hypercalciuria from loss of calcium from the skeleton resulting from inactivity, urinary infection and dehydration. Frequent turning, early mobilization and active treatment of infection can largely prevent this condition [17].

Pathological complications of stones

Renal stones

The most important complication of a stone is obstruction, giving rise to acute or chronic hydronephrosis. When this is further complicated by infection, there may be septicaemia, cortical abscesses, perirenal abscess, erosion into the bowel [18] and xanthogranuloma (see p. 163). Very rarely metaplasia in the urothelium adjacent to a chronic stone leads to squamous cell carcinoma or adenocarcinoma (see p. 210).

Stones in the ureter

If the ureteric calculus is less than 4mm in diameter there is a 92% chance that it will pass spontaneously after a few episodes of ureteric colic [19] and indeed about 60% of all ureteric stones pass spontaneously [20,21]. Nevertheless, even the smallest stones are not without their dangers: when they are causing complete obstruction, there is a risk of septicaemia if the urine is infected because of the backflow of urine into renal veins and lymphatics (see p. 141).

There is also a remote but well-documented risk of reflex renal shutdown from spasm of the contralateral calices and ureter [22].

In the course of time oedema of the wall of the ureter can develop around the stone, however small, which may mimic a urothelial cancer of the ureter (see p. 201).

Stones which get stuck in the ureter for many months may form little pockets past which urine flows without impediment. Sometimes these become infected and erode into adjacent viscera such as the appendix or fallopian tube.

Stones in the bladder

Most stones which are small enough to pass out of the ureter into the bladder will be voided via the urethra. The exception, now rare in the West, occurs in little boys whose urethrae are relatively narrow. Stones that start off in the ureter linger in the bladder, act as a nucleus for the deposition of successive shells of calcium oxalate or struvite and grow so large that it is impossible for them to pass through the urethra.

In the West, bladder stones are only seen in men when there is existing outflow obstruction. In women, there is usually a foreign body at the centre of a stone, e.g. a fragment of a Foley catheter or a non-absorbable suture (Fig. 13.6).

Just as the trauma of a stone gives rise to metaplasia of the urothelium in the kidney, so also in the bladder long-standing calculi may lead to squamous metaplasia and cancer.

Stones in the prostate

These arise in dilated prostatic ducts, usually on a nucleus of corpora amylacea and are often secondarily infected (see p. 378).

Stones in the urethra

Urethral stones are still common in the tropics. The stone travels through the ureter, grows a little in the bladder and then gets stuck at the external urinary meatus. Stones are also seen in urethral diverticula, as in any other undrained pocket of urine (see p. 457).

Clinical features of urinary calculi

Kidney

Pain in the kidney is experienced in the distribution of the dermatomes T9–T11, in the loin radiating down to the testicle and groin. When there is acute dilatation, the pain is colicky: in other circumstances the stone may be entirely silent or cause a vague backache.

Sometimes it is difficult to believe that a small caliceal calculus, without any dilatation, could possibly give rise to pain. Nevertheless, experience shows that removing such a stone may relieve the pain permanently.

Some of the least obtrusive of all stones are the giant staghorn calculi (Fig. 13.7) which are nearly always made of struvite and caused by *Proteus mirabilis*. These stones may be silent, but they are not safe, and the risks of pyonephrosis and sepsis far outweigh the risks even of open surgery, let alone those of combinations of percutaneous nephrolithotomy (PCNL) and extracorporeal shockwave lithotripsy (ESWL) [23,24].

Ureter

Acute ureteric colic strikes without warning. The pain comes in waves. Dysfunction of the overlying intestine — probably caused by extravasation of urine into the retroperitoneal tissues — leads to vomiting and dilatation of the bowel which may mimic intestinal obstruction, and has led to many a mistaken laparotomy.

There is often a trace of blood in the urine passed at the time of the attack.

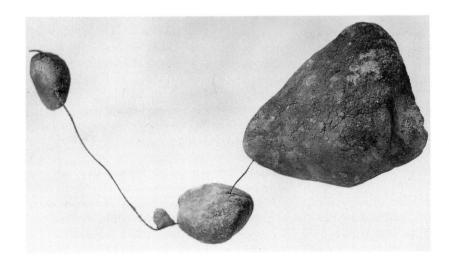

Fig. 13.6 Multiple stones which had formed on a nylon suture in the bladder.

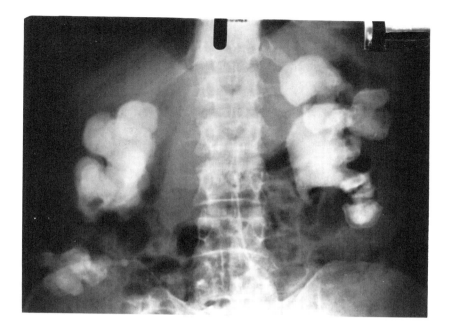

Fig. 13.7 Bilateral giant staghorn calculi: these were almost symptomless in life.

If there is infection in the urine there may be septicaemia with all its sequelae.

Bladder

Stones in the bladder give pain referred typically to the tip of the penis. It is relieved by lying down, and made worse by standing up and moving about. There is frequency and pain on voiding and the last drops of urine are often bloodstained. Most patients with a bladder calculus also have long-standing prostatic outflow obstruction, whose symptoms predominate, the stone being found only by chance in the course of investigation.

Investigations

Investigation of a patient with symptoms suggesting a stone in any part of the urinary tract has three objectives:
1 to make sure that the shadow is indeed a stone;
2 to find out what trouble the stone is causing so that it can be corrected; and
3 to stop it happening again.

Is the shadow really a stone?

In the kidney it is easy to mistake a calcified renal artery aneurysm or calcification in the lymph nodes for a stone. Calcification in the wall of the bladder or ureter in schistosomiasis can resemble a stone (see p. 279) as also may that caused by another extraordinary fluke *Paragonimus westermani* [23].

Phleboliths in the pelvis exactly mimic a calculus, although a computerized tomography (CT) view with contrast medium, or oblique X-rays with a catheter in the ureter, will show the shadow well away from the ureter. A calcified fibroid, teeth in an ovarian dermoid or a large stone in the ureter or prostate may all resemble stones in the bladder (Figs 13.8 & 13.9).

What trouble is the stone causing?

Urography is still the key to the diagnosis of any stone in the urinary tract since most stones are radioopaque, and most obstruction is revealed by dilatation in the urogram.

The catch is the radiolucent stone. For practical purposes these are uric acid stones (Fig. 13.10), although it is better to be aware of xanthine stones in patients who have received protracted treatment for gout, and the excessively rare silicate stones in patients given long courses of magnesium trisilicate for indigestion. The difficulty is quickly solved by ultrasound scan, supplemented where necessary by CT.

If the stone is more than 5 mm in diameter its chance of leaving the renal pelvis or completing its journey down the ureter is so small that it ought to be removed. A small stone in an outlying

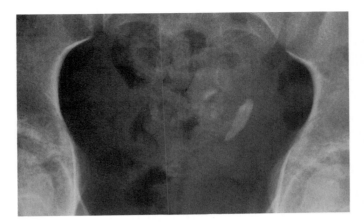

Fig. 13.8 Tooth in an ovarian dermoid, easily mistaken for a stone in the ureter (courtesy of Dr Otto Chan).

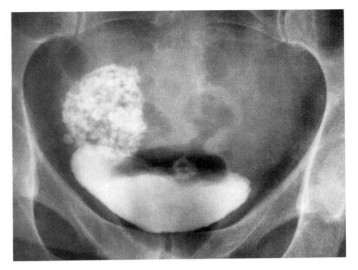

Fig. 13.9 Calcification in an ovarian fibroid, misinterpreted as a calculus in the bladder.

calix, in the absence of infection, can be safely monitored as it may not grow over 20 years.

Renal function

An error may arise if an IVU or isotope scan is performed soon after the onset of ureteric colic when it may show no 'function' in the kidney. The cause of the silent urogram in acute colic is not certain: there may be spasm of the calices and ureter or obstruction to the flow of urine along the nephron but the phenomenon is temporary and completely reversible.

How to stop it happening again

We are told that there are very few pains to compare with that of ureteric colic and patients are anxious to be spared a second episode. The investigations to be performed after a single episode or in the recurrent stone former are as follows.

The first episode

The stone must be analysed wherever possible. A new combination of scanning electron microscopy and X-ray energy dispersive spectroscopy makes it possible to make an accurate identification of the composition of the stone even from the tiny fragments obtained by sieving the urine after ESWL [24].

The urine must be cultured to rule out infection.

The plasma calcium must be measured by an accurate method and, if elevated, it should be measured again in the fasting state. If still elevated, the plasma parathyroid hormone level should be measured. Thought should be given to the possibility that hyperparathyroidism is but one feature of the multiple endocrine syndrome [25]. The localization and removal of parathyroid tumours and hyperplasia should, like cutting for stone, be left to those who specialize in this art.

This will identify all the most important causes of recurrent stone formation: it will detect the cystine stone, the uric acid stone former, the infected struvite stone and the patient whose stones are plainly secondary to some anatomical abnormality in the urinary tract.

The recurrent stone former

For the committed researcher, it is very interesting to know whether a given patient has hypercalciuria or hyperoxaluria, and to decide into which subcategory the patient falls; but if the only therapeutic measure which alters the course of the disease is to drink more water this advice can be given without any expensive investigations.

The traditional 'stone clinic investigations' are as follows.

Two 24-h specimens of urine are measured for calcium and a third specimen is measured 1 week after the patient has been on a diet low in calcium and, to show whether the patient has

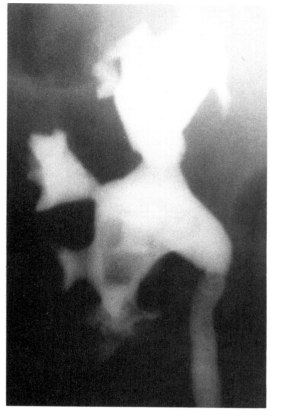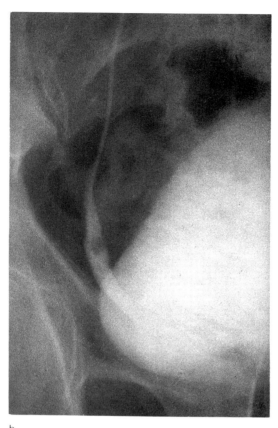

a   b

Fig. 13.10 Radiolucent urate calculi (a) in renal pelvis, and (b) in the right ureter.

absorptive hypercalciuria, this is supplemented by a calcium loading test. Urine calcium is measured after an overnight fast, and again after a dose of calcium gluconate [12].

Hyperoxaluria will be detected in these specimens as will a persistently acid pH which will raise the question of renal tubular acidosis which may call for an acid load test (see p. 59).

If the patient had absorptive hypercalciuria it was customary to place them on a low calcium diet, and give cellulose phosphate to exchange sodium for calcium in the bowel or orthophosphate to increase the amount of pyrophosphate in the urine in the hope that this would inhibit stone formation. If there was a renal leak of calcium, thiazide diuretics were given.

In practice, the low calcium diet carried a risk of osteoporosis [26]: cellulose phosphate lowered the urine magnesium and elevated the urine oxalate and was ineffective [27] — pyrophosphate caused diarrhoea and dehydration. Thiazide diuretics are cheap and safe, so long as care is taken not to allow the patient to drift into hypo-

kalaemia. However, none of these measures prevents the recurrence of calculi. It is far more important to ensure a high output of dilute urine. This being so, one must question the cost-effectiveness of putting the patient through these laborious investigations. This is not to imply that there are no effective measures against stone recurrence: on the contrary, they are valuable in hyperparathyroidism, cystine and uric acid stone disease. For the common problem of hypercalciuria they are remarkably ineffective [27].

Cystine stone. D-penicillamine and N-2-mercaptopropionyl glycine react with cysteine to form soluble compounds (Fig. 13.11), and if used in combination with a high fluid input and measures to alkalinize the urine, may not only prevent stone recurrence but actually dissolve stones *in situ* [28,29].

Uric acid stones. By a high water throughput and keeping the urine pH around 6.5 with a daily

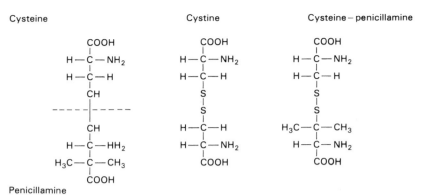

Cysteine

Cystine

Cysteine—penicillamine

Penicillamine

Fig. 13.11 Mechanism whereby penicillamine forms soluble cysteine—penicillamine.

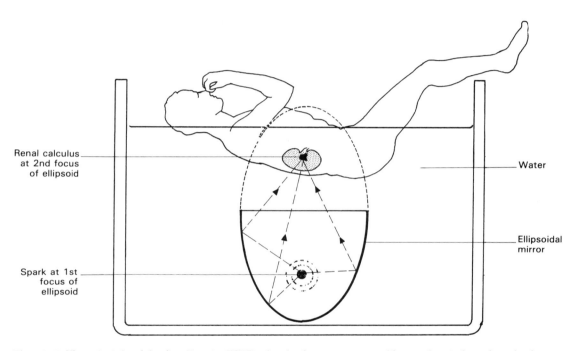

Renal calculus at 2nd focus of ellipsoid

Water

Ellipsoidal mirror

Spark at 1st focus of ellipsoid

Fig. 13.12 The principle of the first Dornier ESWL: the shockwaves generated by an electrical spark at the first focus of an ellipsoidal mirror were reflected onto the second focus where the stones were targeted using X-ray control.

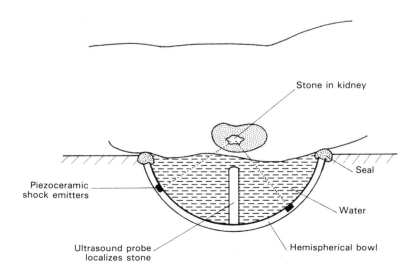

Stone in kidney

Seal

Piezoceramic shock emitters

Water

Ultrasound probe localizes stone

Hemispherical bowl

Fig. 13.13 The principle of piezo-electric lithotripsy: a battery of piezoceramic shock generators are mounted in a hemispherical dish: the shockwaves are focused on the centre of the sphere, where the stones are targeted using ultrasound.

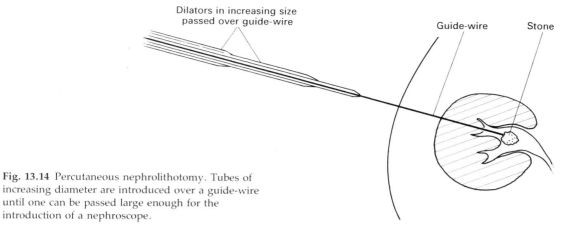

Dilators in increasing size
passed over guide-wire

Guide-wire   Stone

Fig. 13.14 Percutaneous nephrolithotomy. Tubes of increasing diameter are introduced over a guide-wire until one can be passed large enough for the introduction of a nephroscope.

dose of sodium bicarbonate of about 6 g every 24 h, it is possible to avoid subsequent stone formation, and occasionally to dissolve stones *in situ*.

Surgery for stones

For the most part, the management of renal calculi consists of active intervention. The last decade has seen an astonishing revolution in surgical technology, so much that open operations are almost completely outdated, and the surgery of renal and ureteric calculi has become a rare event [30].

The indications for active intervention remain the same: essentially all stones over 5 mm in diameter should be removed. If the stone is causing obstruction, temporary relief can be provided by percutaneous nephrostomy or a double-J stent — the latter by means of a flexible cystoscopy under local anaesthesia.

Once obstruction has been relieved infection is brought under control along the usual lines. Thereafter the management depends upon a judicious combination of ESWL, PCNL and ureteroscopy. These in turn employ a range of new lithotriptors, devices which shatter the calculi into fragments small enough to be extracted or to pass safely down the ureter.

ESWL

The principle of this device is to focus a shock-wave on the calculus. The shock is generated by a spark or an array of piezo-electric emitters (Figs 13.12 & 13.13), and transmitted through the tissues of the body to be focused at the centre of a sphere, or the second focus of an ellipse [31,32].

The stone is localized with ultrasound or X-rays.

There has been much experimental study on the geometry and physics of ESWL [32], as well as on the possible damage it may do to the kidney [33] which suffers splits, intrarenal and occasional extrarenal haemorrhage [34–36]. This may be followed by intrarenal scarring and possible subsequent renal hypertension [37].

PCNL

Having inserted a nephrostomy tube over a

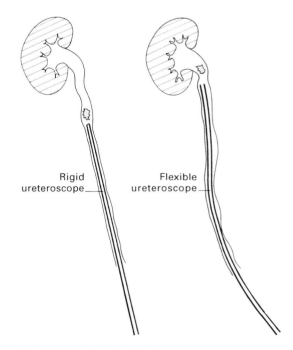

Rigid
ureteroscope

Flexible
ureteroscope

Fig. 13.15 Rigid or flexible fibreoptic ureteroscopes may be passed right up into the renal calices.

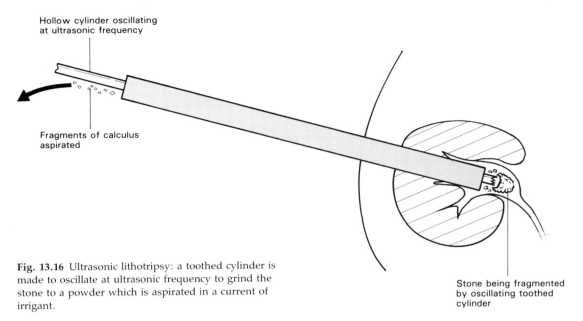

Hollow cylinder oscillating
at ultrasonic frequency

Fragments of calculus
aspirated

Stone being fragmented
by oscillating toothed
cylinder

Fig. 13.16 Ultrasonic lithotripsy: a toothed cylinder is made to oscillate at ultrasonic frequency to grind the stone to a powder which is aspirated in a current of irrigant.

guide-wire, the track is dilated until a 28 Ch sheath can be passed (Fig. 13.14). This is large enough to admit telescopes, forceps and lithotriptors.

Ureteroscopy

The application of the Hopkins rod-lens system to very long thin telescopes made it possible to pass a rigid ureteroscope right up into the renal pelvis (Fig. 13.15). Very thin fibreoptic instruments have the advantage of being flexible. Through these instruments a variety of baskets, based on the original one of Dormia [38] can be used to retrieve stones, or break them up with one of the new lithotriptors.

Ultrasonic probe. A toothed cylinder is made to oscillate at ultrasonic frequency (Fig. 13.16). It grinds the surface of the stone into fine powder which is sucked away in a current of irrigant. If distilled water or glycine is used there is a hazard of dilutional hyponatraemia — the transurethral resection (TUR) syndrome [39] (see p. 1).

Electrohydraulic lithotriptor. A pair of parallel or concentric electrodes connected to a condenser emits a spark in contact with the stone (Fig. 13.17).

Jackhammer. A miniature road-drill is powered by compressed air. Of all the gadgets this appears to be the most effective and versatile. It is

also one of the least costly of these expensive implements [40,41] (Fig. 13.18).

Laser. A pulsed dye laser beam can be passed through a narrow quartz fibre to break up stones. It is particularly appropriate for the ureter, and can be passed along a flexible ureteroscope [42,43] (Fig. 13.19).

Renal calculi

Staghorn calculi

Staghorn calculi can be removed either by repeated ESWL sessions, or a combination of ESWL and PCNL. In most centres the main bulk

Concentric electrode (e.g. URAT 2 etc.)

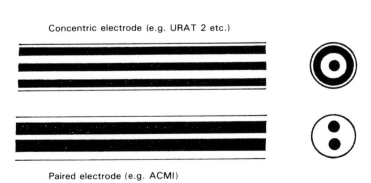

Paired electrode (e.g. ACMI)

Fig. 13.17 Electrohydraulic lithotripsy: concentric or parallel electrodes emit a spark which shatters the stone.

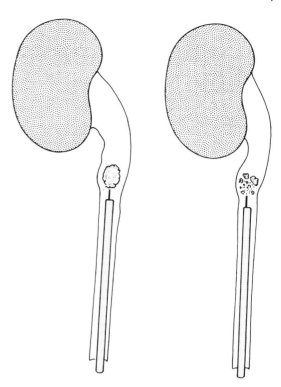

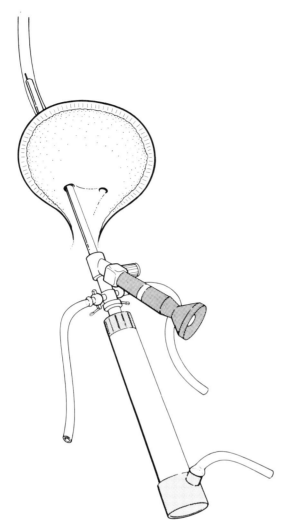

Fig. 13.19 A pulsed dye laser beam may be passed along a flexible quartz fibre to break up a calculus in the ureter.

Fig. 13.18 The Swiss lithoclast: on the principle of the jackhammer probes of varying flexibility may be passed up the ureter or into the renal pelvis to break up a stone.

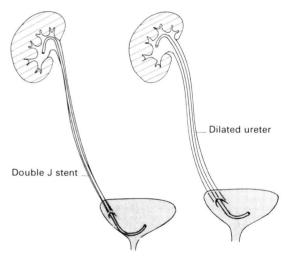

Fig. 13.20 If a double-J stent is left in the ureter, it becomes dilated and allows fragments of stone to pass down.

of the stone is removed by PCNL with the assistance of an appropriate lithotriptor. If the entire kidney can be cleared in one or two sessions this is probably the ideal method [44,45]. A double-J splint in the ureter causes the ureter to dilate, and facilitates the passage of fragments of stone down the ureter (Fig. 13.20).

PCNL is not without its complications, notably from inadvertent perforation of the pleura and colon [46].

It is always wise to allow plenty of time for the fragments to pass before repeating the ESWL [47].

The classical open operation is that of Gil-Vernet [24,48−51]. Through a 12th rib bed

approach, the kidney is mobilized and the renal artery taped (Fig. 13.21). Dissecting between the connective tissue and the muscle of the renal pelvis leads into a plane between the pelvis and

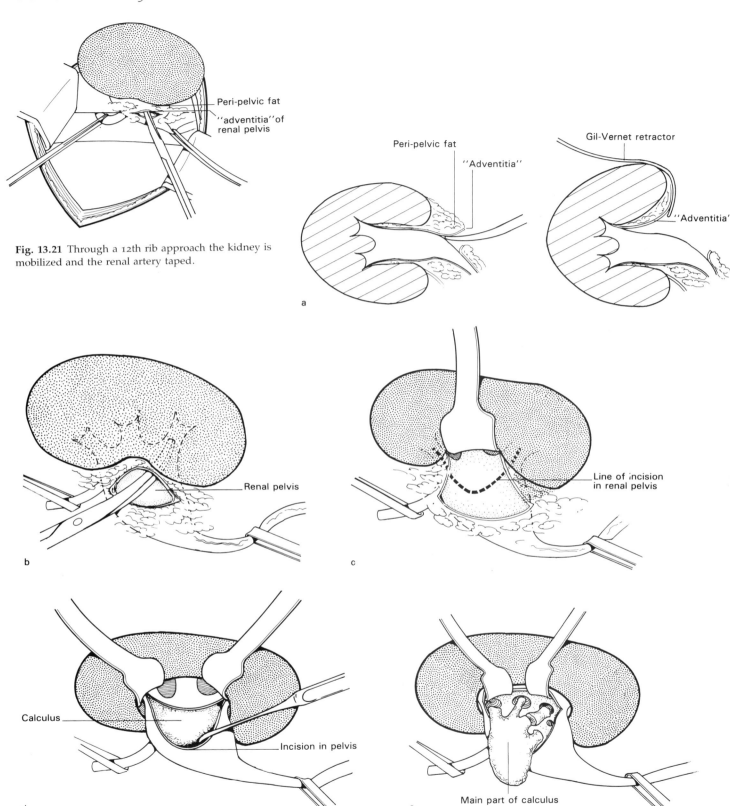

Fig. 13.21 Through a 12th rib approach the kidney is mobilized and the renal artery taped.

Fig. 13.22 Gil-Vernet operation. (a) The bloodless plane between the adventitia of the renal pelvis and its muscle is opened, and the parenchyma retracted (b) to reveal the renal pelvis, (c) which is opened from the upper to the lower calix (d) and the calculus prised out (e).

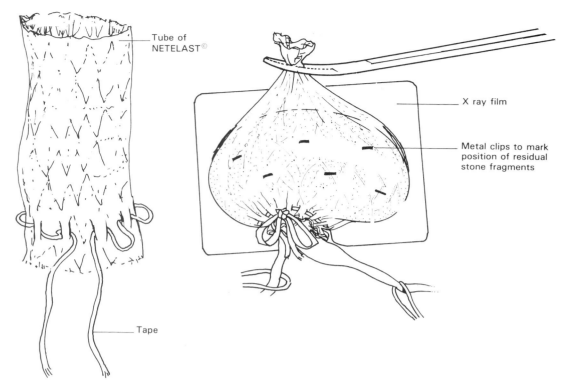

Fig. 13.23 When all the stones are thought to be removed, the kidney is suspended in a Wickham's elastic net stocking so that an X-ray can be taken *in situ*.

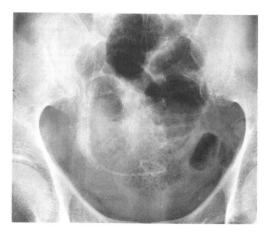

Fig. 13.24 Fragments of stone often queue up in the lower ureter to form a Steinstrasse.

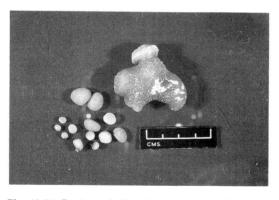

Fig. 13.25 Cystine calculi such as these, which are notoriously difficult to fragment with ESWL, are slippery and very easy to remove with the Gil-Vernet technique.

the sinus fat which can be retracted (Fig. 13.22), allowing a bloodless incision to be made from the superior to the inferior calix. This allows the bulk of the stone to be removed. Outlying mushroom projections into the dilated calices are removed through the caliceal neck, with the aid of a lithotriptor, or through radial incisions in the parenchyma if it is thin. When the parenchyma is thick, the renal artery is occluded and the kidney cooled in sterile ice slush or ice cold irrigant [52]. A coagulum of fibrin can be a useful device to extract outlying fragments from the calices [53]. A small hand-held ultrasound probe is useful in identifying the arcuate vessels so

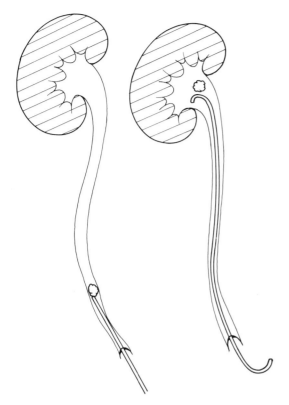

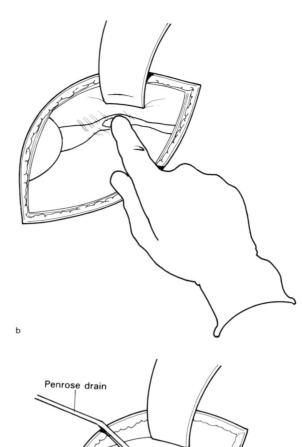

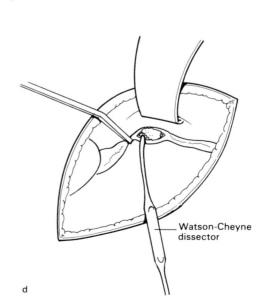

Fig. 13.26 'Push−bang': stones stuck in the ureter may be pushed back into the renal pelvis and there treated with ESWL.

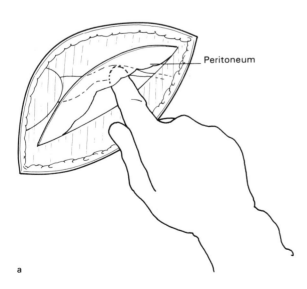

Fig. 13.27 Ureterolithotomy. (a) As soon as the stone is felt behind the peritoneum (b) a sling is passed around it to prevent it slipping up into the kidney. (c) The ureter is incised and (d) the stone prised out.

that these can be avoided when incising the parenchyma [54], and in localizing small fragments of stone. X-rays are taken on the table with a special cone fitted to the X-ray tube [51] (Fig. 13.23).

Smaller renal pelvic calculi

Smaller renal stones are easily dealt with by ESWL or PCNL, the choice being a matter of the availability of the skill and equipment. A double-J stent facilitates the passage of the stone fragments and avoids the discomfort of obstruction by a Steinstrasse (Fig. 13.24).

Cystine stones pose a special problem. The adjuvant use of N-mercaptopropionyl glycine may help reduce the recurrence rate [55]. Experience suggests that the smooth kind of cystine stone is less easy to break up [56], and there may still be a place for open surgery (Fig. 13.25).

Pyelolithotomy uses the same standard 12th rib or vertical lumbotomy approach to the kidney which is mobilized, and the renal artery taped for safety. The renal pelvis is opened in most cases between stay-sutures, the stone lifted out and the incision closed [51].

Ureteric stones

The indications for operating on stones in the ureter have not changed [40], and it is wise to refrain from operating on stones that will pass spontaneously, i.e. those less than 5 mm in diameter. ESWL can be used with modern techniques for most stones, either *in situ* or after pushing them back into the kidney with a ureteric catheter [57,58] (Fig. 13.26).

Stones in the ureter lend themselves particularly well to being fragmented through a ureteroscope [43]. There are risks when these instruments are used in the ureter with major complications, including perforation and late stenosis occurring in 2–9% [42,59,60].

Open ureterolithotomy

This is still sometimes the safest and most certain method for dealing with a stone in the ureter.

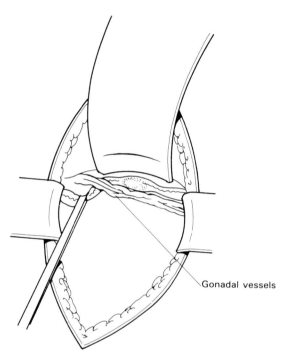

Fig. 13.28 For a stone in the middle third of the ureter be careful not to injure the gonadal vessels.

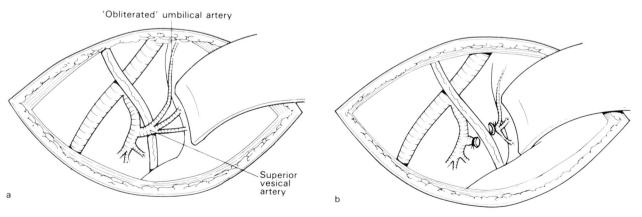

Fig. 13.29 For a stone in the lower end of the ureter the first step (a) is to divide the superior vesical vessels between ligatures to give access (b) to the ureter.

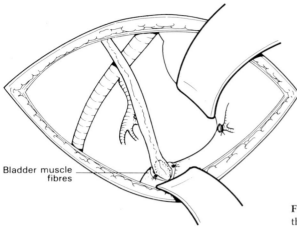

Fig. 13.30 For a stone in the intramural ureter, follow the ureter down by incising the bladder muscle.

For a stone in the upper third of the ureter make a short incision from the tip of the 12th rib forward. Approach the ureter retroperitoneally. Feel for the stone with your finger and pass a silicone rubber sling around the ureter upstream of it. Cut directly down onto the stone and prise it out with a Watson−Cheyne dissector. Close the wound with a drain, but there is no need to close the ureter. It may leak for 2 or 3 days but will heal without a stricture (Fig. 13.27).

In the middle third, a short muscle splitting incision gives excellent access. Take care to separate the gonadal vessels (Fig. 13.28). Otherwise the steps are the same as above.

In the lower third, the secret is to divide the superior vesical pedicle of the vessels first (Fig. 13.29). This liberates the ureter which can now be easily followed right down to the intramural tunnel (Fig. 13.30).

Stones in the bladder

The introduction of the lithotrite 150 years ago may be said to have started modern instrumental urology. The best instruments are still the oldest ones, not forged, but cut from a solid block of steel [61]. The skill of using this historic instrument has now been bypassed by the modern lithotriptors which can be passed down a resectoscope sheath to fragment a calculus in the bladder and the fragments evacuated with an Ellik evacuator. The Mauermayer punch is a most useful device for breaking up residual small fragments.

In boys and in patients with very large stones (Fig. 13.31), it is safer to remove them through a formal open cystotomy because the passage of

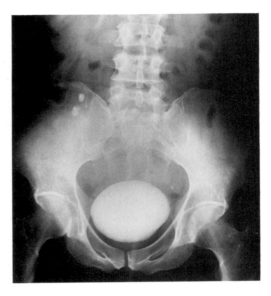

Fig. 13.31 For very large stones in the bladder an open cystotomy is still the safest technique.

urethral instruments is apt to lead to stricture [62].

References

1 Andersen DA (1969) Historical and geographical differences in the pattern of incidence of urinary stones considered in relation to possible aetiological factors, in: Hodgkinson A, Nordin BEC (eds) *Renal Stone Research Symposium*, p. 7. London: Churchill Livingstone.
2 Scott R (1971) The incidence of renal colic in the medical profession in the west of Scotland. *Health Bull (Edin)* 29: 27.
3 Ryall RL (1994) Metabolic aspects of stone disease: graven images and pipe dreams. *Curr Opinion Urol* 4: 223.

4 Gleeson MJ, Griffith DP (1993) Struvite calculi. (review). *Br J Urol* 71: 503.

5 Embon OM, Rose GA, Rosenbaum T (1990) Chronic dehydration stone disease. *Br J Urol* 66: 357.

6 Kavanagh JP, Nishio S, Garside J, Blacklock NJ (1993) Crystallization kinetics of calcium oxalate in fresh, minimally diluted urine: comparison of recurrent stone formers and healthy controls in a continuous mixed suspension mixed product removal crystallizer. *J Urol* 149: 614.

7 Yoshioka T, Koide T, Usunomiya M, Itatani H, Oka T, Sonoda T (1989) Possible role of Tamm—Horsfall glycoprotein in calcium oxalate crystallisation. *Br J Urol* 64: 463—7.

8 Boyce WH, Pool CS, Meschan I, King JS (1958) Organic matrix of urinary calculi. *Acta Radiol* 50: 544.

9 Singer A, Das S (1989) Cystinuria: a review of the pathophysiology and management. *J Urol* 142: 669.

10 Sakhaee K, Poindexter JR, Pak CYC (1989) The spectrum of metabolic abnormalities in patients with cystine nephrolithiasis. *J Urol* 141: 819.

11 Ansari ER, Kazim E, Husain I (1982) Management of the choked ureter in obstructive renal failure due to uric acid lithiasis. *J Urol* 128: 257.

12 Pak CYC (1991) Medical diagnosis of nephrolithiasis, in: Marberger M, Fitzpatrick JM, Jenkins AD, Pak CYC (eds) *Stone Surgery*, pp. 277—91. Edinburgh: Churchill Livingstone.

13 Cochran M, Peacock M, Smith DA, Nordin BEC (1968) Renal tubular acidosis of pyelonephritis with renal stone disease. *Br Med J* 2: 721.

14 Carr RJ (1969) Aetiology of renal calculi: microradiographic studies, in: Hodgkinson A, Nordin BEC (eds) *Renal Stone Research Symposium*, p. 123. London: Churchill Livingstone.

15 Randall A (1937) The origin and growth of renal calculi. *Ann Surg* 105: 1009.

16 Steyn J, Logie NJ (1964) Medullary sponge kidney. *Br J Urol* 36: 482.

17 Comarr AE (1955) A long term survey of the incidence of renal calculosis in paraplegia. *J Urol* 74: 447.

18 Montgomery BSI, Cole RS, Palfrey ELH *et al.* (1988) Spontaneous renocolic fistula secondary to calculous pyonephrosis. *Urology* 31: 147.

19 Sandegaard E (1956) Prognosis of stone in the ureter. *Acta Chir Scand Suppl* 219.

20 Morse RM, Resnick MI (1991) Ureteral calculi: natural history and treatment in an era of advanced technology. *J Urol* 145: 263.

21 Ibrahim AIA, Shetty SD, Awad RM, Patel KP (1991) Prognostic factors in the conservative treatment of ureteric stones. *Br J Urol* 67: 358.

22 Thurston SB, Foord KD (1993) Reflex renal shutdown. *Br J Urol* 71: 233.

23 Lin C-M, Chen S-K (1993) Paragonimus calcified ova mimicking left renal staghorn stone. *J Urol* 149: 819.

24 Bowsher WG, Crocker P, Ramsay JWA, Whitfield HN (1990) Single urine sample diagnosis: a new concept in stone analysis. *Br J Urol* 65: 236.

25 Samaan NA, Ouais S, Ordonez NG, Choksi UA, Sellin RV, Hickey RC (1989) Multiple endocrine syndrome type I. *Cancer* 64: 741.

26 Fuss M, Pepersack T, Bergman P, Hurard T, Simon T, Corvilain J (1990) Low calcium diet in idiopathic urolithiasis: a risk factor for osteopenia as great as in primary hyperparathyroidism. *Br J Urol* 65: 560.

27 Marickar JMF, Rose GA (1985) Relationship of stone growth and urinary biochemistry in long-term follow-up of stone patients with idiopathic hypercalciuria. *Br J Urol* 57: 613.

28 Martin X, Salas M, Labeeuw M, Pozet N, Gelet A, Dubernard JM (1991) Cystine stones: the impact of new treatment. *Br J Urol* 68: 234.

29 Kachel TA, Vijan SR, Dretler SP (1991) Endourological experience with cystine calculi and a treatment algorithm. *J Urol* 145: 25.

30 Rassweilwer J, Koehrmann KU, Alken P (1992) ESWL including imaging. *Curr Opinion Urol* 2: 291.

31 Riehle RA, Newman RC (eds) (1987) *Principles of Extracorporeal Shockwave Lithotripsy.* Edinburgh: Churchill Livingstone.

32 Hunter PT (1987) The physics and geometry pertinent to ESWL, in: Riehle RA, Newman RC (eds) *Principles of Extracorporeal Shockwave Lithotripsy*, pp. 13—27. Edinburgh: Churchill Livingstone.

33 Newman RC (1987) Clinical and experimental effects associated with ESWL, in: Riehle RA, Newman RC (eds) *Principles of Extracorporeal Shockwave Lithotripsy*, pp. 31—41. Edinburgh: Churchill Livingstone.

34 Coptcoat MJ, Webb DR, Kellett MJ *et al.* (1986) The complications of extracorporeal shockwave lithotripsy: management and prevention. *Br J Urol* 58: 578.

35 Donahue LA, Linke CA, Rowe JM (1989) Renal loss following extracorporeal shock wave lithotripsy. *J Urol* 142: 809.

36 Abrahams C, Lipson S, Ross L (1988) Pathologic changes in the kidneys and other organs of dogs undergoing extracorporeal shock wave lithotripsy with a tubeless lithotripter. *J Urol* 140: 391.

37 Shuttleworth KED (1989) Does extracorporeal shockwave lithotripsy cause hypertension? *Br J Urol* 64: 567.

38 Dormia E (1982) Dormia basket: standard technique, observations, and general concepts. *Urology* 20: 437.

39 Sinclair JF, Hutchison A, Baraza R, Telfer ABM (1985) Absorption of 1.5% glycine after percutaneous ultrasonic lithotripsy for renal stone disease. *Br Med J* 291: 691.

40 Schulze H, Haupt G, Piergiovanni M, Wisard M, von Niederhausern W, Senge T (1993) The Swiss lithoclast: a new device for endoscopic stone disintegration. *J Urol* 149: 15.

41 Schmidt A, Rassweiler J, Gumpinger R, Mayer R, Eisenberger F (1990) Minimally invasive treatment of ureteric calculi using modern techniques. *Br J Urol* 65: 242.

42 Bagley DH (1992) Endoscopic laser lithotripsy. *Curr Opinion Urol* 2: 300.

43 McDermott JP, Grove J, Clark PB (1993) Laser lithotripsy with the Candela MDL-2000 laser tripter. *Br J Urol* 71: 512.

44 Dawson C, Whitfield HN (1994) The long term results of treatment of urinary stones (review). *Br J Urol* 74: 397.

45 Dickinson IK, Fletcher MS, Bailey MJ *et al.* (1986) Combination of percutaneous surgery and extra-

corporeal shockwave lithotripsy for the treatment of large renal calculi. *Br J Urol* 58: 581.

46 Vallancien G, Capdeville R, Veillon B, Charton M, Brisset JM (1985) Colonic perforation during percutaneous nephrolithotomy. *J Urol* 134: 1185.

47 Fegan J, Camp LA, Wilson WT, Preminger CM (1993) Treatment philosophy and retreatment rates following piezoelectric lithotripsy. *J Urol* 149: 12.

48 Singh M, Chapman R, Tresidder GC, Blandy JP (1973) The fate of the unoperated staghorn calculus. *Br J Urology* 45: 581.

49 Woodhouse CRJ, Farrell CR, Paris AMI, Blandy JP (1981) The place of extended pyelolithotomy (Gil-Vernet operation) in the management of renal staghorn calculi. *Br J Urol* 53: 520.

50 Wickham JEA (ed.) (1979) *Urinary Calculus Disease.* Edinburgh: Churchill Livingstone.

51 Wickham JEA (ed.) (1984) *Intrarenal Surgery.* Edinburgh: Churchill Livingstone.

52 Marshall V, Blandy JP (1974) Simple renal hypothermia. *Br J Urol* 46: 253.

53 Norris RW, Colvin BT, Kenwright MG, Flynn JT, Blandy JP (1981) *In vitro* studies on optimum preparation of coagulum for surgery of renal calculi. *Br J Urol* 53: 516.

54 Fitzpatrick JM, Murphy DM, Gorey T, Alken P, Thuroff J (1984) Doppler localisation of intrarenal vessels: an experimental study. *Br J Urol* 56: 557.

55 Knoll LD, Segura JW, Patterson DE, Leroy AJ, Smith LH (1988) Long-term follow-up in patients with cystine urinary calculi treated by percutaneous ultrasonic lithotripsy. *J Urol* 140: 246.

56 Bhatta KM, Prien EL, Dretler SP (1989) Cystine calculi — rough and smooth: a new clinical distinction. *J Urol* 142: 937.

57 Cass AS (1992) *In situ* extracorporeal shock wave lithotripsy for obstructing ureteral stones with acute renal colic. *J Urol* 148: 1786.

58 Muller SC, Wilbert D, Thuroff JW, Alken P (1986) Extracorporeal shock wave lithotripsy of ureteral stones, clinical experience and experimental findings. *J Urol* 135: 831.

59 Abdel-Razzak OM, Bagley DH (1992) Clinical experience with flexible ureteropyeloscopy. *J Urol* 148: 1788.

60 Stoller ML, Wolf JS, Hofmann R, Marc B (1992) Ureteroscopy without routine balloon dilatation: an outcome assessment. *J Urol* 147: 1238.

61 Swift-Joly J (1929) *Stone, Calculus Disease of the Urinary Organs.* London: Heinemann.

62 Androulakakis PA (1994) Paediatric stone disease. *Curr Opinion Urol* 4: 213.

Chapter 14: Kidney and ureter — vascular disorders

Renal artery

Congenital anomalies

The underlying pattern of the renal arteries is arranged like the fingers of a hand (Fig. 14.1). There are many variations: two or three of the main branches may spring from a common trunk, and any or all may arise separately from the aorta [1].

Variations on the basic pattern are the rule when the kidney is ectopic. In pelvic or crossed ectopia the segmental vessels may take off from any adjacent artery — aorta, lumbar, common and external iliac arteries [2].

It is very common for the upper segmental vessel to cause an indentation on the neck of the upper calix, an appearance which can be mistaken for a tumour (Fig. 14.2). Very rarely this artery can cause actual obstruction [3].

Haemangioma

It is unclear whether these should be considered to be benign hamartomas or congenital anomalies of the renal arteries. They occur in all sizes, from minute capillary naevi on a papilla, to large arteriovenous malformations (see p. 199).

Clinical features

The main symptom is repeated or persistent haematuria, sometimes accompanied by clot colic. Only with large malformations are there any physical signs: then there may be hypertension and a bruit heard over the loin.

Investigations

The routine investigations for haematuria — IVU, cystoscopy and retrograde urogram — discover blood issuing from one ureter. A large arteriovenous malformation will give a space-occupying mass in the IVU (Fig. 14.3); computerized tomography (CT) and an angiogram (Fig. 14.4) will confirm the diagnosis, but in small angiomas there is no mass and nothing is shown either on the IVU or CT scan. Even an angiogram may fail to detect the source of the bleeding.

Ureteropyeloscopy or percutaneous nephroscopy may show blood issuing out of one of the calices and allow it to be coagulated with the neodymium-yttrium aluminium garnet (YAG) laser or diathermy (Fig. 14.5). Otherwise a partial nephrectomy may be possible [4].

Ask—Upmark kidney

This is a rare deformity of the kidney seen in children with hypertension [5] (Fig. 14.6). The kidney is grossly scarred, like the coarse scarring of reflux nephropathy, but histologically the contracted areas show no inflammation. Instead there are thickened stenosed blood vessels. Its aetiology is unknown but is probably a type of dysplasia.

Traumatic lesions of the renal artery

The renal artery may be avulsed in closed trauma (see p. 121). It is rarely possible to reanastomose the artery but successful cases have been reported where prompt arteriography confirmed the diagnosis and surgical intervention was carried out within hours [6]. Sometimes injury results in dissection of the intima which can be remedied by prompt intervention [7].

Penetrating lesions of the renal artery are a

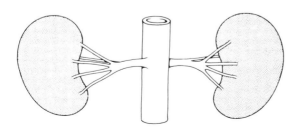

Fig. 14.1 Underlying arrangement of renal artery branches: four anterior and one posterior.

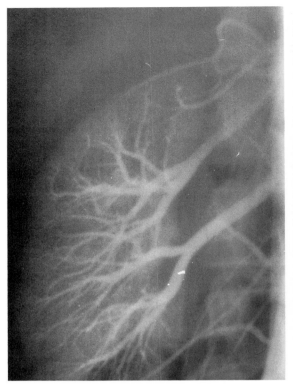

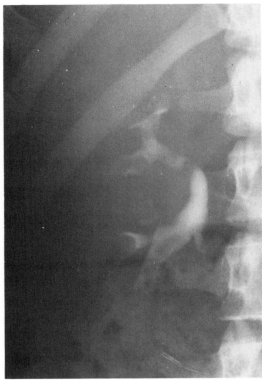

a

b

Fig. 14.2 (a) Arteriogram; (b) Urogram showing upper calix indented by upper pole segmental artery.

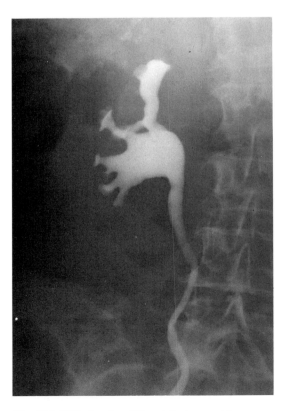

Fig. 14.3 IVU showing filling defect caused by an arteriovenous aneurysm.

common cause of arteriovenous fistula in areas where incidents involving knives are frequent. Elsewhere, the most common cause is renal biopsy and percutaneous renal surgery where the needle or cannula injures part of the wall of a renal vessel and vein. There is more than the usual retroperitoneal haematoma, and within a few weeks the patient develops a thrill and bruit over the loin, sometimes with haematuria [8].

Angiography locates the arteriovenous aneurysm (Fig. 14.7). Small ones may be embolized with metal coils or gelfoam through the angiographic catheter [9]. Larger ones may require partial nephrectomy. Very large arteriovenous fistulae with a large shunt and loss of renal parenchyma require nephrectomy.

Renal artery stenosis

Pathology

Arteriosclerosis

Plaques of atheroma may affect the main renal artery at the junction with the aorta, or along its major branches (Fig. 14.8).

A different pathological process affects

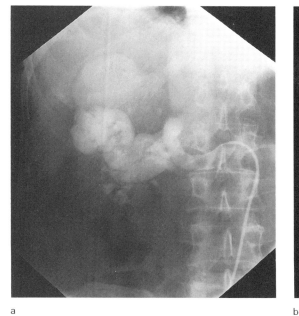
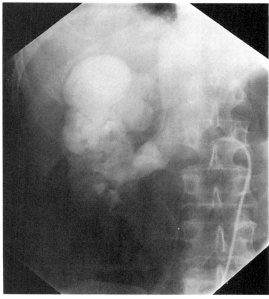

a   b

Fig. 14.4 (a & b) Angiogram showing an arteriovenous aneurysm (courtesy of Mr J.E.A. Wickham).

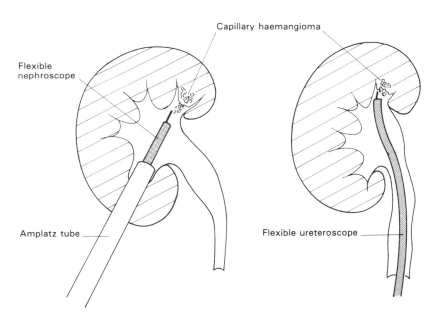

Fig. 14.5 Ureteroscopy or percutaneous nephroscopy may reveal a tiny aneurysm in a calix and allow it to be coagulated with the neodymium-YAG laser.

medium-sized vessels such as the arcuate arteries where the internal elastic lamina is doubled and redoubled — intimal fibroelastic hyperplasia (Fig. 14.9).

A third change — arteriolosclerosis — where hyaline material accumulates just under the intima, is seen in the small afferent arterioles of the glomeruli (see Fig. 14.8).

These pathological processes which may occur singly or together, restrict the flow of blood to the renal parenchyma, and ultimately block it completely. When a segmental artery is blocked there is an infarct of the segment it supplies, and a characteristic atrophy of the full thickness of the cortex and medulla. When smaller branches are occluded, there is a more diffuse loss of parenchyma and an overall shrinkage of the kidney.

Similar changes occur with age and if serial pyelograms have been made one can see the kidneys shrink over the decades (Fig. 14.10). This results in a defect of tubular function — an inability to concentrate urine during the night — resulting in a characteristic nocturnal polyuria (Fig. 14.11) easily mistaken as a symptom of prostatism.

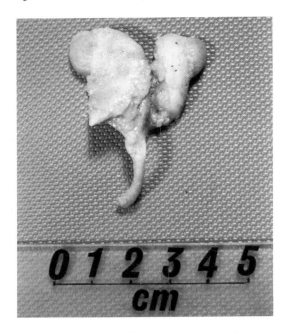

Fig. 14.6 Ask–Upmark kidney, a rare type of dysplasia causing hypertension.

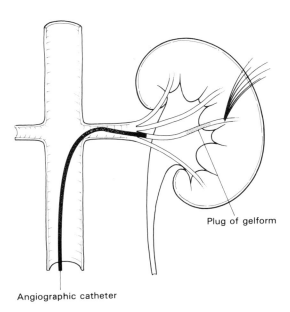

Plug of gelform

Angiographic catheter

Fig. 14.7 A small traumatic arteriovenous aneurysm may be embolized at angiography.

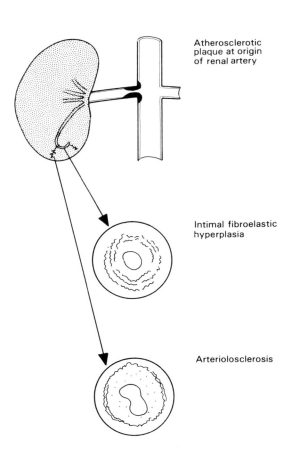

Atherosclerotic plaque at origin of renal artery

Intimal fibroelastic hyperplasia

Arteriolosclerosis

Fig. 14.8 Atheroma and arteriolosclerosis.

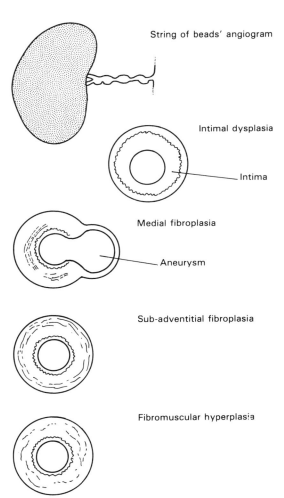

String of beads' angiogram

Intimal dysplasia

Intima

Medial fibroplasia

Aneurysm

Sub-adventitial fibroplasia

Fibromuscular hyperplasia

Fig. 14.9 Fibromuscular dysplasia and hyperplasia.

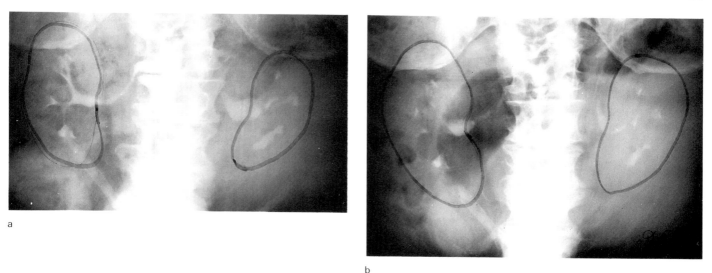

a

b

Fig. 14.10 Tracing of X-rays taken 15 years apart at the age of 66 (left) and 81 (right) in a physician, showing the shrinkage of the kidneys which is seen in old age. (He complained of nocturia but lived to be 92.)

Sickle cell trait

Misshapen sickle cells may give rise to micro-infarction of small vessels in the renal papillae. Painless haematuria is common, but more important is the resulting inability to concentrate urine [10].

Renal artery dysplasia

There is some doubt as to whether this is congenital or acquired: the intima or the media are affected to different degrees.

The intima is affected by patches where it is thickened, alternating with patches where it is unusually thin. This sometimes results in an aneurysmal ballooning of the intima through the wall of the artery. Fibrous tissue is seen just under the adventitia or scattered as if at random, throughout the entire wall of the artery. The result is to convert the artery from a smooth strong cylinder into an irregular perished pipe, here narrowed, there dilated, giving an angiographic appearance of a string of beads (Fig. 14.12).

Pathogenesis of renal hypertension

The lumen of the renal artery must be reduced by some 70% before there is a measurable reduction in blood flow [11] but the pressure gradient across the narrowing may be as much as 40 mmHg [12]. The lowered arterial blood

	Urine output	
May 1	0700 hrs	250 ml
	0905 hrs	50 ml
	1300 hrs	100 ml
	1600 hrs	50 ml
	1900 hrs	100 ml
	2300 hrs	100 ml
May 2nd	0130 hrs	400 ml
	0330 hrs	450 ml
	0500 hrs	400 ml
		1900 ml

Fig. 14.11 Typical urine output chart in an old man without any evidence of outflow obstruction.

pressure leads to reduction in perfusion pressure, glomerular filtration and in the amount of sodium that is filtered. The baroreceptor and macula densa systems release renin [13–15].

Renin is the first in a cascade of enzymes which successively liberate the two active polypeptides — angiotensin II and III — from their inactive globulin carrier 'angiotensinogen' (Fig. 14.13). Both the angiotensins are vasopressors, but in addition angiotensin III causes the adrenal to produce aldosterone.

The amino acid structure of each of these fractions is known, and they can be measured by radioimmunoassay. Every step of this cascade

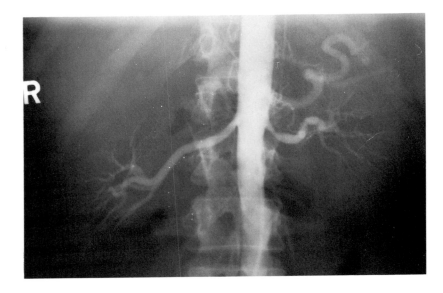

Fig. 14.12 Angiogram showing irregular beading of the left renal artery — fibromuscular dysplasia.

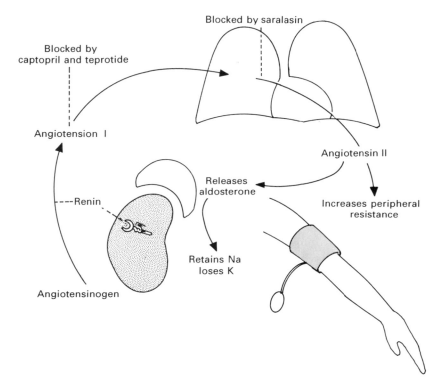

Fig. 14.13 The renin—angiotensin cascade.

has been subjected to intense study which has led to the development of a number of drugs which specifically block particular steps to treat hypertension. Saralasin was one of the first of these agents which blocked angiotensin II. Unfortunately, it also had an agonist effect which could raise the blood pressure to dangerous levels.

Other agents inhibit the conversion of angiotensin I to II. Some occur naturally, e.g. snake venom. Others have been synthesized, e.g. teprotide, captopril, enalapril and enaprilat. One of these (captopril) has a very short action and is useful in the diagnosis of renal hypertension where the plasma renin rises if captropril has been given [12,16—17]. It may precipitate acute renal failure if there is unsuspected renal artery stenosis [18]. The offending kidney can be identified if the renin is measured from each renal vein before and after captopril is given [16,17].

Treatment

Angioplasty

Percutaneous angioplasty is the treatment of first choice: an angioplasty balloon is used to dilate the stenosed part of the renal artery (Fig. 14.14). Review of the results show that the procedure is best in fibromuscular hypoplasia, where it cures 50% of cases, and worst in atheroma where the cure is only 19%. There are some 9% of complications, some of which call for emergency intervention [19]. Fortunately, these cases can still be salvaged [20].

Revascularization

The block between aorta and renal artery may be bypassed with a graft of saphenous vein or internal iliac artery. On the left side the splenic artery can be mobilized and anastomosed directly to the renal artery beyond the stenosis [21−23]. When there is widespread atheroma in the aorta, and occlusion of the splenic artery, autotransplantation may be appropriate. Selecting the most appropriate method calls for experience and judgement. Arterial reconstruction also has a role, not so much with the hope of curing the hypertension, as of preserving renal function and postponing the need for dialysis and transplantation [24].

Nephrectomy

Often the kidney is so shrunken that it is not worth saving, and there are occasions when bilateral nephrectomy and dialysis is the only way to control hypertension.

Embolization

Rather than perform a nephrectomy, many patients have been successfully treated by deliberate embolization of the renal artery or arteries on the diseased side [25].

Renal artery infarction

Small renal infarcts are commonly found at autopsy in older patients as small contracted scars in the renal parenchyma. In younger patients they occur with mitral valve disease, or after open heart surgery. Clinically, there is pain in the loin and sometimes a little haematuria. Urography or DMSA (dimercaptosuccinic

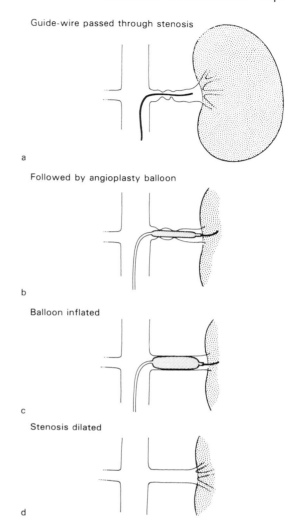

Guide-wire passed through stenosis

a

Followed by angioplasty balloon

b

Balloon inflated

c

Stenosis dilated

d

Fig. 14.14 Angioplasty: the stenosed renal artery is dilated with a balloon.

acid) scans will show the silent segment of parenchyma supplied by a segmental artery (Fig. 14.15). When several segmental arteries are occluded there is a very typical combination of a normal-appearing retrograde urogram, with a dramatic thinning of the renal parenchyma (Figs 14.16 & 14.17).

If acute infarction of the kidney is diagnosed in a patient with suspected renal artery occlusion it is worth operating to attempt to bypass the obstruction because these patients have developed a useful collateral circulation and bypass surgery may preserve renal function and relieve hypertension [26−28].

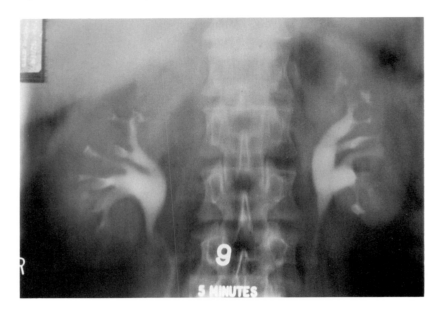

Fig. 14.15 After mitral valvotomy this patient had pain in the left loin with haematuria. Six weeks later this IVU showed absence of the parenchyma of the left lower pole from the infarct.

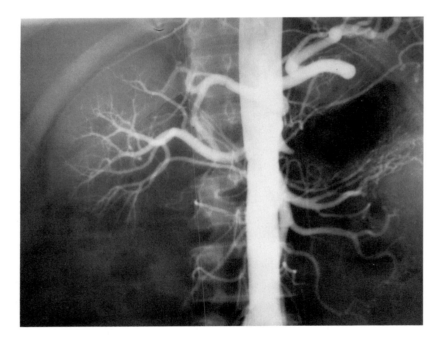

Fig. 14.16 This patient had the sudden onset of hypertension, haematuria and pain in the left loin. The angiogram shows occlusion of the left renal artery: only the upper segmental vessel is spared.

Renal artery aneurysm

Renal artery aneurysms are sometimes found by chance when investigating a patient with hypertension. Others are discovered when they rupture, particularly likely during pregnancy [29,30]. A plain radiograph sometimes shows a characteristic 'ring' due to calcification in the wall of the aneurysm (Fig. 14.18). The kidney on the side of the aneurysm is often smaller than that on the other.

Hypertension is often present, seldom from oversecretion of renin. It increases the risk of rupture of the aneurysm and is an additional reason for intervention. It may be safe not to operate on aneurysms less than 1 cm in diameter, but those over 2 cm should be dealt with without delay [31,32].

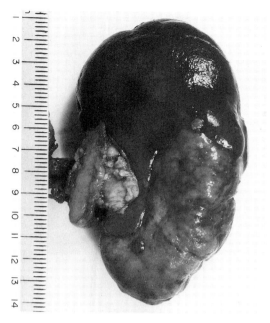

Fig. 14.17 The nephrectomy specimen from the same patient as in Fig. 14.16 showing infarction of most of the kidney: only the upper segment has survived.

Disorders of the renal veins

Congenital anomalies

Every surgeon should be aware of the retroaortic left renal vein. It is a common anomaly, and can cause great difficulty when performing a left nephrectomy for live donor transplantation (see p. 80).

On the right side a persistent post-cardinal vein results in a 'vena cava' which runs in front of the ureter and causes obstruction (see p. 90). The pyelographic appearances are typical and should contraindicate attempts at percutaneous pyelolysis. The open pyeloplasty is easy, and there is no need to attempt to remove the useless segment of ureter from behind the vena cava.

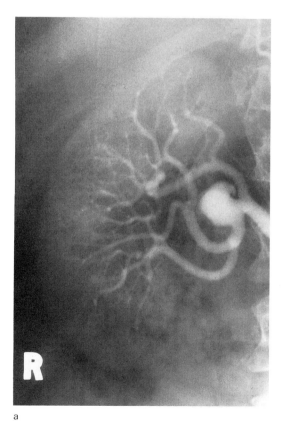

a

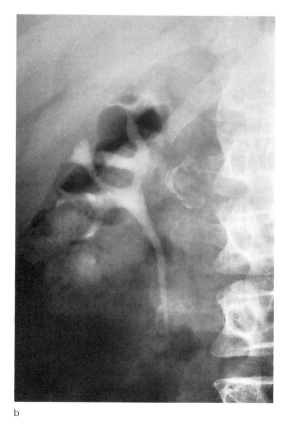

b

Fig. 14.18 (a) Angiogram showing an aneurysm of the right renal artery. (b) Later phase showing a pyelogram, and the ring of calcification in the wall of the aneurysm (courtesy of Mr J.E.A. Wickham).

References

1 Graves FT (1971) *The Arterial Anatomy of the Kidney.* Bristol: Wright.

2 Graves FT (1969) The anatomy of the congenitally deformed kidney. *Br J Surg* 56: 533.

3 Fraley EE (1967) Surgical correction of intrarenal disease. 1. Obstructions of the superior infundibulum. *J Urol* 98: 54.

4 Maddern JP (1967) Surgery of the staghorn calculus. *Br J Urol* 39: 323.

5 Himmelfarb E, Rabinowitz JG, Parvey L *et al.* (1975) The Ask−Upmark kidney. *Am J Dis Child* 129: 1440.

6 Grablowsky OM, Goff JB, Schlegel JU *et al.* (1970) Renal artery thrombosis following blunt trauma: report of four cases. *Surgery* 67: 895.

7 Slavis SA, Hodge EE, Novick AC, Maatman T (1990) Surgical treatment for isolated dissection of renal artery. *J Urol* 144: 233.

8 Heyns CF, van Vollenhoven P (1992) Increasing role of angiography and segmental artery embolization in the management of renal stab wounds. *J Urol* 147: 1231.

9 O'Donnel KF, Pais VM (1976) Arteriovenous aneurysm of kidney after open renal biopsy. *Urology* 7: 305.

10 Forget BC (1988) Sickle cell anemia and associated hemoglobinopathies, in: Wyngaarden JB, Smith LH, Bennett JC (eds) *Cecil Textbook of Medicine 19th.* pp. 888−893 WB Saunders, Philadelphia.

11 Mann FC, Herrick JF, Essex HE *et al.* (1938) The effect on the blood flow of decreasing lumen of a blood vessel. *Surgery* 4: 249.

12 Selkurt EE (1951) The effect of pulse pressure and mean arterial pressure modification of renal hemodynamics and electrolyte and water excretion. *Circulation* 4: 541.

13 Goldfarb DA, Novick AC (1994) The renin-angiotensin system: revised concepts and implications for renal function. *Urology* 43: 572.

14 Davidson RA, Wilcox CS (1992) Newer tests for the diagnosis of renovascular disease. *J Am Med Assoc* 268: 3353.

15 Libertino JA (1993) Renovascular disease. *Curr Opinion Urol* 3: 107.

16 Muller FB, Sealey JE, Case DG *et al.* (1986) The captopril test for identifying renovascular disease in hypertensive patients. *Am J Med* 80: 633.

17 Kaplan NM (1990) The captopril challenge for renovascular hypertension. *Am J Hypertens* 3: 588.

18 Choudhri AH, Cleland JGF, Rowlands PC, Tran TL, McCarty M, Al-Kutoubi MAO (1990) Unsuspected renal artery stenosis in peripheral vascular disease. *Br Med J* 301: 1197.

19 Ramsay LE, Waller PC (1990) Blood pressure response to percutaneous transluminal angioplasty for renovascular hypertension: an overview of published series. *Br Med J* 300: 569.

20 Martinez AG, Novick AC, Hayes JM (1990) Surgical treatment of renal artery stenosis after failed percutaneous transluminal angioplasty. *J Urol* 144: 1094.

21 Novick AC, Straffon RA, Stewart HB *et al.* (1981) Diminished operative morbidity and mortality in renal revascularization. *J Am Med Assoc* 256: 749.

22 Martinez A, Novick AC, Cunningham R, Goormastic M (1990) Improved results of vascular reconstruction in pediatric and young adult patients with renovascular hypertension. *J Urol* 144: 717.

23 Guzzetta PC (1989) Renovascular hypertension in children: current concepts in evaluation and treatment. *J Pediatr Surg* 24: 1236.

24 Novick AC, Textor SC, Bodie B *et al.* (1984) Revascularization to preserve renal function in patients with atherosclerotic renovascular disease. *Urol Clin N Am* 11: 477.

25 Teigen CL, Mitchell SE, Venbrux AC, Christenson MJ, McLean RH (1992) Segmental renal artery embolization for treatment of pediatric renovascular hypertension. *J Vasc Intervent Rad* 3: 111.

26 Schramek A (1973) Survival following late renal embolectomy in a patient with a single functioning kidney. *J Urol* 109: 342.

27 Sheil AGR, Stokes GS, Tiller DJ, May J, Johnson JR, Stewart JH (1973) Reversal of renal failure by revascularisation of kidneys with thrombosed renal arteries. *Lancet* ii: 865.

28 Williams B, Feehally J, Attard AR, Bell PRF (1988) Recovery of renal function after delayed revascularisation of acute occlusion of the renal artery. *Br Med J* 296: 1591.

29 Garritano AP (1957) Aneurysm of the renal artery. *Am J Surg* 94: 638.

30 Harrow BR, Sloane JA (1960) Aneurysm of the renal artery. *J Urol* 81: 10.

31 Martin RS, Meacham PW, Ditesheim JA, Mulherin JL, Edwards WH (1989) Renal artery aneurysm: selective treatment for hypertension and prevention of rupture. *J Vasc Surg* 9: 26.

32 Fleshner NE, Johnston KW (1992) Repair of an autotransplant renal artery aneurysm: case report and literature review. *J Urol* 148: 389.

PART 3
BLADDER

Chapter 15: Structure and function

Comparative anatomy

The bladder, as an entity separate from the cloaca, appeared on the evolutionary scene when fish crawled up onto the land, for there was no need of a bladder in the sea [1–3]. At first it was a water-store, which was later adapted by mammals to serve as an effluent for nitrogenous waste [4].

Other animals developed quite different systems for life on dry land: birds disposed of their nitrogenous waste as semi-solid guano, which saved water and needed no separate urinary bladder.

Embryology

The fetal hind-gut bends round with the curled tail-end of the embryo, in the shape of a hook (Fig. 15.1). The caudal part of the hind-gut remains in communication with the allantois through the urachus and will form the bladder.

The curtain of tissue that descends to separate the bladder from the rectum is the urogenital septum which carries down the lower ends of the Wolffian ducts to open into the bladder, which incorporates them into the trigone (Fig. 15.2).

As the allantois shrinks its lumen becomes a solid cord — the urachus — where vestiges of columnar epithelium link the apex of the bladder to the umbilicus.

When the urogenital septum reaches the perineum the cloacal membrane dissolves to open the urethra and anal canal (Fig. 15.3). In males, the phallic tubercles enlarge and fuse in the midline to form the penis, and the skin progressively rolls in forwards to form the urethra from the opening of the cloacal membrane to the edge of the glands penis (Fig. 15.4). The terminal part of the urethra is a solid cord in the glans which canalizes later on.

Topographical anatomy

The bladder lies in the pelvis anterior to the rectum, posterior to the symphysis pubis. Superiorly, separated by the peritoneum, are coils of small bowel and sigmoid (Figs 15.5 & 15.6).

The lateral relations of the bladder are the fascia of the pelvis, connective tissue containing a rich plexus of veins, beyond which are the obturator internus covered by obturator fascia and the levator ani covered by the pelvic fascia.

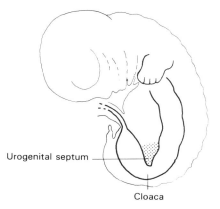

Fig. 15.1 The fetal hind-gut bends round and the urogenital septum descends to separate the bladder from the rectum: the patent urachus keeps the future bladder in continuity with the allantois.

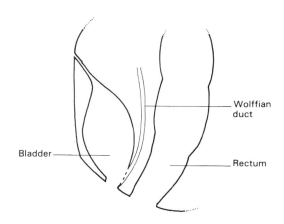

Fig. 15.2 The urogenital septum brings down the Wolffian ducts which will become the ureter.

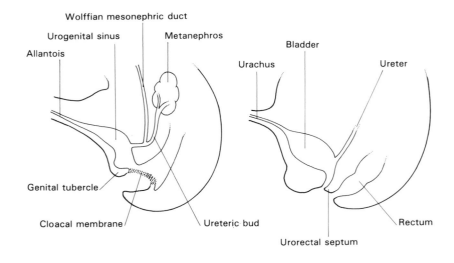

Fig. 15.3 As the urogenital septum reaches the perineum the cloacal membrane dissolves to reveal two openings, the urethra and rectum.

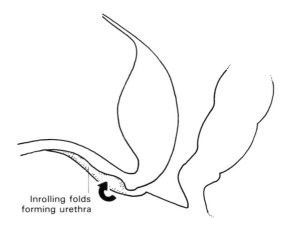

Fig. 15.4 The skin rolls in on either side to form the urethra.

In the loose packing of the pelvic fascia run the superior and inferior vesical, obturator and, in the male, the prostatic vessels (Figs 15.7 & 15.8).

Inferiorly, in the male, there is the prostate over which the base of the bladder forms the trigone, bounded by the interureteric bar and the internal meatus.

Behind the bladder a recess of peritoneum separates it from the rectum: the lowest part of this fold of peritoneum is fused to form the fascia of Denonvilliers.

In the female, the uterus, cervix and vagina lie behind the bladder.

Arteries

The arteries of the bladder are all branches of the internal iliac artery. The superior vesical artery is a branch of the umbilical artery which continues as a more or less obliterated cord in the adult. Two arterial leashes supply the inferior part of the bladder (inferior vesical) and the prostate (prostatic arteries) (Fig. 15.9).

Veins

The veins of the bladder drain into the plexus of Santorini, which communicates with the prostatic and vaginal plexuses, and the internal iliac, ovarian, superior haemorrhoidal and sacral veins, providing a direct route to the bones of the pelvis and vertebrae.

Lymphatics

The lymphatics of the bladder drain to the external and internal iliac nodes and the obturator groups of nodes [5].

Nerves

The bladder receives parasympathetic nerves from the nervi erigentes, and sympathetic fibres from the presacral nerves which follow the branches of the internal iliac artery.

Wall of the bladder

The detrusor of the bladder is made of smooth muscle fibres which weave in and out to form a basket work: distinct layers can only be defined on the trigone and around the bladder neck [6] (Fig. 15.10). Between the muscle bundles are thin strands of connective tissue. Two more muscle bundles sheathe the ureters and continue down

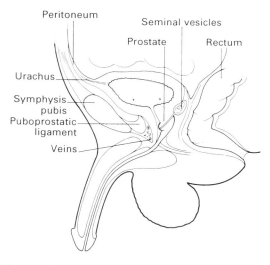

Fig. 15.5 Sagittal section through the male pelvis showing main anatomical relations.

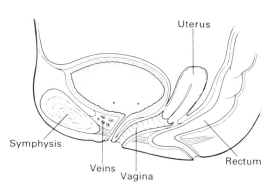

Fig. 15.6 Sagittal section through the female pelvis showing main anatomical relations.

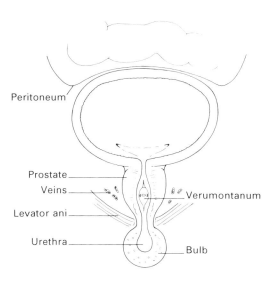

Fig. 15.7 Coronal section through the male pelvis showing main anatomical relations.

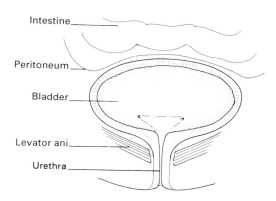

Fig. 15.8 Coronal section through the female pelvis showing main anatomical relations.

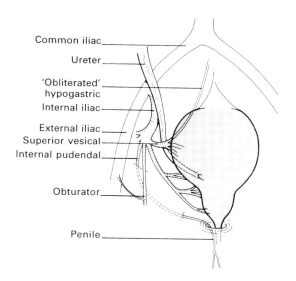

Fig. 15.9 Arterial supply to the male bladder.

to the urethra (Fig. 15.11). There are a few elastic fibres around the bladder neck.

There is a rich lymphatic plexus within the detrusor muscle.

Unlike other viscera, the bladder has no anatomical capsule — outside its muscle the connective tissue is continuous with that around the pelvic veins and fat. Only above, depending on how much the bladder is filled, is there a more or less large patch of peritoneum on its superior surface.

Electron microscopy shows that each detrusor muscle cell is separated from its neighbour by a basal lamina except where they come together and plug in by pegs and sockets (Fig. 15.12) which permit electrical excitation to pass from one cell to another.

The detrusor muscle of the bladder is supplied by three sets of autonomic fibres (Fig. 15.13).

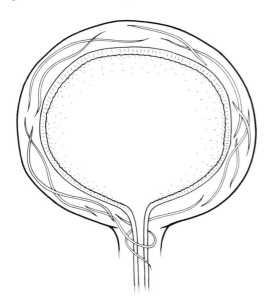

Fig. 15.10 Arrangement of the smooth muscle fibres of the bladder — they swoop from superficial to deep layers and curl around the internal meatus, more like a basket than a series of layers (from [6]).

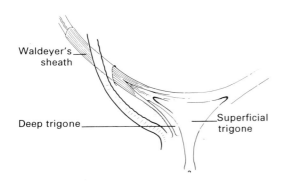

Fig. 15.11 A special sheath of smooth muscle surrounds the lower end of the ureter — Waldeyer's sheath. This is an important part of the antireflux mechanism.

1 Preganglionic autonomic parasympathetic fibres synapse with ganglion cells in the detrusor and stain for acetylcholine esterase.
2 Noradrenergic fibres from the lumbar sympathetic chain and presacral nerve, accompany the arteries of the bladder to synapse with ganglion cells in the pelvic fat.
3 Several other systems of fine nerve fibres, non-adrenergic and non-cholinergic (NANC), have been identified. They stain for various peptides, e.g. vasoactive intestinal polypeptide, substance P, calcitonin gene-related polypeptide, and somatostatin. Their role is unknown at present [7].

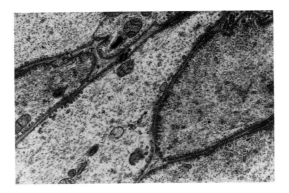

Fig. 15.12 Electron micrograph showing peg-and-socket junctions between cells of the detrusor smooth muscle across which excitation spreads.

Vesicoureteric valve

Leonardo da Vinci first noticed how the ureters entered the bladder through long tunnels which prevented vesicoureteric reflux [8]. These tunnels have a lubricated sleeve of connective tissue which allows the ureters to slide up and down through the detrusor. Outside this sleeve is a sheath of muscle — Waldeyer's sheath — whose muscle fibres run on the surface of the trigone down to the urethra. They have fewer cholinergic nerves and more adrenergic ones than the rest of the detrusor. During micturition they contract to elongate the ureters and prevent reflux [9] (Fig. 15.14).

Bladder neck

In the male, the bladder neck is a collar of smooth muscle which merges distally with the muscular fibres of the prostate (Fig. 15.15). Both are adrenergic and contract on stimulation of the sympathetic nerves [6,10].

In the female, the bladder neck fibres merge obliquely into the wall of the urethra (Fig. 15.16). They are cholinergic rather than adrenergic and play no active part in continence: indeed in normal continent women the bladder neck is often found to be slightly open [11].

Lamina propria

The lamina propria consists of connective tissue of varying thickness. It contains a wispy layer of muscle fibres, which can sometimes lead to errors in interpretation of invasion by bladder cancer. It contains very few lymphatics.

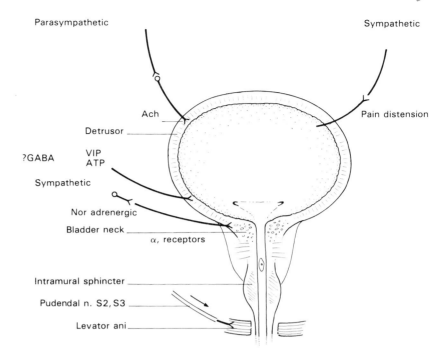

Fig. 15.13 Diagram of efferent and afferent nerves of the bladder (see text for explanation).

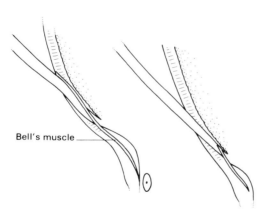

Fig. 15.14 (a & b) The action of Bell's muscle is to draw the ureter down towards the trigone to elongate the antireflux tunnel of the ureter.

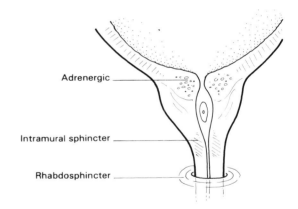

Fig. 15.15 Diagram of the male bladder neck: there is an adrenergic internal sphincter which is normally kept closed.

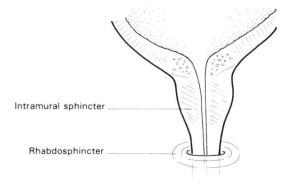

Fig. 15.16 Diagram of the female bladder neck: the bladder neck is not usually closed at rest.

Urothelium

In the empty bladder (Fig. 15.17) the urothelium is some six cells thick though when distended it is only one or two cells thick (Fig. 15.18). Three

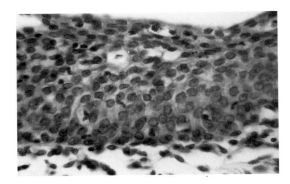

Fig. 15.17 The urothelium in the empty bladder of the dog.

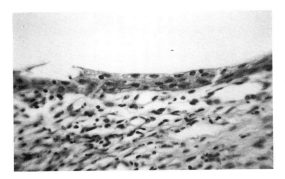

Fig. 15.18 The urothelium in the distended bladder of the dog.

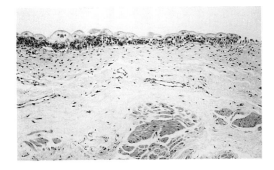

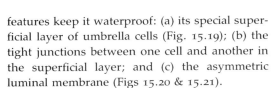

Fig. 15.19 Normal human bladder showing the 'umbrella cells' and the wispy smooth muscle in the lamina propria.

features keep it waterproof: (a) its special superficial layer of umbrella cells (Fig. 15.19); (b) the tight junctions between one cell and another in the superficial layer; and (c) the asymmetric luminal membrane (Figs 15.20 & 15.21).

The surface of the normal human urothelium is thrown into fine wrinkles (Fig. 15.22). In malignancy there is a curious change: instead of wrinkles there are innumerable 'microvilli' (Figs 15.23–15.25).

Some of the cells of the trigone and bladder neck contain cells similar to the chromaffin cells of the bowel. These are the amine precursor uptake and decarboxylation (APUD) vesicles, confirming that this part of the urothelium is derived from the urogenital sinus [6].

Normal function of the bladder

In man, the bladder acts as a reservoir for urine: it does not absorb urine, and the individual gets rid of it when the time and place are convenient, according to social customs.

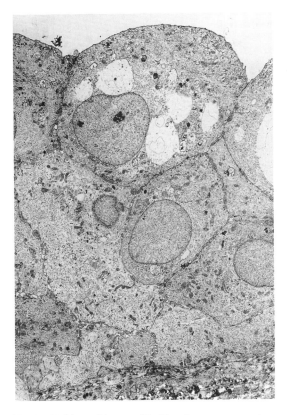

Fig. 15.20 Normal human bladder. Lower power view of normal urothelium with a large surface cell with an asymmetric unit surface membrane. Transmission electron micrograph × 2400 (courtesy of Dr J. Newman).

Although the lining of the bladder is virtually waterproof [12] this is not always so: drugs with a small molecule such as Thiotepa can be absorbed, and when this was first used in large doses bone marrow suppression was reported. Absorption by the bladder may be altered in some diseases, e.g. interstitial cystitis [13].

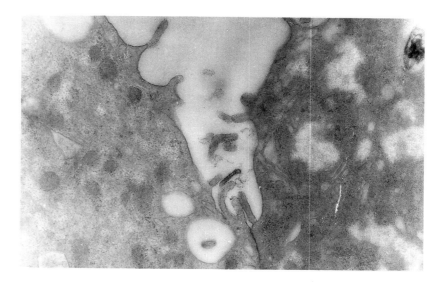

Fig. 15.21 Normal human bladder with two adjacent superficial cells bearing a luminal asymmetric unit membrane. Transmission electron micrograph × 14000 (courtesy of Dr J. Newman).

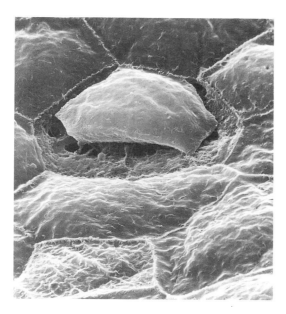

Fig. 15.22 Normal human bladder. Large flat polygonal surface cells with a ridged luminal surface membrane. One cell is in the process of exfoliating. Scanning electron micrograph × 3000 (courtesy of Dr J. Newman).

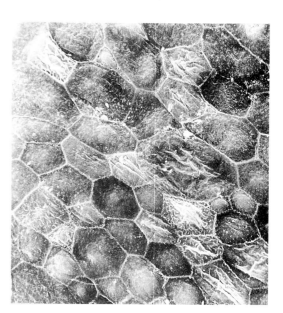

Fig. 15.23 Normal human bladder. Large flat polygonal surface cells with a ridged luminal surface membrane. Scanning electron micrograph × 1000 (courtesy of Dr J. Newman).

The normal bladder fills with urine at a rate which is determined by input via food and drink, and fluid loss in sweat, faeces and respiration. As it fills there is no increase in pressure. A slight sensation of fullness is appreciated by most people when the bladder contains about 250 ml, at which stage there may be a momentary and very slight increase in pressure.

At this stage micturition can normally be postponed for a considerable time, until a stage is reached, in most patients when the bladder contains about 500 ml, when more frequent increases of pressure occur up to 100 cm of water, and the discomfort becomes unbearable, and the patient passes urine. The volume at which this takes place varies considerably from one patient to another.

The underlying neurophysiology of normal micturition is very complex, with sensations from the bladder being represented at the highest levels of the brain.

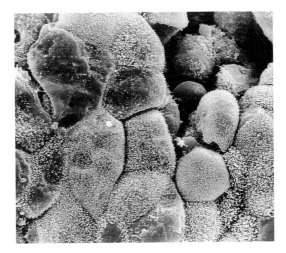

Fig. 15.24 Human bladder tumour surface. The superficial cells have a 'cobblestone' appearance, vary in size and many are covered by pleomorphic microvilli. Scanning electron micrograph × 1300 (courtesy of Dr J. Newman).

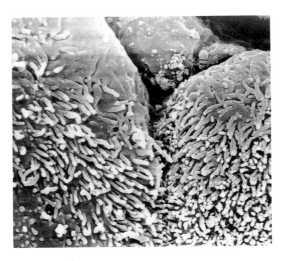

Fig. 15.25 Human bladder tumour surface, showing two adjacent cells covered by tall pleomorphic microvilli. Scanning electron micrograph × 6000 (courtesy of Dr J. Newman).

Spinal reflex arcs for micturition

Afferent impulses from stretch receptors in the bladder pass up in the parasympathetic fibres of the nervi erigentes to the S2 and S3 segments of the spinal cord, which are situated at the level of the T12, L1 intervertebral disc. These afferent fibres synapse with efferent fibres which pass back down the pelvic parasympathetic fibres and stimulate the detrusor muscle fibres, while additional synapses inhibit the action of the anterior horn cells of the pudendal nerve to shut down the action of the striated muscle of the pelvic floor.

The afferent stretch receptors also synapse with sympathetic neurones higher up at T9−L2 from which impulses descend along the sympathetic chain via the presacral nerve, to reach the trigone and internal sphincter where they cause the internal sphincter to relax.

This simple local reflex arc is subject to facilitation and inhibition from centres further up the nervous system, notably one in the pons and another in the frontal lobes. Facilitation causes the contraction of the detrusor and the relaxation of the sphincters to occur when the bladder is less full than usual, e.g. in states of anxiety. Inhibition allows the bladder to become more full than usual, e.g. under the influence of drugs or lesions of the spinal cord.

In the wall of the bladder, the parasympathetic efferent neurones synapse with each other and with postganglionic fibres, as well as with sympathetic fibres carrying impulses destined for the trigone and internal sphincter. The function of these connections is not certain in normal micturition [7] let alone when normal physiology is altered by outflow obstruction [14,15] or old age [16].

This makes the quest for pharmacological control of bladder function inevitably difficult. It is supposed that the main neurotransmitter in the smooth muscle of the internal sphincter and trigone is alpha noradrenaline, while acetylcholine is the neurotransmitter in the muscle of the detrusor. However, in clinical practice anticholinergic drugs are often disappointing when used with the hope of diminishing the force of detrusor contraction, and may not justify their side effects.

References

1 Romer AS, Parsons TS (1977) *The Vertebrate Body*, 5th edn, p. 372. Philadelphia: WB Saunders.
2 Young JZ (1962) *The Life of Vertebrates*, 2nd edn, p. 163. Oxford: Oxford University Press.
3 Hildebrand M (1974) *Analysis of Vertebrate Structure*, p. 303. New York: Wiley.
4 Fraser EA (1950) The development of the vertebrate excretory system. *Biol Rev* 25: 159.
5 Gosling JA, Dixon JS, Humpherson JR (1982) *Functional Anatomy of the Urinary Tract*. London: Gower.

6 Woodburne RT (1960) Structure and function of the urinary bladder. *J Urol* 84: 79.

7 Ambache N, Zar MA (1970) Non-cholinergic transmission by post-ganglionic motor neurones in the mammalian bladder. *J Physiol* 210: 761.

8 Leonardo da Vinci. *Dell' Anatomia.* Fogli: A & B. Cited by Bitker MP (1954) Les uretero-iléo-plasties. *J Urol Néphrol* 60: 473.

9 Dixon JS, Canning DA, Gearhart JP, Gosling JA (1994) An immunohistochemical study of the innervation of the ureterovesical junction in infancy and childhood. *Br J Urol* 73: 292.

10 Learmonth JR (1931) A contribution to the neurophysiology of the urinary bladder in man. *Brain* 54: 147.

11 Versi E (1991) The significance of an open bladder neck in women. *Br J Urol* 68: 42.

12 Jost SP, Gosling JA, Dixon JS (1989) The morphology of normal human bladder urothelium. *J Anat* 167: 103.

13 Chelsky MJ, Rosen SI, Knight LC, Maurer AH, Hanno PM, Riggieri MR (1994) Bladder permeability in interstitial cystitis is similar to that of normal volunteers: direct measurement by transvesical absorption of ^{99m}technetium de-ethylene-triamine-penta-acetic acid. *J Urol* 151: 346.

14 Narayan P, Koney B, Aslam K *et al.* (1995) Neuroanatomy of the external urethral sphincter: implications for urinary continence during radical prostatic surgery. *J Urol* 153: 337.

15 Chapple CR, Milner P, Moss H, Burnstock G (1992) Loss of sensory nerves in the obstructed bladder. *Br J Urol* 70: 373.

16 Malone-Lee J, Wahedna I (1993) Characterisation of detrusor contractile function in relation to old age. *Br J Urol* 72: 873.

Chapter 16: Bladder — congenital abnormalities

Imperfect development of the cloacal membrane

A number of important congenital anomalies arise from imperfect development of the cloacal membrane: of these four are the most significant.

Exstrophy

The cloacal membrane may extend right up to the umbilical cord, separating the pubic bones (Fig. 16.1). When the cloacal membrane disappears the bladder is exposed on the abdominal wall below the umbilicus [1−3] (Figs 16.2 & 16.3). If neglected, the exposed urothelium undergoes intestinal metaplasia and may develop adenocarcinoma [4,5] (Fig. 16.4).

In the male, the urethra is represented by a strip of urothelium on the dorsum of a short broad up-turned penis. The testicles are undescended: inguinal herniae are present (Fig. 16.5). In the female, the clitoris is bifid and the urethra barely present (Fig. 16.6). The anus is displaced anteriorly: its sphincter is weak and the rectum is often prolapsed.

Epispadias

When the cloacal membrane is less extensive (Fig. 16.7), its dissolution leaves a defect in the urethra that may be restricted to the glans or may form a strip along the short curved penis, with a prepuce on the ventral side (Fig. 16.8). If the urinary sphincter is involved the child may be incontinent.

Superior vesical fissure

Here the exstrophy is restricted to the apex of the bladder. The remainder of the bladder is correctly formed (Fig. 16.9).

Cloacal exstrophy

There are many variations on this theme: on either side of the midline there may be an exstrophic half-bladder (Fig. 16.10), each with its ureteric orifice and rudimentary phallus. Between them a length of intestine with two openings represents the ileocaecal region. The upper opening leads into the ileum and dis-

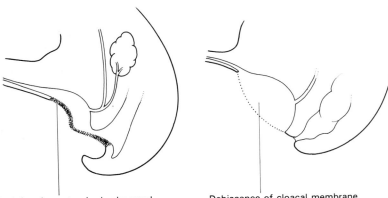

Basic defect in exstrophy is abnormal extension of the cloacal membrane onto lower abdominal wall, preventing fusion of two halves of abdominal wall

Dehiscence of cloacal membrane results in exposure of entire infraumbilical triangle

Fig. 16.1 In exstrophy the cloacal membrane extends right up to the umbilical cord and when it dissolves, the bladder is exposed.

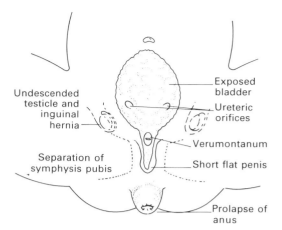

Fig. 16.2 Diagram of the principal features of exstrophy.

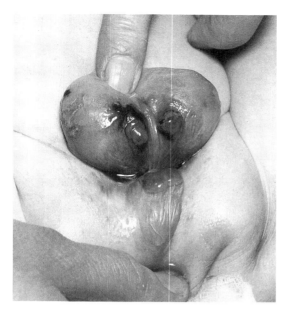

Fig. 16.3 Exstrophy of the bladder in a boy (courtesy of Mr J.H. Johnston).

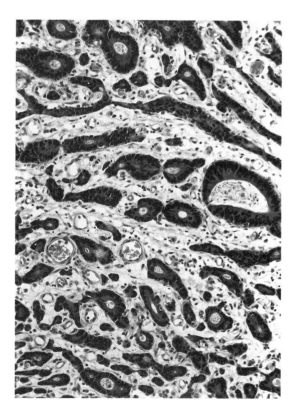

Fig. 16.4 Adenocarcinoma may occur in the chronically exposed bladder of exstrophy, following upon adenomatous metaplasia.

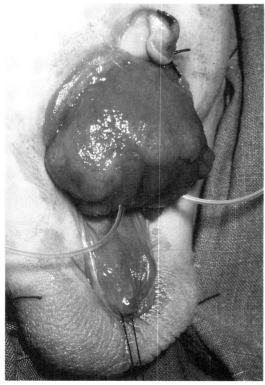

Fig. 16.5 Exstrophy of the bladder (courtesy of Mr Joe Cohen).

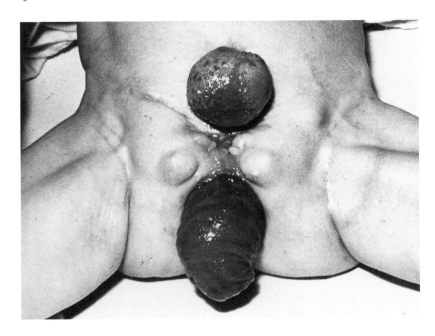

Fig. 16.6 Exstrophy of the bladder in a girl: note complete epispadias, double clitoris and large rectal prolapse (courtesy of Mr J.H. Johnston).

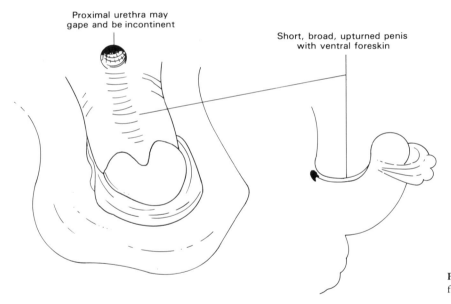

Proximal urethra may gape and be incontinent

Short, broad, upturned penis with ventral foreskin

Fig. 16.7 Diagram of the findings in epispadias.

charges small bowel content; the lower one leads into a loop of large bowel which ends blindly in front of the sacrum. The anus is imperfect and there is usually spina bifida (Fig. 16.11).

Management

These are all rare conditions which should be referred to specialist paediatric urological units dealing with many such cases.

For straightforward exstrophy and epispadias, the earlier the lesion is corrected the better are the results [5–12]. The bladder is mobilized (Fig. 16.12), the ureters are reimplanted through long submucosal tunnels to prevent reflux. The edges of the mobilized bladder and urethra are rolled in to make a new bladder and urethra. The tissues on either side of the bladder neck are mobilized and sewn together. To help closure an osteotomy is performed through the iliac bone just lateral to the sacroiliac joint.

A second operation may be necessary a few years later to achieve continence (Fig. 16.13). In cases operated on early, as many as 50% become

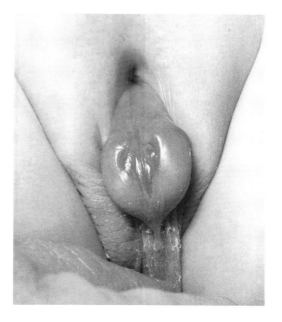

Fig. 16.8 Epispadias in an incontinent boy (courtesy of Mr J.H. Johnston).

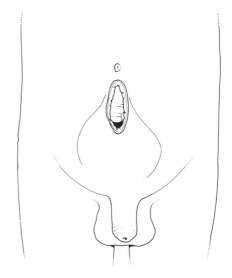

Fig. 16.9 Diagram of the findings in superior vesical fissure.

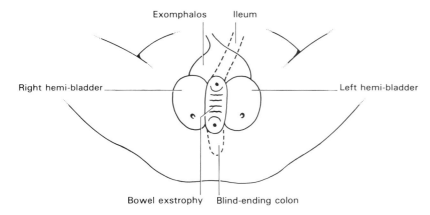

Fig. 16.10 Diagram of the findings in cloacal exstrophy (courtesy of Mr J.H. Johnston).

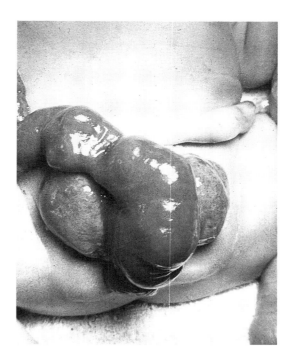

Fig. 16.11 Cloacal exstrophy in a neonate. The bowel exstrophy protrudes between the two halves of the exstrophied bladder, and the ileum has prolapsed through the proximal opening of the bowel (courtesy of Mr J.H. Johnston).

continent. In those who come late, with small, contracted or severely dysplastic bladders, the bladder remnant is excised to prevent cancer, and the ureters are diverted [13] by a continent urinary diversion (see p. 325).

Other cloacal anomalies

These abnormalities are rare: few surgeons have the opportunity to develop expertise. They should be referred to a centre where continuous audit of large numbers tends to improve results.

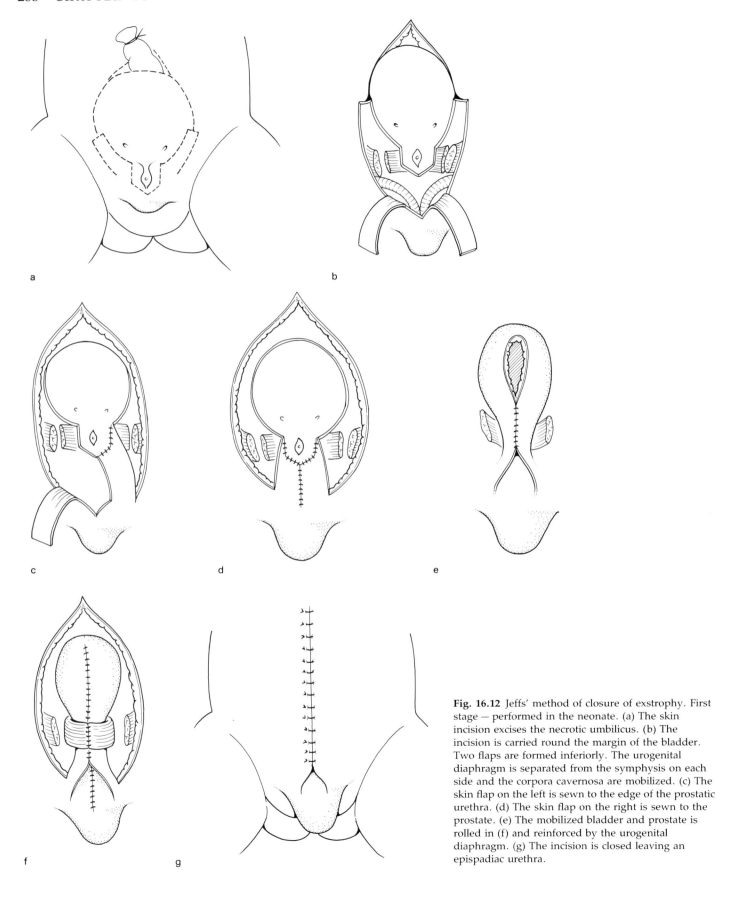

Fig. 16.12 Jeffs' method of closure of exstrophy. First stage — performed in the neonate. (a) The skin incision excises the necrotic umbilicus. (b) The incision is carried round the margin of the bladder. Two flaps are formed inferiorly. The urogenital diaphragm is separated from the symphysis on each side and the corpora cavernosa are mobilized. (c) The skin flap on the left is sewn to the edge of the prostatic urethra. (d) The skin flap on the right is sewn to the prostate. (e) The mobilized bladder and prostate is rolled in (f) and reinforced by the urogenital diaphragm. (g) The incision is closed leaving an epispadiac urethra.

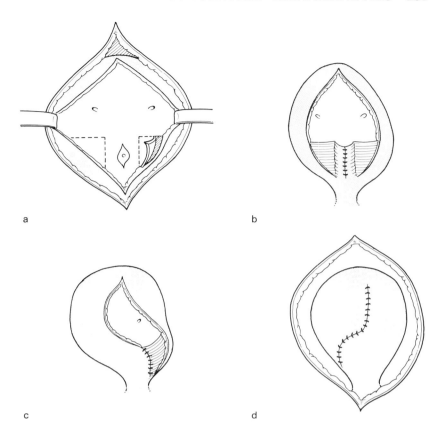

a

b

c

d

Fig. 16.13 Jeffs' method for exstrophy. Second stage — performed at about 3 years. (a) The old incision is reopened. (Not shown here — the ureters are reimplanted to prevent reflux.) A triangle of mucosa is removed on each side exposing the bladder muscle. (b) A tube is formed to make the prostatic urethra. (c) The denuded triangle of bladder is swung across, first on the right side and then on the left (d), to 'double-breast' the new prostatic urethra [7].

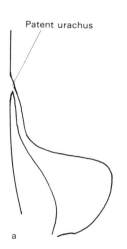

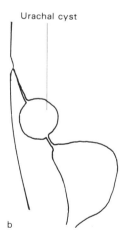

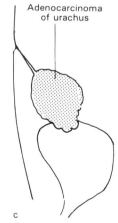

Patent urachus

Urachal cyst

Adenocarcinoma of urachus

a

b

c

Fig. 16.14 Complications of a persistent urachus. (a) It may cause a urinary fistula if associated with outflow obstruction from urethral valves. (b) There may be a midline cyst which may become infected. (c) Carcinoma arising in the urachus presents in the bladder at the apex, and erodes early into the peritoneal cavity.

Other congenital anomalies

Agenesis

Complete agenesis of the bladder usually occurs with other, fatal, multiple deformities.

Hypoplasia

Hypoplasia is associated with epispadias or ectopic ureters opening into the lower urethra. If these abnormalities can be corrected, the bladder usually grows normally.

Duplication

Duplication of the bladder occurs in various forms along with other anomalies whose correction dominates the management [14].

Urachus

If the urachus remains patent and there is an obstruction at the bladder outlet, urine will leak from the umbilicus (Fig. 16.14).

Cysts of the urachus present at any age when they become infected or (rarely) cause ureteric obstruction [15–17]. Carcinoma of the urachus in the adult presents with haematuria. Cystoscopy shows a cherry-sized lump at the air bubble and a much larger mass outside it: biopsy reveals adenocarcinoma (see p. 312).

Congenital diverticula

Most diverticula are secondary to outflow obstruction but a few are truly congenital and have a thick wall containing muscle (Fig. 16.15). Urodynamic studies, which must include measurement of the peak detrusor voiding pressure, rule out any outflow obstruction. They present with urinary infection. Each time the child voids the diverticulum fills up (Fig. 16.16).

If obstruction has been ruled out the diverticulum can be removed and the bladder neck or prostate left alone.

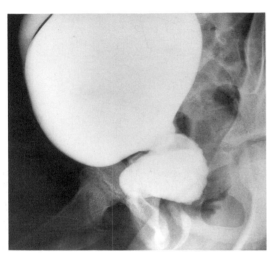

Fig. 16.15 Cystogram showing a congenital vesical diverticulum in a boy aged 5 years (courtesy of Mr J.H. Johnston).

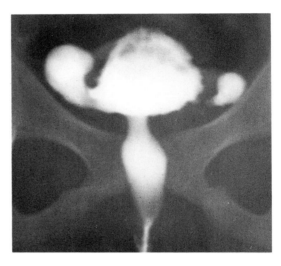

Fig. 16.16 Congenital diverticula, commonly seen in girls (courtesy of Mr J.H. Johnston).

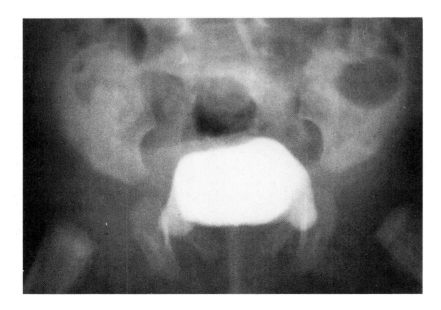

Fig. 16.17 Congenital diverticula protruding into the inguinal canal in a boy — so-called bladder 'ears' (courtesy of Mr J.H. Johnston).

Bladder 'ears'

Innocent protrusions of the bladder are normal in male infants and common in women. In the adult male, they commonly accompany an inguinal hernia into the inguinal canal (Fig. 16.17).

Disorders of development of the sacrum

Sacral agenesis

These are exceedingly rare and represent a variation on the theme of failure of development of the neural canal. The child is born with an absence of most of the sacrum, and a lesion of the cauda equina leading to a neuropathic bladder. The diagnosis is obvious from a plain radiograph of the pelvis, but it is all too easy to miss the absence of the sacrum (Fig. 16.18).

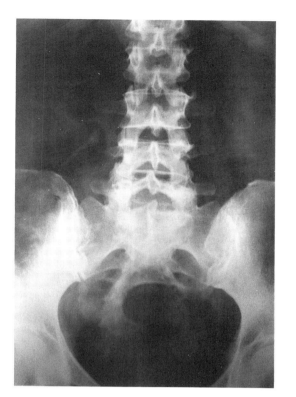

Fig. 16.18 Sacral agenesis associated with neuropathic bladder.

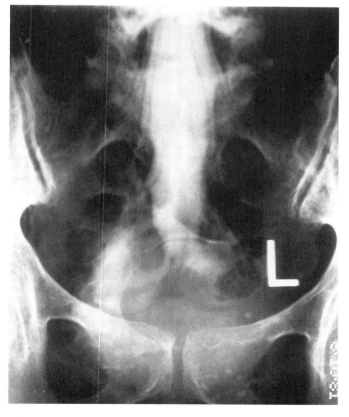

a

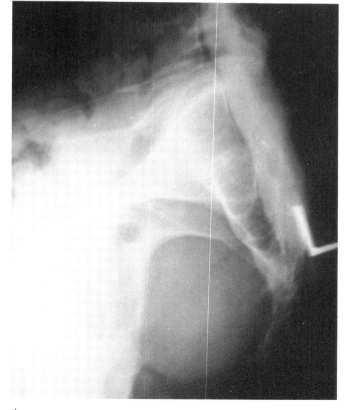

b

Fig. 16.19 A presacral dermoid may deform the bladder and cause mechanical obstruction to defaecation or micturition. (a) Anteroposterior view; (b) lateral view.

Presacral dermoid

A congenital neural canal defect leads to the formation of a dermoid cyst between the sacrum and the rectum. Clinically, they may present with bizarre symptoms, few of which are serious unless the cyst becomes infected. On rectal examination a large mass is found (Fig. 16.19). Surgical intervention is only required if the cyst is causing obstruction or is associated with a cauda equina lesion and carries a high risk of producing a neuropathic bladder even if not already present.

References

1 Johnston HJ (1976) Congenital abnormalities of the bladder and urethra, in: Blandy JP (ed.) *Urology*, vol. 2, p. 619−671. Oxford: Blackwell Scientific Publications.

2 Marshall VF, Muecke EC (1962) Variations in exstrophy of the bladder. *J Urol* 88: 766.

3 Johnston JH, Penn IA (1966) Exstrophy of the cloaca. *Br J Urol* 38: 302.

4 Kandzari SJ, Majid A, Orteza AM, Milam DF (1974) Exstrophy of urinary bladder complicated by adenocarcinoma. *Urology* 3: 496.

5 Davillas N, Thanos A, Liakatas J, Davillas E (1991) Bladder exstrophy complicated by adenocarcinoma. *Br J Urol* 68: 107.

6 Connor JP, Hensle TW, Lattimer JK, Burbige KA (1989) Long-term follow up of 207 patients with bladder exstrophy: an evolution in treatment. *J Urol* 142: 793.

7 Jeffs RD, Lepor H (1986) Management of the exstrophy-epispadias complex and urachal anomalies, in: Walsh PC, Gittes RF, Perlmutter AD, Stamey TA (eds) *Campbell's Urology* 5th Ed. Philadelphia Saunders. 1882

8 Hendren WH (1977) Surgical management of urogenital sinus abnormalities. *J Pediatr Surg* 12: 339.

9 Mollard P, Mouriquand PDE, Buttin X (1994) Urinary continence after reconstruction of classical bladder exstrophy (73 cases). *Br J Urol* 73: 298.

10 Husmann DA, McLorie GA, Churchill BM (1989) Closure of exstrophic bladder: evaluation of factors leading to its success and its importance on urinary continence. *J Urol* 142: 522.

11 Gearhaart JP, Jeffs RD (1989) Bladder exstrophy: increase in capacity following epispadias repair. *J Urol* 142: 525.

12 Husmann, DA, McLorie GA, Churchill BM (1989) Phallic reconstruction in cloacal exstrophy. *Urology* 142: 563.

13 Spence HM, Hoffman WW, Pate VA (1975) Exstrophy of the bladder. 1. Long-term results in a series of 37 cases treated by ureterosigmoidostomy. *J Urol* 114: 133.

14 Abrahamson J (1961) Double bladder and related anomalies: clinical and embryological aspects and a case report. *Br J Urol* 33: 195.

15 Iuchtman M, Rahav S, Zer M, Mogilner J, Siplovich L (1993) Management of urachal anomalies in children and adults. *Urology* 42: 426.

16 Hbuchi T, Miyakawa M (1990) Urachal cysts in the bladder wall. *Br J Urol* 65: 658−9.

17 Collins CN, Sunderland GT, Crossling FT (1990) Urachal cyst: an unusual cause of hydronephrosis. *Br J Urol* 65: 305.

Chapter 17: Bladder — trauma

Closed injury to the bladder

Intraperitoneal rupture of the bladder

Rupture of the bladder without a fracture of the pelvis is classically seen in the elderly drunk who has been injured (Fig. 17.1). The patient seldom remembers the cause and the diagnosis may be difficult because leakage of uninfected hypotonic urine into the peritoneal cavity at first excites little reaction [1,2]. There is no tenderness on palpation: bowel sounds persist. Only a very astute doctor will suspect a vesical injury. When there is any doubt the patient should be admitted for observation.

A cystogram will only show up the tear in the bladder if the bladder is deliberately distended, but a second film taken after the bladder has been emptied may show contrast outside the bladder [3] (Fig. 17.2). At cystoscopy it is so difficult to see the tear because of bleeding that it is seldom worthwhile.

If the diagnosis is made a catheter is left in the bladder and the patient carefully observed [2]. If a pocket of extravasated urine becomes infected, or there is any deterioration in the general condition of the patient, laparotomy will be needed [4].

If the injury is not recognized, the patient gradually develops a chemical peritonitis caused by the escape of urine. The abdomen becomes swollen and tender: bowel sounds disappear. Eventually, there may be fat necrosis and sloughing of omentum and bowel. When in any doubt it is safer to perform a laparotomy and close the rent in the bladder and drain it, for even today these injuries carry a high mortality: in a recent series it was nearly 15% [5].

These patients are often readmitted a few months later with an identical lesion having learned nothing from their previous experience.

Silent rupture of the bladder

After bladder tumours on the dome have been coagulated with diathermy, especially in old people, the coagulated part of the thin wall of the bladder may give way and allow urine to escape into the peritoneum. As with closed injuries the early physical signs are minimal — the urine gives rise to little irritation — and it is only after 2 or 3 days that the patient develops abdominal pain and distension. With prompt catheterization the condition is easily remedied and laparotomy can be avoided.

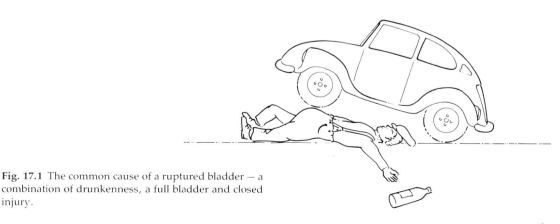

Fig. 17.1 The common cause of a ruptured bladder — a combination of drunkenness, a full bladder and closed injury.

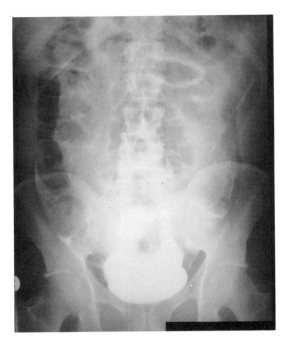

Fig. 17.2 Closed injury to the bladder: cystogram showing extravasation of contrast into the peritoneal cavity.

Catheter trauma

A catheter may be forced through the wall of the bladder, usually one that is already severely contracted. In recent years, it has become a common complication in patients with continent reservoirs which have to be emptied by inter-mittent self-catheterization [6]. The diagnosis is as difficult to make as in the other groups of 'silent' perforation but should always be suspected.

Ether rupture

A diabolically dangerous method for bursting the balloon of a Foley catheter, used to be to inject ether down the side channel. Before it burst, the balloon could rupture the bladder. Ether in the bladder could cause necrosis and even death, and unless great care was taken in every case to wash the bladder out, bits of rubber from the balloon would be left behind on which stones would subsequently form [7].

Bladder rupture in fractures of the pelvis

Some ruptures of the bladder caused by fractures are associated with injuries of the urethra (see p. 460). Others are found when laparotomy is performed for intra-abdominal bleeding (Fig. 17.3). In repairing the bladder, a formal cys-totomy should be made. Fragments of pelvis or even the head of the femur may have to be replaced before the bladder is repaired from within. The ureter should be protected with a catheter. Suprapubic and urethral drainage are provided [1,3].

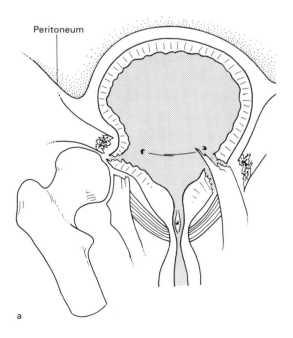

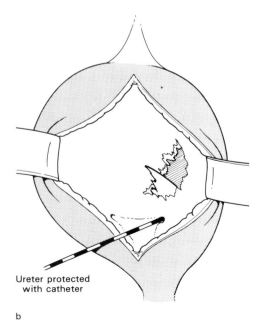

Fig. 17.3 (a) The bladder may be pierced by a fragment of bone. (b) The bladder is opened. The ureters are protected by catheters when repairing the lacerated bladder.

Open injury to the bladder

Operative injury

If the bladder is injured at open operation the laceration is closed there and then with appropriate drainage.

If the injury to the bladder is not noticed at the original operation, e.g. hysterectomy, urine will leak from the vagina a few days later. First, the fluid leaking from the vagina may be shown to be urine by measuring its concentration of urea or creatinine: no other body fluid can have a creatinine concentration greater than that of the plasma [8].

An IVU is done. If the ureter is obstructed it usually means it has been damaged (Fig. 17.4). Cystoscopy is performed and ureterograms are done on both sides to rule out ureteric injury (Fig. 17.5). The fistula between the bladder and vagina is usually obvious and the diagnosis is easy.

The conventional gynaecological teaching is that (a) these fistulae will close of their own accord if the bladder is kept drained continuously for 3 weeks or so; (b) that 2 or 3 months or

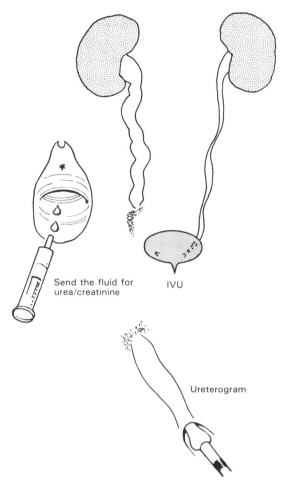

Send the fluid for urea/creatinine

IVU

Ureterogram

Fig. 17.5 It is a wise precaution to perform bilateral ureterograms even when a hole can be seen in the bladder.

more should be allowed to pass before any attempt is made to close them; and (c) that the closure should always be done by the vaginal route [9,10].

Urologists take a completely different view. Few of us have seen patients in whom fistulae have closed spontaneously, but have seen many where the fistula has been allowed to leak for months before anything was done about it.

It is certainly true that very small fistulae can be dealt with by the vaginal route.

Vaginal closure of a vesicovaginal fistula

A small Fogarty or Foley catheter is passed into the fistula, inflated and pulled down. The wall of the vagina is carefully infiltrated with saline and adrenaline, and then the fistula is excised, extending the incision sufficiently to make sure

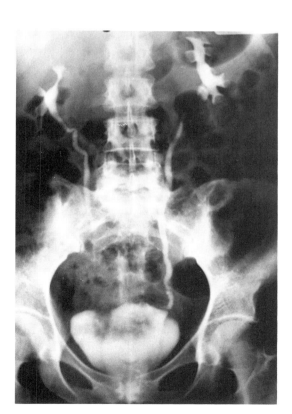

Fig. 17.4 If the IVU shows obstruction it usually means the ureter has been damaged.

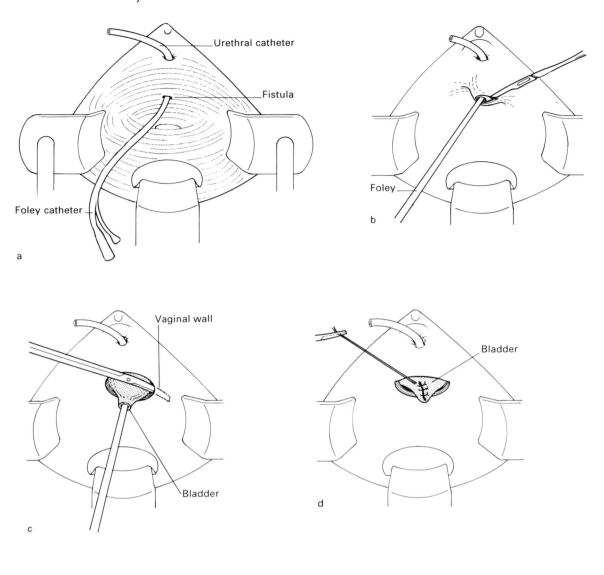

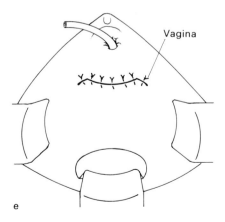

Fig. 17.6 Small vesicovaginal fistulae may be closed per vaginam. (a) A small balloon catheter helps to pull down the fistula which is (b) circumcised and (c) thoroughly mobilized. (d) Then the hole in the bladder is closed in one layer, and (e) covered with a second thick layer of vaginal wall.

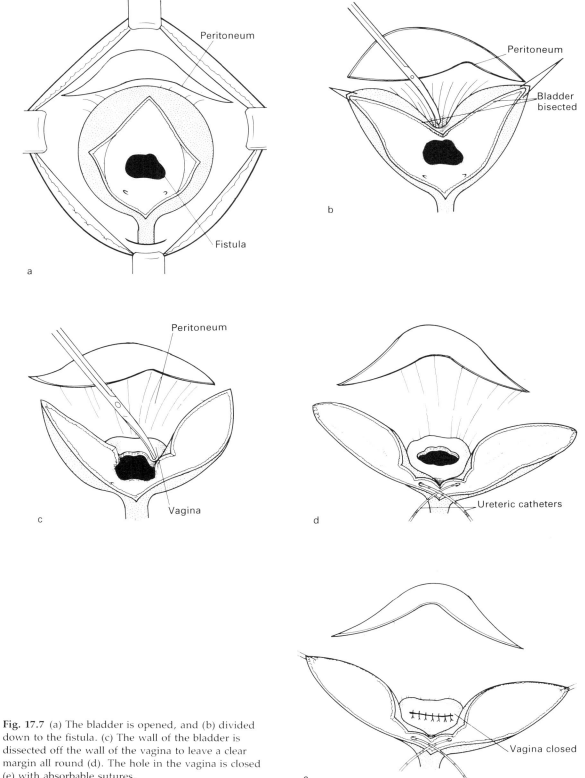

Fig. 17.7 (a) The bladder is opened, and (b) divided down to the fistula. (c) The wall of the bladder is dissected off the wall of the vagina to leave a clear margin all round (d). The hole in the vagina is closed (e) with absorbable sutures.

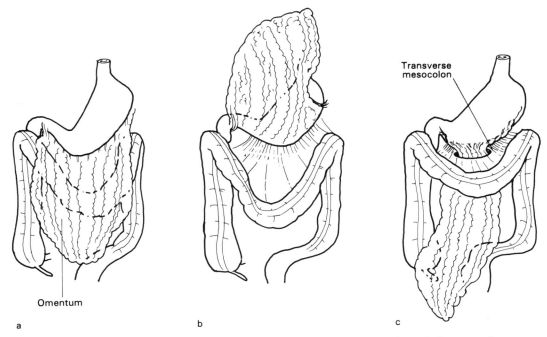

Omentum

a   b   c

Fig. 17.8 (a–c) The omentum is mobilized off the transverse colon and brought through the mesocolon.

that a good thick flap of vaginal wall can be sewn together over it (Fig. 17.6).

Transvesical closure of a vesicovaginal fistula

More often the hole is large, and unless there is sepsis, we disagree with the traditional view that one should wait: on the contrary, we have shown that nothing is lost by early intervention using the following technique [8].

While your cystoscope is in position, pass catheters up each ureter. Then reopen the previous incision whether it is midline or Pfannenstiel. Separate the bowel, stump of the cervix and fallopian tubes from the back of the bladder. Open the bladder between stay-sutures (Fig. 17.7) and divide it in the midline down to the fistula. Carefully separate the edges of the bladder from the vagina and close the hole in the vagina with interrupted 3-0 catgut sutures (Fig. 17.7). A flap of omentum, if necessary mobilized from the transverse mesocolon, is brought down (Fig. 17.8) and sutured over the hole in the vagina (Fig. 17.9). The bladder is now closed, if necessary rotating one half of the bladder over the defect (Fig. 17.10). Each ureter is left splinted with a suitable catheter and the bladder is closed with urethral and suprapubic drainage [8,11].

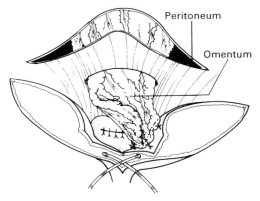

Fig. 17.9 The omentum is sewn over the suture line in the vagina.

Stab wounds

All penetrating injuries demand laparotomy. What is done depends on what is found, the principles being to repair the injuries and provide appropriate drainage, including a catheter in the bladder [12].

Gun-shot wounds

It is necessary to distinguish between gun-shot injuries caused by high and low velocity missiles [12–14].

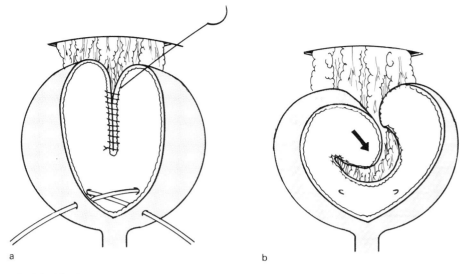

Fig. 17.10 (a & b) The bladder is closed: it may help to rotate one half round to fill the gap.

In both types of injury, if there is any suspicion of trauma to the rectum, a diverting colostomy will avoid the risk of the havoc caused by gas gangrene with its consequent massive loss of tissue [15].

High velocity bullets produce an enormous spherical blast injury with devitalization of all living tissue within its radius. In the few who survive all devitalized tissue must be excised. Primary repair must not be attempted. Free drainage is provided. Delayed primary or secondary suture can be carried out 5—10 days later.

Injuries from low velocity missiles, bullets and shrapnel fragments, call for more conservative debridement but primary closure should not be performed: delayed primary or secondary suture is safer. In bladder injuries the main requirement is to provide free drainage.

References

1 Hayes EE, Sandler CM, Corriere JN Jr (1983) Management of the ruptured bladder secondary to blunt abdominal trauma. *J Urol* 129: 946.
2 Lee JY, Cass AS (1993) Lower urinary and genital tract trauma. *Curr Opinion Urol* 3: 194.
3 Carroll PR, McAninch JW (1983) Major bladder trauma: the accuracy of cystography. *J Urol* 130: 887.
4 Hochberg E, Stone NN (1993) Bladder rupture associated with pelvic fracture due to blunt trauma. *Urology* 41: 531.
5 Renvall S, Nurmi M, Aho A (1989) Rupture of the urinary bladder: a potentially serious condition. *Scand J Urol Nephrol* 23: 185.
6 Rosen MA, Light JK (1991) Spontaneous bladder rupture following augmentation enterocystoplasty. *J Urol* 146: 1232.
7 Gattegno B, Michel F, Thibault P (1988) A serious complication of vesical ether instillation: ether cystitis. *Urology* 139: 357.
8 Blandy JP, Badenoch DF, Fowler CG, Jenkins BJ, Thomas NWM (1991) Early repair of iatrogenic injury to the ureter or bladder following gynecological surgery. *J Urol* 146: 761.
9 Tindall VR (1987) *Jeffcoate's Principles of Gynaecology*, 5th edn, p. 253. London: Butterworths.
10 Clayton SG, Lewis TLT, Pinker G (eds) (1980) *Gynaecology by Ten Teachers*, 13th edn, p. 88. London: Edward Arnold.
11 Wang Y, Hadley HR (1990) Non-delayed transvaginal repair of high lying vesicovaginal fistula. *J Urol* 144: 34.
12 Montie J (1977) Bladder injuries. *Urol Clin N Am* 4: 59.
13 Ochsner TC, Busch FM, Clark BG (1969) Urogenital wounds in Vietnam. *J Urol* 101: 224.
14 Salvatierra O, Rigdon WO, Norris DM, Brady TW (1969) Vietnam experience in 252 urological war injuries. *J Urol* 101: 615.
15 Blandy JP, Singh M (1972) Fistulae involving the adult male urethra. *Br J Urol* 44: 632.

Chapter 18: Bladder — inflammation

Acute cystitis

Acute cystitis is exceedingly common: it affects about 70% of women at one time or another. It is usually caused by an intestinal organism, e.g. *Escherichia coli*, *Klebsiella*, *Proteus mirabilis*, *Streptococcus faecalis*; less often by *Chlamydia trachomatis*, *Neisseria gonorrhoeae* and *Staphylococcus saprophyticus*; and occasionally by viruses, e.g. *herpesvirus hominis* and herpes zoster, and yeasts, e.g. *Candida albicans*.

Microorganisms reach the lining of the bladder through the urine, bloodstream or urethra. Since the female urethra is such a short tube opening into a vagina teeming with organisms, the real question is why every bladder is not always infected. What are the protective mechanisms and why are they breached?

To cause infection bacteria must stick to cells. They stick when a binding molecule on the bacterium (ligand) reacts with a receptor on the host cell [1]. For *Escherichia coli* the ligands stand up from the surface of the cell like the hairs of a caterpillar (Fig. 18.1). The hairs (pili) are antigenically specific for receptors on the epithelial cell surface. Some strains of *E. coli* form only one sort of pili, others may produce several.

Many strains of *E. coli* switch from a piliated to an unpiliated form: this may have disadvantages for the bacteria since the pili not only make them stick to epithelial cells, but also make them susceptible to phagocytosis, leucocytes preferring hairy bacteria.

In the female, the vagina may be colonized

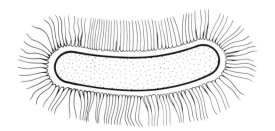

Fig. 18.1 Diagram of a bacterium showing pili. These enable a bacillus to adhere to urothelial cells.

with piliated organisms several days before the clinical onset of infection [2].

Vaginal cells from women who seldom contract urinary infection do not allow pathogenic strains of bacteria to adhere to them, unlike those from women who become frequently infected [3]. Similar differences occur in the mouth and may be determined by the human leucocyte antigen (HLA)-A3 antigen [4]. Adherence of bacteria is by no means the whole story: some strains of *E. coli* never cause urinary infection but can still stick to vaginal cells.

A second defence mechanism in the urinary tract is the protective biofilm of lactobacilli which prevent pathogenic bacilli from reaching the epithelial cells [5–8] — as if all the spaces in a garage have been taken and there is nowhere for the pathogens to park. From time to time this protective layer is breached — empty parking spaces appear. Preliminary trials are in progress using inocula of the correct strain of *Lactobacillus* to prevent recurrent urinary infection in women. Ordinary yoghurt (*L. casei*) will not do.

Clinical features

Sometimes there are obvious predisposing factors: urinary infection may follow a few days after a respiratory infection. Dysuria and frequency may occur shortly after sexual intercourse or a menstrual period. In most women there is no such pattern and attacks begin when least expected.

Stinging and discomfort on urination, with a sensation of incomplete emptying and the need to void frequently, is succeeded by strangury and haematuria, suprapubic and low back pain. Loin pain, fever and shivering usually signify bacterial infection in the kidneys.

There are no physical signs apart from a tenderness over the bladder. The urine is cloudy. If the uncentrifuged urine is inspected via a microscope it will be seen to swarm with white cells at whose edges bacteria can be seen to dance.

Culture of the urine will identify the offending organism and help to choose the appropriate antibiotic. In practice, many women with urinary infection and pus in their urine have what is reported as sterile urine.

A midstream specimen of urine will collect skin organisms as it leaves the urethra in either sex. If the urine is left for several hours these organisms will multiply and give a false impression of infection. If the urine is cultured at once (or is kept refrigerated in the interval) it is possible to distinguish urine that has been contaminated from urine that is truly infected by counting the number of organisms by colony counting. The critical figure is 10^5 colonies per millilitre of urine.

When urine is obtained from a catheter, cystoscope or needle aspiration of the bladder any organisms signify infection. The concept of the colony count only applies to voided urine specimens.

Repeated episodes of infection especially if accompanied by rigors, loin pain or haematuria, demand a complete investigation — intravenous pyelogram (IVP) or ultrasound and cystoscopy to rule out underlying causes of persistent infection, e.g. calculus, foreign body or persistent pockets of undrained urine, which call for appropriate treatment.

We cannot yet influence the rise and fall of the natural protective influences or the way bacteria suddenly become hairy, adherent and pathogenic — the patient should try to keep the system flushed out by drinking and voiding frequently. Advise the patient to have a large glass of water or cup of tea and empty the bladder every 2 h. Since this will not prevent occasional relapses, provide the patients with a small supply of an appropriate antimicrobial, e.g. trimethoprim, sulphonamide, nitrofurantoin, etc. She should take a tablet as soon as she realizes another attack has begun. A single dose may be enough to nip the episode in the bud but it is usually advisable to continue the medication for 24 h [9,10].

If attacks always follow coitus a tablet should be taken immediately afterwards.

If attacks persist in spite of these precautions the old-fashioned remedy of methenamine hippurate can halve the number of relapses without producing resistant organisms [11].

Virus cystitis

In many patients an episode of urinary infection follows an upper respiratory infection. In herpes zoster involving the S2, S3 segments cystoscopy will show a well-defined patch of bladder affected by inflammation, the rest being normal [12]. Virus infections are becoming more common in patients whose immune defences have been weakened by immunosuppressive therapy for transplantation [13,14] or acquired immune deficiency syndrome (AIDS) [15].

Chemical cystitis

Various chemicals have been introduced into the bladder by accident or on purpose, with results that vary from mild irritation to devastating necrosis. Ether was formerly used as a means of exploding the balloons of Foley catheters that would not deflate: if the expansion of the catheter did not rupture the bladder, then the ether could cause chemical necrosis of the bladder that might necessitate cystectomy [16].

Silver nitrate was used for recurrent urinary infections and from time to time gave rise to severe chemical cystitis.

The metabolites of cyclophosphamide, a drug used for leukaemia are excreted in the urine where they may cause mild inflammation or full-thickness necrosis of the entire wall of the bladder with only the ureteric orifices surviving [17]. It can be prevented by diuresis and, if necessary, keeping the bladder empty with a catheter so that the urine metabolites cannot come into contact with the urothelium [18]. Cyclophosphamide damage may also affect the kidneys and ureters [18−20].

The main clinical problem seen with cyclophosphamide cystitis is haemorrhage. On cystoscopy no single bleeding vessel can be seen but the haemorrhage may be persistent and even exsanguinating. Many methods of control have been tried: the oldest being dilute formaldehyde [21,22]. More recently prostaglandin F2 has been tried [23]. Alum irrigation over prolonged periods is claimed to be successful [24], but the author has found it unreliable.

One curious late complication of cyclophosphamide cystitis is leiomyosarcoma of the bladder [25].

Other chemicals which can damage the bladder include acetone [26], and the very same formaldehyde solution that is used to control bleeding in radiation cystitis [27].

Chronic cystitis

Chronic bacterial cystitis

Many women suffer repeated episodes of acute cystitis. Eventually, they become continuous and the patient has constant pain, frequency and dysuria. Cystoscopy shows changes of chronic cystitis: biopsy will show cystitis follicularis or glandularis, or a mixture of both.

These patients are often unusually anxious and kindness and sympathy are no less important in therapy than accurate diagnosis and treatment [28].

Cystitis follicularis

Cystoscopy shows a bumpy mucosa resembling cobblestones (Fig. 18.2). Biopsy shows collections of lymphocytes with germinal follicles in the lamina propria: lymphocytes and plasma cells outnumber the leucocytes (Fig. 18.3). (When these changes are seen in children it demands a very careful follow-up [29].) It is usually seen in elderly women whose urethra has become somewhat stiff and narrow, perhaps from lack of oestrogen stimulation. There is no specific cause for it and to find the responsible organism may need several urine cultures. Diuresis, frequent voiding and a prolonged course of the appropriate antimicrobial agents may be effective. When this fails, a short course of bactericidal antibiotics, if necessary given intravenously, may eradicate the infection. It should be followed up with a prolonged course of a suppressive antibiotic at a lower dose.

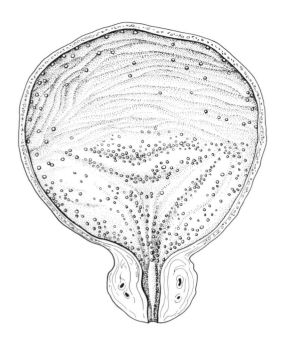

Fig. 18.2 The cystoscopic appearances of cystitis follicularis (courtesy of Dr Frank Marsh).

Cystitis cystica

Biopsy shows von Brunn's nests [30]. They arise when small islands of epithelium become buried and form small vesicles (Fig. 18.4). These have a characteristic cystoscopic appearance — glistening bubbles just under the mucosa, sometimes blackened by the accumulation of haemosiderin. Persistent cystitis cystica may progress to fully developed cystitis glandularis which is premalignant and must be followed with great care [31,32] (Fig. 18.5).

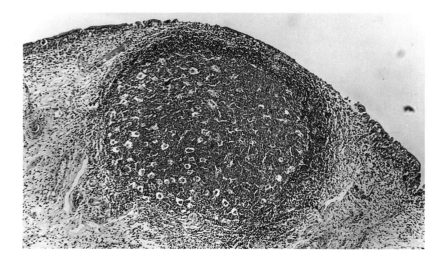

Fig. 18.3 Biopsy of cystitis follicularis showing collections of lymphocytes with a germinal follicle under the urothelium (courtesy of Dr Frank Marsh).

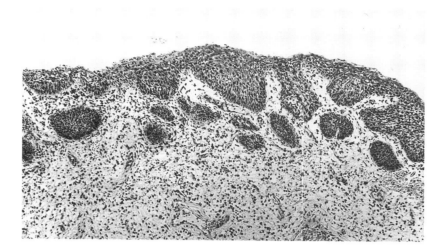

Fig. 18.4 Bladder biopsy showing buried islands of urothelium — the nests of von Brunn.

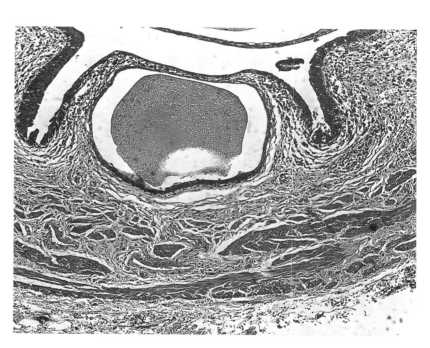

Fig. 18.5 Cystitis cystica (courtesy of Dr R.C.B. Pugh).

Another variation on this theme is nephrogenic adenoma [33]. There may have been a single episode — usually an endoscopic operation — preceding its onset but more often nephrogenic adenoma, like cystitis cystica and cystitis glandularis, are the long-term sequelae of persistent irritation and infection, and are seen with stones or treated tuberculosis (Fig. 18.6).

Eosinophilic cystitis

In this little understood condition the urine is sterile, but cystoscopy shows the bladder to be intensely inflamed and the cause is a matter for conjecture. It has been described in a renal transplant recipient [33] suggesting that some very unusual infective agent — only likely to be seen in an immunosuppressed patient — may be responsible [34]. One case has been reported where it was caused by a patient who ate raw frogs and developed worms that tunneled into the bladder [35]. Usually the cause is unknown. The diagnosis can made by biopsy, which may be performed because the heaped-up inflammatory change looks like cancer [36]. The biopsy shows all layers of bladder crowded with eosinophils (Fig. 18.7).

Innumerable treatments have been tried but

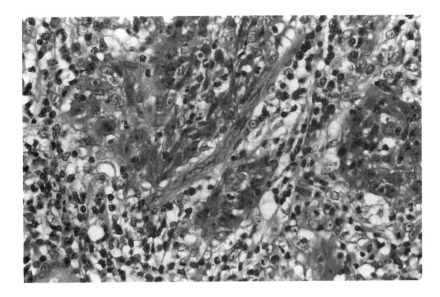

Fig. 18.6 Nephrogenic adenoma (courtesy of Dr Suhail Baithun).

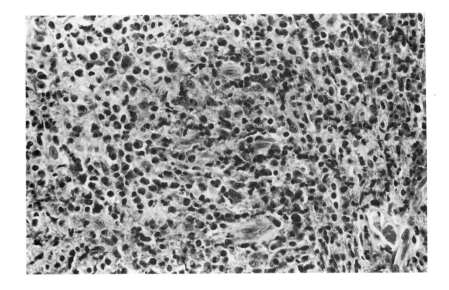

Fig. 18.7 Eosinophilic cystitis (courtesy of Dr Suhail Baithun).

none are reliable. A combination of non-steroidal anti-inflammatory drugs with antihistamines appears to be the most promising [37].

Cystectomy may be required because of ureteric obstruction or contraction of the bladder.

Malacoplakia

In most patients, the symptoms are those of chronic cystitis but no organisms may be found in the urine. Sometimes there is haematuria and cystoscopy shows the characteristic light brown plaques which cannot be distinguished from cancer and demand to be biopsied.

Biopsy shows a granuloma in the epithelium and lamina propria (Fig. 18.8). Within the macrophages there are characteristic Michaelis–Gutmann bodies — tiny calcified spheres built up around bacteria like pearls on a grain of sand in an oyster [38].

When malacoplakia involves the ureter it can cause obstruction, resembling in every way that caused by a urothelial cancer.

Treatment is empirical, but there are theoretical reasons why a combination of trimethoprim and a sulphonamide may be the treatment of choice [39,40].

Malacoplakia is also found in the kidney and testis.

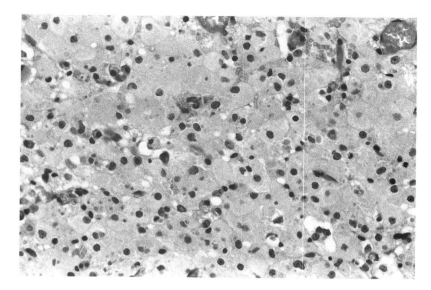

Fig. 18.8 Malacoplakia of the wall of the bladder. The macrophages contain Michaelis—Gutmann bodies (courtesy of Dr Suhail Baithun).

Cystitis emphysematosa

Many intestinal organisms ferment glucose and produce gas. In diabetes, deep-seated infection of the wall of the bladder may cause bubbles of gas to arise with a characteristic appearance [41] (Fig. 18.9). The changes resolve with antibiotic treatment.

Alkaline encrusted cystitis

Infection with *Proteus mirabilis* around an indwelling catheter may invade all the layers of the bladder and deposit calcium salts deep in the muscle (Fig. 18.10). The urothelium is ulcerated and covered with a crust of calcified debris. Bleeding may be profuse [42].

The treatment is by antibiotics and attempts to acidify the urine, which are usually frustrated by the ammonia produced by the *Proteus*.

The end-result is usually a small contracted bladder requiring urinary diversion or cystoplasty.

Tuberculosis

Tuberculosis of the bladder is virtually always associated with renal tuberculosis (see p. 153).

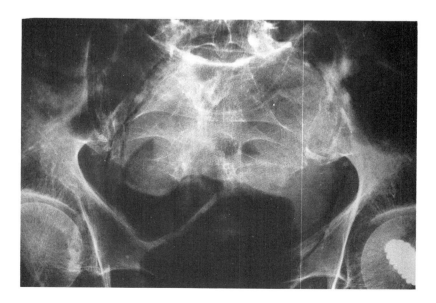

Fig. 18.9 Radiograph showing emphysematous cystitis in a patient with diabetes and a severe urinary infection (courtesy of Dr Otto Chan).

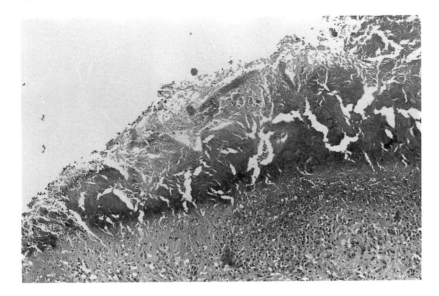

Fig. 18.10 Histological appearance of alkaline encrusted cystitis. All the layers of the bladder are infiltrated with calcified deposits (courtesy of Dr Suhail Baithun).

Clinical features

There is persistent frequency and painful voiding resembling cystitis from any cause. The urine shows many pus cells but is sterile on routine culture.

There are no specific cystoscopic appearances. Classical tubercles are rarely seen, even in the early stages, and any 'tubercles' are more likely to be lymphoid follicles on biopsy. Tuberculosis should be suspected if one ureter is seen to be oedematous and not to move up and down with expulsion of urine. The usual appearance is of generalized redness. Sometimes ulcers are seen: occasionally there is a papillomatous granuloma which resembles a carcinoma and requires biopsy — only then is the right diagnosis made.

Acid- and alcohol-fast bacilli may be found in the urine on Ziehl−Neelsen staining, but it requires culture on Loewenstein−Jensen medium to confirm the presence of *Mycobacterium tuberculosis*. A positive biopsy often speeds up the diagnosis.

Treatment

Treatment should ideally be given in consultation with a chest physician with experience in dealing with tuberculosis. Treatment will involve triple therapy, and requires attention to the possibility of tuberculous lesions elsewhere (see p. 153).

As the granulomas in the bladder respond to treatment, they heal with fibrous tissue and the bladder shrinks until it may have a very small capacity. For such a patient cystoplasty is indicated. If the caecum is used, it makes an excellent substitute for the bladder but because of the risk that it may develop high pressure, and threaten ureteric obstruction, a de-tubularized bladder substitution may be better, at the cost of requiring intermittent self-catheterization [43] (see p. 328).

Chronic interstitial cystitis (Hunner's ulcer)

Hunner reported eight women with symptoms of chronic cystitis, sterile urine, shallow ulcers or stellate scars near the air-bubble, which bled when touched. They all had what he described as a 'granular urethritis' [44,45]. As Hunner's experience grew, so did his disillusion with treatment: nothing did any good [46]. Things are much the same today.

The diagnosis is difficult: the term is usually assigned to a bladder whose urothelium may look normal at first or have a few fine scars. As the bladder is filled under general anaesthesia the patient is obviously stimulated and grunts in a characteristic fashion. As the bladder continues to fill small cracks appear in the epithelium which bleed as the water runs out of the bladder — the typical 'cascade bleeding'.

The cystoscopic appearances so closely imitate carcinoma *in situ* that it is necessary to take mucosal biopsies. The histological appearances are not specific (Fig. 18.11). The urothelium has usually been shed. The underlying lamina propria is full of chronic inflammatory cells,

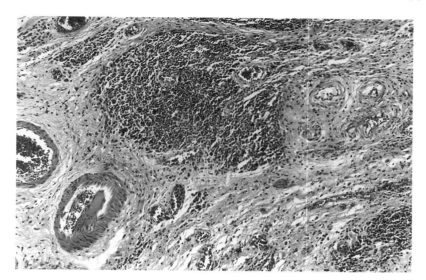

Fig. 18.11 Biopsy from a bladder with interstitial cystitis — Hunner's ulcer. The surface urothelium has been shed. The lamina propria is infiltrated with chronic inflammatory cells including mast cells (courtesy of Dr Suhail Baithun).

among them mast cells, whose granules release histamine [47]. Much importance has been attached to these by some authors, but mast cells are present in 30% of patients with bladder instability and are commonly present in those without interstitial cystitis [48,49].

It seems that whenever a disease has no known cause autoimmunity is blamed: in Hunner's ulcer the offending antigen is bladder muscle [50] or its blood vessels [51]. There is said to be an association with systemic lupus erythematosus, scleroderma and autoimmune thyroiditis [52].

All forms of treatment have been empirical and unsatisfactory. Overdistension of the bladder may give symptomatic relief for up to 6 months [53], as may diathermy of the 'ulcers', instillation of substances thought to affect the waterproofing of the urothelium [54], dimethyl sulphoxide [55], and steroids. Amitriptyline and nifedipine have been found to do good by some, but not by others [56,57]. Indeed the general experience has been that all forms of treatment work in some of the patients some of the time.

Subtotal cystectomy with replacement of the bladder with caecum or de-tubularized bowel does give relief of pain, but not always, and not always for long [58]. In some patients the symptoms return, and in others it is said that similar granulomatous changes appear in the segment of bowel or elsewhere in the intestine [59]. Urinary diversion may be the only solution.

Parasitic diseases of the bladder

Schistosomiasis or bilharziasis

Although the disease was known to the ancient Egyptians [60] its cause was not discovered until 1851 by Theodor Bilharz [61] (Fig. 18.12). Today, it is one of the most serious diseases of mankind affecting over 200 million people — one in 20 of the entire world's population — in Africa, the Middle East, Brazil, Venezuela, Surinam China, the Phillipines, Indonesia, the Mekong delta and Malaysia, and some of the West Indies (Fig. 18.13). In some areas nearly 100% of school-children may be infested [62].

The main species that affect man are *Schistosoma mansoni*, *S. haematobium* and *S. japonicum*: hardly less important are *S. intercalatum*, *S. mattheei* and *S. mekongi*. Each has a complex life cycle (Fig. 18.14) in which there is a sexual generation in humans, and an asexual stage in snails: beside the earliest fossil traces of man are fossils of appropriate snails [63].

The pairs of adult worms, about 1 cm long (Fig. 18.15), live in veins attached by the sucker on the head of the male fluke. They can live for 30 years and lay 400 eggs per day [62]. Any vein can be affected, those of the lamina propria of the bladder being relevant to urologists. The eggs perforate the urothelium, are shed with the urine and hatch in fresh water liberating miracidia (Fig. 18.16). These tiny ciliated creatures are attracted to an appropriate snail which they

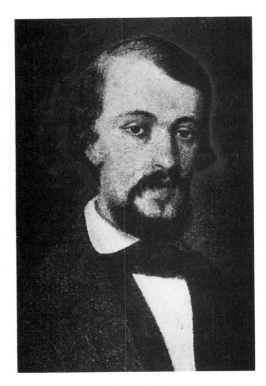

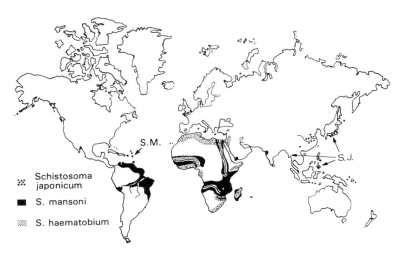

Fig. 18.13 Geographical distribution of schistosomiasis (courtesy of Mr Manmeet Singh).

Fig. 18.12 Theodor Bilharz 1825–1862 (by permission of the Trustees of the Wellcome Museum).

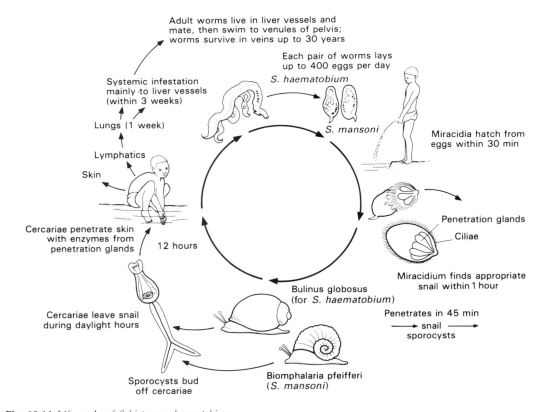

Fig. 18.14 Life cycle of *Schistosoma haematobium*.

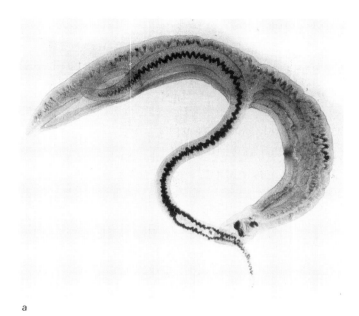

Gynaephoric canal of
male envelops female

Male

Female

Schistosomes
(about 1 cm long)

a

Fig. 18.15 (a & b) Pair of adult schistosome worms
removed from a vein.

b

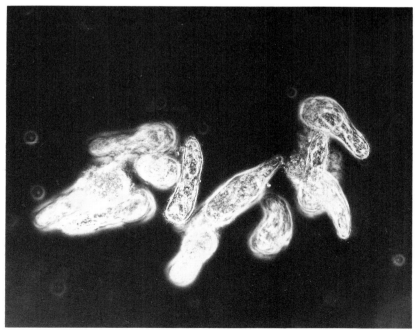

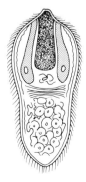

Fig. 18.16 (a & b)
Miracidia (courtesy of
Dr S.W. Attwood).

a

b

invade and there undergo a series of asexual cell divisions eventually forming a cyst which bursts to shed tiny sexual forms of the flukes — the cercariae — into the water (Fig. 18.17). A single snail can shed over 1000 cercariae per hour.

Ten seconds contact between the skin of an adult or child and water containing cercariae allows them to penetrate the skin where they enter the lymphatics and within 24 h may set up an irritation — swimmers' itch — sometimes accompanied by a papular rash which lasts a few days.

Some 2 weeks later the patient may develop symptoms of *Katayama* fever with fever, rigors, sweating, headache, urticaria, cough and facial oedema. This illness may last for up to 3 months, during which the flukes are migrating via the bloodstream to their final destination in veins anywhere in the body — brain, eyes, skin, bowel and bladder.

After about 12 weeks eggs begin to appear in the urine [64]. The diagnosis during the stage of *Katayama* fever is difficult: eosinophilia is conspicuous and immunological tests may be positive [65,66]. Ideally, suspected patients should be followed up and treatment deferred until eggs appear in the urine or stools [67] but modern treatment is so simple and safe that it is often more practical to treat all suspected patients.

Public health and prevention

Sewage systems for urine and faeces would prevent schistosomiasis. In China, clearing irrigation channels and construction of concrete latrines was effective [68]. In parts of the world where water, let alone concrete, are in short supply this is more difficult; moreover the control of *Oncomelania* (the snail host of the Chinese *Schistosoma japonicum*) appears to be easier than that of *Biomphalaria* and *Bulinus* (the snails for *S. mansoni* and *S. haematobium*) [69]. The problem is a political one: until politicians put health before armaments there will be much for surgeons to do.

Pathology

In the pelvis the worm pairs affect the bladder, ureters, seminal vesicles and prostate, with the greatest egg burden being in the bladder [70].

The body reacts to the worms and their eggs by forming a granuloma, mainly in the lamina propria, later amongst the muscle bundles of the detrusor (Fig. 18.18). The eggs secrete a histiolytic

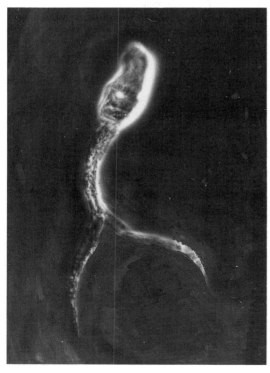

a

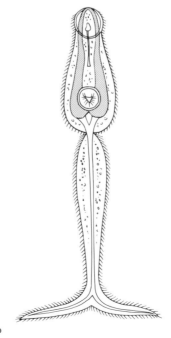

b

Fig. 18.17 (a & b) Cercaria (courtesy of Dr S.W. Attwood).

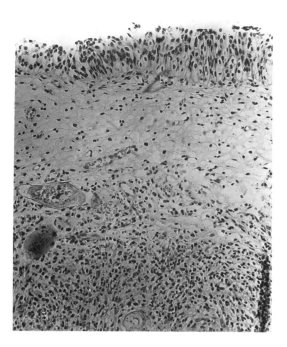

Fig. 18.18 Bilharzia ova in the lamina propria (courtesy of Dr R.C.B. Pugh).

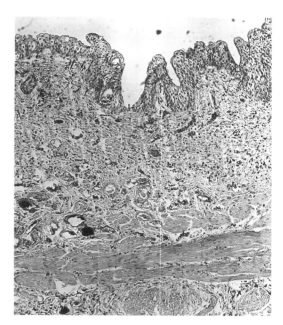

Fig. 18.19 Inflammatory response to calcified ova (courtesy of Dr R.C.B. Pugh).

antigen which evokes a cell-mediated immunological response, attracting eosinophils. The granulomas may project into the lumen of the bladder.

The inflammatory response to the eggs (Fig. 18.19) leads to ischaemia and loss of overlying urothelium, which now undergoes metaplasia, squamous or glandular — changes often made worse by bacterial infection, often with *Salmonella*.

Dead eggs provoke foreign body giant cell reaction and calcification. Healing is succeeded by reinfection, and the repeated cycle of healing, granuloma and ulceration leads to carcinoma *in situ* and overt cancer (Fig. 18.20).

Clinical features

The earliest stages of bilharzial infestation (swimmers' itch and *Katayama* fever) usually go unnoticed and haematuria brings the patient to the doctor. There will be no physical signs.

Investigations

Eggs will be found in the urine, usually the terminal-spined eggs of *Schistosoma haematobium* (Fig. 18.21). Cystoscopy will show minute yellow specks, the bilharzial tubercles, sometimes surrounded by a halo of hyperaemia. Later these

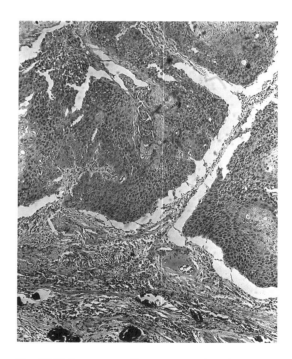

Fig. 18.20 Squamous cell cancer secondary to bilharziasis (courtesy of Dr R.C.B. Pugh).

granulomas enlarge and form polyps which may or may not calcify [70,71]. The intravenous urogram shows characteristic calcification in the bladder, ureters, seminal vesicles and vasa deferentia (Fig. 18.22 & 18.23).

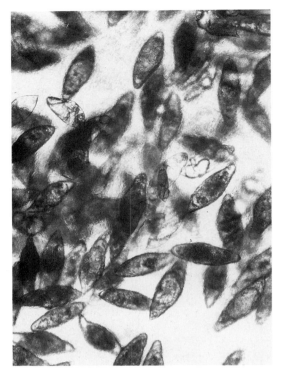

Fig. 18.21 Eggs of *Schistosoma haematobium* from a biopsy of bladder squeezed between two slides.

Elsewhere in the bladder the calcified eggs glisten under the surface like specks of sand (the sandy patches), more obvious from the loss of the vascular pattern of blood vessels in these areas.

Ulceration may extend deep into the tissues outside the bladder, especially anteriorly. Histological features of all the forms of chronic cystitis

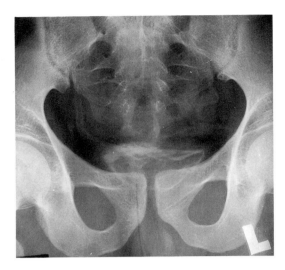

Fig. 18.22 Calcification in the wall of the bladder and ureter in schistosomiasis (courtesy of Mr G. Ravi).

are to be found: cystitis cystica and glandularis, von Brunn's nests, squamous metaplasia and frank leucoplakia.

Treatment

The modern chemotherapy for bilharzia consists of a single dose of Praziquantel, which for safety may be repeated after a month. The local treatment of benign lesions in the bladder consists of transurethral resection of polypi and ulcers [71].

Bladder outflow obstruction

Contracture from healing of granulomas in the bladder neck is often accompanied by weakness

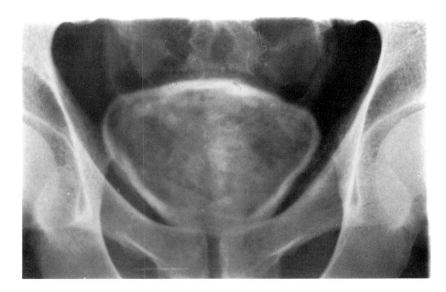

Fig. 18.23 Calcification in the bladder and ureters (courtesy of Professor Aziz Fam).

of the damaged detrusor [72,73]. Calculi often form in the bladder and ureters which are typically calcified and dilated (Fig. 18.24). Scarring draws the ureters onto the trigone calling for caution when resecting the bladder neck [70].

Bilharzial cancer of the bladder

Cancer in bilharziasis has three special features:
1 two-thirds are squamous cell cancers;
2 the age incidence is relatively young (average 46.7 years); and
3 dense fibrosis surrounds the bladder.

Neither transurethral resection nor partial cystectomy is applicable to these large tumours which often present late. There is evidence of impaired T cell function in these patients [74,75]. Total radical cystectomy has been shown to be safe and effective [70]. For those who need the operation a continent diversion is necessary (see p. 327).

Other complications of schistosomiasis

Urethra

Urethral stricture usually involves the bulb and in part may be the result of instrumentation rather than the infestation [70].

Prostate

Secondary infection and prostatitis are common. In the prostate, the ova are distributed throughout the stroma and fibrosis may cause outflow obstruction.

Seminal vesicles

The seminal vesicles are frequently chalked out on the X-ray by the calcified ova. The inflammation can cause haemospermia and painful ejaculation, ova being found in the semen. It may be necessary to remove the vesicles.

Bilharziasis in the female

The uterus, fallopian tubes and ovaries are often involved [76]. Large painful polypi of the urethra and vulva give rise to distressing dyspareunia (Fig. 18.25) Bilharzial fibrosis and ischaemia make repair of obstetrical fistulae more difficult: drug treatment should always be given first [70].

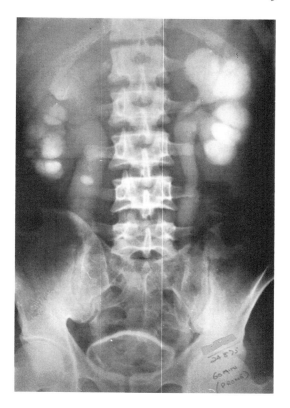

Fig. 18.24 Calcification and dilatation of the ureters (courtesy of Professor Aziz Fam).

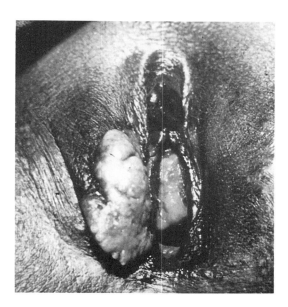

Fig. 18.25 Bilharzial lesion of the vulva — easily confused with carcinoma (courtesy of Mr J. Lawson).

Amoebiasis

Entamoeba histolytica may travel from the bowel into the bladder through a fistula, but more probably is blood-borne. Clinically, it causes cystitis with haematuria and frequency. Cystoscopy shows inflammation, ulceration and polypoid elevations of the urothelium. Balanitis, vaginitis and vulvitis may be complications [77].

Worm infestations

Eustrongylas gigas the legendary 'giant kidney worm' is said to be the largest nematode known to infect humans. Its life cycle is ill-understood. It invades the renal pelvis and destroys the renal parenchyma [78].

Even more bizarre is vesical sparganosis, which is caused by eating raw frogs. The worms make a nest of tunnels in the wall of the bladder causing a mass that must be excised. Antibody titres for *Sparganum* are raised [79].

Burger [80] reported a case of a 23-year-old woman who claimed to have passed a 15 cm 'horsehair worm' *Paragordius esavianus* per urethram.

Catfish

The Carnero or candiru is a catfish 5 cm long and 4 mm wide which is attracted by urine and said to swim up the urethra of unwary people bathing in the Amazon [81].

References

1 Schaeffer AJ (1990) Modifiers of susceptibility to urinary tract infection. *J Urol* 143: 138.
2 Schaeffer AJ, Stamey TA (1977) Studies of introital colonization in women with recurrent urinary infections. IX The role of antimicrobial therapy. *J Urol* 118: 221.
3 Fowler ER, Stamey TA (1977) Studies of introital colonization in women with recurrent urinary tract infections. VII. The role of bacterial adherence. *J Urol* 117: 472.
4 Schaeffer AJ, Radvany RM, Chmiel JS (1983) Human leukocyte antigens in women with recurrent urinary tract infections. *J Infect Dis* 148: 604.
5 Maskell R (1990) Effect on urogenital flora of antibiotic therapy for urinary tract infection. *Scand J Infect Dis* 22: 631–2.
6 Redondo-Lopez V, Cook RL, Sobel JD (1990) Emerging role of lactobacilli in the control and maintenance of the vaginal bacterial microflora. *Rev Infect Dis* 12: 856.
7 Reid G, Bruce AW (1993) Factors influencing the adhesion of uropathogens to the uroepithelium. *Curr Opinion Urol* 3: 21.
8 Hawthorn LA, Reid G (1990) Exclusion of uropathogen adhesion to polymer surfaces by *Lactobacillus acidophilus*. *J Biomed Mater Res* 24: 39.
9 Harbord RB, Gruneberg RN (1981) Treatment of urinary tract infection with a single dose of amoxycillin, co-trimoxazole or trimethoprim. *Br Med J* 283: 1301.
10 Rapoport J, Rees GA, Willmott NJ, Slack RCB, O'Grady FW (1981) Treatment of acute urinary tract infection with three doses of co-trimoxazole. *Br Med J* 283: 1302.
11 Cronberg S, Welin C-O, Henriksson L, Hellsten S, Persson KMS, Stenberg P (1987) Prevention of recurrent acute cystitis by methenamine hippurate: double blind controlled crossover long term study. *Br Med J* 294: 1507.
12 Darget R (1929) Deux cas d'herpes zoster de la vessie. *J Urol (Paris)* 27: 229.
13 Mikuyama K (1989) Hemorrhagic cystitis associated with urinary excretion of adenovirus type 11 following allogeneic bone marrow transplantation. *Bone Marrow Trans* 4: 533.
14 Buchanan W, Bowman JS, Jaffers G (1990) Adenoviral acute hemorrhagic cystitis following renal transplantation. *Am J Nephrol* 10: 350.
15 Lucas SB, Parr DC, Wright E, Papadaki L, Patou G (1989) AIDS presenting as cytomegalovirus cystitis. *Br J Urol* 64: 429.
16 Gattegno B, Michel F, Thibault P (1988) A serious complication of vesical ether instillation: ether cystitis. *Urology* 39: 357.
17 Marsh FP, Vince FP, Pollock DJ, Blandy JP (1971) Cyclophosphamide necrosis of bladder causing calcification, contracture and reflux treated by colocystoplasty. *Br J Urol* 43: 324.
18 Droller MJ, Saral K, Santos G (1982) Prevention of cyclophosphamide-induced hemorrhagic cystitis. *Urology* 20: 256.
19 Efros M, Ahmed T, Choudhury M (1990) Cyclophosphamide-induced hemorrhagic pyelitis and ureteritis associated with cystitis in marrow transplantation. *J Urol* 144: 1231.
20 Levine LA, Richie JP (1989) Urological complications of cyclophosphamide. *J Urol* 141: 1063.
21 Stillwell TJ, Benson RC (1988) Cyclophosphamide-induced hemorrhagic cystitis. A review of 100 patients. *Cancer* 61: 451.
22 Donahue LA, Frank IN (1989) Intravesical formalin for hemorrhagic cystitis; analysis of therapy (review). *J Urol* 141: 809.
23 Shurafa M, Shumaker E, Cronin S (1987) Prostaglandin F2-alpha bladder irrigation for control of intractable cyclophosphamide hemorrhagic cystitis. *J Urol* 137: 1230.
24 Goel AK, Rao MS, Bhagwat AG, Vaidyanathan S, Goswami AK, Sen TK (1985) Intravesical irrigation with alum for the control of massive bladder hemorrhage. *J Urol* 133: 956.
25 Thrasher JB, Miller GJ, Wettlaufer JN (1990) Bladder leiomyosarcoma following cyclophosphamide therapy for lupus nephritis. *J Urol* 143: 119.
26 Kato K, Kitada A, Longhurst PA, Weing AJ, Levin RM (1990) Time-course of alterations of bladder function following acetone-induced cystitis. *J Urol* 144: 1272.
27 Scott MP, Marshall S, Lyon RP (1974) Bladder rup-

ture following formalin therapy for hemorrhage secondary to cyclophosphamide therapy. *Urology* 3: 364.

28 Rees DLP, Faroumand N (1977) Psychiatric aspects of recurrent cystitis in women. *Br J Urol* 49: 651.

29 Hansson S, Hanson E, Hjalmas K *et al.* (1990) Follicular cystitis in girls with untreated asymptomatic or covert bacteriuria. *J Urol* 143: 330.

30 von Brunn A (1893) Ueber drusenahnliche Bildungen in der Schleimhaut des Nierenbeckens, des Ureters und der Harnblase beim Menschen. *Arch Mikr Anat* 41: 294.

31 Jost SP, Dixon JS, Gosling JA (1993) Ultrastructural observations on cystitis cystica in human bladder urothelium. *Br J Urol* 71: 28.

32 Malek RS, Rosen JS, O'Dea MJ (1983) Adenocarcinoma of bladder. *Urology* 21: 357.

33 Molland EA, Trott PA, Paris AMI, Blandy JP (1976) Nephrogenic adenoma: a form of adenomatous metaplasia of the bladder: a clinical and electron microscopical study. *Br J Urol* 48: 453.

34 Horner SA, Weingarten JL (1990) Eosinophilic cystitis in a renal allograft recipient. *J Urol* 144: 342.

35 Oh SJ, Shi JG, Lee SE (1993) Eosinophilic cystitis caused by vesical sparganosis: a case report. *J Urol* 149: 581.

36 Thijssen A, Gerridzen RG (1990) Eosinophilic cystitis presenting as invasive bladder cancer: comments on pathogenesis and management. *J Urol* 144: 977.

37 Motzkin D (1990) Non-steroidal anti-inflammatory drugs in the treatment of eosinophilic cystitis. *J Urol* 144: 1464.

38 Michaelis L, Gutmann C (1902) Ueber einschlusse in blasentumoren. *Z Klin Med* 47: 208.

39 Olmo JMC, Carcamo P, Gaston de Iriarte E, Jimenez F, Martinez-Pineiro L, Martinez-Pineiro JA (1993) Genitourinary malakoplakia. *Br J Urol* 72: 6.

40 Maderazo EG, Berlin BB, Morhardt C (1979) Treatment of malakoplakia with trimethoprimsulfamethoxazole. *Urology* 13: 70.

41 Katz DS, Aksoy E, Cunha BA (1993) *Clostridium perfringens* emphysematous cystitis. *Urology* 41: 458.

42 Letcher HG, Matheson NM (1935) Encrustation of the bladder as a result of alkaline cystitis. *Br J Surg* 23: 716.

43 Gil-Vernet JM (1965) The ileocolic segment in urological surgery. *J Urol* 94: 418.

44 Hunner GL (1914) A rare type of bladder ulcer in women. *Trans South Surg Gyn Assoc* 27: 247.

45 Hunner GL (1915) A rare type of bladder ulcer in women: report of cases. *Boston Med Surg J* 172: 660.

46 Hunner GL (1930) Neurosis of the bladder. *J Urol* 24: 567.

47 Christmas TJ, Rode J, Milroy EJG, Turner-Warwick RT (1989) Mast cells in interstitial cystitis: their site of action? *Neurourol Urodynam* 8: 394.

48 Messing EK (1994) Interstitial cystitis (editorial). *J Urol* 151: 355.

49 Moore KH, Nickson P, Richmond DH, Sutherst JR, Manasse RP, Helliwell TR (1992) Detrusor mast cells in refractory idiopathic instability. *Br J Urol* 70: 17.

50 Silk MR (1970) Bladder antibodies in interstitial cystitis. *J Urol* 103: 307.

51 Witherow RO'N, Gillespie L, McMullen L, Goldin RD, Walker MM (1989) Painful bladder syndrome — a clinical and immunopathological study. *Br J Urol* 64: 158.

52 Parivar F, Bradbrook RA (1986) Interstitial cystitis. *Br J Urol* 58: 239.

53 Badenoch AW (1971) Chronic interstitial cystitis. *Br J Urol* 43: 718.

54 Parsons CL, Benson G, Childs SJ, Hanno P, Sant GR, Webster G (1993) A quantitatively controlled method to study prospectively interstitial cystitis and demonstrate the efficacy of pentosanpolysulfate. *J Urol* 150: 845.

55 Perez-Marrero R, Emerson LE, Feltis JT (1988) A controlled study of dimethyl sulfoxide in interstitial cystitis. *J Urol* 140: 36.

56 Hanno PM, Buehler J, Wein AJ (1989) Use of amitryptiline in the treatment of interstitial cystitis. *J Urol* 141: 846.

57 Fleischmann JD, Huntley HN, Shingleton WB, Wentworth DB (1991) Clinical and immunological response to nifedipine for the treatment of interstitial cystitis. *J Urol* 146: 1235.

58 Nielsen KK, Kromann-Andersen B, Steven K, Hald T (1990) Failure of combined supratrigonal cystectomy and Mainz ileocecocystoplasty in intractable interstitial cystitis: is histology and mast cell count a reliable predictor for the outcome of surgery? *J Urol* 144: 255.

59 MacDermott JP, Charpied CG, Tesluk H, Stone AR (1990) Recurrent interstitial cystitis following caecocystoplasty: fact or fiction? *J Urol* 144: 37.

60 Miller RL, Armelagos GJ, Ikram S, De Jonge N, Krijger FW, Deelder AM (1992) Palaeoepidemiology of schistosome infection in mummies. *Br Med J* 304: 555—6.

61 Bilharz T (1852) Fernere Beobachtungen über das die Pfortader des menschen bewohnende Distomum hämatobium, und sein Verhältniss ze gewissen pathologischen Bildungen. *Z Wiss Zool* 4: 72.

62 Webbe G (1981) Schistosomiasis: some advances. *Br Med J* 283: 1104.

63 Wright CA (1971) *Flukes and Snails*. London: Allen & Unwin.

64 Stuiver PC (1984) Acute schistosomiasis (*Katayama* fever). *Br Med J* 288: 221.

65 Tosswill, JHC, Ridley DS (1986) An evaluation of the ELISA for schistosomiasis in a hospital population. *Trans Roy Soc Trop Med Hyg* 80: 435.

66 Davis A (1986) Recent advances in schistosomiasis. *Q J Med* 58: 95.

67 Chapman PJC, Wilkinson PR, Davidson RN (1988) Acute schistosomiasis (*Katayama* fever) among British air crew. *Br Med J* 297: 1101.

68 Smith AJ (1974) Public health in China. *Br Med J* 2: 492.

69 Nelson GS (1972) Immunological control of schistosomiasis. *Br Med J* 4: 172.

70 Ghoneim MA (1984) Bilharziasis: the lower genitourinary tract, in: Husain I (ed.) *Tropical Urology and Renal Disease*, pp. 261—80. London: Churchill Livingstone.

71 Chatelain C (1977) *La Bilharziose Uro-génitale*. Paris: Masson.

72 Koraitim M (1973) A new concept of bilharzial bladder neck obstruction: the triple mechanism. *J Urol* 79: 393.

73 Ibrahim AIA, Patil KP, El Tahir MI, Shetty SD, Anandan N (1991) Bilharzial vesicoureteric reflux and bladder neck stenosis: fact or fiction? *Br J Urol* 68: 582.

74 Raziuddin S, Shetty S, Ibrahim A, Patil K (1990) Activated CD4-positive T-lymphocytes and impaired cell-mediated immunity in patients with carcinoma of the urinary bladder with schistosomiasis. *Cancer* 65: 931.

75 Raziuddin S, Shetty S, Ibrahim A (1991) T cell abnormality and defective interleukin-2 production in patients with carcinoma of the urinary bladder with schistosomiasis. *J Clin Immunol* 11: 103—13.

76 Kardorff R, Traore M, Doehring-Schwerdtfeger E, Vester U, Ehrich JHH (1994) Ultrasonography of ureteric abnormalities induced by *Schistosoma haematobium* infection before and after praziquantel treatment. *Br J Urol* 74: 703.

77 Thomas FD (1936) *Entamoeba histolytica* involvement of urinary tract. *Urol Cut Rev* 40: 199.

78 Lisboa JA (1945) Eustrongylus renal Humana. *Brazil Med* 59: 101.

79 Oh SJ, Chi JG, Lee SE (1993) Eosinophilic cystitis caused by vesical sparganosis: a case report. *J Urol* 149: 581.

80 Burger R (1972) *Paragordius esavianus* passed per urethram. *J Urol* 108: 469.

81 Herman JR (1973) Candiru: urinophilic catfish. *Urology* 1: 265.

Chapter 19: Bladder — tumours

Aetiology

The incidence of bladder cancer has risen slowly in recent decades both in the United States and Britain (Fig. 19.1). It occurs twice as often in white men as in black: four times more in men than in women [1−3].

Many aetiological factors are known to cause cancer of the bladder [2]. On a worldwide scale bilharziasis (see p. 279) is far the most important. Cigarette smoking is an important cause although the incidence of bladder cancer does not parallel that in the lung. Smokers who develop bladder cancer may be unable to detoxify the tobacco-tar carcinogens from want of N-acetyl transferase in the liver [4].

In a part of Taiwan where a toxic substance in the water leads to ischaemia of the lower limb, there is an increased incidence of bladder cancer [5].

Industrial carcinogens have been known to cause bladder cancer since 1895 when Rehn first observed it in aniline dye workers [6]. Hueper traced the carcinogen to 2-naphthylamine in 1938 [7,8].

In the rubber industry 1- and 2-naphthylamine and benzidine were indicted [9] and it was made a prescribed industrial disease. Occupational cancers of the bladder may have a long latency interval of up to 40 years between exposure to the carcinogen and the development of cancer, so that it is often difficult to prove the association

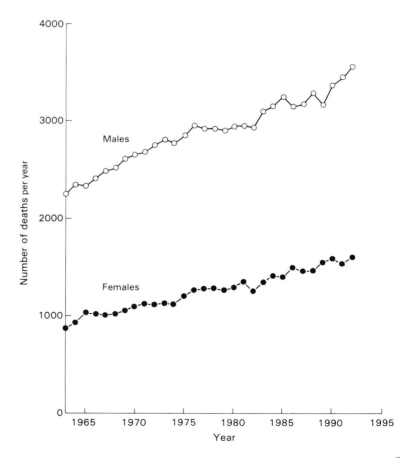

Fig. 19.1 Deaths from cancer of the bladder in England and Wales (from the Registrar General, Office of Population Census and Surveys).

even if a patient can remember the names of the chemicals to which exposure occurred [10].

The chemical industry stopped using 1- and 2-naphthylamine in 1940, the rubber and electrical cable industry 10 years later. In gasworks, coal tar and the fumes from coke ovens and retort houses continued to contain 2-naphthylamine until 1960 when gas was no longer made from coal.

The occupation of other patients may also be relevant [10].

1 rat-catchers (alpha naphthylthiourea contaminated with 2-naphthylamine);
2 textile workers (carcinogenic dyes);
3 polyurethane plastics industry — car bumpers and soles of shoes (methylene-*bis*-orthochloroaniline (MBOCA);
4 laboratory workers (benzidine);
5 leather work;
6 printing (used car oil);
7 aluminium refining;
8 machine turning (mineral oil);
9 lorry drivers (diesel);
10 hairdressers (dyes);
11 amateur anglers (maggots stained with chrysoidin).

Saccharin caused bladder cancer in rats but there has been no increase in diabetics who consume a lot of saccharin [11]. Coffee by itself seems to be safe, unless combined with smoking [12]. Dispute continues over the risk of analgesic consumption [13].

In experimental animals nitrosamines produce cancer of the bladder: they are formed from substances in everyday use, e.g. tobacco alkaloids, and liberated from bacteria in the bladder and bowel (Fig. 19.2). Vitamin C blocks nitrosamine formation and vitamin A prevents them causing bladder cancer in rats [1,9].

Viruses may play a role in the causation of bladder cancer which is three times more common in men who have viral condylomata acuminata. The human papillomavirus was recovered in 16 out of 18 examples of bladder tumour [14].

One significant association has been reported in neuropathic bladders, especially in those who come to treatment for end-stage renal failure. One should have a high index of suspicion in such patients who often have a long history of chronic urinary infection and chronic cystitis [15].

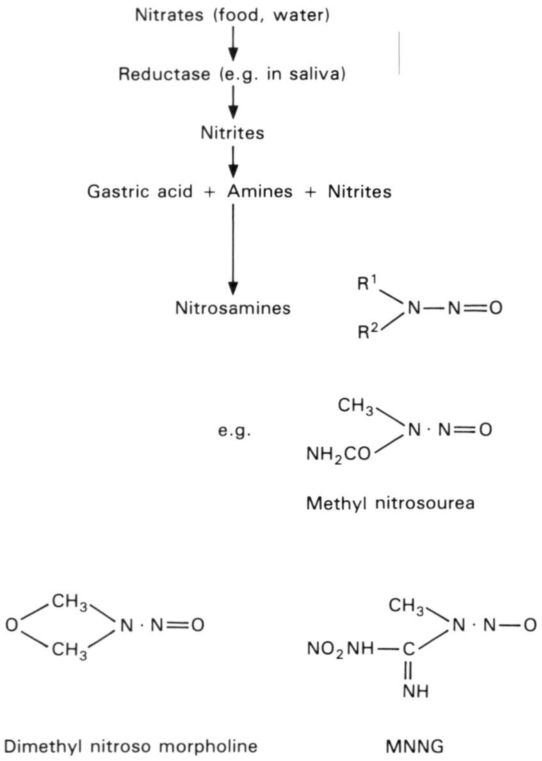

Fig. 19.2 Formation of nitrosamines in urine.

Pathology

Benign tumours of the bladder

Papilloma

Whether this exists is a matter for dispute. Most urologists have a healthy suspicion of so-called papilloma, and regard it as one end of a spectrum of more or less malignant urothelial tumours. By definition it has a single layer of cells, which have no malignant cytological features, and an intact basement membrane (Fig. 19.3).

Inverted papilloma

This is a rare tumour which seldom causes haematuria and is often found by chance on cystoscopy where it resembles a sebaceous cyst in the skin — smooth, pale and rounded. It has a characteristic histological appearance (Fig. 19.4). Like papilloma, it should be regarded with suspicion and followed up carefully.

Haemangioma

Occurring in all sizes, these may cause more or

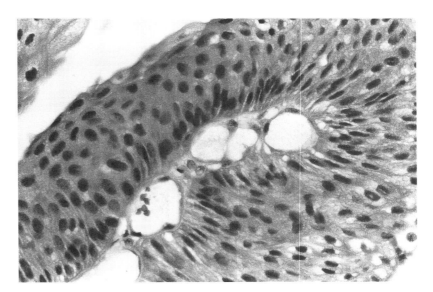

Fig. 19.3 Papilloma of the bladder — a rare tumour. It has the normal thickness of urothelium showing no malignant cytological features and an intact basement membrane (courtesy of Dr Suhail Baithun).

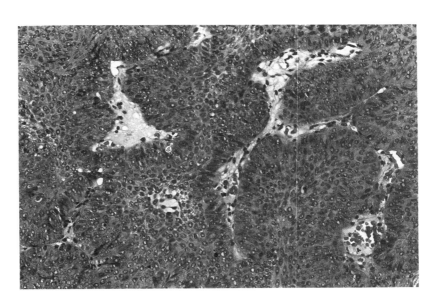

Fig. 19.4 Inverted papilloma of the bladder (courtesy of Dr Suhail Baithun).

less profuse haemorrhage. On cystoscopy they appear as an angry collection of veins, often confined to one side of the bladder. They respond very well to coagulation with diathermy or the neodymium-yttrium aluminium garnet (YAG) laser [16].

Malignant tumours of the bladder

Most bladder tumours arise from transitional epithelium (urothelium), but it is prone to undergo metaplasia to squamous or columnar epithelium, and so squamous cancer and adeno-carcinoma are also seen. Repeated irritation, e.g. from infection, stricture, bilharziasis or stone, can give rise to either type of metaplasia. There

is a regular sequence of changes — cystitis cystica with von Brunn's nests, glandular metaplasia or nephrogenic adenoma and finally adenocar-cinoma — characteristic of neglected exstrophy. The urachus is normally lined by columnar epithelium and most, but not quite all, urachal cancers are adenocarcinomas.

Macroscopic appearances

At cystoscopy carcinoma *in situ* may appear entirely normal or at worse, slightly injected, resembling ordinary bacterial cystitis. Other car-cinomas take one of three forms: (a) a papillary growth; (b) a solid nodule; or (c) an ulcer (Fig. 19.5). In general, the less differentiated the

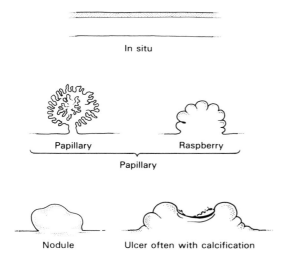

In situ

Papillary   Raspberry
        Papillary

Nodule   Ulcer often with calcification

Fig. 19.5 Like cancer anywhere, a bladder cancer can take one of three macroscopic forms — a papillary growth, a solid nodule or an ulcer.

tumour, the more solid and ulcerated it becomes. Bladder tumours are often multiple and sometimes associated with urothelial tumours of the kidney pelvis and ureter.

Grade

Bladder cancers are classified into three grades G1, G2 and G3 [17] (Fig. 19.6). Flow cytometry gives a more objective measure of ploidy [18].

Stage

The Union International Contre le Cancer (UICC) [17] system is used worldwide but its most recent revision of 1992 has yet to be adopted by most urologists (Fig. 19.7). In the new revision the following stages are used:
- **Ta**: No invasion of lamina propria.
- **Tis**: Flat carcinoma *in situ*.
- **T1**: Invasion of lamina propria.
- **T2**: Invasion of superficial muscle.
- **T3a**: Invasion of deep muscle.
  T3b: Invasion of fat (i) microscopically; or (ii) macroscopically.
- **T4a**: Invasion of prostate, uterus, vagina.
  T4b: Invasion of pelvic wall, abdominal wall.
Certain important points about the TNM nomenclature must be appreciated if one is to compare the results of treatment in different centres.

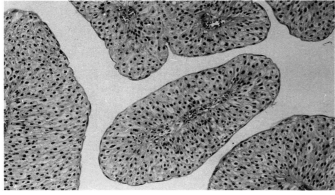

a

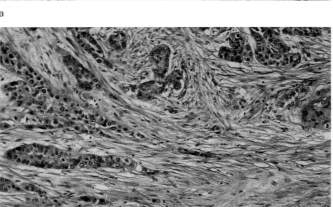

c

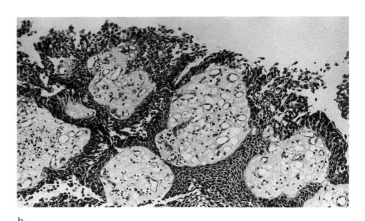

b

Fig. 19.6 Three grades of bladder cancer: (a) grade 1, well differentiated; (b) grade 2, intermediate differentiation; and (c) grade 3, undifferentiated tumour invading muscle (courtesy of Dr E.A. Courtauld).

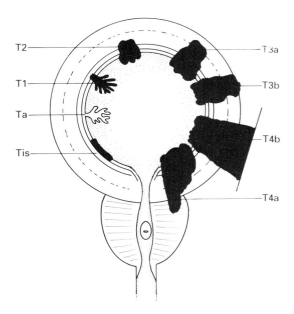

Fig. 19.7 UICC system of staging of bladder cancer (see text for further details).

When the entire bladder is available to the pathologist, e.g. after total cystectomy, the stage is allocated the prefix P. When only a cystoscopic biopsy is available, the prefix is pT. When only cystoscopic assessment, but no biopsy is available, the prefix is T.

In evaluating the N stage, the pathologist who is provided with the nodes removed at radical cystectomy will often find tumour that was missed in the computerized tomography (CT) scan. These differences introduce errors when attempts are made to compare the results of treatment by cystectomy versus radiotherapy or chemotherapy (see below). It is also necessary to be aware that there may be considerable inter-observer error in assigning G grade and T stage to the same samples of bladder cancer [19,20].

Carcinoma in situ (Tis)

When the urothelium is flat, without any papillary processes, there is a continuous spectrum between normal urothelium, atypia and carcinoma *in situ* [21] and the distinction between them is subjective and open to error [22] (Fig. 19.8). They share one important feature: although the cells making up carcinoma *in situ* may be anaplastic, they have not yet penetrated the basement membrane. Carcinoma *in situ* may occur on its own (primary), or in a part of the bladder some way from an exfoliative tumour (secondary).

Ta

These are papillary tumours which have not penetrated the basement membrane [17] (Fig. 19.9). Most of these tumours are G1, and have an excellent prognosis, but it is important to watch out for the rare G3 tumours which do very badly (see below) [23].

T1

Here the tumour has penetrated the basement membrane, and its cells are invading the lamina propria. This step in invasion significantly worsens the prognosis [24] (Fig. 19.10).

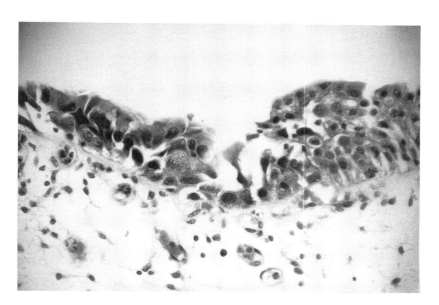

Fig. 19.8 Carcinoma *in situ* (courtesy of Dr E.A. Courtauld).

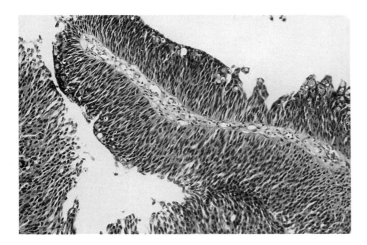

Fig. 19.9 Ta. The well-differentiated cells have not penetrated the basement membrane (courtesy of Dr E.A. Courtauld).

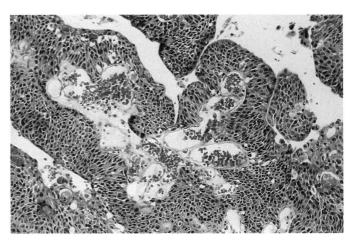

Fig. 19.10 pT1. The tumour cells have penetrated the basement membrane (courtesy of Dr E.A. Courtauld).

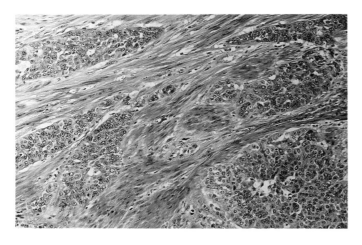

Fig. 19.11 pT2. The superficial muscle is invaded by tumour (courtesy of Dr E.A. Courtauld).

T2

The tumour has invaded the detrusor muscle and has access to its rich lymphatic plexus. The prognosis is even worse [24] (Fig. 19.11).

T3

The distinction between T2 and T3 stems from the classical study on the survival of patients after total cystectomy by Jewett and Strong (1946) [25]. They found that if the tumour had invaded more than half-way through the detrusor muscle the patients had a worse prognosis. In fact there were only 15 cases with muscle invasion in this study, and only one with metastases: slender evidence for a generalization which has dominated urological thinking. In fact it is impossible to define a half-way line in the formalin-fixed specimen let alone in life and there is little dif-

ference in the prognosis between T2 and T3 tumours [24]. The important step is invasion of muscle, rather than how far the tumour has gone into it (Fig. 19.12).

T4

Once the tumour has passed through the wall of the bladder it has free access to the fat and connective tissue around the bladder (Fig. 19.13), since the only biological barrier to its spread is the peritoneum on its vault and the double layer of peritoneum (the fascia of Denonvilliers) posteriorly. Bladder cancers only invade the rectum or peritoneum very late in the course of the disease. The rest of the bladder has no capsule, and once the cancer has penetrated the muscle it is into the perivesical fat, lymphatics and veins.

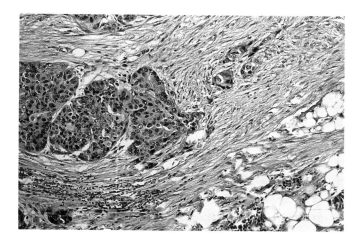

Fig. 19.12 pT3. The deep layers of the muscle are invaded by tumour (courtesy of Dr E.A. Courtauld).

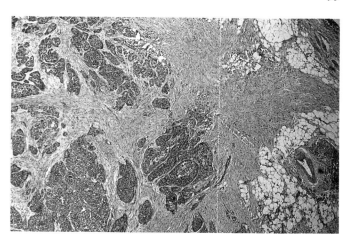

Fig. 19.13 pT4. The tumour is invading adjacent viscera (courtesy of Dr E.A. Courtauld).

Spread of bladder tumours

Direct spread

Bladder cancer spreads directly through the perivesical fat into adjacent bowel, uterus and bone. It also spreads across the wall of the bladder probably by direct implantation — 'kiss cancer' [26].

Urine-borne spread

Tumours may be carried down the urethra and implanted onto abrasions caused by the passage of urethral instruments and are often implanted near the air-bubble presumably because particles of tumour are carried there at the time of transurethral resection [26].

Lymphatic permeation

Spread by lymphatic permeation and embolism carries the tumour to the regional nodes along the branches of the internal iliac artery, and from there along the paraortic nodes.

Haematogenous spread

Blood-borne spread by veins is a late event in bladder cancer, but from time to time is seen even in well-differentiated and apparently superficial tumours which unexpectedly give rise to pulmonary or other distant metastases.

Prostatic route

Once a bladder cancer has invaded the prostate it can spread by lymphatics and veins directly into the bone marrow of the pelvis, femora and lumbar vertebrae (see p. 370).

Squamous cell cancer

Squamous cell cancers arise in areas of urothelium that have undergone metaplasia [27] as is usual in bilharziasis. Elsewhere, it is preceded by leucoplakia which almost invariably goes on to cancer [28–30]. (This needs to be distinguished from the 'vaginal metaplasia' which is a normal finding on the trigone of many women and is not premalignant.) Squamous cell cancer (Fig. 19.14) has a notoriously bad prognosis, and is relatively resistant to radiation [31].

Adenocarcinoma

The urachus is the fetal allantois, a continuation of the hind-gut. It is usually lined by columnar epithelium and almost invariably gives rise to adenocarcinoma [32–34] (Fig. 19.15).

Elsewhere in the bladder, adenocarcinoma arises in areas of urothelium that have undergone metaplasia through the intermediate stage of cystitis cystica and cystitis glandularis [35]. It is almost inevitable in neglected exstrophy (see p. 287) but all cases of cystitis glandularis and nephrogenic adenoma including those found in association with pelvic lipomatosis should be carefully followed up.

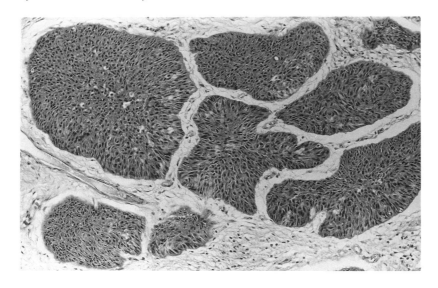

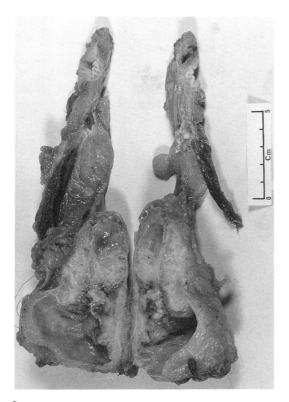

a

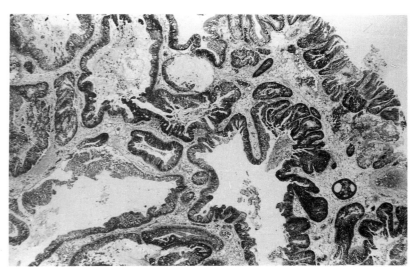

b

Fig. 19.14 Squamous cell cancer of the bladder (courtesy of Dr Suhail Baithum).

Fig. 19.15 (a) Macroscopic view of carcinoma of the urachus, and (b) histology of adenocarcinoma arising in the urachus (courtesy of Dr Suhail Baithum).

If there is any doubt as to the origin of an adenocarcinoma in the bladder, immunohisto-logical methods will identify its origin, e.g. from prostate, by immunoperoxidase staining for prostatic-specific antigen.

Other types of metaplasia are also rarely encountered in the bladder. They may include sarcomatoid and microcytic features, as well as the formation of bone and cartilage. One of the most significant of these variations in terms of sensitivity to radiation is the appearance of trophoblastic elements which express human chorionic gonadotrophin [36] (see p. 307).

Other tumours

Pheochromocytoma

This gives the characteristic history of paroxysmal hypertension during micturition [37]. There are raised levels of vanillylmandelic acid and catecholamines. The tumour can be exactly localized by [131]iodine-meta-iodobenzyl guanidine (MIGB) (see p. 628). The treatment is by local excision, with all the usual precautions when operating for pheochromocytoma. Local recurrence is common.

Rhabdomyosarcoma

This presents with painful frequency in children and until recently was almost uniformly fatal (Figs 19.16 & 19.17). It is localized by CT scanning. It is important to be aware of its existence, and make sure the child is referred to a specialist paediatric urological centre where today a survival rate of 55% may be obtained by a combination of systemic chemotherapy and radiation, and the bladder can be preserved in more than half of these cases [38].

Leiomyosarcoma

This is even less common. It has been reported following cyclophosphamide therapy for lupus nephritis and Hodgkin's disease [39].

Clinical features

The chief symptom of bladder cancer is haema-

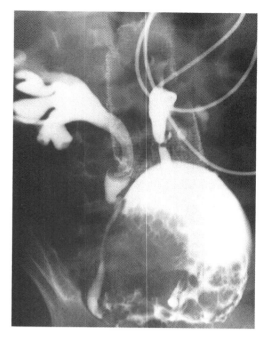

Fig. 19.16 Rhabdomyosarcoma of the bladder (courtesy of Mr R.H. Whitaker).

turia, either noticed by the patient or detected by routine testing of the urine. It is the presenting symptom in 80% of patients. In about 15%, the symptoms are frequency and dysuria which suggest ordinary bacterial cystitis and suspicion is only aroused when sterile pyuria is discovered. The remaining 5% have a variety of symptoms including anaemia, uraemia or distant metastases [40].

There are seldom any physical signs. In late

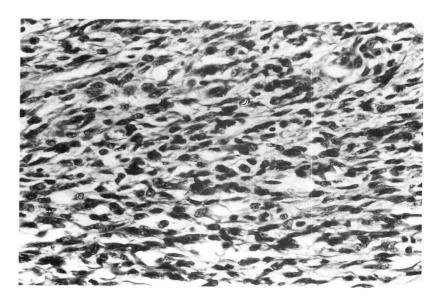

Fig. 19.17 Histology of rhabdomyosarcoma of the bladder.

cases induration may be felt on rectal examination, or in the suprapubic region.

Investigations

Urine cytology

Urine for cytology must be fixed otherwise autolysis of the cells will make features of cancer more difficult to recognize [41]. A roughly equal volume of 10% formalin is added to the freshly passed urine (Fig. 19.18).

The cytologist looks for an increased nuclear/cytoplasm ratio or clumps of multinucleate cells. Single cells shed from a well-differentiated tumour cannot be differentiated from cancer, but a complete frond can be distinguished from a well-differentiated papillary tumour. False positive findings occur when the urothelium has been injured, e.g. by a stone, and mitotic cells are detached from the growing edge at the site of repair.

An objective method of detecting nuclear enlargement is provided by flow cytometry of the cells in the urine (Fig. 19.19).

Intravenous urogram

Until recently, it was the invariable rule that every patient with haematuria should have an IVU. This may show filling defects in the bladder film or obstruction to a ureter (Figs 19.20 & 19.21). Obstruction to the ureter usually but not always signifies invasion of the muscle [42].

Ultrasound

Ultrasound scanning of the kidneys and bladder is beginning to replace the IVU: in expert hands even small bladder tumours can be detected by this method (Fig. 19.22). However it still does not exclude with certainty tumours in the renal pelvis or ureters [43,44].

CT scanning

A CT scan (Fig. 19.23) may show very large pelvic lymph nodes, but is unreliable in assessing the stage of a bladder tumour [45,46].

Magnetic resonance imaging (MRI)

The main advantage claimed for this technique is in staging bladder tumours, since it may be able to distinguish between oedema and infiltrating cancer [47] (Fig. 19.24). It is, however, dauntingly expensive.

Cystoscopy

Unless a tumour has been shown by the urogram or the ultrasound the next investigation for haematuria is cystoscopy. The flexible cystoscope [48–50] now allows a quick and painless examination in the clinic (Fig. 19.25). Very small tumours can be coagulated there and then with

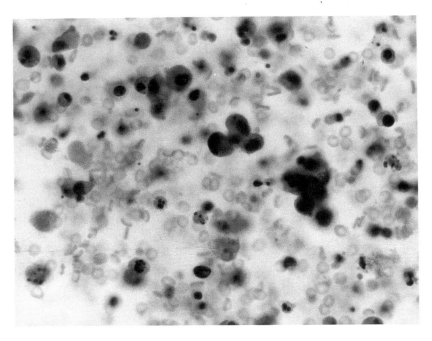

Fig. 19.18 Cytology of cells from the urine showing features of cancer.

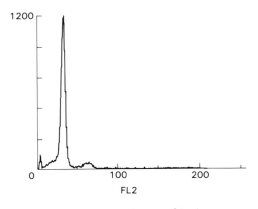

Fig. 19.19 Flow cytometry gives an objective measure of ploidy of populations of cells shed in urine; these are mainly diploid (large peak) with a few cells in mitosis (right).

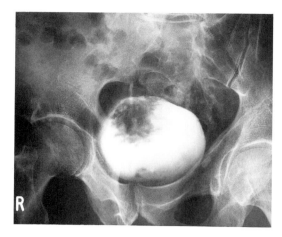

Fig. 19.20 IVU showing filling defect of the bladder typical of a papillary carcinoma.

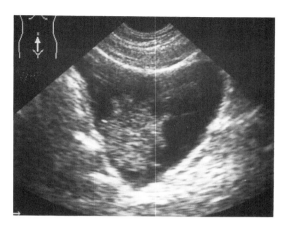

Fig. 19.22 Ultrasound scan of a bladder tumour.

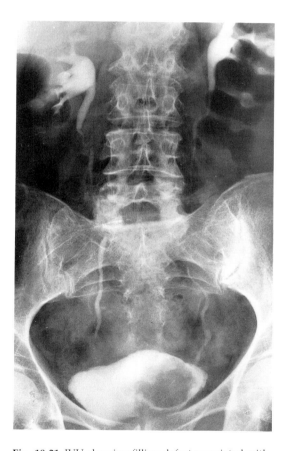

Fig. 19.21 IVU showing filling defect associated with obstruction of the ureter, usually indicating that the tumour has invaded the bladder wall.

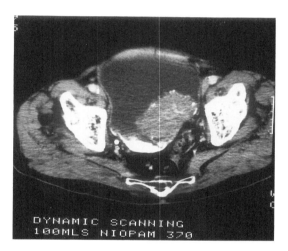

Fig. 19.23 CT showing invasion of pelvic lymph nodes from a bladder cancer (courtesy of Dr Otto Chan).

the neodymium-YAG laser [51] (Fig. 19.26), after which a biopsy still gives adequate morphology to permit accurate grading and staging of the tumour.

Larger tumours require cystoscopy under anaesthesia at which the tumour is resected, and bimanual examination is performed with the patient relaxed to assess depth of invasion of the muscle.

Resection for grading and staging

Precaution — if the tumours are situated on the lateral wall of the bladder near the base there is a

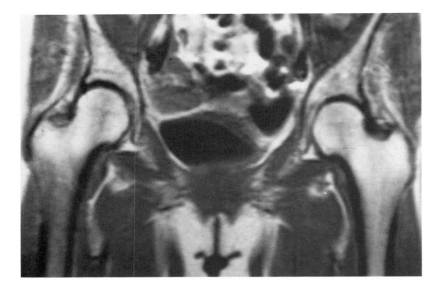

Fig. 19.24 MRI showing bladder tumour (courtesy of Dr Michael Kellett).

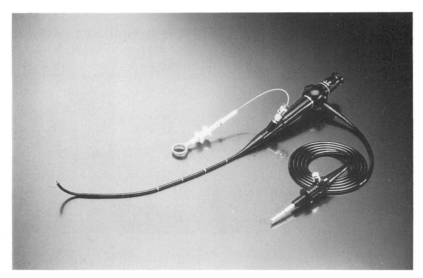

Fig. 19.25 Flexible cystoscope.

risk of obturator nerve stimulation. Use as low a current as possible or have the patient paralysed (see p. 10).

Small tumours may be removed with a single stroke of the resectoscope loop, taking a complete divot of underlying detrusor muscle (Fig. 19.27).

For larger tumours where more bleeding is to be expected an irrigating resectoscope will provide a better view and keep bladder filling constant so that the tumour does not continually retreat from the resectoscope.

In resecting a larger bladder tumour one should keep to a regular plan [52]. The first step is to find the edge of the stalk by trimming away the overhanging bush at one side (Fig. 19.28). Once

the edge has been found, the base of the stalk is coagulated with the roly-ball electrode, to seal the vessels in the stalk: the rest of the resection then becomes relatively bloodless.

The resection is continued by following the edge of the stalk all round carrying the strokes of the resectoscope from the periphery towards the centre, to keep the margin of the stalk cleanly cut and prevent the bush from overhanging. Eventually, all the bush will have been removed. The chips are now evacuated and sent to the laboratory in formalin labelled 'tumour bush'.

A second deliberate resection is then performed of the base of the stalk to sample the deeper layers of muscle. This tissue is sent

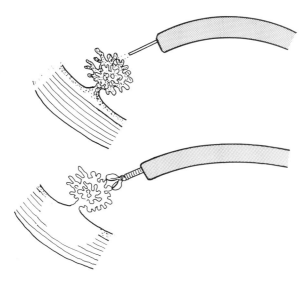

Fig. 19.26 Small tumour recurrences can be coagulated with the neodymium-YAG laser through the flexible cystoscope. A biopsy may be taken afterwards.

separately labelled as 'tumour stalk' to help the pathologist stage the tumour (Fig. 19.29). The base is thoroughly coagulated with the roly-ball to seal off blood vessels and destroy any malignant cells that may have been left behind. Haemostasis must be complete.

After resecting a small tumour a catheter is not necessary, but for larger ones it is wise to leave an irrigating catheter in place for 24 h.

Complications. Small perforations of the detrusor are of little consequence so long as haemostasis has been obtained. A little extravasation of irrigant will soon reabsorb and so long as the catheter is draining freely no untoward complication need be expected.

Perforations into the peritoneal cavity require laparotomy to allow the hole in the bladder to be closed and make sure any diathermy injury to adjacent bowel has been found and repaired.

Very large papillary tumours

When there are papillary tumours that seem to fill the whole bladder, the first attempt to resect them may be very difficult because bleeding makes it impossible to see what one is doing. With modern illumination and the irrigating resectoscope this situation has become rare, and the need for Helmstein's technique seldom arises. Nevertheless it is worth keeping it in mind [53,54].

Helmstein's technique

Use continuous epidural anaesthesia which can be topped up from time to time. Epidural anaesthesia has the effect of reducing blood pressure significantly, which is desirable. Attach a rubber balloon to a catheter with a side arm to a pressure monitor (Fig. 19.30). Inflate the balloon with glycine until the pressure is midway

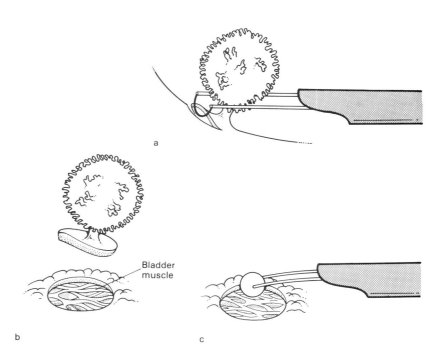

Fig. 19.27 (a & b) A small papillary tumour can be removed with a divot of underlying muscle with a single stroke of the resectoscope. (c) The base is coagulated.

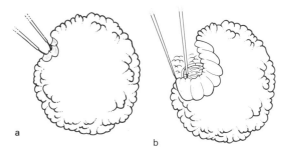

Fig. 19.28 To reach the stalk of a larger tumour the overhanging bush must be resected (a), then the stalk can be coagulated (b).

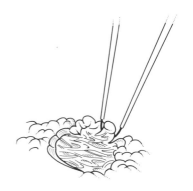

Fig. 19.29 After removing the bush, the stalk is resected and sent separately to assist in staging the tumour.

between the systolic and diastolic blood pressure, and leave it at this pressure for 6 h. At the end of the period of inflation an irrigating catheter is left in the bladder for 4–5 days to wash out the

necrotic debris. After 2–3 weeks a second cystoscopy will show that the bulk of the tumour has disappeared, leaving only the stumps of their stalks behind (Fig. 19.31), which can then be resected down to muscle for proper staging.

Large solid tumours

There is little point in attempting to resect a large solid tumour completely since some permutation of radiation, chemotherapy or cystectomy is going to be needed. A few deep bites should be resected from the rolled edge of the tumour for the purpose of staging and grading (Fig. 19.32).

Tumours in diverticula

When performing a cystoscopy for haematuria in a bladder with diverticula it is most important to get a good look inside each of them. Cancer inside a diverticulum causes oedema and redness of the edge of the opening and may close it up completely. Always make sure by bimanual examination that there is no induration and confirm this by ultrasound and CT scan (Fig. 19.33).

Field biopsies

Except when the tumour is obviously very large and invasive it is wise to acquire four quadrant biopsies from the urothelium, elsewhere using cup forceps, to detect carcinoma *in situ*. Only a

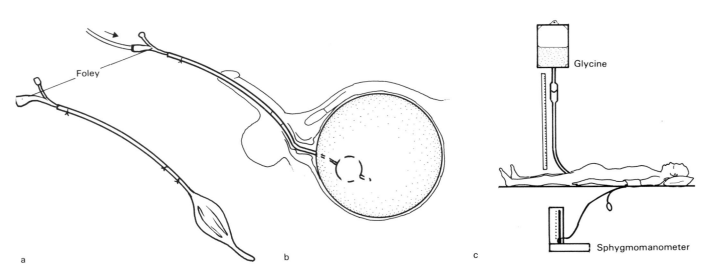

Fig. 19.30 Helmstein's balloon technique. A rubber balloon is attached to a foley catheter (a) and distended with glycine until a pressure is reached which is 10 cmH$_2$O greater than the diastolic blood pressure (b), and left there for 6 h (c).

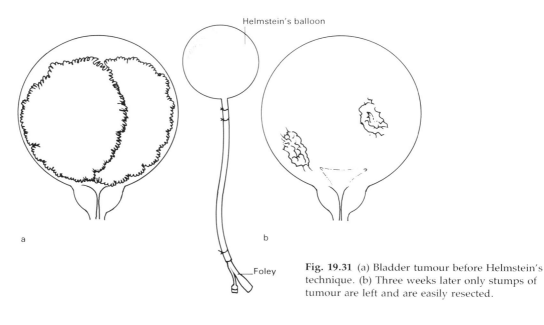

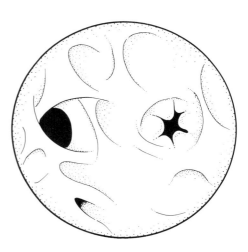

Fig. 19.31 (a) Bladder tumour before Helmstein's technique. (b) Three weeks later only stumps of tumour are left and are easily resected.

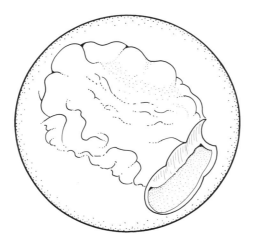

Fig. 19.32 A deep bite is taken from the edge of a large solid tumour to identify the grade and stage of the tumour.

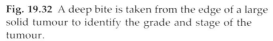

Fig. 19.33 Oedema around the opening of a diverticulum is very suspicious of a tumour inside. If you cannot see inside a diverticulum, arrange for an ultrasound or CT scan.

tiny piece of tissue is needed. After taking biopsies, coagulate the site of biopsy to stop bleeding.

Treatment

Superficial bladder tumours

More than 80% of bladder tumours are superficial Ta or T1 and can be managed by endoscopic means. All must be carefully followed up and it is important that the record system notes the site, grade and T stage of each recurrence, and how many there have been. There are many versions of this follow-up chart (Fig. 19.34) including computerized versions [24].

Exceptions to this rule are superficial G3 tumours, whether *in situ* or papillary. These have such a deadly prognosis that they are handled much more aggressively [55,56]. The G3 papillary tumours are treated as if they were already invading the muscle and will be discussed below, as will the special problem of carcinoma *in situ*.

Follow-up

It is usual to follow the majority of the well-differentiated superficial tumours by check cystoscopy with the flexible cystoscope at regular and lengthening intervals so long as there are only a few solitary recurrences. With increasing experience with ultrasound scanning of the bladder it is likely that in many cases cystoscopy will be replaced by ultrasound scanning [43,50].

Any recurrent tumours are biopsied and resected or coagulated with laser or diathermy [57].

When tumours recur often, and in large num-

bers, then adjuvant intravesical chemotherapy is given after resecting or coagulating the tumours.

Adjuvant intravesical chemotherapy

Thiotepa

The first of many agents to be shown to be useful in lessening the number and frequency of recurrences was Thiotepa [58,59], an alkylating agent which crosslinks nucleic acids and proteins. The main side effect is marrow suppression. This is dose related and can be avoided by giving 30 mg on alternate days for three doses, checking the platelet count each intervening day [58]. It is effective in reducing the numbers of recurrences in about 50% of patients, and is a useful and

Fig. 19.34 Chart used for recording tumour recurrences, named (with affection) the 'Harrygram' after Mr H.R. England.

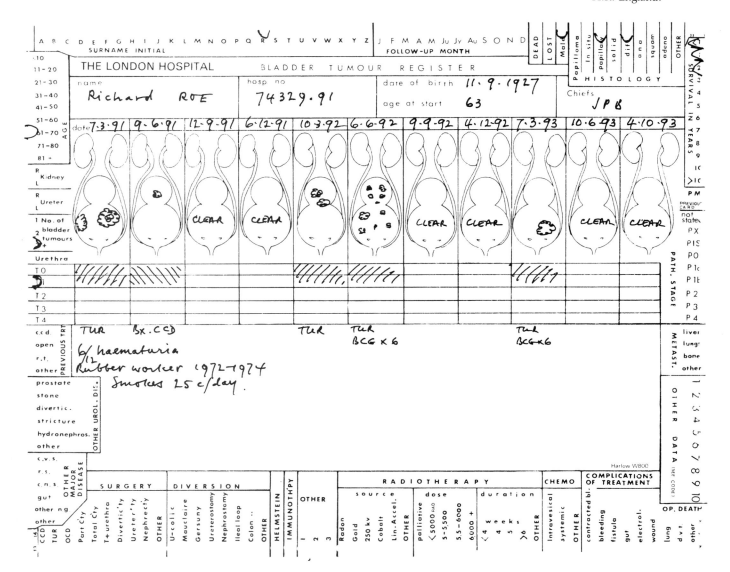

inexpensive first line of treatment in the patient with multiple or frequent recurrences.

Ethoglucid

Ethoglucid (Epodyl) is also an alkylating agent. It has a larger molecule and less risk of marrow toxicity from absorption. Its response rate is similar to Thiotepa but it causes a more or less painful cystitis [60,61].

Mitomycin C

This is much more expensive, has an even higher molecular weight, and less risk of absorption, but it can cause severe skin rashes if not handled with scrupulous care. It has a response rate similar to that of Thiotepa and Epodyl, and may work where they fail [62–64]. A very characteristic calcification is seen at the site of biopsies [65].

Doxorubicin (Adriamycin)

This gives a response rate similar to Mitomycin, but with more chemical cystitis. Where the bladder has been biopsied a similar calcification is seen [66–67].

Epirubicin

This is a similar agent, with less risk of causing marrow suppression [68]. In short, there is very little difference in the efficacy of all these chemotherapeutic agents: they all work some of the time, and if one fails, another might succeed [69].

Intravesical immunotherapy

Bacille Calmette—Guérin (BCG)

BCG was introduced by Morales [70] with the intention of producing an immune response to bladder tumours. It quickly proved to be very effective in some centres, less so in others — a difference which proved to be due to variations in the five or more methods used to attenuate the tubercle bacillus [71–74]. There are also differences in the doses which have been used.

Toxicity with BCG includes miliary tuberculosis, tuberculous cystitis and hepatitis. If recognized, each of these complications responds promptly to triple drug therapy but there have been fatalities [74,75]. It is reassuring for the patient to know that the best response often occurs in those who have had the most severe side effects.

There is a somewhat larger proportion of useful responses after BCG than intravesical chemotherapy and a complete response may continue for 5 years or more. As with chemotherapy, some patients do not respond. For BCG this may be because their urothelium lacks the blood group precursor T antigen, which acts as a receptor for the BCG. If this is confirmed it will become possible to spare these patients a useless course of treatment [76].

One small note of caution has been sounded by the report that the growth and spread of second primary malignancies may be accelerated by BCG [77].

Interferon and interleukin-2

In view of the long held suspicion that bladder tumours may be started off by infection with a type of papillomavirus [78–79], it seemed possible that interferon, which is so effective against other viral infections, might be useful in treating bladder tumours but the results have been disappointing [80]. Intravesical interleukin-2 seems capable of causing tumour regression but the dose required makes this an expensive option.

Radiotherapy

Radiation therapy has seldom been used for superficial tumours. Colloidal intravesical yttrium was formerly used with impressive results [81] but teletherapy has generally given poor results in multiple tumours unless they are undifferentiated (G3) [82].

Phototherapy

Many have welcomed the concept of sensitizing bladder cancers with some agent such as haematoporphyrin, and then illuminating with light of appropriate wavelength and brightness, to kill the cancers and spare the normal bladder wall. It is still a most exciting concept, and still in the developmental stage. At present its usefulness is limited by the damage and fibrosis which are inflicted on normal bladder tissue [83].

If BCG and chemotherapy have failed to suppress multiple recurrences, cystectomy is the best option for those few patients with well-differentiated tumours which are too numerous or extensive to resect. Radiation is futile and so the patient can be offered a continent urinary diversion (see p. 325).

Carcinoma in situ

The treatment of carcinoma *in situ* is contentious. There is an influential school of thought which regards this condition as being so dangerous, and the patient so likely to develop invasion and metastases, that total cystectomy is justified as soon as the diagnosis has been made [83–86].

The contrary view is that it is worth attempting to cure this field change by chemotherapy or immunotherapy [87–91] provided the patient is kept under careful supervision.

In a small series, systemic cyclophosphamide was found to give complete and sometimes long-lasting remission [90]. However, great caution is necessary in following up cases of carcinoma *in situ*. Not only is it necessary to take repeated field biopsies of the bladder urothelium, but from time to time it is necessary to biopsy the prostate as well. If the *in situ* change affects the urothelium of the prostatic ducts, the outlook is much worse and cystectomy should be considered.

Tumour invading muscle — T2, T3

This is one of the most controversial topics in modern urology: it concerns tumours with a very poor prognosis, most of which are anaplastic (G3) and many of which have already spread into the regional lymph nodes.

Thirty years ago, the prognosis for radical total cystectomy for tumours that had invaded muscle was so poor [92] that attempts were made to improve the results by adjuvant radiation therapy. Historical comparison of the results at the beginning of these decades with those towards the end appeared to show benefit from radiation therapy [93], but of course there had been many improvements in the technique of cystectomy, in anaesthesia and in pre- and postoperative care.

There was always a price to be paid for any apparent advantage to be gained from radiation: it left the bowel relatively ischaemic and the surgical tissue planes were obliterated by radiation fibrosis. Some patients had severe radiation enteritis. For these reasons many surgeons gave up radiation therapy altogether, and obtained results which were no worse for doing without it [94,95].

Avoiding radiation therapy made it possible to offer the patient a continent reservoir without the additional hazards that followed radiation, i.e. intestinal ischaemia and failure of anastomoses (see p. 325).

Over the same period, other centres continued to use radiation as the first line of treatment, noting that the bladder cancers would sometimes disappear completely after radiotherapy and not return. Since it was impossible to predict whether the tumour would respond or not, all patients with invasive bladder cancers were offered radiation, and cystectomy was reserved for those whose tumours failed to respond, or returned — the so-called salvage cystectomy.

Several careful prospective randomized trials were then set up in order to compare cystectomy after a limited dose of preoperative radiation versus radical radiotherapy with salvage cystectomy reserved for the non-responders [96,97]. There was no difference in the overall results.

A more thoughtful analysis of the data showed that the overall figures concealed two populations of invasive transitional cell bladder cancers: (a) those which responded at once to the course of radiation; and (b) those which did not. The responders had a 5-year survival rate approaching 70%; the non-responders only 17% [98]. These findings were repeated in a further series [99] (Fig. 19.35) and confirmed by others [100–102].

Only half of the tumours show a complete response to radiotherapy. This means that in some centres radiation is being given to half the patients — at the price of delaying cystectomy — without benefit. In other centres, cystectomy is being performed needlessly in half the patients who could have responded to radiotherapy.

The problem was how to choose the responders from the non-responders without a trial of radiotherapy. Conventional histological criteria show virtually all these tumours to be G3, and the usual histological criteria could not distinguish responders from non-responders.

However, recently it appeared that tumours which show a nil or partial response to radiotherapy also stain for beta human chorionic gonadotrophin (HCG) (Fig. 19.36), show squamous metaplasia [103] and lose the ability to express class I HLA (human leucocyte antigen) antigens [104,105]. These are fundamental biological features of tissues, such as the human

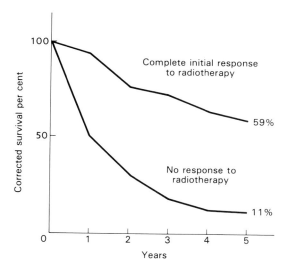

Fig. 19.35 Corrected survival rate of T3 bladder tumours showing two populations, those who did and those who did not respond to radiotherapy (redrawn from [102]).

trophoblast, which can escape immune surveillance, and it is tempting to speculate that these features may have a more profound significance than merely a want of response to radiation.

Except possibly when the histology shows squamous metaplasia and beta HCG there is no clear survival advantage between a trial of radiation with the option of salvage cystectomy, a limited dose of radiation followed by cystectomy, or radical cystectomy alone.

Nevertheless, two serious criticisms of radiotherapy remain: first, that its side effects cause an unacceptable morbidity. This is not the case [106]. Second, continent diversion becomes so much more hazardous if the bowel has been previously irradiated that many surgeons would consider it an absolute contraindication. This remains an important issue.

Neodymium-YAG laser for T2—T4 tumours

After a thorough resection the underlying tissue can be destroyed with diathermy or the neodymium-YAG laser, the latter producing a more controlled layer of coagulation [107] (Fig. 19.37). The technique, which is still under trial, offers an alternative method of treatment for elderly and unfit patients for whom cystectomy is not an option.

Systemic chemotherapy for invasive bladder cancer

It is an axiom in oncology that chemotherapeutic agents are only effective in combination if they have given a significant response when used alone. In bladder cancer, few systemic agents have shown any efficacy when used alone.

Methotrexate as an adjuvant to cystectomy with or without radiotherapy was useless: as was *cis*-platinum when used in a two-centre combined trial [108]. Combinations of vinblastine, platinum and bleomycin have shown promise in the short term and are still being evaluated [109–112]. They seem to have an advantage in deferring the onset of late distant

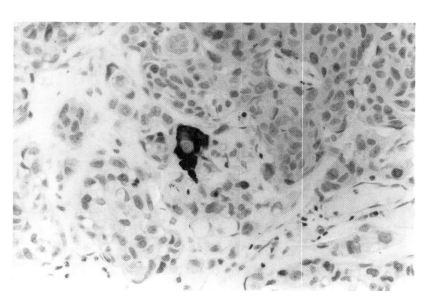

Fig. 19.36 Immunoperoxidase staining for beta HCG, positive findings signify lack of responsiveness to radiotherapy and a poor prognosis (courtesy of Dr Jo Martin).

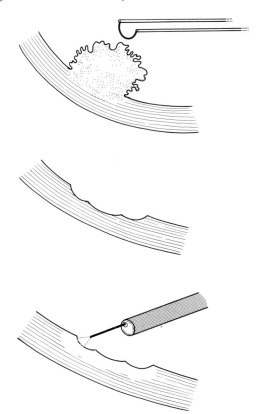

Fig. 19.37 Coagulation of a tumour with the neodymium-YAG laser.

metastases after cystectomy for cancers with positive lymph nodes [113].

Partial cystectomy

Partial cystectomy is seldom indicated in transitional cell cancer of the bladder, local recurrence being almost inevitable because of widespread premalignant field changes, and alternative treatments have replaced this operation in the last 20 years. It is, however, indicated in carcinoma arising in the urachus or in a diverticulum where the technique is described below.

Total cystectomy

Preliminary staging node dissection

If it is agreed that total cystectomy is futile in the presence of positive lymph nodes, then as with carcinoma of the prostate, there are advantages in performing a sampling node dissection with a minimally invasive laparoscopic method at a preliminary sitting. This allows the nodes to be carefully examined by paraffin section before deciding on the cystectomy [114] (see p. 417).

Technique

Through a long midline incision adhesions are separated. The peritoneum is divided to mobilize the caecum and mesentery (Fig. 19.38). The bowel is packed away from the pelvis. The incision in the peritoneum is continued anteriorly to separate the bladder from the symphysis and allow the bladder to be retracted medially. If not already done, a bilateral node dissection is performed taking the lymph nodes medial to the common and external iliac artery (Fig. 19.39). The nodes are sent for frozen section. In patients with severe bladder symptoms it may be necessary to go ahead with a palliative cystectomy even when the nodes are positive, though in general alternative methods of treatment will be preferred.

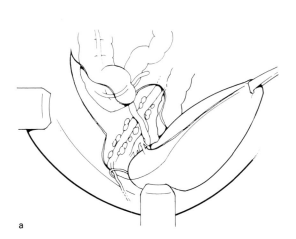

a

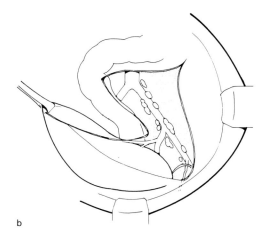

b

Fig. 19.38 (a & b) The peritoneum is mobilized on either side to reveal the bifurcation of the aorta and the iliac vessels with their lymph nodes.

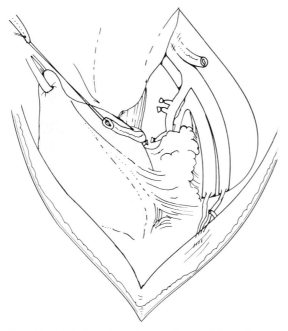

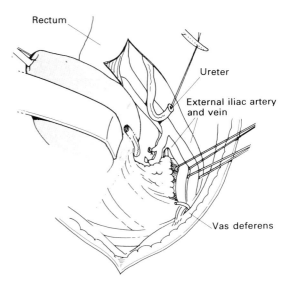

Fig. 19.40 The common and internal iliac vessels are cleaned.

Fig. 19.39 The lymph nodes are dissected from the iliac vessels.

If the decision is made to proceed with the cystectomy, the internal iliac artery is cleaned on one side and all its medial branches are ligated and divided one after the other (Figs 19.40 & 19.41). The ureters are divided and marked with stay-sutures. The same procedure is repeated on the other side.

Retracting the bladder upwards, the fat is carefully cleaned from the puboprostatic ligaments to define the retropubic veins which are meticulously taken up by suture ligature and divided (Fig. 19.42). If one plans to retain the urethra (e.g. in a solitary tumour without carcinoma *in situ*), the neurovascular bundles of Donker may be pushed down and laterally, without compromising the dissection and may preserve penile erection in men [115] (Fig. 19.43).

Lifting the bladder upwards and depressing the rectum, the plane of cleavage between the layers of Denonvilliers' fascia is opened, and the dissection carried down behind the prostate and seminal vesicles, keeping clear of the rectum (Fig. 19.44).

In multifocal tumours the urethra should always be removed [116,117]. In single tumours that are not associated with field changes of carcinoma *in situ*, the urethra can be divided distal to the prostate and marked with stay-

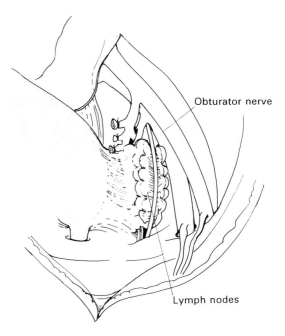

Fig. 19.41 The sleeve around the obturator nerve must be slit open to dissect off the lymph nodes.

sutures if a continent reservoir is planned (see p. 326).

If the urethra is to be removed a second midline incision is made in the perineum (Fig. 19.45). The corpus spongiosum is separated from the corpora cavernosa piecemeal, until the entire corpus spongiosum has been removed by turning the penis inside out (Fig. 19.46).

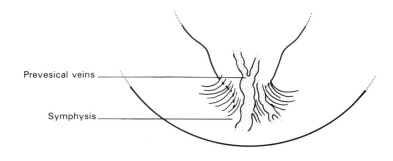

Prevesical veins

Symphysis

Fig. 19.42 The dorsal veins are defined and divided.

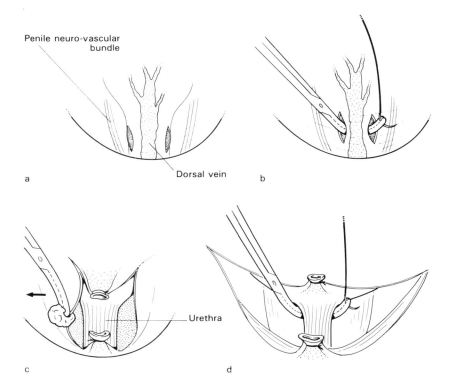

Penile neuro-vascular
bundle

Dorsal vein

a   b

Urethra

c   d

Fig. 19.43 To spare the neurovascular bundle to the penis, (a) the fascia is incised on either side of the dorsal veins. (b) The veins are ligated. (c) The neurovascular bundles are displaced laterally and posteriorly to reveal the urethra (d).

The dissection of the membranous urethra is easiest from the perineum. In front, the bulbar arteries can be seen and ligated before being divided (Fig. 19.47), as are the two dorsal arteries of the penis on either side of its dorsal vein. Once this has been done, each side of the membranous urethra is freed by dividing the tough fascial bands on each side. Finally, the urethra is pulled upwards, while one finger either side of the midline depresses the rectum, and throws into prominence the rectoprostatic ligament which is divided close to the prostate (Fig. 19.48). The membranous urethra is now free, and is drawn up into the pelvis, allowing the prostate to be separated from the rectum under vision.

The specimen is now free. The rest of the operation is determined by the choice of urinary diversion to be employed in the particular case (see p. 320).

Postoperative care

To achieve good results with total cystectomy great care must be taken over every detail of management [118]. A prolonged period of ileus is to be expected during which aspiration via a gastrostomy is much more comfortable for the patient than a nasogastric tube. Every precaution must be taken with wound closure to prevent infection and to prevent deep vein thrombosis.

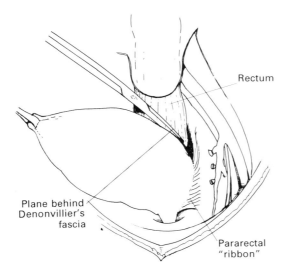

Fig. 19.44 The bladder is pulled up, and the plane between the layers of fascia of Denonvilliers is opened between the bladder and rectum.

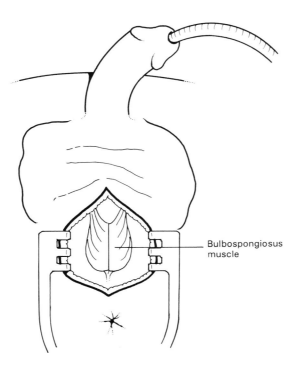

Fig. 19.45 Urethrectomy. A midline incision is made in the perineum.

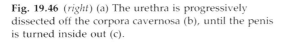

Fig. 19.46 (*right*) (a) The urethra is progressively dissected off the corpora cavernosa (b), until the penis is turned inside out (c).

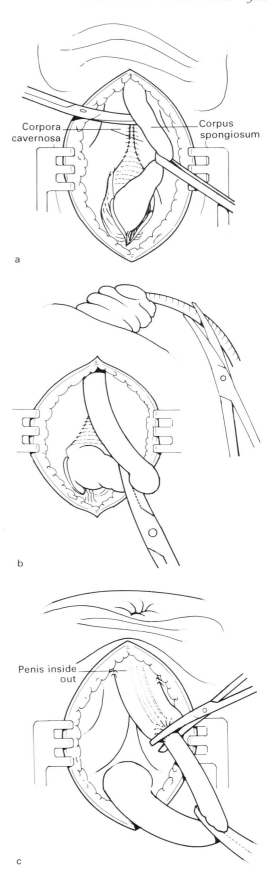

a

b

c

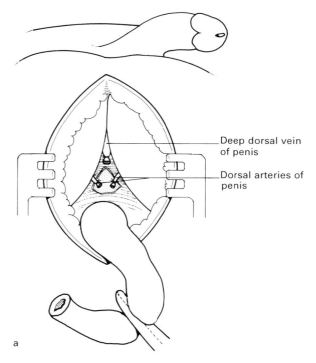

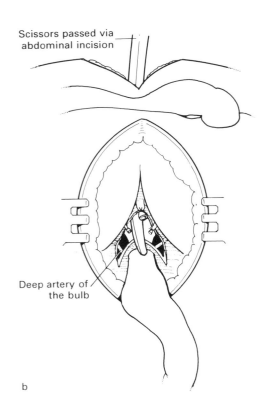

Fig. 19.47 The dorsal arteries and vein (a), and the bulbar arteries (b) are divided.

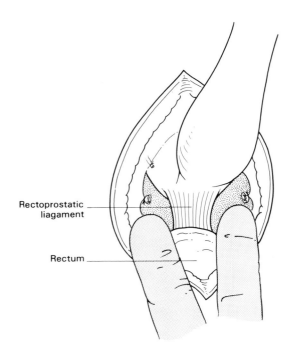

Fig. 19.48 The rectum is pushed down with two fingers to display the rectoprostatic ligament which is divided.

Squamous cell carcinoma

Squamous cell cancer is almost never diagnosed before it has invaded deeply into the wall of the bladder.

The squamous cell cancer that occurs as a sequela of chronic bilharziasis is said to be unresponsive to radiation treatment. Those with the most experience of this condition treat it by radical total cystectomy [119] with excellent results.

Bilharziasis (see p. 279) is endemic in countries where the standard of living is poor and few patients can afford urostomy appliances even if they would stick on in conditions of heat and moisture. Ghoneim and Kock have evolved a continent ureterosigmoidostomy which avoids reflux. The pressure in the reservoir is lowered by adding on a de-tubularized patch of small bowel [120] (see p. 326).

In Europe, where squamous cancer is not associated with bilharziasis it is also somewhat radioresistant, and total cystectomy is advised for cases with muscle invasion. Adjuvant radiation may diminish the chance of local recurrences [31,121]. The diagnosis of squamous cell cancer is usually obvious at cystoscopy — there is a thick dead white crust of keratin, and the urine has a characteristic and unforgettable stink.

Carcinoma of the urachus

This rare carcinoma presents with haematuria. On cystoscopy a cherry-red swelling is seen in the vault near the air-bubble. Bimanual palpation always shows a much larger mass outside the bladder than the lump seen on cystoscopy (Fig. 19.49). Biopsy shows adenocarcinoma [122].

Through a midline incision the skin and anterior rectus sheath are separated (Fig. 19.50) and then a wedge-shaped *en bloc* excision is performed of all the tissues from the umbilicus downwards and outwards to the obliterated

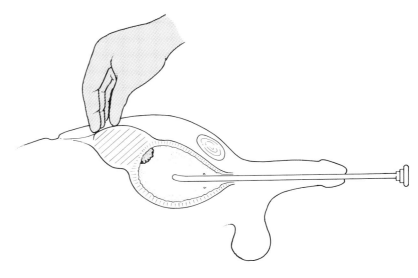

Fig. 19.49 A carcinoma of the urachus forms a mass outside the bladder much larger than the little cherry which is seen through the cystoscope.

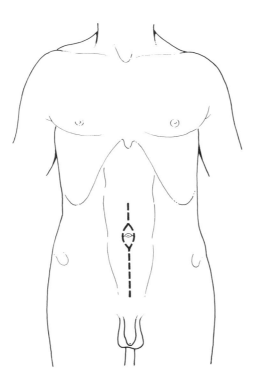

Fig. 19.50 The incision for carcinoma of the urachus includes the umbilicus.

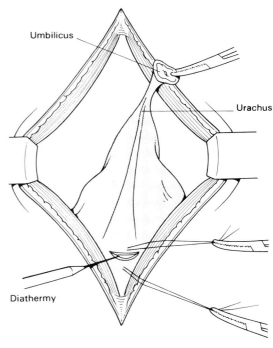

Fig. 19.51 Most of the bladder, urachus and the wedge of tissue extending to the obliterated hypogastric arteries on either side, is removed *en bloc*. The bladder is opened well away from the tumour.

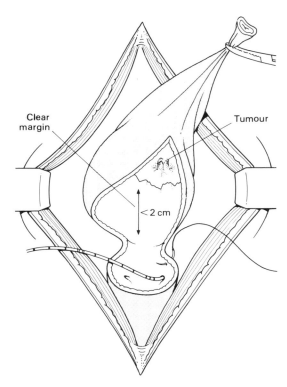

Fig. 19.52 Only a narrow rim of bladder is left around the trigone. The ureters are marked with catheters.

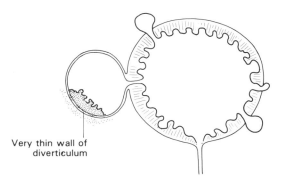

Fig. 19.53 Carcinoma in a diverticulum. The wall is always so thin that invasion has usually occurred.

hypogastric arteries (Fig. 19.51). This broad wedge of tissue is taken down to the trigone, leaving only a rim, perhaps 1 cm wide, well clear of the dome of the bladder (Fig. 19.52). This is closed over a catheter. It was shown over 80 years ago [123] that the bladder will regenerate to a normal capacity from this rim of trigone within a few weeks. There is no need to perform a total cystoprostatectomy or to enlarge the bladder with ileum or colon.

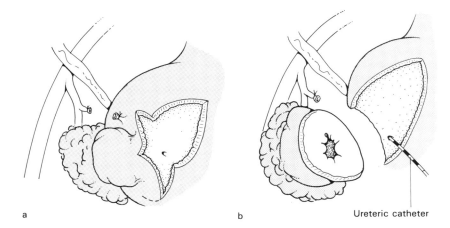

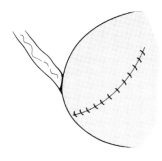

Fig. 19.54 Carcinoma in a diverticulum. (a) The bladder is opened well clear of the diverticulum. (b) The ureter is marked with a catheter, and a wide ellipse of bladder taken *en bloc* with the diverticulum, the extravesical fat, and the lymph nodes along the internal iliac vessels. (c) The bladder is closed.

Cancer in a diverticulum

The wall of a diverticulum is so thin that a tumour has only to penetrate the lamina propria and it has gone through its wall (Fig. 19.53). For this reason tumours in diverticula have a sinister reputation, and even a small and apparently superficial one calls for wide partial cystectomy.

Through an adequate midline incision the superior vesical artery on the side of the diverticulum is divided between ligatures to allow the lateral wall of the bladder to be rolled forwards. The bladder is opened and ureteric catheters are placed in both ureters to protect them. A wide cuff of bladder is removed including the orifice of the diverticulum (Fig. 19.54). The diverticulum itself is removed together with all its surrounding fat and the internal iliac and obturator lymph nodes. The bladder is closed with drainage.

A postoperative course of radiotherapy and/or chemotherapy is given in all those (the majority) who are found to have spread outside the bladder.

References

1 Doll R, Peto R (1981) The causes of cancer: quantitative estimates of avoidable risks of cancer in the United States today. *J Natl Canc Inst* 66: 1191.

2 Silverman DT, Hartge P, Morrison AS, Devesa SS (1992) Epidemiology of bladder cancer. *Hematol Oncol Clin N Am* 6: 1.

3 Ross RK, Paganini-Hill A, Henderson BE (1988) Epidemiology of bladder cancer, in: Skinner DG & Lieskovsky G (eds) *Diagnosis and Management of Genitourinary Cancer*, pp. 23–31. Philadelphia: WB Saunders.

4 Mommsen S, Sell A, Barford N (1982) N-acetyltransferase phenotypes of bladder cancer patients in a low risk population. *Lancet* ii: 1228.

5 Chiang HS, Guo HR, Hong CL, Lin SM, Lee EF (1993) The incidence of bladder cancer in the black foot disease endemic area in Taiwan. *Br J Urol* 71: 274.

6 Rehn L (1895) Blasengeschwultse bei fuchsinarbeitern. *Arch Clin Chir* 50: 588.

7 Hueper WC, Wiley FH, Wolfe HD (1938) Experimental production of bladder tumors in dogs by administration of beta-naphthylamine. *J Industr Hyg Toxicol* 20: 46.

8 Bennett DA (ed.) (1976) *Tumours of the Bladder in the Chemical Industry: a Study of their Causes and Prevention*. Chemical Industries Association.

9 Case RAM, Hosker ME (1954) Tumour of the urinary bladder as an occupational disease in the rubber industry in England and Wales. *Br J Prev Soc Med* 8: 39.

10 Hendry WF, Blandy JP, Glasham RW *et al.* (1988) Occupational bladder cancer: a guide for clinicians. *Br J Urol* 61: 183.

11 Rothwell K (1992) *The Interaction of Smoking and Workplace Hazards: Risks to Health*. WHO Publications, Geneva.

12 Momas I, Daures JP, Festy B, Bontoux J, Gremy F (1994) Bladder cancer and black tobacco cigarette smoking: some results from a French case-control study. *Eur J Epidemiol* 10: 599.

13 Fokkens W (1979) Phenacitin abuse related to bladder cancer. *Environ Res* 20: 192.

14 Sigurgeirsson B, Lindelof B, Eklung G (1991) Condylomata acuminata and risk of cancer: an epidemiological study. *Br Med J* 303: 341.

15 Yaqoob M, McClelland P, Bell GM, Ahmad R, Bakran A (1991) Bladder tumours in paraplegic patients on renal replacement therapy. *Lancet* 338: 1554.

16 Smith JA (1990) Laser treatment of bladder hemangioma. *J Urol* 143: 282.

17 Hermanek P, Sobin LH (1992) *International Union against Cancer TNM Classification of Malignant Tumours*, 4th edn, 2nd revision. Berlin: Springer.

18 Masters JRW, Camplejohn RS, Parkinson MC, Woodhouse CRJ (1989) DNA ploidy and the prognosis of stage pT1 bladder cancer. *Br J Urol* 64: 403.

19 Ooms ECM, Anderson WAD, Alons CL, Boon ME, Veldhuizen RW (1983) Analysis of the performance of pathologists in the grading of bladder tumors. *Hum Pathol* 14: 140.

20 Abel PD, Henderson D, Bennett MK, Hall RR, Williams G (1988) Differing interpretations by pathologists of the pT category and grade of transitional cell cancer of the bladder. *Br J Urol* 62: 339.

21 Tannenbaum M, Romas NA, Droller MJ (1988) The pathobiology of early urothelial cancer, in: Skinner DG, Lieskovsky G (eds) *Diagnosis and Management of Genitourinary Cancer*, p. 55. Philadelphia: WB Saunders.

22 Richards B, Parmar MKB, Anderson CK *et al.* (1991) Interpretation of biopsies of 'normal' urothelium in patients with superficial bladder cancer. *Br J Urol* 67: 369.

23 Abel PD, Hall RR, Williams G (1988) Should pT1 transitional cell cancers of the bladder still be classified as superficial? *Br J Urol* 62: 235.

24 Hendry WF, Rawson NSB, Turney L, Dunlop A, Whitfield HN (1990) Computerisation of urothelial carcinoma records: 16 years experience with the TNM system. *Br J Urol* 65: 583.

25 Jewett HJ, Strong GH (1946) Infiltrating carcinoma of the bladder: relation of depth of penetration of the bladder wall to incidence of local extension and metastases. *J Urol* 55: 366.

26 Page BH, Levinson VB, Curwen MP (1978) The site of recurrences of non-infiltrating bladder tumours. *Br J Urol* 50: 237.

27 Tannenbaum SI, Carson CC, Tatum A, Paulson DF (1983) Squamous carcinoma of the urinary bladder. *Urology* 22: 597.

28 Jones MA, Bloom HJG, Williams G, Trott PA, Wallace DM (1980) The management of squamous cell carcinoma of the bladder. *Br J Urol* 52: 511.

29 Morgan RJ, Cameron KM (1980) Vesical leukoplakia. *Br J Urol* 52: 96.

30 Roehrborn CG, Teigland CM, Spence HM (1988) Progression of leukoplakia of the bladder to squamous cell carcinoma 19 years after complete

urinary diversion. *J Urol* 140: 603.

31 Swanson DA, Liles A, Zagars GK (1990) Preoperative irradiation and radical cystectomy for stages T2 and T3 squamous cell carcinoma of the bladder. *J Urol* 143: 37.

32 Thomas DG, Ward AM, Williams JL (1971) A study of 52 cases of adenocarcinoma of the bladder. *Br J Urol* 43: 4.

33 Herr HW (1994) Urachal carcinoma: the case for extended partial cystectomy. *J Urol* 151: 365.

34 Sheldon CA, Clayman RV, Gonzalez R, Williams RD, Fraley EE (1984) Malignant urachal lesions. *J Urol* 131: 1.

35 Gill HS, Dhillon HK, Woodhouse CRJ (1989) Adenocarcinoma of the urinary bladder. *Br J Urol* 64: 138.

36 Iles RK, Chard T (1991) Human chorionic gonadotropin expression by bladder cancers: biology and clinical potential. *J Urol* 145: 45.

37 Higgins PM, Tresidder GC (1966) Phaeochromocytoma of the urinary bladder. *Br Med J* 2: 274.

38 Broecker BH, Plowman N, Pritchard J, Ransley PG (1988) Pelvic rhabdomyosarcoma in children. *Br J Urol* 61: 427.

39 Thrasher HB, Miller GJ, Wettlaufer JN (1990) Bladder leiomyosarcoma following cyclophosphamide therapy for lupus nephritis. *J Urol* 143: 119.

40 Wallace DM (1959) Tumours of the bladder, in: Smithers D (ed.) *Neoplastic Disease at Various Sites*, vol. 2. Edinburgh: Churchill Livingstone.

41 Schoonees R, Gamarra MG, Moore RH, Murphy GP (1971) The diagnostic value of urinary cytology in patients with bladder carcinoma. *J Urol* 106: 693.

42 Pereira JH, Towler JM (1990) Ten cases of transitional cell carcinoma of bladder causing ureteric obstruction. *Br J Urol* 66: 628.

43 Davies AH, Cranston D, Meagher T, Fellows GJ (1989) Detection of recurrent bladder tumours by transrectal and abdominal ultrasound compared with cystoscopy. *Br J Urol* 64: 409.

44 Spencer J, Lindsell D, Mastoakou I (1990) Ultrasonography compared with intravenous urography in the investigation of adults with haematuria. *Br Med J* 301: 1074.

45 Voges GE, Tauschke E, Stöckle M, Alken P, Hohenfellner R (1989) Computerized tomography: an unreliable method for accurate staging of bladder tumors in patients who are candidates for radical cystectomy. *J Urol* 142: 972.

46 Nurmi M, Katevuo K, Puntala P (1988) Reliability of CT in preoperative evaluation of bladder carcinoma. *Scand J Urol Nephrol* 22: 125.

47 Persad R, Kabala J, Gillatt D, Penry B, Gingell JC, Smith PJB (1993) Magnetic resonance imaging in the staging of bladder cancer. *Br J Urol* 71: 566.

48 Blandy JP, Fowler CG (1986) Lower tract endoscopy. *Br Med Bull* 42: 280.

49 Fowler CG, Badenoch DF, Thakar DR (1984) Practical experience with flexible fibrescope cystoscopy in outpatients. *Br J Urol* 56: 618.

50 Davies AH, Mastorakou I, Dickinson AJ *et al.* (1991) Flexible cystoscopy compared with ultrasound in the detection of recurrent bladder tumours. *Br J Urol* 67: 491.

51 Fowler CG, Boorman LS (1986) Outpatient treatment of superficial bladder cancer. *Lancet* i: 38.

52 Blandy JP, Notley RG (1993) *Transurethral Resection*, 3rd edn. London: Heinemann.

53 Helmstein K (1972) Treatment of bladder carcinoma by a hydrostatic pressure technique. *Br J Urol* 44: 434.

54 England HR, Rigby C, Shepheard BGF, Tresidder GC, Blandy JP (1973) Evaluation of Helmstein's distension method for carcinoma of the bladder. *Br J Urol* 45: 593.

55 Jenkins BJ, Nauth-Misir RR, Martin JE, Fowler CG, Hope-Stone HF, Blandy JP (1989) The fate of G3 pT1 bladder cancer. *Br J Urol* 64: 608.

56 Birch BRP, Harland SJ (1989) The pT1 G3 bladder tumour. *Br J Urol* 64: 109.

57 Manyak MJ (1993) Photodynamic therapy for superficial bladder carcinoma. *Curr Opinion Urol* 3: 220.

58 Oravisto KJ (1972) Optimal intravesical dosage of Thiotepa in the prophylaxis of recurrent bladder papillomatosis. *Scand J Urol Nephrol* 6: 26.

59 England HR, Flynn JT, Paris AMI, Blandy JP (1981) Early multiple-dose adjuvant Thiotepa in the control of multiple and rapid T1 tumour neogenesis. *Br J Urol* 53: 588.

60 Robinson MRG, Shetty MB, Richards B *et al.* (1977) Intravesical Epodyl in the management of bladder tumors: combined experience of the Yorkshire Urological Cancer Research Group. *J Urol* 118: 972.

61 Mufti GR, Virdi JS, Hall MH (1990) Long-term follow-up of intravesical Epodyl therapy for superficial bladder cancer. *Br J Urol* 65: 32.

62 Tolley DA, Hargreave TB, Smith PH *et al.* (1988) Effect of intravesical Mitomycin C on recurrence of newly diagnosed superficial bladder cancer: interim report from the Medical Research Council subgroup on superficial Bladder Cancer (Urological Cancer Working Party). *Br Med J* 296: 1759.

63 Soloway MS (1985) Treatment of superficial bladder cancer with intravesical Mitomycin C: analysis of immediate and long-term response in 70 patients. *J Urol* 134: 1107.

64 Neild VS, Sanderson KV, Riddle PR (1984) Dermatitis due to mitomycin bladder instillations. *J Roy Soc Med* 77: 610.

65 Drago PC, Badalament RA, Lucas J, Drago JR (1989) Bladder wall calcification after intravesical Mitomycin C treatment of superficial bladder cancer. *J Urol* 142: 1071.

66 Oosterlink W, Kurth KH, Schroeder F *et al.* (1993) A prospective European Organization for Research and Treatment of Cancer Genitourinary Group randomized trial comparing transurethral resection followed by a single intravesical instillation of Epirubicin or water in single stage Ta, T1 papillary carcinoma of the bladder. *J Urol* 149: 749.

67 Kurth KH, Schroeder FH, Tunn U *et al.* (1984) Adjuvant chemotherapy of superficial transitional cell bladder carcinoma: preliminary results of a EORTC randomised trial comparing doxorubicin hydrochloride, ethoglucid and transurethral resection alone. *J Urol* 132: 258.

68 Cerosimo RJ, Hong WK (1986) Epirubicin: a review of the pharmacology, clinical activity and adverse effects of an adriamycin analogue. *J Clin Oncol*

4: 425—31.

69 Bouffioux C, Denis L, Oosterlink W *et al.* (1992) Adjuvant chemotherapy of recurrent superficial transitional cell carcinoma: results of a EORTC randomised trial comparing intravesical instillation of Thiotepa, doxorubicin and cisplatin. *J Urol* 148: 287.

70 Morales A (1984) Long-term results and complications of intracavitary bacillus Calmette—Guérin therapy for bladder cancer. *J Urol* 132: 457.

71 Sarosdy MF, Lamm DL (1989) Long-term results of intravesical bacillus Calmette—Guérin therapy for superficial bladder cancer. *J Urol* 142: 719.

72 Kelley DR, Ratliff TR, Catalona WJ *et al.* (1985) Intravesical bacillus Calmette—Guérin therapy for superficial bladder cancer: effect of BCG viability on treatment results. *J Urol* 134: 48.

73 Morales A, Nickel JC, Wilson JWL (1992) Dose-response of bacillus Calmette—Guérin in the treatment of superficial bladder cancer. *J Urol* 147: 1256.

74 Deresiewicz RL, Stone RM, Aster JC (1990) Fatal disseminated mycobacterial infection following intravesical bacillus Calmette—Guérin. *J Urol* 144: 1331.

75 Rawls WH, Lamm DL, Lowe BA *et al.* (1990) Fatal sepsis following intravesical bacillus Calmette—Guérin administration for bladder cancer. *J Urol* 144: 1328.

76 Dow JA, di Sant'Agnese PA, Cockett ATK (1989) Expression of blood group precursor T antigen as a prognostic marker for human bladder cancer treated by bacillus Calmette—Guérin and interleukin-2. *J Urol* 142: 978.

77 Khanna OP, Chou RH, Son DL *et al.* (1988) Does bacillus Calmette—Guérin immunotherapy accelerate growth and cause metastatic spread of second primary malignancy? *Urology* 31: 459.

78 Mevorach RA, Cos LR, di Sant'Agnese PA, Stoler M (1990) Human papillomavirus type 6 in grade I transitional cell carcinoma of the urethra. *J Urol* 143: 126.

79 Rovere GQD, Oliver RTD, McCance DJ, Castro JE (1988) Development of bladder tumour containing HPV type 11 DNA after renal transplantation. *Br J Urol* 62: 36.

80 Galvani D, Griffiths SD, Cawley JC (1988) Interferon for treatment: the dust settles (review). *Br Med J* 296: 1554.

81 Alcock CJ, Durrant KR, Smith JC, Fellows GJ (1986) Treatment of multiple superficial transitional cell carcinoma of the bladder with intravesical yttrium-90. *Br J Urol* 58: 287.

82 Quilty PM, Duncan W (1986) Treatment of superficial (T1) tumours of the bladder by radical radiotherapy. *Br J Urol* 58: 147.

83 Benson RC, Kinsey JH, Cortese DA, Farrow GM, Utz DC (1983) Treatment of transitional cell carcinoma of the bladder with hematoporphyrin derivative phototherapy. *J Urol* 132: 1090.

84 Hudson MA, Herr HW (1995) Carcinoma *in situ* of the bladder. *J Urol* 153: 564.

85 Wolf H, Melsen F, Pedersen SE, Nielsen KT (1994) Natural history of carcinoma *in situ* of the urinary bladder. *Scand J Urol Nephrol Suppl* 157: 147.

86 Jakse G, Putz A, Feichtinger J (1989) Cystectomy:

the treatment of choice in patients with carcinoma *in situ* of the bladder? *Eur J Surg Oncol* 15: 211.

87 Harland SJ, Charig CR, Highman W, Parkinson MC, Riddle PR (1992) Outcome in carcinoma *in situ* of bladder treated with intravesical bacille Calmette—Guérin. *Br J Urol* 70: 271.

88 Stricker PD, Grant ABF, Hosken BM, Taylor JS (1990) Topical Mitomycin C therapy for carcinoma *in situ* of the bladder: a follow-up. *J Urol* 1432: 34.

89 Mukjamel E, deKernion JB (1989) Conservative treatment of diffuse carcinoma *in situ* of the bladder with repeated courses of intravesical therapy. *Br J Urol* 64: 143.

90 Jenkins BJ, England HR, Fowler CG *et al.* (1988) Chemotherapy for carcinoma *in situ* of the bladder. *Br J Urol* 61: 326.

91 Betton PR, Herr HW, Whitmore WF *et al.* (1989) Intravesical bacillus Calmette—Guérin therapy for *in situ* transitional cell carcinoma involving the prostatic urethra. *J Urol* 141: 853.

92 Whitmore WF, Marshall VF (1962) Radical total cystectomy for cancer of the urinary bladder: 230 consecutive cases five years later. *J Urol* 87: 853.

93 Whitmore WF (1980) Integrated irradiation and cystectomy for bladder cancer. *Br J Urol* 52: 1.

94 Skinner DG, Lieskovsky G (1984) Contemporary cystectomy with pelvic node dissection compared to preoperative radiation therapy plus cystectomy in management of invasive bladder cancer. *J Urol* 131: 1069.

95 Jacobi GH, Klippel FF, Hohenfellner R (1983) Funfzehn Jahre Erfahrung mit der radikalen Cystecktomie ohne praeoperative Radiotherapie beim Harnblasenkarzinom. *Aktuel Urol* 14: 63.

96 Wallace DM, Bloom HJG (1976) The management of deeply infiltrating (T3) bladder carcinoma: controlled trial of radical radiotherapy versus pre-operative radiotherapy and radical cystectomy (first report). *Br J Urol* 48: 587.

97 Bloom HJG, Hendry WF, Wallace DM, Skeet RG (1982) Treatment of T3 bladder cancer: controlled trial of preoperative radiotherapy and radical cystectomy versus radical radiotherapy. *Br J Urol* 54: 136.

98 Blandy JP, England HR, Evans SJW *et al.* (1980) T3 bladder cancer — the case for salvage cystectomy. *Br J Urol* 52: 506.

99 Blandy JP, Tiptaft RC, Paris AMI, Oliver RTD, Hope-Stone HF (1985) The case for definitive radiotherapy and salvage cystectomy. *World J Urol* 3: 94.

100 Shearer RJ, Chilvers CED, Blook HJG, Bliss JM, Horwich A, Babiker A (1988) Adjuvant chemotherapy in T2 carcinoma of the bladder. A prospective trial: preliminary report. *Br J Urol* 62: 558.

101 Abratt RP, Wilson JA, Pontin AR, Barnes RD (1993) Salvage cystectomy after radical irradiation for bladder cancer — prognostic factors and complications. *Br J Urol* 72: 756.

102 Jenkins BJ, Caulfield MJ, Fowler CG *et al.* (1988) Reappraisal of the role of radical radiotherapy and salvage cystectomy in the treatment of invasive (T2/T3) bladder cancer. *Br J Urol* 62: 343.

103 Jenkins BJ, Martin JE, Baithun SI, Zuk RJ, Oliver RTD, Blandy JP (1990) Prediction of response to radiotherapy in invasive bladder cancer. *Br J Urol* 65: 345.

104 Moutzouris G, Hannopoulos D, Barbatis C, Zaharof A, Theodorou C (1993) Is beta-human chorionic gonadotrophin production by transitional cell carcinoma of the bladder a marker of aggressive disease and resistance to radiotherapy? *Br J Urol* 72: 907.

105 Nouri AME, Smith MEF, Crosby D, Oliver RTD (1990) Selective and non-selective loss of immuno-regulatory molecules (HLA-A,B,C antigens and LFA-3) in transitional cell carcinoma. *Br J Cancer* 62: 603.

106 Lynch WJ, Jenkins BJ, Fowler CG, Hope-Stone HF, Blandy JP (1992) The quality of life after radical radiotherapy for bladder cancer. *Br Urol* 70: 519.

107 McPhee MS, Arnfield MR, Tulip J, Lakey WH (1988) Neodymium-YAG laser therapy for infiltrating bladder cancer. *J Urol* 140: 44.

108 Studer UE, Bacchi M, Biedermann C *et al.* (1994) Adjuvant cisplatin chemotherapy following cystectomy for bladder cancer: results of a prospective randomized trial. *J Urol* 152: 81.

109 Sternberg C, Arena MG, Calabresi F *et al.* (1993) Neoadjuvant M-VAC (methotrexate, vinblastine, doxorubicin and cisplatin) for infiltrating transitional cell carcinoma of the bladder. *Cancer* 72: 1975.

110 Chersi D, Stewart LA, Parmar MKB *et al.* (1995) Does neoadjuvant cisplatin-based chemotherapy improve the survival of patients with locally advanced bladder cancer: a meta-analysis of individual patient data from randomized clinical trials. *Br J Urol* 75: 206.

111 Stockle M, Meyenburg W, Wellek S *et al.* (1992) Advanced bladder cancer (stages pT3b, pT4a, pN1 and pN2) improved survival after radical cystectomy and three adjuvant cycles of chemotherapy. Results of a controlled prospective trial. *J Urol* 148: 302.

112 Waehre H, Ous S, Klevmark B *et al.* (1993) A bladder cancer multi-institutional experience with total cystectomy for muscle-invasive bladder cancer. *Cancer* 72: 3044.

113 Chauvet B, Brewer Y, Felix-Faure C, Davin JL, Vincent P, Reboul F (1993) Combined radiation therapy and cisplatin for locally advanced carcinoma of the urinary bladder. *Cancer* 72: 2213.

114 Bowsher WC, Clarke A, Clarke DG, Costello AJ (1992) Laparoscopic pelvic node dissection. *Br J Urol* 70: 276.

115 Tomic R, Sjodin J-G (1992) Sexual function in men after radical cystectomy with or without urethrectomy. *Scand J Urol Nephrol* 26: 127.

116 Beahrs JR, Fleming TR, Zincke H (1984) Risk of local urethral recurrence after radical cystectomy for bladder cancer. *J Urol* 131: 264.

117 Stöckle M, Gokcebay E, Riedmiller H, Hohenfellner R (1990) Urethral tumor recurrences after radical cystoprostatectomy: the case for primary cysto-prostatourethrectomy. *J Urol* 143: 41.

118 Frazier HA, Robertson JE, Paulson DR (1992) Complications of radical cystectomy and urinary diversion: a retrospective review of 675 cases in two decades. *J Urol* 148: 1402.

119 Ghoneim MA, Ashamallah AG, Hammady S, Gaballah MA, Soliman HS (1979) Cystectomy for carcinoma of the bilharzial bladder: 138 cases 5 years later. *Br J Urol* 51: 541.

120 Ghoneim MA, Kock NG, Lycke G, El-Din ABS (1987) An appliance-free, sphincter-controlled bladder substitute: the urethral Kock pouch. *J Urol* 138: 1150.

121 Swanson DA, Liles A, Zagars GK (1990) Preoperative irradiation and radical cystectomy for stages T2 and T3 squamous cell carcinoma of the bladder. *J Urol* 142: 37.

122 Beck AD, Gaudin HJ, Bonham DG (1970) Carcinoma of the urachus. *Br J Urol* 42: 555.

123 Fenwick EH (1911) *The Indications for Widely Resecting the Bladder Walls in Vesical Growths*. London: Adlard.

Chapter 20: Urinary diversion

History

The long history of urinary diversion begins, it is said, with Franco, who created an artificial urinary fistula in 1556 [1]. Later Petit (1770) made a nephrostomy for calculous pyonephrosis [1]. Any kind of external fistula requires either an indwelling tube or a suitable external collecting appliance, and none were really suitable until the invention of the adhesive bag in 1950. The most extreme example of an external fistula was exstrophy, for which life with collecting devices was so miserable that it led Simon to attempt the first ureterosigmoidostomy, being led to this bold step by the consideration that: 'patients whose bladder, after the operation of lithotomy, opens into the rectum, acquire a certain control over the fluid contents of that bowel, by means of both sphincters ani' [2]. Using special catheters armed with sharp stylets, he passed seton sutures from ureters into the rectum and tied them tightly. His patient became dry, but within a year both ureters became 'choked with calculous concretions' [3] and he died. Shortly afterwards, in 1851, Lloyd attempted the same procedure, but perforated the peritoneum and the patient died 10 days later [4]. These two complications were to bedevil urinary diversion for another century.

Fistulae

Nephrostomy

Deliberate external fistulae are still useful, the most common being the percutaneous nephrostomy for temporarily relieving upper tract obstruction. For more permanent nephrostomy a larger tube that can be changed at regular intervals is needed, and for this Tresidder's technique [5] is still the best (Fig. 20.1): it allows the replacement catheter to be drawn in by the old one. The complications of permanent nephrostomy are inevitable infection and calculus

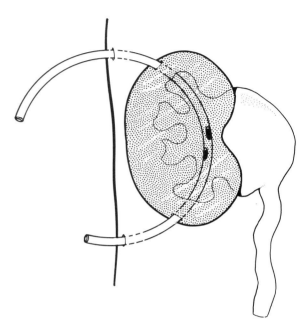

Fig. 20.1 Tresidder's method of nephrostomy. This enables the tube to be changed at regular intervals.

formation, so that it is today only used when all other methods are inappropriate.

Ureterostomy

Ureterostomy is also a method of diversion to be used only in the last resort: when the ureter is wide it can be split, everted and brought to the skin like an ileostomy (Fig. 20.2). For ureters of more normal calibre there is a tendency for the stoma to undergo stenosis, which a double-Z plasty may partly avoid (Fig. 20.3). Ureterostomy *in situ* [6] can be a useful emergency diversion (Fig. 20.4) so long as the curve from ureter to skin is very smooth; otherwise it will be impossible to change the tube.

Suprapubic cystostomy

The most simple and useful temporary diversion is the suprapubic cystostomy, commonly used in

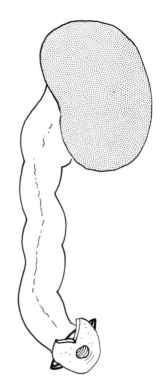

Fig. 20.2 Ureterostomy when the ureter is dilated.

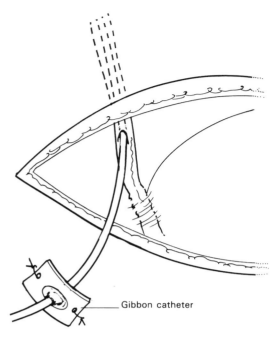

Fig. 20.4 Ureterostomy *in situ*.

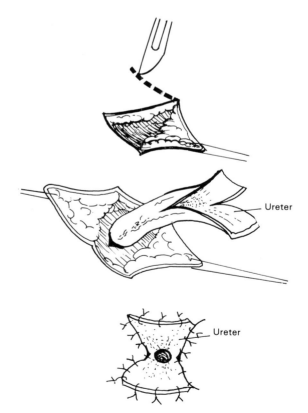

Fig. 20.3 Double-Z plasty for ureterostomy with an undilated ureter.

retention of urine where a urethral catheter is difficult to pass. The technique is very simple (Fig. 20.5). If the cystostomy has to remain in for a longer period and a larger tube is needed, the fine track can be dilated using percutaneous nephrolithotomy equipment, or a formal suprapubic cystostomy performed. Such cases are nearly always men who have undergone previous surgery when the peritoneum is apt to be stuck to the symphysis, and great care is needed in finding the bladder (Fig. 20.6). A permanent suprapubic cystostomy is an uncomfortable permanent diversion, always complicated by infection and calculi and there are usually better alternatives.

One of these is suprapubic vesicostomy. It is seldom indicated. A tube is made of bladder like a Boari flap and brought up to the skin (Fig. 20.7). If the track of the tube passes sufficiently obliquely through the abdominal wall, it will be continent and the patient can then empty the bladder by intermittent self-catheterization at will. It has a place in some neuropathic bladders when the bladder neck is closed or spastic.

Ureterosigmoidostomy

For a century after Simon, surgical efforts were devoted to eliminating the dangers of ascending

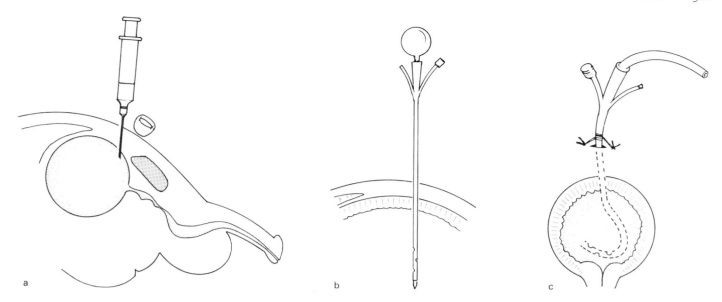

Fig. 20.5 (a–c) Suprapubic cystostomy.

infection and leakage from ureterosigmoidostomy. Innumerable techniques were devised for performing the ureterosigmoidostomy [7] but it was not until a direct elliptical mucosal anastomosis was combined with an antireflux tunnel that the problem was solved [8,9].

Then there appeared a new complication, hitherto overshadowed by the operative risks of ureterosigmoidostomy. Physiologists had long been aware that if enough urine was absorbed by the intestine, it could eventually lead to renal tubular damage [10,11], but the complication was thought to be very rare [12,13]. Then, in 1950 Ferris and Odel published their long-term follow-up of 124 patients and found that no fewer than 62% had developed severe acidosis [14]. Others confirmed these findings. Urological wards were full of patients with the severe symptoms of this condition. It took several years before its pathogenesis was understood.

The biochemical changes were due to two factors: first and foremost was absorption of urine. Since normal urine is acidotic to the plasma by one-third too much chloride, this absorption at a milli-equivalent for milli-equivalent rate can cause hyperchloremia, and the real problem is how much absorption occurs [15].

The second factor was renal function. If renal tubular function was perfect, it could cope with the acidosis. But when continued absorption of urine or damage from ascending infection and obstruction began to impair tubular function,

then acidosis would appear. This explained why it took so long for acidosis to develop in patients who started off with good kidneys [16].

Once the hazards of acidosis were appreciated, surgeons welcomed other alternatives to ureterosigmoidostomy. Nevertheless the method still has a place, e.g. when the patient has a good anal control, good renal function and a relatively short life expectancy [17]. There are a number of good techniques, but the 'combined method' of Leadbetter is still the standard one (Fig. 20.8).

The follow-up must include careful monitoring of the patient's biochemical status, and if hyperchloraemic acidosis develops, a daily supplement of sodium bicarbonate should be given. In view of the late risk of cancer of the colon, every patient who has had a ureterosigmoidostomy for more than 10 years should undergo an annual colonoscopy.

Intestinal conduits

The ileal conduit was developed in occupied France during World War II. The French surgeons were glad to explain their new techniques to the surgeons in the liberating forces. The techniques could not gain wide acceptance until an effective adhesive appliance for ileostomy was introduced in 1950. The operation was first described in the English literature by Bricker [18] (sadly, without any acknowledgement of priority to the French). The ileal conduit soon replaced ureterosigmoidostomy. It avoided acidosis, reflux and

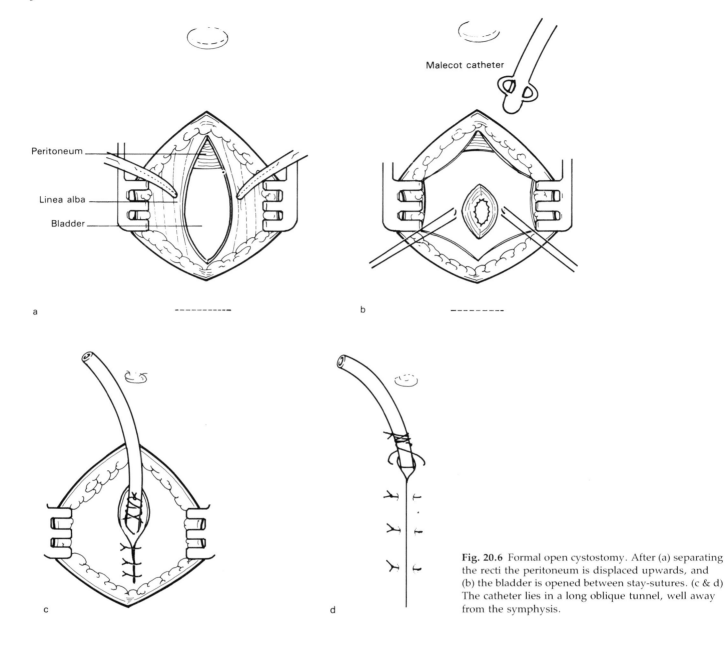

Peritoneum

Linea alba

Bladder

a

Malecot catheter

b

c

d

Fig. 20.6 Formal open cystostomy. After (a) separating the recti the peritoneum is displaced upwards, and (b) the bladder is opened between stay-sutures. (c & d) The catheter lies in a long oblique tunnel, well away from the symphysis.

infection: above all it was much safer. It was virtually free from the hazards of urinary leakage: if urine did leak, it would escape more easily through the lumen of the ileum than through a drain. This was especially valuable during an era when radiotherapy was being increasingly used in the treatment of bladder cancer, after which ureterosigmoidostomy carried a formidable mortality [19].

There were a number of useful simplifications of the original French/Bricker method of making an ileal conduit, notably the simple anastomosis of Wallace [20]. Using this technique the ileal

loop became the diversion of choice. It requires attention to detail.

As much care should be given in choosing the right site for the appliance as is given to the operation itself. The site of the stoma is chosen after the patient has worn an appliance, filled with water, when sitting, lying down and with his or her clothes on. Care must be taken to avoid placing the site of the stoma on a scar, skin crease or where the belt is usually tightened.

After bowel preparation a length of ileum is selected with a good blood supply, from an unirradiated area (Fig. 20.9). Having isolated the

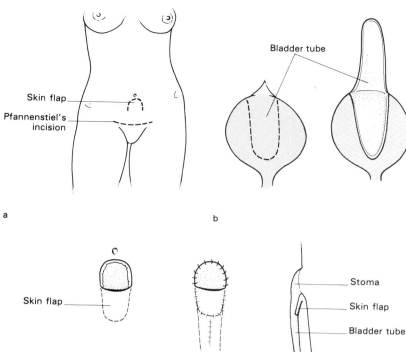

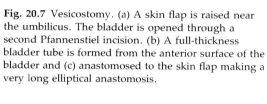

Fig. 20.7 Vesicostomy. (a) A skin flap is raised near the umbilicus. The bladder is opened through a second Pfannenstiel incision. (b) A full-thickness bladder tube is formed from the anterior surface of the bladder and (c) anastomosed to the skin flap making a very long elliptical anastomosis.

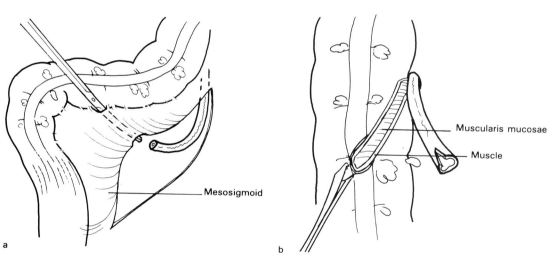

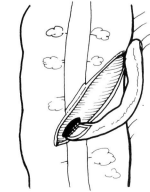

Fig. 20.8 Leadbetter's technique of ureterosigmoidostomy. (a) The ureter is brought between the layers of the mesosigmoid. (b) A tunnel is made for the ureter through the muscle of the colon. (c) An elliptical anastomosis is made between the spatulated ureter and colonic mucosa. The muscle is closed over the ureter: to prevent closing it too tightly a catheter is placed alongside the ureter while the stitches are tied.

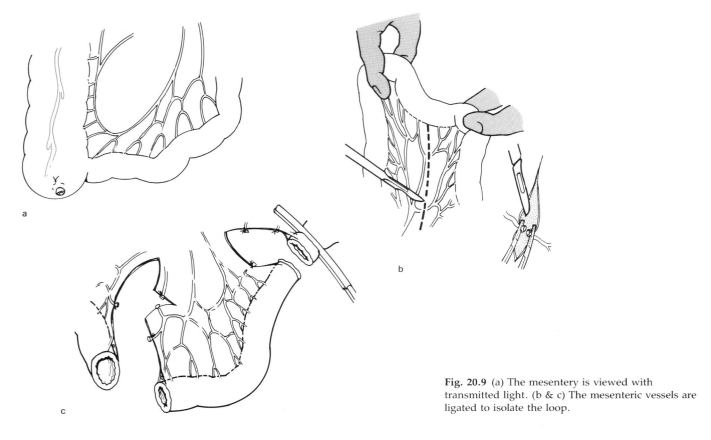

Fig. 20.9 (a) The mesentery is viewed with transmitted light. (b & c) The mesenteric vessels are ligated to isolate the loop.

loop, an end-to-end anastomosis is performed (Fig. 20.10). The ureters are spatulated and anastomosed together to form a common stoma which is then sewn to the open end of the bowel (Fig. 20.11). It saves anxiety if the ureters are intubated for a few days.

Colonic conduits

From time to time it is convenient to make a conduit out of a suitable length of the large bowel, e.g. the sigmoid after pelvic exenteration. Exactly the same principles are used [21,22]. There are no special advantages or disadvantages in using large rather than small bowel. Urinary absorption and the risk of reflux is identical.

The follow-up of patients with either type of intestinal conduit should include regular monitoring of their electrolytes, especially when there is already some impairment of renal function. In addition, ultrasound or urography is necessary to detect dilatation of the loop or of the

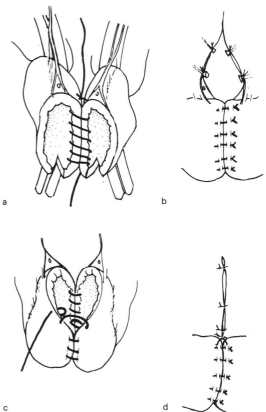

Fig. 20.10 (*right*) (a–d) The ends of the ileum are anastomosed together.

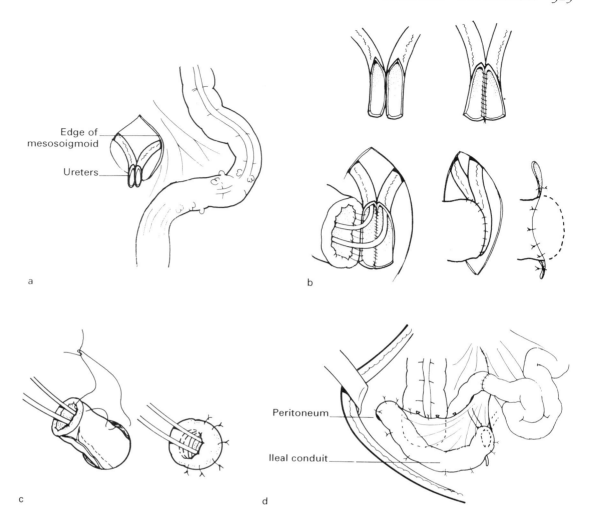

Edge of mesosoigmoid

Ureters

a

b

Peritoneum

Ileal conduit

c

d

Fig. 20.11 (a) The ends of the ureters are spatulated and sewn together, and anastomosed to one end of the isolated ileal loop (b). The other end is brought out on the skin as an ileostomy (c & d).

upper tracts. Stones are a frequent long-term complication of intestinal conduits.

Continent urinary reservoirs

Despite the safety of the ileal conduit, many patients disliked their urinary stoma and, however good the appliance, it was always likely to leak or come unstuck at the least convenient moment. Compared with the best of the ureterosigmoidostomy results there were serious drawbacks. The problem was how to make ureterosigmoidostomy more safe.

Mauclaire's operation

One way was to use the rectosigmoid as a reservoir, but divert the faeces through a proximal colostomy [23] (Fig. 20.12). To many patients a 'dry' colostomy was more acceptable than a

urinary stoma. Mauclaire's operation limited the surface area of colon so that there was less reabsorption of urine [24], and the urine in the rectum, though never sterile, had far fewer organisms when the faecal stream had been diverted. Mauclaire's operation had its advocates, but it never became popular, nor was it entirely free from the risk of acidosis [25−28].

Gersuny's operation

A modification of Mauclaire's operation without an abdominal colostomy had been attempted by Gersuny in 1899 [29] with a fatal outcome. It was tried again with success by Marion in 1910 [30]. The object was to bring Mauclaire's colostomy out through the sphincter of the anus, using the plane between the rectal mucosa and muscle. Although often revived, the possible complications were daunting. Retraction of the anal

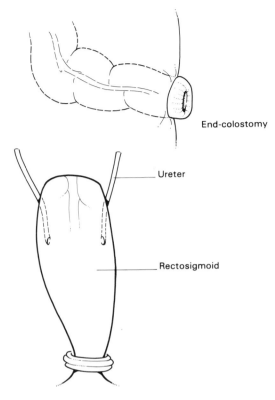

Fig. 20.12 Mauclaire's operation.

colostomy meant that even the more successful cases tended to end up with a common cloaca for urine and faeces [31−34].

The Mansoura diversion

In Egypt, incontinence means social ostracism and adhesive appliances are expensive and unreliable in the hot climate. Ghoneim, working with Kock, has devised an ingenious modification of Mauclaire's operation which offers the patient a capacious urinary reservoir, prevents reflux of urine even in ureters that have been damaged by bilharziasis, and employs an intussusception valve which keeps the urine in the rectum and out of the rest of the colon, so limiting the absorbent surface area [35] (Fig. 20.13).

Continent pouches

There had been attempts from the turn of the century [36,37] to use the right colon as a reservoir. Bricker, Eiseman, Gilchrist and Merricks [38−40] developed a technique that was claimed to give a capacious reservoir with a continent ileal stoma which could be emptied by periodic intermittent self-catheterization (Fig. 20.14).

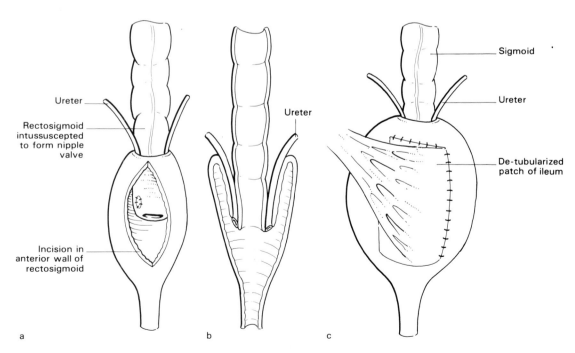

Fig. 20.13 The Mansoura diversion. (a) The sigmoid is intussuscepted to form a non-return valve. (b) The ureters are led down between the layers of the intussuscepted bowel to prevent reflux. (c) An isolated patch of ileum is added to the rectosigmoid to give extra capacity.

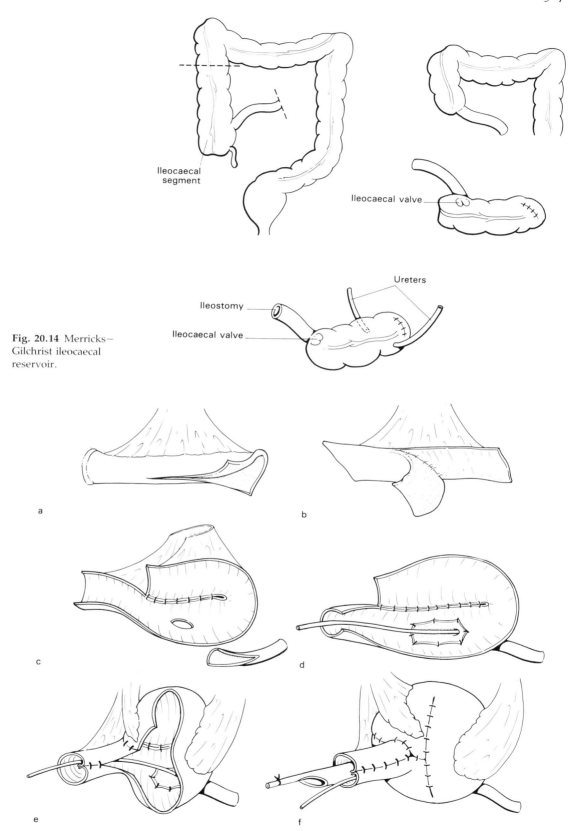

Fig. 20.14 Merricks–Gilchrist ileocaecal reservoir.

a

b

c

d

e

f

Fig. 20.15 (a–f) A reservoir is made from ileum stripped of its mucosa. Urothelium grows out from the implanted ureter to reline the reservoir.

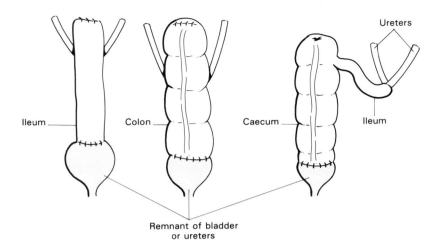

Ileum

Colon

Caecum

Ileum

Ureters

Remnant of bladder
or ureters

Fig. 20.16 A simple length of ileum, colon or ileum and colon were added onto the trigone after subtotal cystectomy.

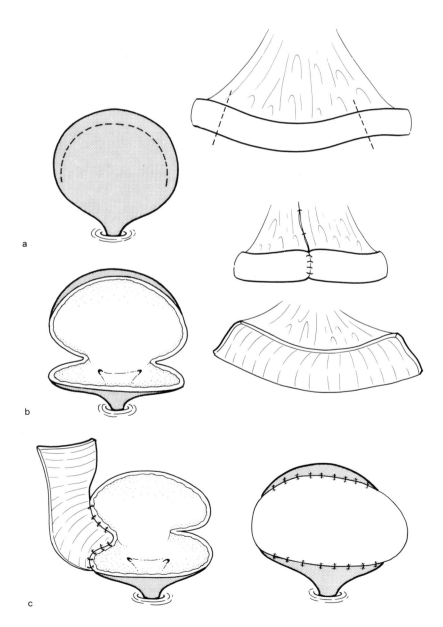

a

b

c

Fig. 20.17 Clam cystoplasty. (a) The bladder is opened in the coronal plane and a length of ileum is isolated. (b) The ileum is opened and sewn into the bladder (c) to give extra volume and lower the pressure.

Couvelaire [41] was critical of the method 'Elle n'a rien d'une vessie, ni la continence, ni la miction'. Nor was it free from the complications of acidosis, ascending infection and calculus formation.

Regenerated bladders

As early as 1911, Fenwick had noted the astonishing capability of regeneration in the human bladder after subtotal cystectomy for cancer [42], recalling the earlier observations in the dog by Tizzoni and Foggi [43]. This led to a series of hopeful attempts to get a bladder to regenerate from the divided stumps of the urethra and ureters over a plastic mould [44], or by encouraging urothelium to reline a 'bladder' made of bowel stripped of its absorbent mucosa [45] (Fig. 20.15). In fact these experiments produced something similar to a bladder in the dog, but as soon as the moulds were removed they underwent contraction, and had no clinical application.

De-tubularized bowel pouches

The earliest attempts to enlarge the bladder with bowel were performed for bladders that had undergone contracture from tuberculosis or interstitial cystitis. Different segments of intestine were used, including colon, small intestine and caecum (Fig. 20.16). Spontaneous contractions of the bowel, especially the caecum, would result in incontinence of urine especially at night, but a more serious consequence of these uninhibited contractions was that they generated such a high pressure that there would be ureteric reflux and obstructive nephropathy.

These could be avoided if the bowel were 'de-tubularized', i.e. opened out and sewn into the bladder as a flat patch. The uncoordinated bowel contractions would not generate any pressure: indeed, such a patch could be used in 'clam cystoplasty' to overcome deliberately raised bladder pressure in patients with vesical detrusor instability [46−49] (Fig. 20.17).

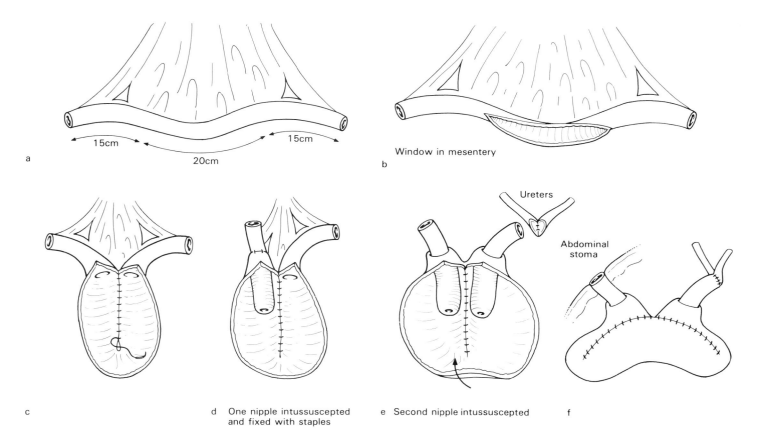

Fig. 20.18 Kock's pouch. (a) A 45 cm length of ileum is isolated and (b) the middle 20 cm opened out. (c−e) The ileum at each end is intussuscepted to form an antireflux nipple, which is secured with staples. (f) One end forms the stoma, the other is anastomosed to the ureters. The middle portion is formed into a reservoir.

As a result of this discovery, it became possible to devise a new kind of pouch or bladder enlargement with a very low pressure — so low indeed that it would not take much pressure on the outlet to maintain continence (Fig. 20.18). Continence was usually at the expense of needing self-catheterization, and occasional spontaneous rupture [50].

Although Kock had first developed this pouch as a faecal reservoir for patients undergoing colectomy for ulcerative colitis, the idea was quickly adapted as a urinary reservoir. At first the stoma was led out on the skin: later it was anastomosed to the urethra as a true substitute for the bladder [51].

Since only a very low pressure was needed to keep in the urine one could make use of an artificial sphincter, a loop of ileum, plicated ileum or the appendix.

The ingenuity of its enthusiasts knew no bounds and every conceivable permutation and combination of every part of the gastrointestinal tract was used to provide low pressure continent substitutes for the bladder [52–55] (Fig. 20.19). The multiplicity of these techniques and their innumerable modifications shows that none of

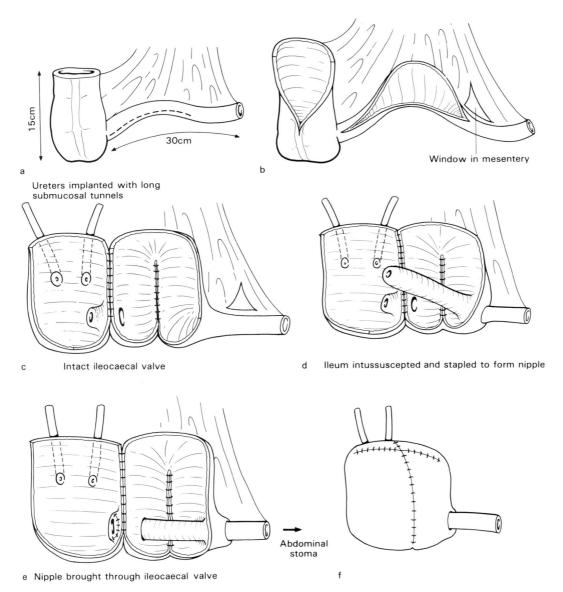

Fig. 20.19 (a–f) The Mainz pouch. A 30 cm length of ileum and caecum are isolated. One end of the ileum is intussuscepted and brought through the ileocaecal valve as a long antireflux nipple. The ureters are implanted into the caecum with long submucosal tunnels. The rest of the ileum is sewn onto the caecum to give a low-pressure reservoir. The pouch may be joined to the skin or to the urethra.

them are yet perfect. Preoperative radiation to the bowel rules them out.

The two problems that remain a challenge are how to prevent reflux up the ureters, and how to maintain continence. In the Kock pouch, reflux from the reservoir to the ureters is prevented by an ileal intussusceptum which forms a long nipple-like valve. Continence of urine is achieved by a second intussusceptum valve on the efferent limb of ileum.

In Camey's technique, reflux is prevented by a submucosal tunnel similar to the classical Leadbetter valve in ureterocolic anastomosis [56] (Fig. 20.20). Mitrofanoff [55,57] uses the appendix, where present, as a long narrow stoma, joining it to the skin or the urethra. At the umbilicus it is invisible [58]. Others use plicated ileum to provide continence [59].

None of these ingenious operations is without its dangers and difficulties. Even in experienced hands about 30% of the operations have to be revised several times before they are right.

The metabolic complication of hyperchloraemic acidosis was at first thought to be negligible. It is being seen with increasing frequency, for the same reason that it went unnoticed for so long after ureterosigmoidostomy. There is no reason to suppose that it will not become more common in future [60–66].

Calculi have been reported, as would seem inevitable, when metal staples have been used to form the antireflux nipples, e.g. in the Kock pouch, or when Marlex and similar non-absorbable material was used to keep the nipple in position [67].

When such a long length of terminal ileum is excluded from the gastrointestinal tract there is a theoretical possibility of vitamin B_{12} deficiency so that a regular haematological check should form part of the follow-up [68].

Whether these pouches will be prone to cancer remains a worrying question. It took 20 years of experience with ureterosigmoidostomy before the risk of colonic cancer came to light [69].

References

1 Crowley RT, Swigart LL (1960) Urinary diversion. *Am J Med Sci* 240: 232.
2 Simon J (1852) Ectropia vesicae. *Lancet* ii: 568.
3 Simon J (1855) Congenital imperfection of the urinary organs treated by operation. *Trans Path Soc Lond* 6: 256.
4 Lloyd J (1851) Ectrophia vesicae: absence of the anterior walls of the bladder. Operation: subsequent death. *Lancet* ii: 370.
5 Tresidder GC (1957) Nephrostomy. *Br J Urol* 29: 130.
6 Walsh A (1967) Ureterostomy *in situ*. *Br J Urol* 39: 744.
7 Hinman F, Weyrauch HM (1936) A critical study of the different principles of surgery which have been used in uretero-intestinal implantation. *Trans Am Assoc Genitourin Surg* 29: 15.
8 Weyrauch HM (1956) Landmarks in the development of ureterointestinal anastomosis. *Ann Roy Coll Surg Engl* 18: 343.
9 Leadbetter WF, Clarke BG (1955) Five years experience with ureteroenterostomy by the 'combined' technique. *J Urol* 73: 67.
10 Baird JS, Scott R, Spencer RD (1917) Studies on the transplantation of the ureters into the intestines. *Surg Gynecol Obstet* 24: 482.
11 Bollmann JL, Mann FC (1927) Nitrogenous constituents of blood following the transplantation of the ureters into different levels of the intestine. *Proc Soc Exper Biol Med* 24: 923.
12 Boyd JD (1931) Chronic acidosis secondary to ureteral implantation. *Am J Dis Child* 42: 367.
13 Jewett HJ (1944) Uretero-intestinal implantation in two stages for cancer of bladder: modification of original technique and report on 33 cases. *J Urol* 52: 536.
14 Ferris DO, Odel HM (1950) Electrolyte pattern of the blood after bilateral ureterosigmoidostomy. *J Am Med Assoc* 142: 634.
15 Stamey TA, Scott WW (1957) Ureteroileal anastomosis. *Surg Gynecol Obstet* 104: 11.
16 Hopewell J (1959) The hazards of uretero-intestinal anastomosis. *Ann Roy Coll Surg Engl* 24: 159.
17 Stöckle M, Becht E, Voges G, Riedmiller H,

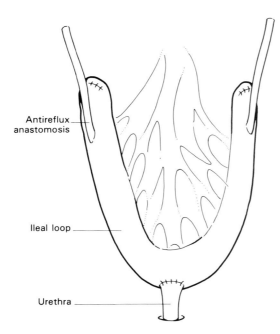

Fig. 20.20 Camey's operation. The ureters are anastomosed through a long submucosal tunnel to each end of the loop of ileum which is anastomosed to the stump of the urethra after cystectomy.

Antireflux anastomosis

Ileal loop

Urethra

Hohenfellner R (1990) Ureterosigmoidostomy: an outdated approach to bladder exstrophy? *J Urol* 143: 770.

18 Bricker EM (1950) Bladder substitution after pelvic evisceration. *Surg Clin N Am* 30: 1511.

19 Higgins PM, Hamilton RW, Hope-Stone HF (1966) The hazards of total cystectomy after supervoltage irradiation of the bladder. *Brit J Urol* 38: 311.

20 Wallace DM (1966) Ureteric diversion using a conduit: simplified technique. *Brit J Urol* 38: 522.

21 Turner-Warwick RT (1960) Colonic urinary conduits. *Proc Roy Soc Med* 53: 1032.

22 Mogg RA (1967) Urinary diversion using the colonic conduit. *Br J Urol* 39: 687.

23 Mauclaire M (1895) De quelques essais de chirurgie expérimentale applicables au traitement de l'exstrophie de la vessie et des anus contre nature complèxes. *Ann Mal Org Génitourin* 13: 1080.

24 Hayward RH, Wakim KG, ReMine WH, Grindlay JH (1961) An experimental study of the role of the colonic mucosa in hyperchloremic acidosis. *Surg Gynecol Obstet* 112: 357.

25 Pyrah LN (1960) Implantation of the ureters into an isolated rectosigmoid bladder. *Proc Roy Soc Med* 53: 1027.

26 Brunschwig A, Daniel W (1960) Pelvic exenteration operations with summary of 66 cases surviving more than 5 years. *Ann Surg* 151: 571.

27 Paull DP, Hodges CV (1955) The rectosigmoid colon as a bladder substitute. *J Urol* 74: 360.

28 Wallace DM (1961) Maydl's operation. *Proc Roy Soc Med* 54: 383.

29 Gersuny R (1898) *Wien Klin Wschr* 11: 990.

30 Heitz-Boyer M, Hovelacque A (1912) Création d'une nouvelle vessie et un nouvel urètre. *J Urol Néphrol* 1: 237.

31 Lowsley OS, Johnston TH, Rueda A (1953) A new operation for diversion of the urine with voluntary control of feces and urine. *J Int Coll Surg* 20: 457.

32 Johnson TH (1956) Further experiences with a new operation for urinary diversion. *J Urol* 76: 380.

33 Duhamel B (1957) Création d'une nouvelle vessie par exclusion du rectum et abaissement rétro-rectal et transanal du colon. *J Urol Nephrol* 63: 925.

34 Comte H, Bottou M, Ouradou J (1961) Onze cas de véssie rectale avec abaissement trans-sphincterien du sigmoide chez l'adulte et leurs résultats. *Mem Acad Chir* 87: 553.

35 Ghoneim MA, Ashamallah AK, Mahran MR, Kock NR (1992) Further experience with the modified rectal bladder (the augmented and valved rectum) for urine diversion. *J Urol* 147: 1252.

36 Verhoogen J, de Grauewe A (1909) La cystectomie totale. *Folia Urol* 3: 629.

37 Makkas M (1910) Zur Behandlung der Blasenektopie. Umwandlung des ausgeschalteten Coecum zur Blase und der Appendix zur Urethra. *Zentralbl Chir* 37: 1073.

38 Bricker EM, Eiseman B (1950) Bladder reconstruction from cecum and ascending colon following resection of pelvic viscera. *Ann Surg* 132: 77.

39 Gilchrist RK, Merricks JW, Hamlin HH, Rieger IT (1950) Construction of a substitute bladder and urethra. *Surg Gynecol Obstet* 90: 752.

40 Merricks JW, Gilchrist RK (1957) Follow-up on operation for urinary bladder reconstruction. *Arch*

Surg 74: 780.

41 Couvelaire R, Magder E, Auvert J, Moulonguet A, Pinaire J (1961) La place du greffon intestinal dans la traitement des tumeurs de la vessie. *J Urol Néphrol* 67: 441.

42 Fenwick EH (1911) *The Indications for Widely Resecting the Bladder Walls in Vesical Growth.* London: Adlard.

43 Tizzoni G, Foggi A (1888) Die Wiederherstellung der Harnblase: experimentelle Untersuchungen. *Zentralbl Chir* 15: 921.

44 Bohne AW, Osborne RW, Hettler PT (1955) Regeneration of the urinary bladder in the dog following total cystectomy. *Surg Gynecol Obstet* 100: 259.

45 Blandy JP (1961) Ileal pouch with transitional epithelium and anal sphincter as a continent urinary reservoir. *J Urol* 86: 749.

46 Bohne AW, Urwiller KL, Aarmento DF (1961) Vesicoureteral reflux. *J Urol* 86: 548.

47 Fenn N, Conn IG, German KA, Stephenson TP (1992) Complications of clam enterocystoplasty with particular reference to urinary tract infection. *Br J Urol* 69: 366.

48 George VK, Russell GL, Shutt A, Gaches CGC, Ashken MH (1991) Clam ileocystoplasty. *Br J Urol* 68: 487.

49 Kockelbergh RC, Tan JBL, Bates CP, Bishop MC, Dunn M, Lemberger RJ (1991) Clam enterocystoplasty in general urological practice. *Br J Urol* 68: 38.

50 Rosen MA, Light JK (1991) Spontaneous bladder rupture following augmentation enterocystoplasty. *J Urol* 146: 1232.

51 Skinner DG, Leiskovsky G, Boyd SD (1988) Continent urinary diversion. A five and a half year experience. *Ann Surg* 208: 377.

52 Goldwasser B, Barrett DM, Benson RC (1986) Bladder replacement with use of a detubularized right colonic segment: preliminary report of a new technique. *Mayo Clin Proc* 61: 615.

53 Thuroff JW, Alken P, Riedmiller H, Jacobi GH, Hohenfellner R (1988) One hundred cases of Mainz pouch: continuing experience and evolution. *J Urol* 140: 283.

54 Weidner W, Jarrar K, Rothauge CF (1988) Ileum-pouch-neobladder without stoma for urinary diversion after cystoprostatectomy. *Urology* 31: 107.

55 Mitrofanoff P, Bonnet O, Annoot MP, Bawab F, Grise P (1992) Continent urinary diversion using an artificial urinary sphincter. *Br J Urol* 70: 26.

56 Le Duc A, Camey M, Teillac P (1987) An original antireflux ureteroileal implantation technique: long term follow-up. *J Urol* 137: 1156.

57 Mitrofanoff P (1980) Cystostomie continente trans-appendiculaire dans le traitement des vessies neurologiques. *Chir Ped* 21: 297.

58 Monfort G, Guy JM, Morrisson-Lacombe G (1984) Appendicovesicostomy: an alternative urinary diversion in the child. *Eur Urol* 10: 361.

59 Woodhouse CRJ, Macneily AE (1994) The Mitrofanoff principle: expanding upon a versatile technique. *Br J Urol* 74: 447.

60 Duckett JW, Lotfi A-H (1993) Appendicovesicostomy (and variations) in bladder reconstruction. *J Urol* 149: 567.

61 Noble JR, Mata JA, Humble RL, Culkin DJ (1990) Maxi-pouch — a new technique for ileal conduit

conversion to continent urinary reservoir. *J Urol* 143: 116.

62 Mitchell ME (1990) Long prospects and problems of continent urinary diversions. *J Urol* 143: 370.

63 McDougal WS (1992) Metabolic complications of urinary intestinal diversion. *J Urol* 147: 1199.

64 Rowland RG, Rink RC (1994) Bladder augmentation and substitution cystoplasty, including continent diversion. *Curr Opinion Urol* 4: 205.

65 Akerlund S, Delin K, Kock NG, Lycke G, Philipson BM, Volkmann R (1989) Renal function and upper urinary tract configuration following urinary diversion to a continent ileal reservoir (Kock pouch): a prospective 5–11 year follow-up after reservoir construction. *J Urol* 142: 964.

66 Fisch M, Wammack R, Muller SC, Hohenfellner R (1993) The Mainz pouch II (sigma rectum pouch). *J Urol* 149: 258.

67 Ginsberg D, Huffman JL, Lieskovsky G, Boyd S, Skinner DG (1991) Urinary tract stones: a complication of the Kock pouch continent urinary diversion. *J Urol* 145: 956.

68 Steiner MS, Morton RA, Marshall FF (1993) Vitamin B_{12} deficiency in patients with ileocolic neo-bladders. *J Urol* 149: 255.

69 Nurse DE, McCrae P, Stephenson TP, Mundy AR (1988) The problems of substitution cystoplasty. *Br J Urol* 61: 423.

Chapter 21: Bladder — disorders of function

Many disorders of bladder function result from easily recognizable conditions like prostatic enlargement or urinary infection. Sometimes the underlying cause is less obvious and a neurological cause may be proven or suspected. In either case, the range of symptoms with which the patient can present are rather limited: they can be assigned to abnormalities in the two functions of the urinary bladder. Hesitancy, poor stream and inability to void to completion represent a failure of the bladder's emptying function while failure of urine storage gives urgency, frequency of micturition and incontinence.

Urodynamic investigations produce numerical results which have been the source material of a generation of urological dissertations leaving a literature disproportionate to the contribution of urodynamic studies to everyday urology. The enthusiasts emphasize the precision of a urodynamic diagnosis, highlighting the discrepancy between the symptoms which patients report and the actual abnormalities shown by the tests [1]. However, few patients will suffer at the hands of the minimalist who reserves urodynamic investigations for those in whom there is a genuine diagnostic doubt.

Urinary incontinence

The International Continence Society (ICS) has attempted to standardize the terminology used to describe bladder function and dysfunction [2]. Urinary incontinence is defined as 'a condition where involuntary loss of urine is a social or hygienic problem and is objectively demonstrable'. Extraurethral incontinence is loss of urine through a channel other than the urethra, e.g. vesicovaginal and ureterovaginal fistulae which are dealt with elsewhere (see p. 355).

Urinary incontinence is further subdivided into stress incontinence, urge incontinence and overflow incontinence. Reflex incontinence is due to abnormal reflex activity in the spinal cord without a sensation of urgency. Urodynamic studies are indicated when the type of incontinence is not clear on clinical grounds.

Frequency—volume recording

As a first step, it may help for the patients to keep a diary recording their urinary frequency, the volume passed and any episodes of incontinence. If possible, this should be related to fluid intake. By noting the precautions taken to avoid wetness, the diary can give a picture of the disability which the incontinence causes. Though frequency—volume charts are useful, it may take a good deal of time to explain what is needed and a well-motivated patient to get an accurate record. Diaries are particularly valuable to engage the interest of adolescents with nocturnal bedwetting. They are also a useful way to diagnose patients whose nocturia results from an inability to concentrate urine at night — a common finding in old age and early heart failure.

A small degree of stress incontinence is common in up to 50% of healthy women and many men report dribbling of urine after micturition. Most of these people do not require treatment and the urine output diary can help to identify those who do.

Pad testing

If a person is soaking one or more sanitary pads each day, they have significant incontinence which usually needs further investigation. The amount of urine loss can be assessed objectively by a pad test for which the patient is issued with a supply of plastic bags and enjoined to save all pads used over a period of days. The pads are then collected centrally for weighing. This type of investigation is burdensome for the patient and is rarely used outside of research studies.

Measurement of post-micturition residual urine

The post-micturition residual urine is the volume of urine which remains in the bladder when the person considers micturition to be complete. A residual urine is characteristically seen in established bladder outflow obstruction or when there is detrusor failure. The presence of a significant residual urine in the context of prostatic enlargement signals the imminence of complications of chronic urinary retention, including superadded acute retention. In spinal cord disease, e.g. multiple sclerosis, it may indicate functional outflow obstruction due to a failure of the normal coordination of sphincter opening and detrusor contraction during micturition (detrusor—sphincter dyssynergia). True detrusor failure is most often due to end-stage chronic retention but can also follow a lower motor neurone lesion to the S_2-S_4 parasympathetic outflow such as that which follows major surgery in the pelvis.

Urethral catheterization provides an indisputable measure of the residual urine volume but the risk of introducing infection precludes it unless a catheter is to be passed for some other reason. Transabdominal ultrasound will provide an image of the bladder and a reasonable approximation of the residual volume can be calculated from measurements taken from the scan.

The residual volume can vary between voids and the accuracy of the estimate depends upon the mathematical formula used to calculate it. However, most would accept a residual of 100 ml as abnormal after voiding, especially if the same result was recorded on more than one occasion.

Urine flow rate

The rate of urine flow depends upon the expulsive force developed by the detrusor and the outflow resistance during micturition. Both factors can be affected by psychological factors and flow rate measurements on a voided volume of less than about 150 ml are unreliable [3]. A uroflow measurement will usually give a graphic

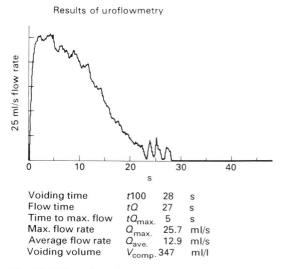

Results of uroflowmetry

Voiding time	$t100$	28	s
Flow time	tQ	27	s
Time to max. flow	$tQ_{max.}$	5	s
Max. flow rate	$Q_{max.}$	25.7	ml/s
Average flow rate	$Q_{ave.}$	12.9	ml/s
Voiding volume	$V_{comp.}$	347	ml/l

Fig. 21.1 Normal uroflow measurement.

read-out which presents the pattern of flow, its maximum ($Q_{max.}$) and average ($Q_{ave.}$) rate as well as the total volume of urine passed ($V_{comp.}$) (Fig. 21.1). A single flow measurement should be treated with caution but most normal men should be able to produce a maximum peak flow of 15 ml/s or more. A maximum flow of less than 10 ml/s is usually taken as unequivocally abnormal. A normal flow rises to a peak which is sustained for most of the void. Infravesical obstruction produces a flattened curve (Fig. 21.2) which is said to have a box shape when the obstruction is caused by urethral stricture. Obstructed voiding due to failure of sphincter relaxation typically gives a pattern of intermittent flow (Fig. 21.3). This picture is seen in the detrusor—sphincter dyssynergia of neurological

Fig. 21.2 The flattened curve of infravesical obstruction (a) with prostatic hyperplasia. (b) with a urethral stricture.

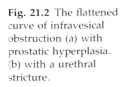

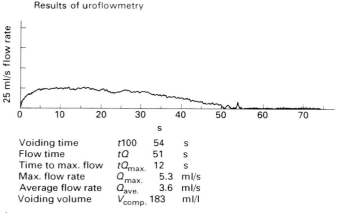

Results of uroflowmetry

Voiding time	$t100$	54	s
Flow time	tQ	51	s
Time to max. flow	$tQ_{max.}$	12	s
Max. flow rate	$Q_{max.}$	5.3	ml/s
Average flow rate	$Q_{ave.}$	3.6	ml/s
Voiding volume	$V_{comp.}$	183	ml/l

(a)

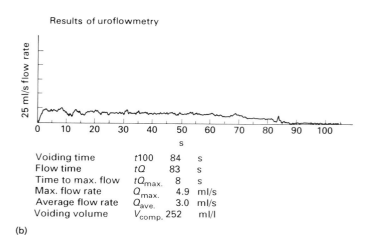

Results of uroflowmetry

Voiding time	$t100$	84	s
Flow time	tQ	83	s
Time to max. flow	$tQ_{max.}$	8	s
Max. flow rate	$Q_{max.}$	4.9	ml/s
Average flow rate	$Q_{ave.}$	3.0	ml/s
Voiding volume	$V_{comp.}$	252	ml/l

(b)

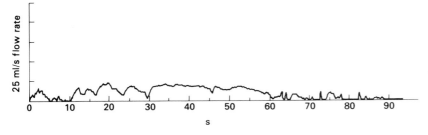

Results of uroflowmetry

Voiding time	$t100$	88	s
Flow time	tQ	72	s
Time to max. flow	$tQ_{max.}$	19	s
Max. flow rate	$Q_{max.}$	9.4	ml/s
Average flow rate	$Q_{ave.}$	4.9	ml/s
Voiding volume	$V_{comp.}$	354	ml/l

Fig. 21.3 Obstructed voiding caused by failure of sphincter relaxation: note the intermittent flow.

disease as well as the rather less well-explained failure of voluntary relaxation of the external sphincter which afflicts some men especially when they attempt to void in public places.

The urine flow rate is normally greater in women who may be able to generate maximum rates in excess of 25 ml/s. Flow rate measurement is less commonly performed in women. It is reduced when there is a true urethral stenosis. In some women, obstructed voiding is associated with abnormal electromyographic activity in the urethral rhabdosphincter and may be seen with a syndrome of urgency and urinary frequency [4].

Filling cystometry

Compliance is the change in intravesical pressure which occurs with a given change in volume (ml/cmH$_2$O). There is very little increase in the pressure within the normal bladder as it fills, i.e. compliance is very high. There is a cessation of detrusor activity possibly mediated in part by the sympathetic nervous system. At some point which depends upon the filling rate, the subject becomes aware of a sensation from the bladder. This first sensation is succeeded by an urge to void which can be suppressed even though it is associated with a transient rise in intravesical pressure. Further bladder filling is uncomfortable.

The technique of filling cystometry varies but the principle is simple. A catheter is used to fill the bladder while intravesical pressure is measured by means of a second catheter. A pressure line in the rectum measures variations in intra-abdominal pressure which are electronically subtracted from the intravesical pressure to give a graphic read-out of the so-called detrusor pressure (Fig. 21.4). The patient voids

before the procedure. There is dispute as to whether the residual urine should be drained and measured at this stage but most prefer to fill on top of the residual urine. Formerly in some centres, carbon dioxide gas was used to fill the bladder: although this was quicker, it was considered less physiological than sterile water or radioopaque contrast medium.

During the filling study the patient is asked to report sensations from the bladder. The volume at which the first sensation is felt and that when there is an urge to void are taken as important measures of bladder sensation. The pressure trace is scanned to detect rises in pressure which reflect abnormal detrusor contractions. The onset of these contractions may be affected by the rate of filling and the temperature of the filling fluid, and patients may be asked to perform other manoeuvres, e.g. to cough or to change position, in order to provoke them. If they occur, the patient is asked to attempt to suppress them, and a note is made as to whether this is possible.

Abnormalities of the filling cystometrogram

Sensory frequency

Even if patients are carefully selected for filling cystometrography because they have unexplained urgency and frequency with or without incontinence, the detrusor pressure trace is often normal, with an end filling pressure of less than 15 cmH$_2$O and no abnormal detrusor contractions. A proportion of these patients report their first sensation and urge to void at a smaller filling volume than would be expected: they are labelled as suffering from 'sensory urgency'. Since this may be the result of intravesical pathology, a cysto-

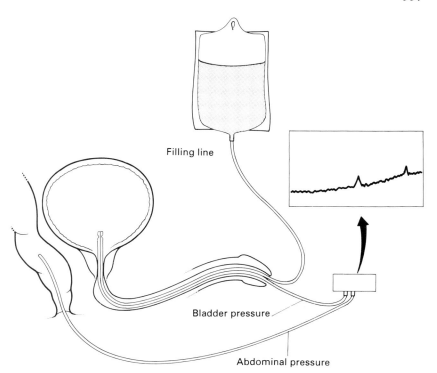

Fig. 21.4 Cystometry. Intra-abdominal pressure is measured in the rectum and is subtracted from the pressure measured in the bladder to give the detrusor pressure.

scopy is always indicated. If there is no bladder lesion, the term might be taken to imply a hypersensitivity of the bladder, but no adequate explanation of the pathophysiology of this condition has ever been offered.

Detrusor instability and detrusor hyperreflexia

Uninhibited detrusor contractions cannot be suppressed and give rise to detrusor pressures of over 15 cmH$_2$O (Fig. 21.5). They are said to demonstrate 'detrusor instability' when the patient cannot be found to have any neurological disease: when there is neurological disease they are said to show 'detrusor hyperreflexia' [2]. If the urethral sphincter cannot cope with the high intravesical pressure, which may exceed 80 cmH$_2$O, the patient will be wet.

Poor detrusor compliance

Sometimes the detrusor pressure shows a steady rise during filling to reach an end filling pressure greater than 15 cmH$_2$O (Fig. 21.6). This may be due to the 'small bladder syndrome' from fibrosis after radiotherapy or extensive bladder surgery. On other occasions, it is seen against a background of neurological disease, especially of the lower segments of the spinal cord. It is then more difficult to explain other than by failure of the normal bladder compliance mechanism which is thought to be neurally mediated.

Voiding pressure studies

In a very few patients it is impossible to tell whether they have obstruction from a measurement of flow rate and post-micturition residual volume. In these patients it may be useful to measure the detrusor pressure as the patient voids. In men, the upper limit of normal voiding pressure is 60 cmH$_2$O and in women it is 40 cmH$_2$O. In those with outflow obstruction the voiding pressure may be as high as 80 cmH$_2$O and may or may not be associated with a low flow [5]. There is a tendency for the urethral pressure line to be expelled during voiding and in order to get a true measurement it may be necessary to insert a line through a suprapubic needle.

Videocystometry

If X-ray fluoroscopic equipment is available, important anatomical information can be obtained by using water-soluble X-ray contrast medium to fill the bladder. This will demonstrate the saccules, the thickened bladder wall, and the 'fir-tree' appearance of the high pressure neuropathic

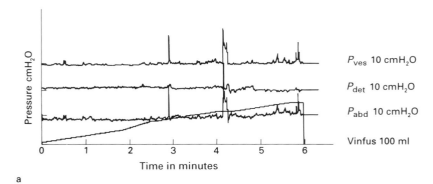

P_ves 10 cmH₂O
P_det 10 cmH₂O
P_abd 10 cmH₂O
Vinfus 100 ml

Time in minutes

a

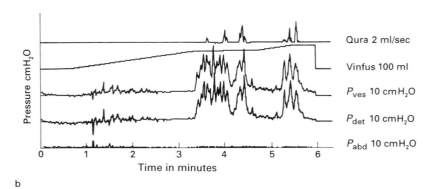

Qura 2 ml/sec
Vinfus 100 ml
P_ves 10 cmH₂O
P_det 10 cmH₂O
P_abd 10 cmH₂O

Time in minutes

b

Fig. 21.5 Filling cystometrogram. (a) Normal: spikes of intra-abdominal pressure occur during coughing. (b) Uninhibited detrusor contractions cause a rise in detrusor pressure which cannot be suppressed.

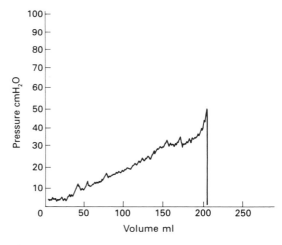

Fig. 21.6 Filling cystometrogram: poorly compliant detrusor.

bladder (Fig. 21.7). In stress incontinence, weakness of the supportive tissues around the bladder neck will be evident by descent of the pelvic floor during coughing while at the same time the contrast may enter the urethra to give 'beaking' (Fig. 21.8) or frank incontinence.

Uroflow, filling and voiding cystometry, with or without video, along with measurement of the post-micturition residual urine volume are

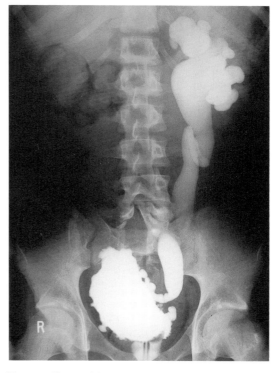

Fig. 21.7 Fir tree bladder with reflux on the left side.

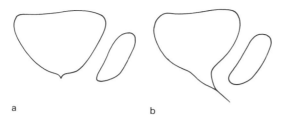

Fig. 21.8 Tracing of cystogram showing 'beaking'.

the elements of a standard urodynamic study. Other investigations including urethral pressure profilometry and the fluid bridge test for stress incontinence are research tools which are insufficiently standardized for general use. Improvements in ultrasound technology mean that the urethra can now be scanned during voiding, and 'dynamic ultrasonography' can give similar information to fluoroscopy without exposure to ionizing radiation [6].

Neural control of bladder function

The neurobiology of human continence is complex and poorly understood [7]. The interleaved fibres of bladder smooth muscle encircle the bladder neck in males. This is the so-called internal sphincter or bladder neck mechanism, which is well supplied with sympathetic nerve endings (see p. 251). It is often sufficient to maintain continence if the external sphincter mechanism has been destroyed, but its role in the maintenance of normal continence is uncertain. The bladder neck contracts during seminal emission and damage to the pelvic sympathetic nervous system leads to retrograde ejaculation. In women, the internal sphincter is much less easily demonstrable [8] and continence does not depend upon a competent bladder neck [9].

The intramural external sphincter is composed of striated muscle fibres which lie within the urethral wall. This muscle extends for approximately 2 cm distal to the prostate in a man and is anatomically separate from the muscle of the pelvic floor through which this part of the membranous urethra passes (see p. 251). In women almost the whole of the urethra has striated sphincter muscle within its wall (see p. 252). The striated muscle of the external sphincter (also known as the rhabdosphincter) is made up of type 1, slow-twitch fibres and has remarkable electrophysiological properties [8]. Unlike skeletal muscle, which is electrically silent at rest, an electromyogram (EMG) of the urethral sphincter muscle has a steady background of tonic activity which persists even during sleep and light anaesthesia. This reflects the function of the muscle which is to keep the pressure within the urethra above the intravesical pressure while the bladder is filling. When the intravesical pressure rises during coughing and sneezing, there is a reflex contraction of the external sphincter with an increase in EMG activity. The EMG becomes silent as the sphincter relaxes before the onset of the detrusor contraction as micturition starts. When voiding has finished the detrusor stops contracting and sphincter tone returns.

Both the detrusor and the intramural external urethral sphincter are innervated by parasympathetic nerves whose cell bodies are in segments S2—S4 of the spinal cord, in the conus which lies approximately at the level of the L1 vertebra. Preganglionic fibres destined to synapse in ganglia near or in the bladder wall go in the cauda equina to exit through the appropriate sacral foramina. They then follow the pelvic nerves, an ill-defined nervous plexus which courses over the pelvic viscera and the side wall of the pelvis to reach the vesical plexus. Here the parasympathetic (excitatory) neurones synapse with each other and with postganglionic fibres, and probably make connections with adrenergic (probably inhibitory) fibres which have come with the hypogastric plexus from T11—L2 segments of the spinal cord. The integration of the autonomic nervous system at this level is still a matter for speculation, as is the role of the 'non-adrenergic non-cholinergic' (NANC) neuropeptides such as gamma-aminobutyric acid (GABA) and vasoactive intestinal peptide (VIP) which can be demonstrated especially in the region of the bladder neck [10].

Bladder sensation is mediated by bare endings in the suburothelial nervous plexus. They send afferent fibres which join the spinal cord via the pelvic, pudendal and hypogastric nerves. Urethral sensation seems to travel mainly via the pudendal nerve along with proprioceptive input from the pelvic floor [11].

Control of micturition

Normal micturition depends upon an orderly sequence of striated muscle relaxation, sustained detrusor smooth muscle contraction and sphincter contraction. The neural mechanisms which control this sequence have been extensively investigated in experimental animals but much remains obscure. Two levels of central nervous system (CNS) integration are recognized. Onuf's nucleus is a collection of cell bodies in the lower spinal cord, and there is a switching centre in the pons. It appears that the complex act of micturition is mediated by supraspinal reflexes which pass through the pontine centre (Fig. 21.9). This long reflex arc is very vulnerable to interruption during its course up and down the length of the spinal cord [12]. This explains the frequency of bladder dysfunction when the cord is damaged by direct trauma or by multiple sclerosis. The role of segmental reflexes is uncertain: they seem to become prominent when the supraspinal reflexes become inoperative and they may mediate detrusor hyperreflexia [12].

Neurophysiological investigations

The peripheral nerve fibres which control bladder function are non-myelinated and take an ill-defined course deep within the pelvis. This makes

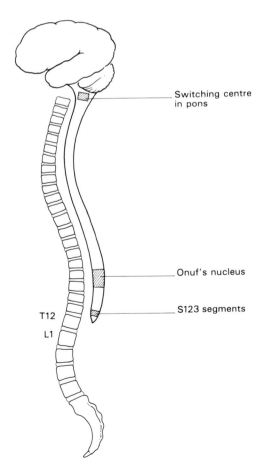

Fig. 21.9 Diagram of the reflex pathways of the bladder.

Switching centre in pons

Onuf's nucleus

S123 segments

T12

L1

them difficult to study by conventional neurophysiological methods which measure the velocity of propagation of action potentials in myelinated nerves. Researchers have used various strategies to circumvent this difficulty, but their data have proved complex to obtain or to interpret [13].

External sphincter EMG

Many of the machines used to record the pressure traces for cystometrography have a channel which can be used to sample EMG recorded from surface electrodes placed on the skin of the perineum. In practice, such recordings are rarely made because the circumstances of cystometrography are inappropriate for EMG recording which requires relaxation of the patient and electrical silence. The signal obtained is liable to be contaminated with input from skeletal muscles other than those of the pelvic floor and sphincter.

A more precise but more technically demanding method is to use a concentric needle electrode to sample the activity in the intramural external sphincter muscle. With care and skill, the needle can be introduced from the perineum in a man or the anterior vaginal wall in a woman. The sphincter muscle is located by monitoring the audio signal obtained from the electrode tip, which gives a characteristic fast clicking sound when the needle is in the sphincter. This clicking represents the tonic electrical activity in muscle motor units in the sphincter. It increases as additional units are recruited when the patient strains.

The electrical activity of individual motor units in the sphincter can be captured electronically so that they can be analysed. If the nerves supplying the muscle have been damaged, each surviving nerve sprouts additional axons to reinnervate more deprived muscle fibres than before and so the EMG of reinnervated striated muscle has a characteristic complexity (Fig. 21.10).

In addition to being used to detect sphincter reinnervation, concentric needle EMG can also be used to detect grossly abnormal discharges within the muscle which appear to be associated with a failure of sphincter relaxation [14].

Bulbocavernosus reflex

The bulbocavernosus reflex is the contraction of the bulbocavernosus muscle which occurs when a stimulus is applied to the penis or the clitoris. Measurement of the latency of this response (the

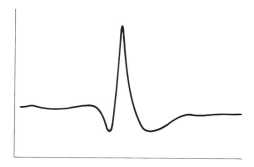

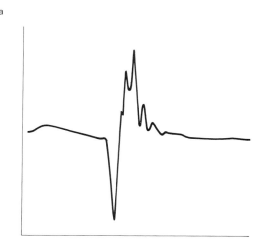

Fig. 21.10 (a) The normal EMG compared with that of reinnervated muscle (b).

delay between the application of the stimulus and the contraction of the muscle) is one of a number of methods which have been used to quantify 'sacral evoked responses' [15]. The average reflex latency of around 35 ms is said to be increased in lower motor neurone disorders but there is considerable overlap between normal and abnormal. The technique has the merit of being easy to perform but assessment of a reflex mediated by myelinated fibres can have only indirect relevance to the investigation of disorders of innervation by the autonomic nervous system.

Stress incontinence

Patients with stress incontinence complain of urinary leakage when intra-abdominal pressure rises: so-called 'giggle incontinence' affects young girls, but the patient is more commonly a parous middle-aged woman with urinary loss on coughing, sneezing or abdominal straining. This may be due to isolated weakness of the external

sphincter itself, though this is difficult to measure directly and difficult to correct.

More commonly there is lack of support for the whole bladder neck region. This is easier to demonstrate clinically, and treatments for stress incontinence aim to increase support for the bladder neck. In parous females, stress incontinence is thought to be due to neuromuscular damage to the pelvic floor during childbirth though the precise mechanism is in dispute: some consider that traumatic denervation of the sphincter itself is the important element; others think that damage to the fibroconnective tissue which supports the bladder neck is the primary abnormality [16].

Incontinence occasionally occurs soon after delivery but more often there is a delay until the birth injury is compounded by the decrease in overall muscular strength which occurs with ageing. Stress incontinence in men is much less common and is almost always associated with known injury to the sphincter (typically after transurethral resection of the prostate) or its nerve supply. Isolated sphincter damage is less common in women, but may follow urethrotomy, operation for a urethral diverticulum or a failed sling operation for stress incontinence. Indeed, repeated operations for stress incontinence can lead to gross scarring of the urethra which may be indistinguishable from the 'drain-pipe urethra' occasionally seen after radical surgery and radiotherapy for carcinoma of the cervix.

Investigations

The first step is to establish that there is leakage during abdominal straining. In most but not all cases, there will be a demonstrable gush of urine from the urethra when the woman coughs or strains — a positive 'stress test'. In some women the history of stress incontinence is clear, but in others symptoms suggesting urgency or urinary frequency confuse the picture. Indeed, the smooth muscle contractions which characterize detrusor instability may be precipitated by coughing or changes in posture, making it impossible to be sure of the diagnosis from the symptoms alone.

Because the treatment of stress incontinence and urge incontinence are quite different, it is very important to distinguish between the two. In stress incontinence there is an incomplete urethral closure mechanism which the ICS define as one which allows leakage in the absence of detrusor contraction [2]. Under these circumstances leakage (genuine stress incontinence) may occur whenever intravesical pressure exceeds intraurethral pressure. This implies that a cystometrogram is necessary to rule out the presence of unstable bladder contractions before a diagnosis of genuine stress incontinence can be made. A videocystometrogram will also demonstrate the radiographic signs of stress incontinence, i.e. bladder neck descent, 'beaking' and leakage of contrast medium during coughing or abdominal straining. An alternative is to use dynamic ultrasound to demonstrate the abnormality of the bladder neck.

Treatment

Patients with stress incontinence are often overweight and it is usual to urge them to reduce. This may be enough to cure very mild leakage and it will certainly make the patient a better operative risk but usually the attempt at dieting fails and serves only to delay definitive treatment.

Pelvic floor exercises are designed to strengthen the muscles of the pelvic floor. The patient is taught to contract the appropriate pelvic muscles and given a programme of regular exercise to improve their strength. Various aids are available to instruct and motivate the patient: electrical stimulation may help to identify the correct muscles to contract, and practice keeping weighed cones in the vagina against gravity may give a sense of progress and achievement. Pelvic floor exercises certainly have a place in the management of men who suffer stress incontinence after transurethral resection of the prostate, which is often transitory, and if nothing else the exercises help to sustain morale while spontaneous improvement occurs. It has been claimed that up to 70% of women with stress incontinence can be improved by pelvic floor exercises [17]. However, such results are only possible with great commitment on the part of the patient and the therapist.

Surgery

Where there is a significant degree of urethrocele accompanying a mild degree of stress incontinence, it is sensible to consider referral to a gynaecologist for an anterior vaginal (Manchester) repair because this may be sufficient to cure the leakage (Fig. 21.11). In most women, however, the urologist will aim to increase bladder neck support and at the same time decrease bladder neck and urethral mobility. An artificial urethral sphincter may be considered in men with incontinence that is established to be due to sphincter weakness, and perhaps in a few women who remain incontinent after successful surgery to support the bladder neck.

Operations to support the bladder neck

There are a number of operations which broadly aim to support the bladder neck and to prevent its descent during abdominal straining. A super-

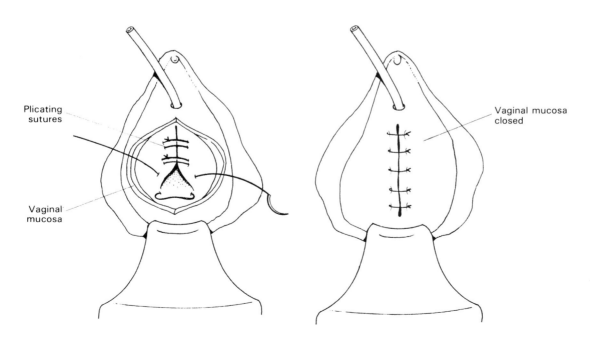

Plicating sutures

Vaginal mucosa

Vaginal mucosa closed

Fig. 21.11 Principles of anterior colporrhaphy.

ficially attractive approach is to pass a non-absorbable tape as a sling behind the bladder neck and to anchor its ends to the anterior abdominal wall or pectineal ligament. Unfortunately, this sling has a tendency to work its way through the part of the urinary tract which it is intended to support, and the method ought to be abandoned. Millin's sling procedure makes ingenious use of the rectus fascia, and may have a place when all else has failed. For most women a colposuspension, an operation which makes use of the anterior vaginal wall as a hammock to support the bladder neck, is the operation of choice.

Anterior colposuspension

The principle of colposuspension is best demonstrated by the Birch operation. After a mandatory cystoscopy to rule out intravesical pathology — including non-absorbable material from previous misguided sling operations — a urethral catheter is inserted. The retropubic space is exposed through a Pfannenstiel or lower midline incision.

Unless there is much scarring from previous surgery, the connective tissue on either side of the bladder neck can be swept laterally by gentle blunt dissection (Fig. 21.12). A few friable veins may need to be diathermied but bleeding is seldom a problem. As the space on either side of the bladder neck is developed posteriorly,

the anterior vaginal wall comes into view as a pinkish-white fibromuscular structure in the depths of the wound. If an assistant flexes two fingers anteriorly within the vagina they can be palpated on either side of the catheter balloon (Fig. 21.13).

The connective tissue is carefully cleaned until enough of the anterior vaginal wall comes into view to place the stitches used in the repair. The assistant's fingers in the vagina provide a guide for a series of interrupted absorbable sutures placed deeply into vaginal tissue. The sutures are taken through a suitable piece of the pectineal fascia on the back of the pubis (Fig. 21.14). The assistant lifts the anterior vaginal wall towards the pubis to help in siting these fascial sutures and to allow them to be tied without tension or bow-stringing (Fig. 21.15). Two or three sutures on either side of the bladder neck are enough to secure the ends of the vaginal hammock and to excite the fibrous reaction which is probably essential to the longer term success of the repair. The wound is closed in the usual way with or without a tube to drain the retropubic space created by the dissection. Postoperatively, it is usual to leave the urethral catheter for 1 week.

In the past, the patient was encouraged to

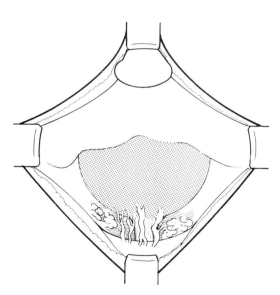

Fig. 21.12 Anterior colposuspension. Through a Pfannenstiel incision the connective tissue and fat on either side of the bladder neck is swept laterally by gentle blunt dissection.

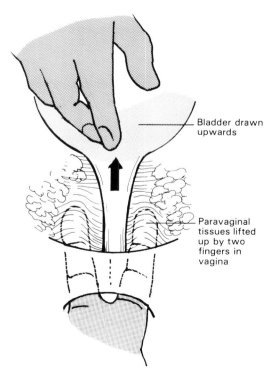

Bladder drawn upwards

Paravaginal tissues lifted up by two fingers in vagina

Fig. 21.13 Two fingers of the assistant lift up the vaginal wall.

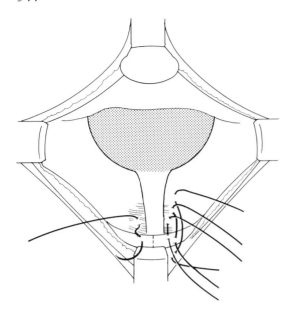

Fig. 21.14 Strong absorbable sutures are placed between the vaginal wall and the pectineus fascia behind the pubis.

remain in bed for the first few days after the operation. A change in surgical philosophy, and the need to maximize the use of hospital beds, has led to earlier mobilization with no proven ill effect on the results of colposuspension.

Endoscopic bladder neck suspension

This term is used here to encompass a range of eponymous procedures (Stamey, Raz, Peyrera) whose common aim is to reproduce the effect of a Birch anterior colposuspension without the need for open surgery. The ends of the anterior vaginal wall hammock are supported by long non-absorbable sutures which run from the vaginal walls to the rectus sheath. In the method described by Stamey, the sutures were placed using specially designed long needles passed from the vagina to the anterior abdominal wall. The ends of the suture were buttressed like tension sutures to prevent them cutting out. These buttresses had to be buried in the vaginal wall, and had a tendency to become infected and cause abscesses and troublesome discharge.

Stamey's imitators have used similar needles but have tended to simplify the procedure by omitting the buttresses. What follows is the author's version which illustrates the principles and has the advantage of being extremely simple to perform (Fig. 21.16). A urethral catheter is inserted after cystoscopy. A 0.5 cm stab incision is made in the midline just above the pubis. A Stamey needle is inserted through the puncture, pulled to one side, and passed through the anterior rectus sheath about 1 cm to one side of the midline. The needle is then passed along the back of the pubis aiming at the operator's finger in the vagina, and well to the side of the urethral catheter. When the tip of the needle is felt, the finger is withdrawn, and the needle pushed through the anterior wall of the vagina. It is

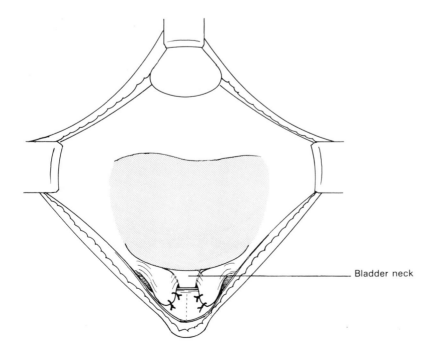

Bladder neck

Fig. 21.15 The sutures are tied, forming a vaginal hammock for the bladder neck.

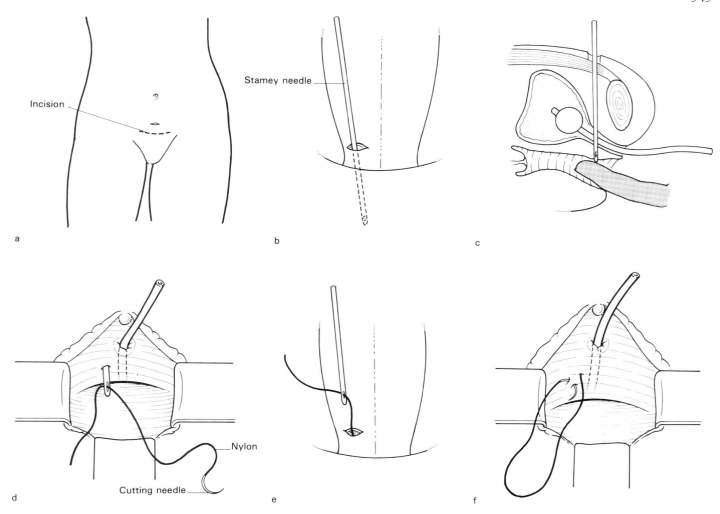

Fig. 21.16 Endoscopic bladder neck suspension. (a–c) The Stamey needle is inserted through a 5 mm skin puncture, pulled laterally and passed close to the back of the pubis to the finger placed in the vagina; (d & e) the needle is threaded with a nylon suture. (f) Two bites are taken through the vaginal wall.

threaded with the free end of a strong monofilament nylon suture on a curved cutting needle.

The Stamey needle is withdrawn and the nylon is pulled out of the puncture wound. The anterior vaginal wall is then exposed with a retractor, and two or three turns are taken through its full thickness with the cutting needle, which is then cut off. The Stamey needle is passed down again about 1 cm lateral to the first pass: the nylon is threaded again into the eye of the Stamey needle and drawn up through the puncture (Fig. 21.17). The same procedure is repeated on the other side.

At this stage, it is important to re-examine the bladder to check that the sutures have not transfixed it. In this event — which is not uncommon — they must be removed and replaced: this does not cause long-term effects and is preferable to injury to the inguinal vessels which may occur if the needles are passed too far laterally. The operation is completed by tying the ends of the nylon sutures where they emerge through the abdominal stab incision. It is somewhat difficult to judge how tightly they should be tied, but it is reassuring to know that it does not seem to be essential to know the precise tension. One should aim to prevent the bladder neck from descending during straining rather than to pull it up at rest.

A 'stab' suprapubic catheter allows progress towards normal voiding to be monitored postoperatively. The suprapubic catheter is clamped after a day or two and removed if voiding occurs. If the sutures have been tied too tightly it may be necessary to leave the catheter in place for a time. Very occasionally, it may be necessary to dilate the urethra if resumption of voiding is unduly delayed.

Millin's sling

The initial stages of Millin's operation resemble those of an anterior colposuspension, but a

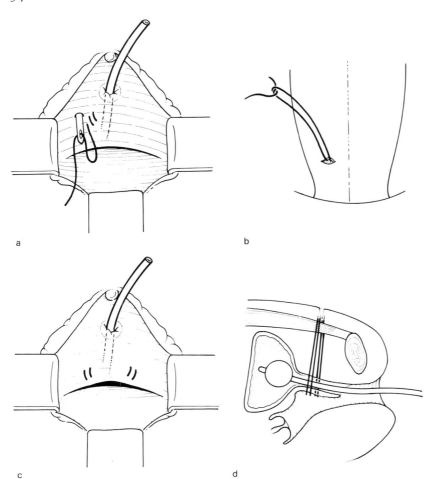

a

b

c

d

Fig. 21.17 (a−c) The Stamey needle is passed again, emerging 1 cm to the side of the first track, grasps the nylon, and withdraws it. The same procedure is repeated on the other side. (d) After checking with the cystoscope that the sutures have not passed through the bladder, the sutures are tied. A suprapubic catheter is left *in situ*.

Pfannenstiel incision is essential. The space on either side of the bladder neck is developed and the dissection continued in the plane between urethra and anterior vaginal wall so that a suitable curved instrument can be passed posterior to the bladder neck (Fig. 21.18). The sling is fashioned by cutting a strip of anterior rectus sheath parallel to the Pfannenstiel incision (Fig. 21.19). This strip of fascia remains attached at one end, the other end being taken through the rectus muscle and behind the bladder neck (Fig. 21.20). The free end of the fascial strip is sutured to the pectineus fascia on the back of the pubis with absorbable sutures (Fig. 21.21). The wound is drained and closed in the usual way.

Choice of operation

The choice of operation for stress incontinence is controversial. Formal anterior colposuspension seems to give better long-term results in most hands. Up to 60% of patients will be cured in the medium term by an endoscopic bladder neck

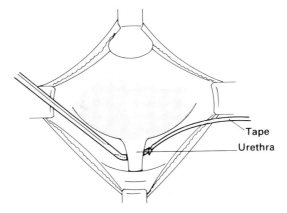

Tape

Urethra

Fig. 21.18 A right angled forceps is passed behind the bladder neck.

suspension which leaves little or no scarring and requires a shorter hospital stay. Unless the longer term results of Stamey-type procedures are shown to be very much worse it seems reasonable to offer this in the first instance, to perform an

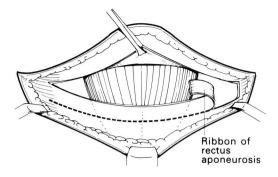

Fig. 21.19 A ribbon of fascia is taken from the rectus aponeurosis.

Ribbon of
rectus
aponeurosis

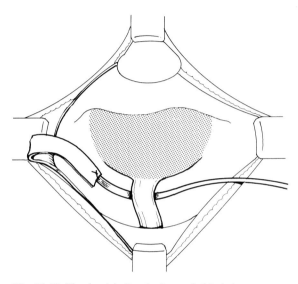

Fig. 21.20 The fascial sling is drawn behind the bladder neck.

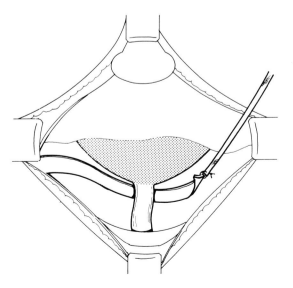

Fig. 21.21 The free end of the sling is sutured to the pectineal fascia behind the pubis.

anterior colposuspension for those in whom this fails, and to keep the Millin sling in reserve [18].

Artificial urethral sphincter

The indications for an artificial urethral sphincter are limited and most urologists will never implant one. Given the present state of technology it is probably right that these operations are performed in specialized centres which can accumulate the necessary experience and constantly audit their results.

In essence, an artificial sphincter may be considered for a patient with sphincter weakness incontinence which can be managed in no other way. Bladder instability is not by itself a contra-indication but may need surgical treatment in its own right [19].

Post-prostatectomy incontinence is more common in those who have pre-existing detrusor instability. Even when there is evidence of significant sphincter weakness, continence may recover spontaneously up to a year after surgery. Many patients can be managed by an external collecting device, and for elderly or infirm patients this may be the best option. An artificial sphincter may be offered to men who are fit for surgery but disabled by continuing sphincter weakness incontinence. In women the most common indication is failure of all other treatments for stress incontinence.

There are several artificial urethral sphincters of which only the Brantley—Scott device has stood the test of time: the Kaufman and Rosen devices are now redundant. The implantation of a Brantley—Scott sphincter, while simple in concept, requires meticulous attention to detail, and the reader is referred elsewhere for a full description [19].

The sphincter will only be implanted after full urodynamic assessment and cystourethroscopy. The artificial sphincter works by applying occlusive pressure with a fluid-filled cuff encircling a convenient part of the bladder outflow. This may be the bladder neck or in men, the bulbar urethra. Pressure in the cuff and urethral occlusion is maintained by fluid from a pressure-regulating inflation balloon. To open the sphincter for voiding, the cuff is deflated by a manually operated pump which transfers fluid from the cuff to the balloon (Fig. 21.22). The pump is implanted in the scrotum or labium majus. Refilling of the cuff and reapplication of occlusive pressure to the urethra occurs spontaneously by slow flow of fluid from the reservoir balloon.

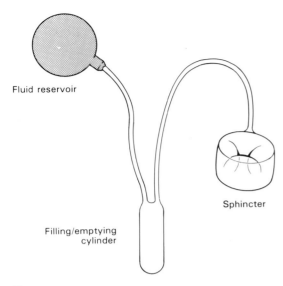

Fig. 21.22 Brantley—Scott incontinence device.

For a well-selected individual an artificial sphincter may be the only chance for continence, and this should not be denied. However, even in the most experienced hands there may be complications from failure of the device, infection and erosion, particularly when there has been urethral damage caused by previous unsuccessful surgery.

Urge incontinence

The ICS defines urge incontinence as the involuntary loss of urine associated with a strong desire to void. Urgency occurs when there is overactivity of the detrusor (motor urgency) or hypersensitivity of the bladder (sensory urgency). It is not always associated with incontinence.

Motor urgency

Motor urgency is associated with unstable contractions of the detrusor which can be demonstrated while the patient is attempting to inhibit micturition during the filling phase of the cystometrogram. As we have seen, this type of instability may result from an interruption of the supraspinal reflexes which control bladder function — the detrusor is 'hyperreflexic'. More often, the instability has no obvious neurological cause, but may in some cases be associated with bladder outflow obstruction. The detrusor instability responsible for urgency in patients with prostatic disease is indistinguishable from hyperreflexia. Clinical examination and pressure—flow studies may be needed to make a diagnosis.

Sensory urgency

A diagnosis of sensory urgency will be made if there is urgency without detrusor instability. The patient may report the first sensation at a smaller filling volume than normal, and the maximum volume to which the bladder can be comfortably filled may be smaller. Cystoscopy is essential to rule out an intravesical cause such as infection, interstitial cystitis or carcinoma — especially carcinoma *in situ*. In a few cases there appears to be a heightened awareness of sensation from the bladder without any obvious structural or functional cause. The mechanism by which this occurs is obscure and it may represent one extreme of the range of normal bladder awareness. Such patients may be difficult to treat in a logical way: empirical therapy is the norm.

Some women with sensory urgency respond, at least temporarily, to urethral dilatation and may be labelled as suffering from the 'urethral syndrome': others may benefit from a regime of bladder drill to 'retrain' the bladder: still others seem to benefit from long-term low dose antibiotics. Whether any of these treatments do anything other than allow time for spontaneous improvement is uncertain.

Treatment

It will usually be clear from the cystometrogram whether there is motor or sensory frequency. If there is motor frequency, i.e. there are unstable contractions during the filling phase, the next step is to look for a cause.

Urgency, urge incontinence and bladder outflow obstruction

In men past middle age, bladder outflow obstruction due to prostatic enlargement is the most common culprit. If the flow rate is normal, it may be necessary to do pressure—flow studies to confirm the diagnosis. A high pressure (over $40\,cmH_2O$) with low flow indicates obstruction. Removing the obstruction by means of prostatectomy will cure the instability in some patients, but the results are often delayed and disappointing.

An association between functional voiding obstruction and detrusor instability has also been described in women but its prevalence is yet to be determined.

When there is no bladder outflow obstruction, the next step is to distinguish those with a definable neurological cause (i.e. detrusor hyperreflexia) from the much larger number with idiopathic detrusor instability. In practice, urological symptoms are rarely the first manifestation of neurological disease other than multiple system atrophy, and in most cases the underlying neurological defect is all too evident.

Bladder drill

Disabled patients may be incontinent because they are too immobile to respond effectively to their urinary urgency. Detrusor instability is often related to bladder volume and a regime of frequent toiletting may be enough to prevent wetness. Others may simply need to have a commode or toilet made more easily available. Behavioural training can also help, though it would be overoptimistic to expect the 90% success rate claimed by some of its advocates. The patient is taught mental strategies to delay micturition in the hope that this will 'retrain' the bladder. Bladder training does not work if the patient has a neurological disease but may be worth trying when there is a mild degree of incontinence due to idiopathic instability.

Drug treatment

Drugs are commonly used to treat urgency, frequency and incontinence due to detrusor instability. Unfortunately, none are reliably effective and all have potentially troublesome side effects. They act by modifying the activity of the parasympathetic nerve supply to the detrusor with or without some membrane-stabilizing effect on the smooth muscle itself.

Probanthine is an anticholinergic drug which is cheap and appears to be safe. It has been supplanted in urological practice by oxybutinin which has a more potent anticholinergic effect on the bladder and some membrane-stabilizing effect as well. Terodiline was similarly effective but was withdrawn because it was cardiotoxic. All these drugs cause drowsiness, blurring of vision, dry mouth and constipation among other side effects which are intolerable to many of those who take them.

Neuro-urology

The basic aims of management of the neuropathic bladder are to minimize the risk of renal damage by preventing high pressure within the system and to improve symptoms by suppressing detrusor hyperreflexia. A limited range of treatment options are available and, in practice, investigation can be confined to simple tests which help to establish failure of bladder emptying and its consequences, and those which demonstrate the presence of bladder instability. Surgery has a small place in the management of patients with progressive neurological disease. It is generally reserved for those patients in whom medical management fails to stop a deterioration of renal function or for those with particularly disabling symptoms which cannot be controlled by medical means.

Spinal cord injury

After serious spinal cord injury there is a variable period during which the bladder is acontractile — 'spinal shock'. Usually, reflex activity of the detrusor returns within days or weeks, although in a minority it is lost for ever. Why this should be is unknown. Poor bladder emptying after spinal injury may be due to detrusor—sphincter dyssynergia or poorly sustained detrusor contraction. Even when dyssynergia is suspected, attempts to improve bladder emptying by sphincterotomy do not always work. This has led to the suggestion that there may be additional 'occult' lesions at the sacral level which cause poor detrusor contractility though these are difficult to demonstrate neurophysiologically [20]. Certainly, damage to the lowest part of the spinal cord, conus or cauda equina, causes a mixture of upper and lower motor neurone defects with an unpredictable effect on bladder function.

It was formerly common to catheterize patients during the period of spinal shock. Because of the risks of infection most patients are now managed by intermittent catheterization until reflex voiding is established. If chronic catheterization is indicated, a suprapubic is better than a urethral catheter.

Tethered cord

A tethered cord is one of the possible consequences of spinal dysraphism. Symptoms usually occur as the child grows and bladder problems may be delayed into adult life when they may be difficult to diagnose. Low back pain is common and there will be radiographic evidence of lumbosacral spina bifida. Urodynamic studies may show either a small hyperreflexic bladder or a large capacity acontractile one. Neurosurgical intervention may abolish pain, but bladder function may not improve.

Neurologists see many patients in whom a diagnosis of 'idiopathic detrusor instability' is made in the absence of any overt neurological defect. How vigorously such patients should be investigated to exclude a tethered cord remains to be established [21].

Cauda equina lesions

Damage to the sacral roots S2–S4, either within the spinal canal or extradurally, results in a lower motor neurone disorder of bladder function: the bladder becomes atonic, or hypotonic if the denervating injury is partial [22]. Bladder compliance may also be reduced.

Although normal sensation of bladder stretch is lost, some awareness of pain may still be present due to afferent sympathetic pathways travelling with the hypogastric nerves. The striated urethral sphincter may be denervated and weakened. Stress incontinence is common.

Central protrusion of lumbar discs (L2–L3: L3–L4) are a common cause of damage to the cauda equina. Cauda equina lesions may also result from trauma, spinal metastases or intradural tumours. An unusual and poorly understood cauda equina syndrome can also occur in long-standing ankylosing spondylitis.

Multiple sclerosis

In multiple sclerosis, plaques of demyelination occur throughout the CNS and it is not surprising that they can disrupt the nervous pathways for bladder control or that bladder problems should be very common [23]. Demyelination in the spinal cord is probably the major cause of impaired bladder control.

The commonest symptoms are frequency and urgency of micturition due to hyperreflexic detrusor contractions. Urge incontinence occurs if the hyperreflexic contractions are very strong, if the pelvic floor has been denervated by stretch injury in childbirth, or if the patient is unable to reach a toilet in time because of immobility.

Patients may also find it difficult to start micturition because bulbospinal pathways are interrupted. Hesitancy is not uncommon but retention is unusual. Detrusor–sphincter dyssynergia causes the stream to be interrupted or to stop prematurely.

A hyperreflexic detrusor is the commonest finding in urodynamic studies of those with multiple sclerosis, though most studies also report a variable incidence of hyporeflexic or areflexic bladders. Interruption of pathways between the pontine micturition centre and the sacral cord would be expected to produce hyperreflexia: hyporeflexia and areflexia are less easy to explain.

It has been taught that a urodynamic assessment of these patients is essential in planning correct management [24]. This is a counsel of perfection: in practice, the treatment options are usually limited to treating hyperreflexia by drugs and improving bladder emptying by catheterization, the need for which is usually apparent from less vigorous investigations.

Upper tract damage leading to renal impairment seems to be less common in multiple sclerosis than spinal cord trauma possibly because low detrusor compliance is present less often. In men, it is probably advisable to perform a renal ultrasound to look for upper tract dilatation every 3–4 years but this may be unnecessary in women.

Tropical spastic paraplegia

Tropical spastic paraplegia due to meningoencephalitis follows infection by the retrovirus HTLV-1. As might be expected in a spinal cord disorder, urinary symptoms are a common feature. Patients have frequency, urgency and urge incontinence. Urodynamic investigations show a combination of disorders [25].

Parkinson's disease

Parkinson's disease can involve the neural mechanisms which control bladder function and frequency and urgency are common [26]. Most urodynamic studies have shown a high incidence of detrusor hyperreflexia possibly resulting from loss of inhibition exerted by the basal ganglia on the pontine micturition centre. Unfortunately, clinical studies have shown no consistent change in detrusor hyperreflexia despite a therapeutic response to either levodopa [27] or apomorphine [28].

The external sphincter is also abnormal in Parkinson's disease: this may be a bradykinesia of sphincter relaxation.

Bladder symptoms in Parkinson's disease are difficult to manage. The most taxing problem arises when the patient is an elderly man whose outflow obstruction may well be due to his prostate. As yet there is no sure way to resolve this problem though urine flow rates measured before and after apomorphine may help. Patients with Parkinson's disease do badly after surgery [29]. Reducing hyperreflexia with drugs and alleviating incomplete bladder emptying by intermittent catheterization should probably be considered first.

Multiple system atrophy

Multiple system atrophy was originally thought to be an uncommon condition presenting predominantly with orthostatic hypertension and autonomic failure. The disorder is now recognized as having protean manifestations [30]. It can present either with features of the Shy—Drager syndrome, cerebellar ataxia or atypical parkinsonism. Disturbances of continence and micturition invariably accompany the other neurological changes in the Shy—Drager syndrome and may be the presenting symptom.

Urodynamic investigations of patients with the Shy—Drager syndrome have demonstrated detrusor hyperreflexia, loss of the micturition reflex and large residual urines, but no evidence of detrusor—sphincter dyssynergia [31]. A decrease in bladder compliance may be marked in advanced cases. Denervation of the sphincters may be demonstrated electromyographically. The picture of bladder dysfunction observed in a patient is produced by various deficits and may alter considerably with progression of the disease.

Systematic analysis of sphincter electromyography is now used to distinguish patients with multiple system atrophy who present with atypical parkinsonism, from those with idiopathic Parkinson's disease. This is important because a mistaken diagnosis of bladder outflow obstruction due to prostatic enlargement often leads to a prostatectomy early in the course of the disease and leaves many of these men incontinent. Prostatectomy destroys the bladder neck and the denervation which occurs in multiple system atrophy means that continence can no longer by maintained by the rhabdosphincter. Since patients may have several years of active life before becoming disabled by the progress of their disease it is clearly important to recognize this entity and avoid surgery. Post-micturition residuals in these patients may be between 200 and 400 ml so that bladder dysfunction can be greatly improved by the patient learning to perform intermittent self-catheterization. Because unstable contractions may also be a feature, particularly in the early stages of the disease, treatment with oxybutinin can have a beneficial effect.

Urinary retention in women

Urinary retention in women is uncommon. Unless a positive diagnosis is made, the unfortunate sufferer is likely to be labelled as suffering from a hysterical conversion syndrome.

The anatomy of the female outflow tract is such that some women are able to void by relaxing the sphincter and pelvic floor musculature, without a significant rise in detrusor pressure. Difficult or obstructed voiding is highly abnormal. Certain possible mechanisms should be considered:

1 Urethral strictures may result from trauma during parturition or be associated with vulval atrophy in the elderly. They are rare.
2 Detrusor—sphincter dyssynergia may cause urinary retention but clinical signs and symptoms of spinal cord disease will almost always be evident, e.g. signs in the lower limbs and detrusor hyperreflexia. Retention of urine is very rarely the first and only symptom of multiple sclerosis.
3 Loss of contractility of the detrusor muscle due to injury of the S3/S4 roots can result in bladder denervation, an atonic bladder and urinary retention. Recently, a detrusor myopathy has been described but is probably very uncommon [32].
4 The most common cause of retention in young women is a condition which until recently was thought to be psychogenic. Urethral sphincter electromyography reveals abnormal myotonic-like activity (so-called complex repetitive discharges and decelerating bursts) which seem to impair relaxation of the sphincter. These women have no symptoms of sacral root lesion or autonomic disturbance: anal sphincter control is normal and they have no disturbance of perineal sensation. There may be an association with polycystic ovaries [4]. If the diagnosis is made by single fibre electromyography, the patient can be spared a fruitless round of consultations and investigations. Unfortunately, treatment remains difficult, and most of these women have to be taught intermittent self-catheterization.

Medical treatment of impaired bladder emptying

When urological causes for impaired emptying have been excluded, the cause of significant residual urine in patients with neurological diseases is usually due either to deficient detrusor contraction or to detrusor—sphincter dyssynergia. In patients with spinal cord disease both factors may operate. Attempts to stimulate detrusor contraction or sphincter relaxation by drugs are largely futile. Where there is sphincter weakness manual expression of the bladder contents by suprapubic pressure (Credé's manoeuvre) may be possible. However, this may lead to dilatation of the upper urinary tract and many patients end up requiring some mechanical form of bladder drainage.

Intermittent catheterization

Intermittent catheterization has transformed the management of neurogenic bladder disorders. The method was originally described as an aseptic procedure performed by medical staff [33] but was shown by Lapides to be equally safe using a clean but non-sterile technique [34]. Clean intermittent self-catheterization is equally applicable to children and the elderly [35,36].

The frequency of catheterization is often best determined by the patients themselves, but in general the volumes drained on each occasion should be less than 500 ml. A nurse specialist or continence advisor is normally responsible for providing information and teaching the technique. Learning is more difficult for females and a mirror is useful at first. The majority master the method with adequate advice and training even if they greet the prospect with expressions of revulsion.

Benefit from self-catheterization depends on the volume of urine that can be held within the bladder before incontinence occurs. A weak urethral sphincter or severe detrusor hyperreflexia will reduce the functional capacity of the bladder. Urinary infection is a surprisingly infrequent complication of this procedure. By draining the residual urine from the bladder, the incidence of symptomatic urinary infection may actually be reduced although asymptomatic bacteriuria may be a more frequent finding. Manual dexterity is an important factor and may determine a patient's ability to carry out clean intermittent self-catheterization, but good eyesight does not seem to be essential. Many patients find it helpful to talk to another patient who has already mastered the technique.

Chronic indwelling catheter

For some patients, poor hand function and the want of a suitable carer, may make clean intermittent catheterization impossible. It may be unsuitable for patients whose main bladder disorder is hyperreflexia but for these patients an add-on 'clam' cystoplasty using opened-out bowel, may lower the pressure inside the bladder despite the detrusor contractions and make intermittent catheterization feasible. This is especially valuable in children with the neuropathic bladders that occur with spina bidifa (see p. 328).

There remain some patients for whom an indwelling catheter is the only means of ensuring adequate urinary drainage and personal hygiene.

The main complications of long-term catheterization are leakage alongside the catheter, intermittent blockage and chronic urinary infection. Stone formation may occur in association with the presence of the catheter and infection. Treatment of infection with antibiotics and antiseptic washouts is unlikely to be complete and may lead to colonization of the urinary tract with resistent organisms. Bypassing around the catheter is common, usually as a result of uninhibited detrusor contractions. Logically, one may attempt to manage this with anticholinergic medication, but seldom with much success. The use of increasingly bigger balloons only worsens the detrusor instability, and large catheters result eventually in a grossly patulous urethra.

Suprapubic catheterization

Recently, there has been a renewed interest in the traditional method of suprapubic catheterization [36]. An indwelling suprapubic catheter offers effective urinary diversion which is less liable to expulsion or bypassing. Some patients may need a 'clam' cystoplasty: others need an operation to occlude the urethra especially when the bladder neck has been destroyed by an indwelling catheter.

Surgery for the neurogenic bladder

When symptoms due to hyperreflexia have failed to respond to drugs and have become intolerable, or there is any suggestion of high pressure damage to the kidneys, a cystoplasty should be considered whereby a de-tubularized patch of bowel is let into the wall of the bladder to reduce the pressure (see p. 328).

Pouch reservoirs and continent diversions are all associated with a significant incidence of serious complications and there are some patients for whom this is not suitable. For them, when intermittent catheterization has proved to be impossible and an indwelling catheter does not work, there is a place for urinary diversion by means of a simple ileal conduit (see p. 325).

References

1 Abrams P, Feneley RCL (1978) The significance of the symptoms associated with bladder outflow obstruction. *Urol Int* 33: 171.

2 Abrams P, Blaivas JG, Stanton SL, Andersen JT (1988) The standardisation of terminology of lower urinary tract function. *Scand J Urol Nephrol* 114: 5.

3 Torrens M (1987) Urodynamics, in: Torrens M, Morrison JFB (eds) *The Physiology of the Lower Urinary Tract*, p. 277. London: Springer.

4 Fowler CJ, Christmas TJ, Chapple CR *et al.* (1988) Abnormal electromyographic activity of the urethral sphincter, voiding dysfunction, and polycystic ovaries: a new syndrome? *Br Med J* 297: 1436.

5 McGuire EJ (1992) The role of urodynamic investigation in assessment of benign prostatic hypertrophy. *J Urol* 148: 1133.

6 Mouritzen L, Rasmussen A. (1993) Bladder neck mobility evaluated by vaginal ultrasonography. *Br J Urol* 71: 166.

7 Burnstock G (1990) Innervation of bladder and bowel, in: Bock G, Whelan J (eds) *Neurobiology of Incontinence*, p. 2. Chichester: CIBA Foundation/John Wiley.

8 Gosling J, Dixon JS, Critchley HOD *et al.* (1981) A comparative study of the human external sphincter and periurethral levator muscles. *Br J Urol* 53: 35.

9 Versi E (1991) The significance of an open bladder neck in women. *Br J Urol* 68: 42.

10 Burnstock G (1986) The changing face of autonomic neurotransmission. *Acta Physiol Scand* 126: 67.

11 Morrison JFB (1987) Sensations arising from the lower urinary tract, in: Torrens M, Morrison JFB (eds) *The Physiology of the Lower Urinary Tract*, p. 89. London: Springer.

12 de Groat WC (1990) Central neurol control of the lower urinary tract, in: Bock G, Whelan J (eds) *Neurobiology of Incontinence*, p. 27. Chichester: CIBA Foundation/John Wiley.

13 Kiff ES, Swash M (1984) Normal proximal and delayed distal conduction in the pudendal nerves of patients with idiopathic (neurogenic) faecal incontinence. *J Neurol Neurosurg Psychiatr* 47: 820.

14 Fowler CJ, Kirby RS, Harrison MJG, Milroy EJG, Turner Warwick RT (1984) Individual motor unit analysis in the diagnosis of disorders of urethral sphincter innervation. *J Neurol Neurosurg Psychiatr* 47: 637.

15 Galloway NTM, Chisholm GD, McInnes A (1985) Patterns of significance of the sacral evoked response (the urologist's knee jerk). *Br J Urol* 57: 145.

16 Snooks SJ, Setchell M, Swash M, *et al.* (1984) Injury to innervation of pelvic floor sphincter musculature in childbirth. *Lancet* i: 546.

17 Hahn I, Milsom I, Fall M, Ekelund P (1993) Long term results of pelvic floor training in female stress urinary incontinence. *Br J Urol* 72: 421.

18 O'Sullivan DC, Chilton CP, Munson KW (1995) Should Stamey colposuspension be our primary surgery for stress incontinence? *Br J Urol* 75: 457.

19 Mundy AR (1993) *Urodynamic and Reconstructive Surgery of the Lower Urinary Tract*, p. 61. Edinburgh: Churchill Livingstone.

20 Lucas MG, Thomas D (1989) Lack of relationship of conus reflexes to bladder function after spinal cord injury. *Br J Urol* 63: 24.

21 Galloway NTM, Tainsh J (1985) Minor defects of the sacrum and neurogenic bladder dysfunction. *Br J Urol* 57: 154.

22 Pavlakis AJ, Siroky MB, Goldstein I (1983) Neuro-urologic findings in conus medullaris and cauda equina injury. *Arch Neurol* 40: 570.

23 Betts CD, Fowler CJ, Fowler CG (1991) Multiple sclerosis and urinary dysfunction. *Neurol Urodyn* 10: 358.

24 Blaivas JG, Bhimani G, Labib MB (1979) Vesico-urethral dysfunction in multiple sclerosis. *J Urol* 122: 342.

25 Shibasaki H, Endo C, Kuroda Y *et al.* (1988) Clinical picture of HTLV-1 associated myelopathy. *J Neurol Sci* 87: 15.

26 Murnaghan GD (1961) Neurogenic disorders of the bladder in parkinsonism. *Br J Urol* 33: 403.

27 Fitzmaurice H, Fowler CJ, Rickards D (1985) Micturition disturbances in Parkinson's disease. *Br J Urol* 57: 652.

28 Christmas TJ, Kempster PA, Chapple CR *et al.* (1990) Role of subcutaneous apomorphine in parkinsonian voiding dysfunction. *Lancet* ii: 1451.

29 Staskin DS, Vardi Y, Siroky MA (1988) Post-prostatectomy incontinence in the parkinsonian patient: the significance of poor voluntary sphincter control. *J Urol* 140: 117.

30 Bannister R (1984) *Autonomic Failure*. Oxford: Oxford University Press.

31 Kirby R, Fowler CJ, Gosling J *et al.* (1986) Urethro-vesical dysfunction in progressive autonomic failure with multiple system atrophy. *J Neurol Neurosurg Psychiatr* 49: 554.

32 Martin J, Sobeh M, Swash M, Nicols C, Baithun SI, Jenkins BJ (1993) Detrusor myopathy: a cause of detrusor weakness with retention. *Br J Urol* 71: 235.

33 Guttman L, Frankel H (1966) The value of intermittent catheterisation of traumatic paraplegia and tetraplegia. *Paraplegia* 4: 63.

34 Lapides J, Diokno AC, Lowe BS *et al.* (1974) Follow up on unsterile, intermittent self-catheterisation. *J Urol* 126: 119.

35 Webb RJ, Lawson AL, Neal DE (1990) Clean intermittent self-catheterisation in 172 adults. *Br J Urol* 65: 20.

36 Barnes DG, Shaw PJR, Timoney AG, Tsokos N (1993) Management of the neuropathic bladder by suprapubic catheterisation. *Br J Urol* 72: 169.

Chapter 22: Fistulae and sinuses

Principles and definitions

A fistula is an abnormal communication between two epithelial surfaces — usually between one hollow viscus and another, or with the skin. A sinus is an abnormal track leading to the exterior. Fistulae and sinuses tend to heal spontaneously. They persist for one or more of the following reasons (Fig. 22.1):

1 There is obstruction to the viscus, e.g. to the ureter or urethra, downstream to the opening of the fistula.

2 The fistula or sinus has been present for so long that the track is lined by epithelium.

3 The fistula or sinus contains or leads down to a foreign body (e.g. a non-absorbable suture or a calculus).

4 The underlying cause is a chronic granuloma, e.g. tuberculosis, xanthogranuloma, actinomycosis, Behçet's syndrome, Wegener's granuloma or, in the perineum, Crohn's disease.

5 The tissues have been rendered ischaemic by previous radiotherapy.

6 The fistula or sinus leads down to a cancer.

Complications

A fistula leading from the urinary tract to the skin will leak urine. This may be intermittent or continuous according to the site of the internal opening of the fistula. The urine is often cloudy from infection and resembles lymph or serous fluid but the diagnosis can easily be made by measuring its content of urea or creatinine — only urine can have a concentration of these substances greater than that of plasma.

If the communication is between the bowel and the urinary tract the main danger is from infection by faecal organisms which may be lethal.

If there is a large surface area of granulation tissue in contact with the urine as it escapes from a fistula, or if the urine enters the bowel, then urine will be absorbed, and lead to hyperchloraemic acidosis.

Calcification occurs around chronic fistulae and stones often form in them.

Pathology

A number of congenital fistulae occur which involve the bladder as in exstrophy, a persistent urachus or an ectopic ureter. These are dealt with elsewhere (see pp. 256−263) but it is wise to remember that they can present in adult life [1].

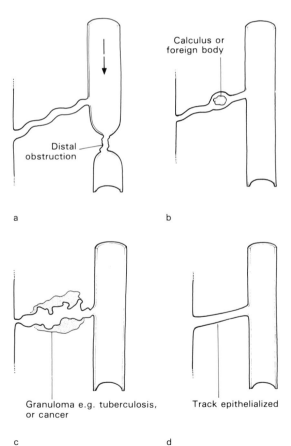

Fig. 22.1 Causes for persistence of a fistula or sinus.
(a) Obstruction to a viscus downstream of the fistula.
(b) Stone or foreign body, e.g. suture in the track.
(c) Granuloma, e.g. tuberculosis or cancer in the track.
(d) The track has become lined with epithelium.

Investigations

Measurement of the plasma electrolytes may show hyperchloraemic acidosis. Microscopic examination of the urine may show vegetable or striated muscle fibres in the deposit. Gas from the bowel may show up the ureter and renal pelvis. Usually the diagnosis is confirmed radiologically by a sinogram, a fistulogram, a cystogram or gastrografin enema. It may be helpful to use the old-fashioned method of giving indigo—carmine intravenously to colour the urine blue, and when a fistula between the lymphatics and the urinary tract is suspected the 'Sudan sandwich' — containing the dye Sudan 3 — will stain the urine pink [2].

Sinuses

Persistent sinuses after operations on the urinary tract are nearly always due to the use of non-absorbable suture material or metal clips. One particularly difficult type is seen when the renal vessels have been ligated with non-absorbable material at nephrectomy in the presence of infection, e.g. in calculi or pyonephrosis. The sinus typically tracks up and down the psoas muscle

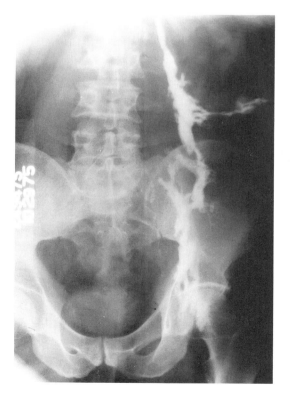

Fig. 22.2 Sinogram leading along a psoas abscess to non-absorbable sutures on the site of a nephrectomy.

and may even point in the groin to resemble a femoral hernia (Fig. 22.2). Attempts to deal with the sinus by drainage and antibiotics are always followed by relapse: the only way to cure the condition is to reopen the old incision, reflect the bowel and remove the offending material.

Persistent sinuses after operations on the kidney may also be caused by tuberculosis or actinomycosis [3] — and the diagnosis only made by sending pus from the sinus for culture.

Fistulae

Kidney

A rare group of fistulae occur between the renal pelvis and the gastrointestinal tract [4−13]. The underlying cause is usually infection caused by a calculus, leading to a perinephric abscess, often complicated by xanthogranuloma. Transitional cell carcinoma may also give rise to such a fistula. The presentation is that of a painful mass in the loin, accompanied by fever. X-rays may show gas in the renal pelvis. Radical surgical excision of the involved kidney and bowel can give a permanent cure.

Ureter

Fistulae between the ureter and the vagina are well-recognized complications of hysterectomy and other pelvic operations [14,15]. Today, it is becoming accepted that prompt diagnosis followed by prompt repair using a Boari flap gives the best results (see p. 128) [16].

Fistulae have also been described between the ureter and the fallopian tube or uterus [17]. Whatever the cause of the fistula, the ureter is usually obstructed, and the clinical picture is complicated by pain in the loin and the complications of obstruction and infection in the upper tract. When the lesion has been neglected and the diagnosis is made only after several months, the kidney may be hopelessly damaged by obstruction and necessitate nephrectomy.

Fistulae may occur between the ureter and colon or small intestine, occasionally between the ureter and appendix, from which urine enters both the colon and ileum. The main clinical problem arises from absorption of urine leading to hyperchloraemic acidosis. The situation may be complicated by infection, especially if there is a large collection of urine in communication with a source of infection.

A particular clinical picture is seen when the

ureter communicates with the fallopian tube or uterus — a very rare condition which has been seen when a stone has ulcerated from the ureter into the fallopian tube. If in addition there is diabetes, the picture can be further complicated by gas formation in the upper tract [17].

Bladder

Vesicovaginal fistulae which occur after neglected obstructed childbirth and operations on the pelvis and uterus have been dealt with elsewhere (see p. 268). Fistulae between bladder and recto-sigmoid are relatively common and a fistula into the ileum is seen as an uncommon complication of Crohn's disease.

One specially dangerous type of fistula follows radiation. The pathological process here is ischaemia from radiation arteritis, and any attempt at repair demands the introduction of new healthy tissue, e.g. omentum, gracilis or non-irradiated bowel.

Vesicocolic fistula

In Britain about half of the vesicocolic fistulae are caused by cancer of the sigmoid, the other half arise from diverticulitis, when an abscess around a diverticulum bursts into the bladder [18,19]. Very rarely, the fistula involves the appendix, presumably in consequence of an appendix abscess bursting into the bladder [20] (Figs 22.3–22.6).

At first there is a severe cystitis, often with

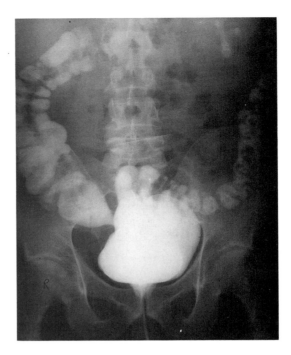

Fig. 22.4 Fistula between appendix, sigmoid and bladder (courtesy of Editor, *British Journal of Urology*).

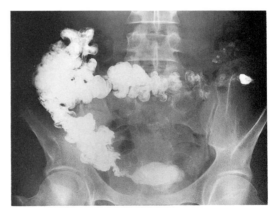

Fig. 22.5 Fistula between terminal ileum and bladder in Crohn's disease.

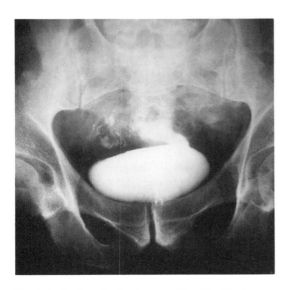

Fig. 22.3 Vesicocolic fistula caused by diverticular disease of the colon.

haematuria and more or less systemic illness. In time the cystitis becomes less severe, with intermittent exacerbations. The patient often notices bubbles in the urine like soda-water, but curiously only admits this bizarre symptom when the question is directly put. Examination may reveal tenderness or a mass over the descending colon and sigmoid. The urine will contain profuse faecal organisms, vegetable and striated muscle fibres.

At cystoscopy it is often very difficult to see the fistula, which is usually on the posterior wall of the bladder. It is often concealed by oedema.

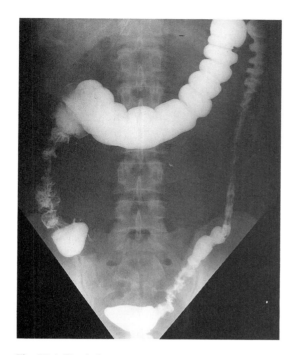

Fig. 22.6 Fistula between sigmoid and bladder caused by carcinoma of the sigmoid colon.

Pressure over the suprapubic region may cause pus to issue like toothpaste from the fistula, and occasionally faeces and gas are seen to emerge.

A cystogram may show the communication, but the pressure in the sigmoid is usually much greater than that in the bladder so that the fistula is usually better seen with a contrast enema.

The differential diagnosis between cancer and diverticular disease requires colonoscopy and biopsy.

The treatment then depends on the severity of the inflammation in the pelvis. The classical method was to perform a diverting colostomy, wait 3–6 weeks, and then carry out a colonic resection. Today, with antibiotics and a more effective and precise preoperative diagnosis, the affected bowel can usually be resected and anastomosis performed in a single stage without the need for any colostomy. Once the affected bowel has been removed, the hole in the bladder is closed with absorbable sutures and a catheter left indwelling for 5 or 6 days.

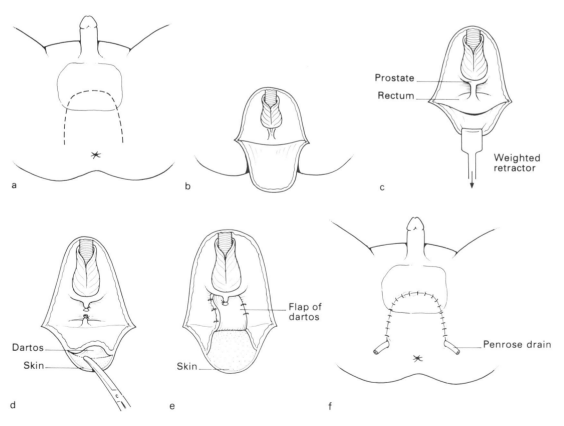

Fig. 22.7 Closure of fistula between rectum and prostate. (a) A full thickness scrotal flap is formed. (b) The bulbar urethra is exposed. (c) The plane is opened between prostate and rectum to expose the fistula track. (d) The fistula is divided between ligatures and a flap of dartos muscle separated from the scrotal skin. (e) The flap of dartos if sutured between the divided ends of the fistula, and (f) the scrotal flap is replaced with drainage.

Vesicoileal fistulae

These uncommon fistulae can pose a difficult diagnostic problem, while their subsequent treatment calls for all the skills of the gastro-enterologist, for whom the management of Crohn's disease poses an everyday, if difficult challenge.

Vesicouterine fistula — Youssef's syndrome

In this unusual condition the patient develops intermittent haematuria at the time of the menstrual period, raising the differential diagnosis of endometriosis. Otherwise there are few symptoms [21—23].

Urethra

Most fistulae involving the male urethra arise from periurethral abscesses complicating strictures (see p. 478). Fistulae between the prostatic urethra and rectum occur after prostatectomy usually for cancer, where difficulty has been encountered in removing tissue from the posterior part of the gland, or in locating the landmarks at transurethral resection.

The main hazard of these fistulae is from faecal infection and a diverting colostomy may be urgently needed. There is a choice of methods for closing fistulae between urethra and rectum. For small low fistulae in the region of the prostate and bulbar urethra, a ∩-shaped scrotal flap gives access to the fistula, and after dividing it a plug of dartos is detached from the skin flap and used to reinforce the closure (Fig. 22.7).

For larger low fistulae the full thickness mucosal flap technique of Parks [25] is used (Figs 22.8 & 22.9). For those that occur higher in the recto-sigmoid, especially when there has been radiation injury, Parks' pull-through operation is better (Figs 22.10—22.14). The sigmoid is mobilized, if necessary after liberating the splenic flexure and descending colon. The full thickness of mucosa is stripped out of the rectum down to the dentate line, and the sigmoid drawn through and sutured to the rectal mucosa at the edge of the anus. This preserves the rectal sphincters and propriocep-

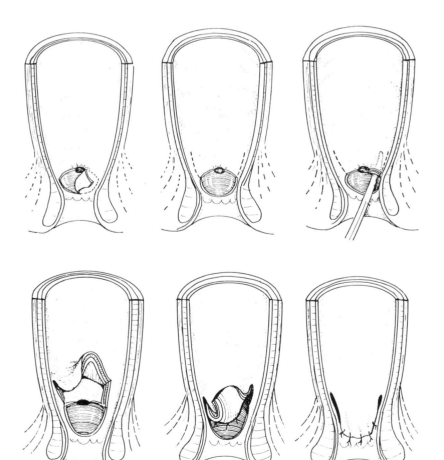

Fig. 22.8 Parks' operation for large low fistulae between prostatic urethra and anal canal. Through an anal retractor, an ellipse of mucosa is removed below the fistula exposing the circular muscle of the rectum. A proximal flap is developed using the full thickness of the rectal wall.

Fig. 22.9 The flap of rectal wall is brought down to cover the hole and sutured to the rectal mucosa.

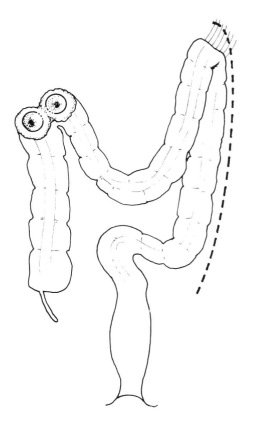

Fig. 22.10 Parks' pull-through operation for large high fistulae. A protecting double-barrelled colostomy is made and the left side of the colon mobilized.

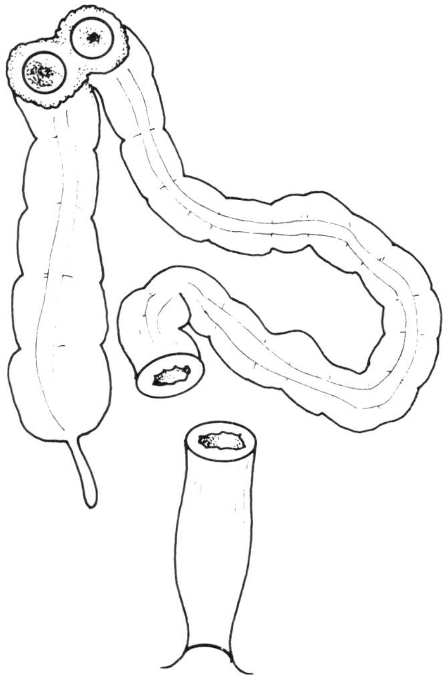

Fig. 22.11 The sigmoid is divided at the rectosigmoid junction.

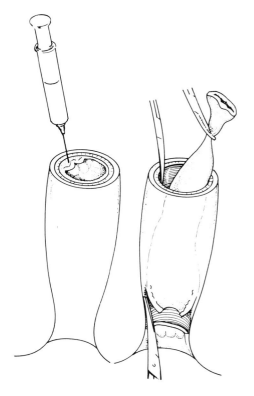

Fig. 22.12 With the help of saline−adrenaline injections a cylinder of the mucosa of the rectum is separated from the muscular wall well distal to the fistula.

tive sensation, while closing the hole with full thickness bowel.

Arterial fistulae

Fistulae between the aorta and ureter, or common iliac artery and ileal loop [14,26] are sometimes encountered after urological operations such as ureterolysis, radical salvage node dissection for testis tumours, and total cystectomy with diversion. The diagnosis is sometimes made only when there has been a catastrophic haemorrhage, but if appropriate investigations are performed at an early stage when there is a warning haemorrhage, steps can sometimes be taken to correct the damage. Wherever possible, it is necessary to avoid the use of non-absorbable prosthetic material when repairing the damage to the large vessel or, if this is unavoidable, then it should be protected by omentum.

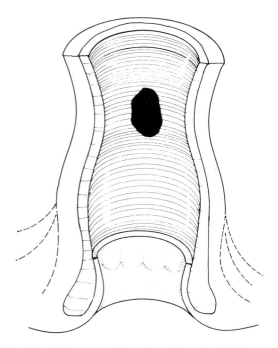

Fig. 22.13 No attempt is made to close the fistula.

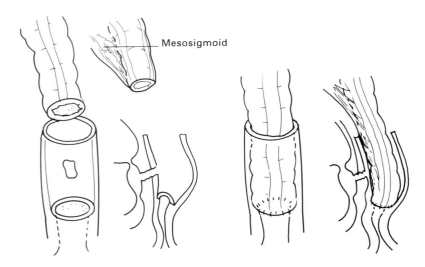

Fig. 22.14 The sigmoid is drawn down through the sleeve of rectum and sutured to the mucosa inside the anus. The mesosigmoid lies against the fistula.

References

1 MacNeily AE, Koleitat N, Kirulata HG, Homsy YL (1992) Urachal abscesses, protean manifestations, their recognition and management. *Urology* 40: 530.

2 Marsden PD (1993) Obstructive lymphatic filariasis. *Br Med J* 306: 136.

3 Morgan RJ, Molland EA, Blandy JP (1977) Renal actinomycosis. *Eur Urol* 3: 307.

4 Bissada NK, Cole AT, Fried FA (1973) Reno-alimentary fistula: an unusual urological problem. *J Urol* 110: 273.

5 Dunn M, Kirk D (1973) Renogastric fistula: case report and review of the literature. *J Urol* 109: 785.

6 Hoare EM (1973) Duodeno-ureteric fistula. *Br J Surg* 60: 407.

7 Kuss R, Truelle A, Jardin A (1972) Fistule pyelo-duodenale. *J Urol Nephrol* 78: 906.

8 McDougal WS, Persky L (1972) Traumatic and spontaneous pyelo-duodenal fistulas. *J Trauma* 12: 665.

9 Lande G (1970) Appendicovesical fistula. *T Norsk Legefor* 90: 704.

10 Lockhart-Mummery HE (1958) Vesico-intestinal fistula. *Proc Roy Soc Med* 51: 1032.

11 Op den Orth JO (1969) A radiologically demonstrated fistula between the common bile duct and the right renal pelvis. *Radiol Clin Biol (Basel)* 38: 402.

12 Smith PJB, Williams RE, Dedombal AT (1972) Genitourinary fistulae complicating Crohn's disease. *Br J Urol* 44: 657.

13 Gil-Salom M, Oron-Alphente J, Ruiz-del Castillo J, Chuan-Nuez P, Carretero-Gonsalez P (1989) Nephrobronchocutaneous fistula. *Br J Urol* 64: 652.

14 Blasko F-J, Saladie J-M (1991) Ureteral obstruction and ureteral fistulas after aortofemoral or aortoiliac by-pass surgery (review). *J Urol* 145: 237.

15 Bazeed M, Nabeeh A, El-Kenawy M, Ashamalla A (1995) Urovaginal fistulae: 20 years' experience. *Eur Urol* 27: 34.

16 Blandy JP, Badenoch DF, Fowler CG, Jenkins BJ, Thomas NWM (1991) Early repair of iatrogenic injury to the ureter or bladder after gynecological surgery. *J Urol* 146: 761.

17 Christmas TJ, Badenoch DF (1988) Pneumonephrosis due to a Fallopian tube/ureteric fistula. *Br J Urol* 62: 187.

18 Firfer R, Maganini RJ (1970) Colovesical fistula due to colon diverticulitis. *Amer J Proctol* 21: 206.

19 Hughes ESR (1965) Diverticulitis with vesico-colic fistula. *Austr New Zeal J Surg* 34: 188.

20 Marshall VR, Molland EA, Blandy JP (1975) Appendico-vesico-colic fistula. *Br J Urol* 47: 544.

21 Youssef AF (1960) *Gynecological Urology.* Springfield, Illinois: Charles C Thomas.

22 Medeiros AD, Guimaraes MV (1973) Youssef's syndrome: a case report. *J Urol* 109: 828.

23 Hache L, Pratt JH, Cook EN (1966) Vesicouterine fistula. *Mayo Clin Proc* 41: 150.

24 Blandy JP, Singh M (1972) Fistulae involving the adult male urethra. *Br J Urol* 44: 632.

25 Tiptaft RC, Motson RW, Costello AJ, Paris AMI, Blandy JP (1983) Fistulae involving rectum and urethra: the place of Parks' operations. *Br J Urol* 55: 711.

26 Beaugié JM (1971) Fistula between external iliac artery and ileal conduit. *Br J Urol* 43: 450.

PART 4
PROSTATE

Chapter 23: Prostate — structure and function

Anatomy

Comparative anatomy

In mammals, the urethra has sets of secretory glands opening into it at different levels between the bladder and the external meatus. In mammals with a mating season, these glands enlarge or shrink along with other secondary sexual features. John Hunter observed 'in the mole the prostate gland in winter is hardly discernible, but in the spring becomes very large and is filled with mucus' [1].

Hunter examined many other species [2] of which specimens are preserved in the Hunterian Museum of the Royal College of Surgeons [3]. The mammalian prostate may be diffuse (goat, sheep, hippopotamus, whale and marsupials), or collected in a body with distinct lobes (dog or man), or it may be a mixture of both (rodents) [4].

Because of this extreme variability, it is necessary to be wary of falling into the trap of seeing similarities between organs that are in fact entirely different, e.g. the prostate of dog and man, which differ fundamentally in their anatomical origin, their histology, their response to hormones, and the benign swellings which arise in them [4]. The same reservations apply to using terms such as 'lobe' and 'capsule' [5].

Our closest mammalian kin are the primates. Here we find variations on a common underlying theme [6,7] (Fig. 23.1). There are two distinct 'prostates' — cranial and caudal — shaped like croissants rather than doughnuts. There is a gap between them for the vasa deferentia and common ejaculatory ducts to enter the urethra on either side of the verumontanum which also contains the vestige of the fused Müllerian ducts — the utriculus masculinus.

Just downstream of the caudal prostate is the external sphincter: it is made of two muscular components — unstriated and striated — which are both cephalad and distinct from the levator ani sheet of the pelvic floor.

In man, the cranial prostate fits into the caudal prostate like an egg in an egg-cup (Fig. 23.2); both prostates are deficient in front where glandular tissue is replaced by a fibromuscular septum [5] (Fig. 23.3).

Embryology

The prostate forms in the mesenchyme of the urogenital septum which separates the primitive hind-gut into the bladder and rectum. The thin film which covers the convexity of the hind-gut — the cloacal membrane — dissolves to leave gaps in front of and behind the urogenital septum — urethra and anus (see p. 248). Running down in this septum are the Müllerian and Wolffian ducts and the ureteric buds (Fig. 23.4).

In the sixth week of fetal life, when the Sertoli cells of the developing testis secrete the Müllerian inhibitory factor, the fused Müllerian ducts disappear except for a tiny sac — the utriculus masculinus which is like a volcanic crater on the summit of the verumontanum.

About a week later, testosterone from the newly forming Leydig cells testis [8,9] causes buds of urethral epithelium to sprout into the mesenchyme above and below the verumontanum. Formerly, this ingrowth or urothelial buds was thought to follow the pattern of the lobes of the adult prostate [10] but this is no longer accepted [11,12].

Maturation of the prostate

In early fetal life, the mesenchyme of the prostate differentiates into fibrous tissue and muscle but there are few glandular elements. At birth, the prostate has an outer zone of circular muscle fibres, a middle zone of longitudinal fibres and an inner zone of fibrous tissue. Soon after birth (Fig. 23.5), glandular elements bud out from the posterior wall of the urethra each side of the verumontanum, and displace the urethra forwards (Fig. 23.6). This arrangement persists until puberty when the prostate enlarges in every

363

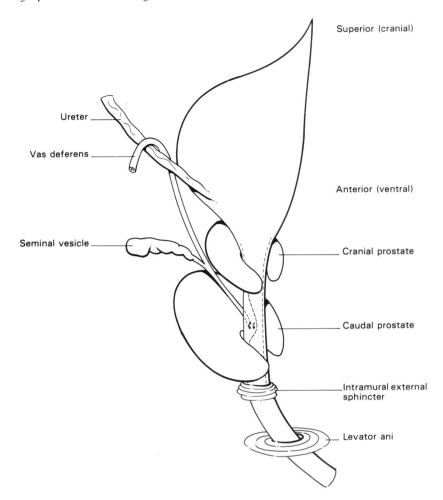

Superior (cranial)

Ureter

Vas deferens

Anterior (ventral)

Seminal vesicle

Cranial prostate

Caudal prostate

Intramural external sphincter

Levator ani

Fig. 23.1 The fundamental 'blueprint' of the primate prostate. There are two distinct prostates, cranial and caudal between which pass the ejaculatory ducts. Note also the two distinct parts to the external sphincter.

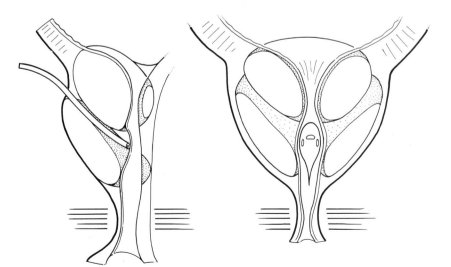

Fig. 23.2 In man, the cranial prostate is fitted into the caudal prostate like an egg in an egg-cup.

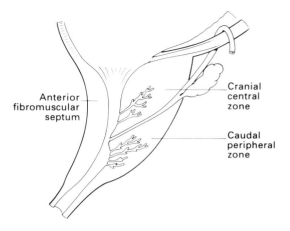

Fig. 23.3 The gap in the front of the prostate in man is filled by a fibromuscular septum.

direction and elongates the urethra [13,14] (Fig. 23.7).

At about the age of 40, small nodules of hyper-

plastic acini and muscle begin to appear in the inner zone of the gland (Fig. 23.8). These nodules grow and coalesce to become the benign nodular hyperplasia of old age.

The normal pattern of growth and development of the prostate gland depends on testosterone. It is prevented by castration before puberty. To become activated, testosterone must be converted to dihydrotestosterone by the enzyme 5-alpha reductase within the prostatic cells. Eunuchs and males with the rare inborn error of metabolism which deprives them of 5-alpha reductase do not develop a prostate [15,16].

Topographical anatomy

In the young adult male, the prostate is about the size of a chestnut, weighing 10–15 g. The urethra bends slightly as it passes through the gland

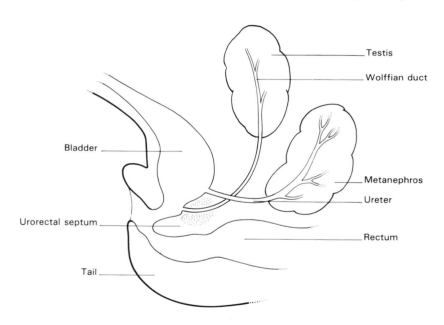

Fig. 23.4 The prostate begins to form in the mesenchyme of the urogenital septum in the vicinity of the opening of the Wolffian ducts.

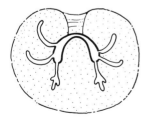

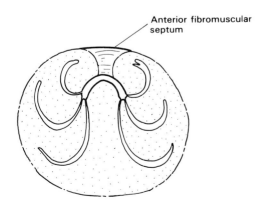

Fig. 23.5 The prostatic ducts grow (a) back, out and round from either side of the verumontanum, and (b) displace the urethra forwards.

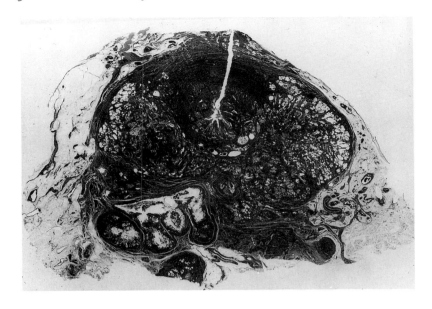

Fig. 23.6 Transverse section through prostate showing the fan-shaped arrangement of ducts and the anterior fibromuscular septum.

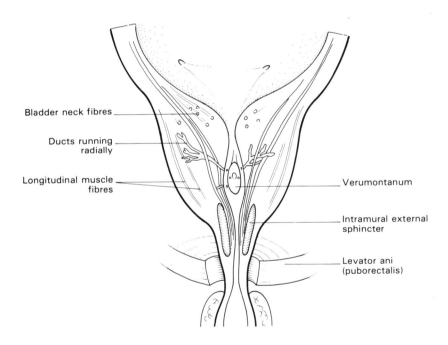

Bladder neck fibres

Ducts running radially

Longitudinal muscle fibres

Verumontanum

Intramural external sphincter

Levator ani (puborectalis)

Fig. 23.7 Diagram of structure of normal adult prostate. There is a stroma made of smooth muscle and fibrous tissue, into which run the prostatic ducts and acini.

(Fig. 23.9). The prostate is thin in front (the fibromuscular septum) where it is devoid of acini. The openings of the prostatic ducts are found along the posterior half of the prostatic urethra, and the glands curve round on either side. There is virtually no glandular tissue in the midline anteriorly.

Most of the normal adult gland lies behind the urethra. It is separated into an inner cranial and an outer caudal zone by the entry of the ejaculatory ducts. The innermost part of the inner cranial prostate is termed the paraurethral zone.

Cranial to the prostate are the trigone, ureters and base of the bladder: behind lie the seminal vesicles and vasa deferentia. The two layers of peritoneum that form the fascia of Denonvilliers separate the prostate and vesicles from the rectum behind. Anteriorly lie the deep veins of the penis and the symphysis pubis.

Posterolateral to the prostate are the neuro-vascular bundles which supply the corpora cavernosa of the penis [17] (Fig. 23.10).

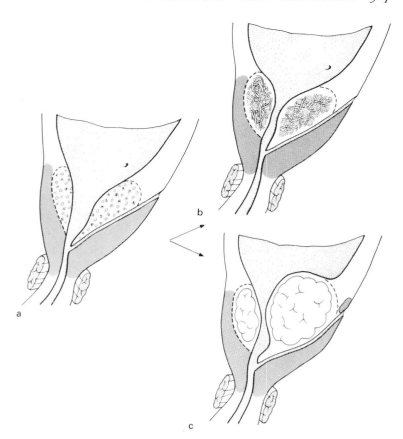

Fig. 23.8 (a) Around the age of 40 nodules of hyperplastic acini and muscle begin to appear in the inner zone which may (b) form a ring of muscle, or (c) a bulky mass of 'adenoma'.

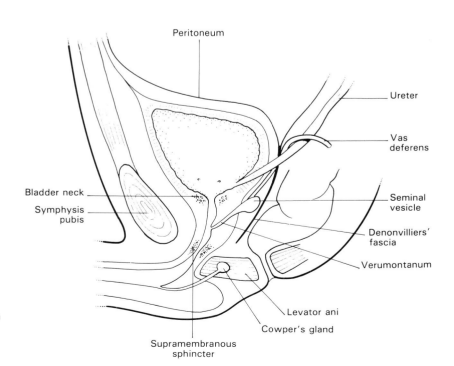

Fig. 23.9 Sagittal section through the prostate showing anatomical relations.

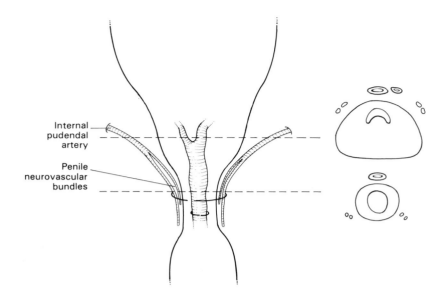

Fig. 23.10 Diagrammatic cross-sections through the prostate at two levels showing the situation of the neurovascular bundles to the penis.

Arteries

The prostate has a rich blood supply entering the gland in two main leashes on either side from the superior vesical branches of the internal iliac artery [18]. To the urologist they are familiar as the 2 and 10 o'clock, and 5 and 7 o'clock arteries (Fig. 23.11).

Veins

A profuse venous network drains into the plexus of Santorini in the pelvis, which communicates with the obturator and internal iliac veins, as well as with the bones of the pelvis, vertebrae and upper third of each femur, so affording an easy route for the spread of infection or cancer.

Lymphatics

The lymphatics of the prostate retrace the course of the obturator and iliac arteries but like the veins, they also communicate directly with the bone marrow of the vertebrae, pelvis and femora. Lymphatics also accompany the little neuro-vascular bundles which enter the gland together with their sleeve of fat through the thin layer of connective tissue — the so-called anatomical capsule. Around the nerves are other tissue spaces — the perineural spaces — distinguished from lymphatics because they are not lined with endothelium. Cancer cells readily spread along either route (Fig. 23.12).

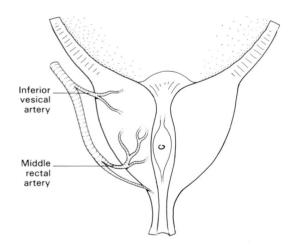

Fig. 23.11 (a) The main arterial supply to the prostate from the inferior vesical and middle rectal arteries. (b) At TURP the main vessels are to be expected at 10, 2, 5 and 7 o'clock.

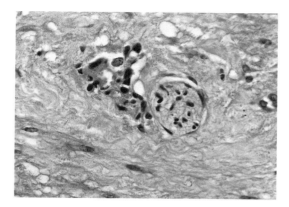

Fig. 23.12 Perineural spaces among the neurovascular bundles which penetrate the capsule of the prostate (courtesy of Dr Suhail Baithun).

Nerves

The prostate receives sympathetic and parasympathetic nerve fibres which pierce the thin capsule along with the fine branches of the arteries [19]. These nerves end on alpha$_1$ receptors on muscle fibres, alpha$_2$ receptors on blood vessels, cholinergic receptors on the acini, and a rich system of vasoactive intestinal polypeptide (VIP) and amine precursor uptake and decarboxylation (APUD) nerves whose function is still a mystery [20,21].

Capsule of the prostate

There are three separate entities which share this term, to the continuing confusion of urologists.

Anatomical capsule. To anatomists this is the film of fibrous tissue which surrounds the gland. Unlike the tough capsule of the kidney or liver, this is no more than the continuation of the connective tissue surrounding the prostate and the pelvic veins (Fig. 23.13). At operation when this thin layer with its veins is swept aside the finger touches glandular tissue [22].

Capsule at open prostatectomy. In the early days of prostatectomy after the adenoma was enucleated from its 'shell' with the finger, at first it was thought that the entire prostate had been removed from within its anatomical capsule [23]. Before long the error was recognized, and it became clear that the 'shell' left behind was a layer of compressed prostatic tissue, often containing adenomatous nodules [24] (Fig. 23.14).

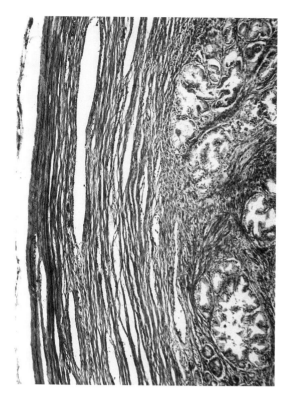

Fig. 23.13 Section through the edge of the normal prostate. Note the absence of a clear 'capsule' — the connective tissue around the prostate is continuous with that of the surrounding veins and fat (courtesy of Mr Basil Page).

Capsule at transurethral resection. Thirty years later with the introduction of transurethral resection the term 'capsule' was given to the lacy tissue which could be recognized at transurethral resection (TUR) [24] (Fig. 23.15). The skill of TUR rested on being able to remove all the adenoma without perforating this supposed 'capsule' outside which lay fat and veins. Again, this was an error: the capsule recognized during TUR consists of a thin layer of prostatic tissue outside which are the prostatic veins and fat. The layer of tissue is in fact thinner than the wire of the resectoscope loop [24].

Physiology

Exocrine function of the prostate

Little is known of the function of the prostate and what we think we know is suspect, being derived mainly from observations on laboratory animals whose prostate has biologically very little to do with that of man. Hardly any studies

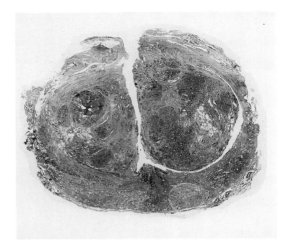

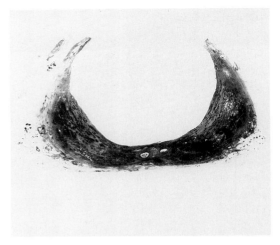

Fig. 23.14 The 'capsule' left behind at open prostatectomy is the compressed outer shell of caudal prostate, often containing adenomatous nodules and sometimes cancer (courtesy of Mr Basil Page and the Editor of the *British Journal of Urology*).

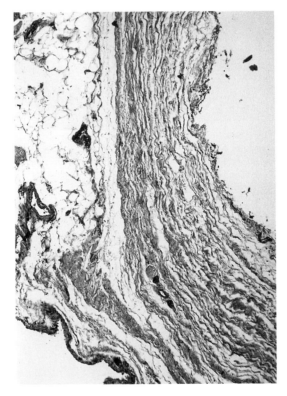

Fig. 23.15 The 'capsule' which is identified during TURP is the thin layer of connective tissue outside the prostate proper (courtesy of Mr Basil Page and the Editor of the *British Journal of Urology*).

have been made on the prostate of primates [25,26]. Estimates of its contribution to the volume of semen vary from 1.6 to 12% [26]. A number of biochemically active substances have been recovered from the prostatic fluid of animals: spermine, prostaglandin, transaminase, acid and alkaline phosphatase, fibrinolysins and zinc, but nothing is known of their physiological purpose [26].

Prostatic acid phosphatase (PAP)

There is a family of enzymes which hydrolyse phosphatic esters under acid conditions. Some are found in the spleen and other organs [27]. At least nine isoenzymes can be separated by electrophoresis — one of these is specific for the prostate and was labelled PAP [28].

Measurement of this enzyme by its action on a substrate is relatively imprecise but is still widely used. Radioimmunoassay gives more precision, but has been superseded by prostate-specific antigen (PSA) [29]. It should be noted that useful as these are in urology, they tell us nothing of the physiological function of the prostate.

Prostate-specific antigen (PSA)

PSA is a glycoprotein found only in the secretory cells of the prostatic acini and in no other tissue of the body [30]. Its serum level depends on the quantity of prostatic tissue present: hence it is elevated in benign hyperplasia and much more so in prostatic cancer. It is measured by radio-immunoassay in the serum and identified by immunoperoxidase staining on histological section, thus clearly identifying metastases that have arisen from the prostate. In prostatic cancer, it enables its response to treatment to be monitored [31]. It tells us nothing about the normal physiological function of the prostate [32,33].

Hormone receptors

Hormone receptors for testosterone have been found in the caudal prostate of the macaque monkey but they do not help in predicting response to hormone treatment of cancer in man [34,35].

Prostate and sphincters

At the neck of the bladder there is a ring of $alpha_1$ adrenergic smooth muscle mixed up with prostatic acini and fibrous tissue (Fig. 23.16). In middle age, this ring of muscle, often referred to as the 'bladder neck', although distorted by adenoma, remains under the influence of $alpha_1$ agonists. Stimulation of the presacral nerve causes it to contract. $Alpha_1$ blockers cause it to relax [36,37].

Caudal to the verumontanum, there is a second sphincter which is the key landmark in TUR. It is sometimes called the 'supramembranous sphincter' but a better term for it is 'intramural external sphincter' [38]. It is contained in the few millimetres of tissue immediately surrounding the urethra and is quite distinct from the striated pubococcygeal part of the levator ani [38]. During operations on the bulbar urethra, e.g. resection for cancer or repair of a ruptured posterior urethra, this intramural external sphincter can be clearly seen above and moving independently from the hiatus in the levator ani sheet (Fig. 23.17).

The intramural sphincter has two components: (a) an inner sleeve of smooth muscle which is continuous with that of the prostate (and thought to be supplied by $alpha_1$ adrenergic nerves); and (b) an outer layer of striated muscle

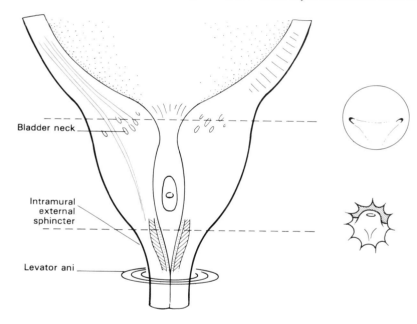

Fig. 23.16 The three components of the sphincter of the prostate. The bladder neck is made up of alpha-adrenergic smooth muscle mixed with prostatic acini and some fibrous tissue.

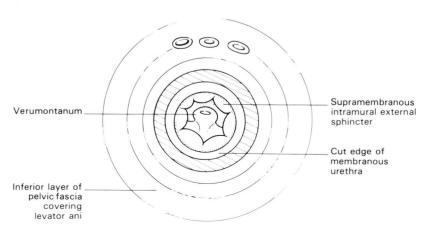

Fig. 23.17 At urethrectomy or urethroplasty the ring of the levator ani can be seen to be quite distinct from the supramembranous sphincter which is part of the wall of the membranous urethra — hence 'intramural sphincter'.

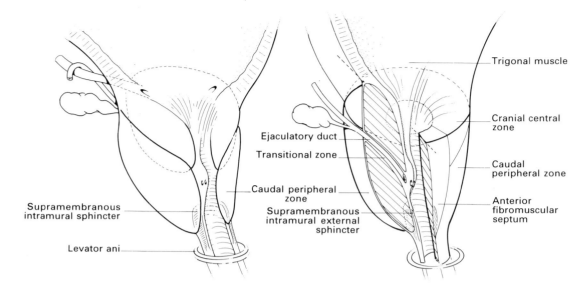

Fig. 23.18 Schematic view of the prostate showing the situation of the supramembranous intramural sphincter.

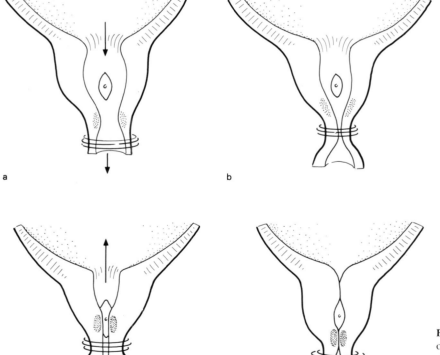

Fig. 23.19 (a) During micturition all the sphincters are open. (b) On completion of voiding the rhabdosphincter closes. (c) Then the intramural sphincter closes and the prostatic urethra milks back the urine. (d) Finally, the bladder neck closes and the external sphincter relaxes.

(Fig. 23.18), a special striated muscle made up of small cells, classified as the slow-twitch type which have the property of maintaining contraction for long periods [39]. Electron microscopy shows these small slow-twitch fibres to have a high content of lipid and mitochondria which makes them able to maintain contraction for a long period.

Every urologist should appreciate how small and vulnerable is this precious sleeve of muscle on which continence in the male depends after operations on the bladder neck or prostate.

At the beginning of normal micturition the bladder neck relaxes and at the same time the detrusor contracts. When the bladder is empty, the external sphincter closes first and the prostatic urethra is emptied by milking back the small quantity of urine it contains into the bladder, and then the bladder neck closes (Fig. 23.19).

Both components of the intramural sphincter are innervated by pelvic splanchnic nerves.

Prostate and ejaculation

The ejaculatory ducts open either side of the verumontanum. At the moment of ejaculation, the bladder neck closes (under sympathetic stimulation) and prevents retrograde flow of semen into the bladder. If the bladder neck has been cut, the sympathetic nerves have been divided or the alpha$_1$ drive to the bladder neck has been blocked by medication, then semen will leak back into the bladder producing a more or less 'dry ejaculation'.

References

1 Palmer JF (1835) (ed.) *The Works of John Hunter*. London: Longman.

2 Griffiths J (1890) Observations on the prostate in man and the lower animals. Part 2. *J Anat* 24: 27.

3 *Descriptive catalogue of the physiological series in the Hunterian Museum of the Royal College of Surgeons of England*, Part 1, 1970, pp. 273—9. London: Churchill Livingstone.

4 Price D, Williams-Ashman HG (1961) The accessory reproductive glands of animals, in: Young WC, Corner GW (eds) *Sex and Internal Secretions*, 3rd edn, vol. 1, p. 366. Baltimore: Williams & Wilkins.

5 McNeal JE (1983) Relationship of the origin of benign prostatic hypertrophy to prostatic structure of man and other mammals, in: Hinman F (ed.) *Benign Prostatic Hypertrophy*, p. 152. New York: Springer.

6 Hill WCO (1935—1966) *Primates. Comparative Anatomy and Taxonomy*, 6 vols. Edinburgh: Edinburgh University Press.

7 Blandy JP, Lytton B (1986) What is the prostate and what is it for? in: Blandy JP, Lytton B (eds) *The Prostate*, pp. 1—11. London: Butterworths.

8 Siitery PK, Wilson JD (1974) Testosterone formation and metabolism during male sexual differentiation in the human embryo. *J Clin Endocrinol Metab* 38: 113.

9 Cunha GR, Fujii H, Neubauer BL, Shannon JM, Sawyer L, Reese BA (1983) Epithelial—mesenchymal interactions in prostatic development, I. Morphological observations on prostatic induction by urogenital sinus mesenchyme in epithelium of the adult rodent urinary bladder. *J Cell Biol* 96: 1662.

10 Lowsley OS (1912) The development of the human prostate gland with reference to the development of other structures at the neck of the urinary bladder. *Amer J Anat* 13: 299.

11 McNeal JE (1989) Anatomy and embryology, in: Fitzpatrick JM, Krane RJ (eds) *The Prostate*, pp. 3—9. London: Churchill Livingstone.

12 McNeal JE (1969) Regional morphology and pathology of the prostate. *Amer J Clin Pathol* 49: 347.

13 Griffiths J (1989) Observations on the anatomy of the prostate. *J Anat* 23: 374.

14 Semple JE (1963) Surgical capsule of the benign enlargement of the prostate. *Br Med J* 2: 1640.

15 Yokoyama M, Seki N, Tamai M, Takeuchi M (1989) Benign prostatic hyperplasia in a patient castrated in his youth. *J Urol* 142: 134.

16 Imperato-McGinley J, Guerrero L, Gautier T, Peterson RE (1974) Steroid 5 alpha-reductase deficiency in man: an inherited form of male pseudohermaphroditism. *Science* 186: 1213.

17 Donker PJ, Droes JTPM, van Ulden BM (1976) Anatomy of the musculature and innervation of the bladder and urethra, in: Williams DI, Chisholm GD (eds) *Scientific Foundations of Urology*, vol. 2, p. 32. London: Heinemann.

18 Flocks RH (1937) The arterial distribution within the prostate gland: its role in transurethral prostatic resection. *J Urol* 37: 524.

19 Villers AM, McNeal JE, Redwine EA, Freiha FS, Stamey TA (1989) The role of perineural space invasion in the local spread of prostatic adenocarcinoma. *J Urol* 142: 763.

20 James S, Chapple CR, Phillips MI *et al.* (1989) Autoradiographic analysis of alpha-adrenoceptors and muscarinic cholinergic receptors in the hyperplastic human prostate. *J Urol* 142: 438.

21 Jones DR, Griffiths GJ, Parkinson MC *et al.* (1989) Comparative histopathology, microradiography and per-rectal ultrasonography of the prostate using cadaver specimens. *Br J Urol* 63: 508.

22 Sattar AA, Noel JC, Wespes E, Schulman CC (1994) Prostatic capsule: fact or fiction? *XIth Congress, European Association of Urology*, 13—16 July, Berlin. Abstract No. 464, p. 243.

23 Freyer PJ (1900) A new method of performing prostatectomy. *Lancet* i: 744.

24 Page BH (1980) The pathological anatomy of digital enucleation for benign prostatic hyperplasia and its application to endoscopic resection. *Br J Urol* 52: 111.

25 Zuckerman S (1938) The effects of prolonged oestrogenic stimulation on the prostate of the rhesus monkey. *J Anat* 72: 264.

26 Mann T (1963) *Biochemistry of Semen and of the Male Reproductive Tract*. London: Methuen.

27 Kutscher W, Wolbers H (1915) Prostatphosphatase. *Zeitschr Physiol Chem* 236: 237.

28 Yam LT, Li CY, Lam KW (1980) The non-prostatic acid phosphatases in the male accessory sex gland, in: Hafex ESE, Spring Mills E (eds) *Human Reproductive Medicine*, vol. 4, p. 183. Amsterdam, Elsevier.

29 Bruce AW, Mahan DE (1986) Acid phosphatase: its estimation and clinical significance, in: Blandy JP, Lytton B (eds) *The Prostate*, pp. 147—62. London: Butterworth.

30 Wang MC, Valenzuela LD, Murphy GP (1979) Purification of a human prostate-specific antigen. *Invest Urol* 17: 159.

31 Babayan RK (1989) Diagnosis and methods of staging prostatic carcinoma, in: Fitzpatrick JM, Krane RJ (eds) *The Prostate*, pp. 273–80. Edinburgh: Churchill Livingstone.

32 Schoonees R, De Klerk JN, Murphy GP (1966) Correlation of prostatic blood flow with ^{65}zinc activity in intact, castrated and testosterone-treated baboons. *Invest Urol* 6: 476.

33 Kerr WK, Kerestec AG, Mayoh H (1960) Distribution of zinc within the human prostate. *Cancer* 13: 550.

34 Ghanadian R, Auf G, Chisholm GD, O'Donoghue EPN (1978) Receptor proteins for androgens in prostatic disease. *Br J Urol* 50: 567.

35 Ghanadian R (1989) Hormone receptors in the prostate, in: Fitzpatrick JM, Krane RJ (eds) *The Prostate*, pp. 11–17. London: Churchill Livingstone.

36 Learmonth J (1913) A contribution to the neurophysiology of the urinary bladder. *Brain* 54: 147.

37 McGuire EJ (1986) Functional changes in prostatic obstruction, in: Blandy JP, Lytton B (eds) *The Prostate*, pp. 23–32. London: Butterworth.

38 Gosling JA, Dixon JS, Humpherson RR (1982) *Functional Anatomy of the Urinary Tract*. London: Gower.

39 Gosling JA, Dixon JS, Critchley HOD, Thompson SA (1981) A comparative study of the human external sphincter and periurethral levator ani muscles. *Br J Urol* 53: 35.

Chapter 24: Prostate — inflammation

Acute prostatitis

Aetiology

Before the development of antibiotics, acute prostatitis was a dreaded complication of haematogenous sepsis. Even today, acute prostatitis may
be preceded by dental or upper respiratory infection, especially in diabetics and neonates [1].
More often there is evidence of infection in the
urinary tract, and the offending organism is
usually *Escherichia coli*, *Klebsiella* or *Pseudomonas*,
which may be recovered from urine or blood.

Clinical features

Malaise and fever, sometimes with rigors, are
followed by pain in the perineum and difficulty
and discomfort on urination, and sometimes
acute retention of urine. There may be haematuria. On rectal examination the prostate is
swollen and tender. There may be an excess of
pus cells in the urine (Fig. 24.1).

Treatment

Pending the result of bacterial sensitivities one
may start with a combination of gentamycin and
cinoxacin. If acute retention develops, suprapubic cystostomy is preferable to urethral instrumentation which may provoke septicaemia or
epididymitis. After about a week of broad
spectrum antibiotics it is wise to continue with a
4-week course of trimethoprim.

Complications

Epididymitis may follow within hours or days of
the onset of acute prostatitis. An abscess may
form in the prostate and if neglected, may rupture

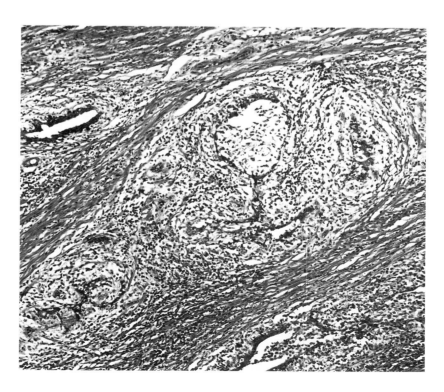

Fig. 24.1 Microscopic appearance of acute prostatitis. The acini are filled with pus and the surrounding tissue contains round cells and polymorphs (courtesy of Dr J.K. Oates).

into the rectum. To avoid a fistula it is better to drain the abscess into the urethra using a resecto-scope loop [2] (Fig. 24.2).

Recurrent acute prostatitis

Recurrent episodes of acute prostatitis are common and should respond to the usual treatment — a few days of a broad spectrum anti-biotic such as gentamycin or cinoxacin, followed by a long course of trimethoprim.

Chronic prostatitis

Chronic bacterial prostatitis

Chronic infection of the prostate is common after urethral surgery and is an almost constant feature of urethral strictures. Crystals or carbon particles added to the urine will find their way into the prostatic ducts by intraprostatic reflux [3,4] and this is often demonstrated in urethro-grams performed for stricture surgery (Fig. 24.3). Chronic prostatic infection is inevitable where there is an indwelling catheter, and is one of the principal hazards of this form of drainage in paraplegia.

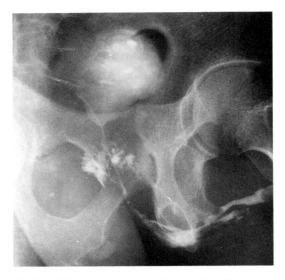

Fig. 24.3 Urethrograms often show reflux of contrast into the ducts of the prostate upstream of a stricture.

Clinical features

The clinical features of chronic bacterial prosta-titis are seldom specific: some have relapsing episodes of frequency and painful voiding. On examination, the prostate feels 'boggy' and may

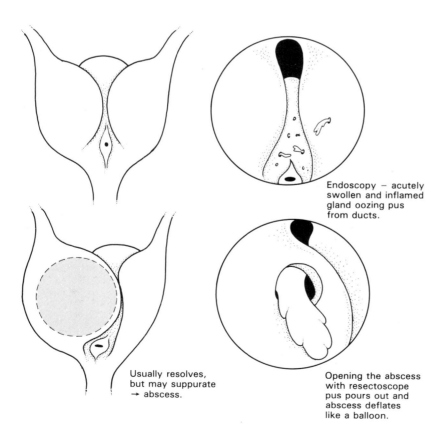

Endoscopy — acutely swollen and inflamed gland oozing pus from ducts.

Usually resolves, but may suppurate → abscess.

Opening the abscess with resectoscope pus pours out and abscess deflates like a balloon.

Fig. 24.2 Endoscopy during acute prostatitis shows a red, swollen gland with pus oozing from the ducts. An abscess forms a tense swollen mass which should be incised with the resectoscope loop so that pus drains into the urethra.

be tender on palpation. Calculi are often present in the radiograph, usually multiple and small (Fig. 24.4) but occasionally very large, and protruding into the lumen or the urethra or up into the bladder [5] (Fig. 24.5).

Investigations

It can be difficult to make the diagnosis of bacterial prostatitis if the urine is not infected. Culture of the fluid expressed from the urethra by prostatic massage is the traditional method, but is open to the error of contamination of this fluid by urethral organisms. Often microscopy and counting of the number of white cells per millilitre is performed in the first 10 ml of urine passed immediately after prostatic massage, and compared with the mid stream urine using a

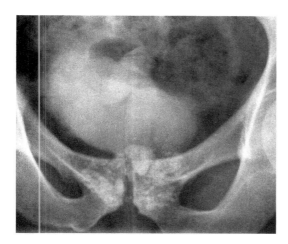

Fig. 24.4 Multiple small calculi are common in the prostate.

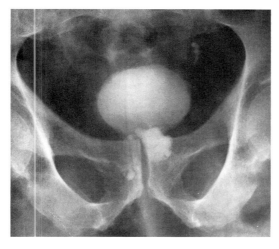

Fig. 24.5 Occasionally a large stone may fill one half of the prostate.

counting chamber [6]. A more sophisticated version of this test is as follows [6,7]:

1 The first 10 ml of voided urine (VB1) are cultured. They are thought to yield the innocent commensal organisms from the anterior urethra.
2 The midstream urine is then cultured (VB2) and is thought to show organisms present in the bladder.
3 Prostatic massage is performed and the expressed secretions cultured.
4 A third specimen of urine (VB3) passed immediately after prostatic massage is thought to carry organisms derived from the prostate itself. To make a diagnosis of bacterial prostatitis there should be 10 times more organisms in the prostatic secretions and VB3 than in VB1 or VB2.

Culture of the semen is rarely helpful: the bulk of the semen comes from the seminal vesicles anyway, and organisms cultured may have come from the urethra. Microscopy may be misleading, since immature sperms resemble pus cells.

Treatment

Antimicrobial agents can only penetrate the alkaline tissue of the prostate if they are themselves bases — hence the role of trimethoprim and cinoxacin [8]. In clinical practice, improvement often follows treatment with what should, in theory, be inappropriate agents such as the tetracyclines.

Tuberculous prostatitis

Most urologists will encounter this rare entity only once or twice in their careers. By the time it is diagnosed, the prostate has a characteristic endoscopic appearance, rather like a hollowed out hydronephrosis [9]. Biopsy of the shell of tissue remaining will give the diagnosis. Tuberculous prostatitis is usually associated with tuberculosis in the seminal vesicles, epididymes and vasa. A cold abscess may point in the perineum and form a fistula into the rectum [10–12]. Treatment with the usual antituberculous combination chemotherapy produces a complete resolution of the granuloma, but leaves the prostate curiously empty (see p. 160).

Brucellosis

Even more rare than tuberculosis, but a close mimic of this condition, is brucellosis which causes a chronic granuloma with patchy calcification [13]. It is also associated with epididymitis.

Other granulomas

The genitourinary tract is often involved in Behçet's syndrome and the prostate is often inflamed along with the urethra [14]. The prostate has also been the primary site for the onset of Wegener's granulomatosis [15] and malacoplakia [16].

Abacterial prostatitis

One cause of the absence of bacteria may be error in performing the localizing tests described above or, more often, previous treatment of the patient with antimicrobial agents. Special culture methods are required in order to identify fungi, *Mycoplasma* or *Chlamydia trachomatis*. Where *Chlamydia* is suspected it is often easier to give the patient 2 weeks of tetracycline. Because of this unsatisfactory system of diagnosis, the entity of non-bacterial prostatitis merges inexorably into the picture of prostatodynia. As with all inflammations for which no microorganism can be found responsible, it is tempting to look for an immunological cause, and antibody deposition has been found in some cases of abacterial prostatitis [17]. In others, resection of the tissue shows multiple eosinophils, suggesting some parasitic infection, but no specific parasite is ever found.

Prostatodynia

A large number of men complain of low back pain, discomfort in the perineum and frequency of micturition. Sometimes the pain is intense, and has features resembling proctalgia fugax in which there is spasm of the striated muscle of the floor of the pelvis. Rectal examination is difficult and painful. Urodynamic studies using electromyography may show failure of relaxation of the pelvic floor [18].

Investigations

Transrectal ultrasound reveals such a wide variation in the texture of the normal prostate that it is necessary to be very cautious before accepting this as evidence for some organic cause of pain in the prostate. There are an equal number of innocent variations from the normal anatomy of the seminal vesicles, and it is most unwise to attribute vague pain in the perineum to any of these [17] (see p. 615).

Often a borderline value for the prostate-specific antigen further confuses the clinical picture in these patients.

A careful and sympathetic history is probably the best investigation: it often elicits a psychosomatic problem, of which tension in the perineum is but a manifestation of more serious tensions elsewhere. Some sexual misdemeanour, real or imagined, and treatment of a supposed infection, often confirms the patient's suspicion that he has 'caught something' and deserves to be punished. Early referral of such a patient to a psychiatrist can prevent endless investigations and courses of futile treatment for a condition he has not got.

There are also men whose symptoms are equally severe and often related to violent exercise. No evidence of infection can be found. On attempting to pass a flexible cystoscope they are unable to relax their external sphincter and touching it with the tip of the instrument brings on the pain. Whatever its cause, this condition seems fortunately to be self-limiting, but it is useful to know that the discomfort is relieved by rectal suppositories of non-steroidal anti-inflammatory agents such as diclofenac.

Treatment of chronic prostatitis

Transurethral resection

Unless the patient has been clearly shown to have obstruction, with a restricted flow rate and a raised intravesical voiding pressure, it is most unwise to perform any kind of surgery on these patients, clinical experience showing again and again that it only makes them worse. The histology of the tissue shows only fibrosis (Fig. 24.6).

Thermotherapy

The marked subjective improvement in symptoms reported in most controlled trials with transrectal or transurethral hyperthermia for benign enlargement have been interpreted to suggest that heat may have a numbing effect on prostatic sensory nerves. If this is confirmed, it might be found to give relief to patients with chronic prostatitis and prostatodynia.

Haemospermia

Haemospermia is a very common symptom, and in nearly every case no cause will be found for it. But, before reassuring the patient, a careful

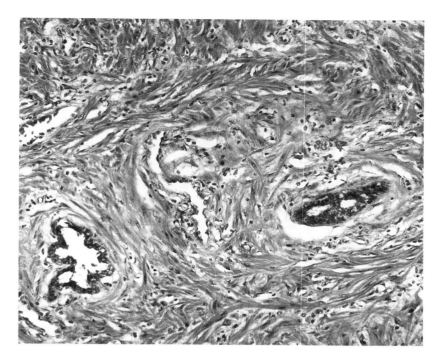

Fig. 24.6 Histology in chronic prostatitis: the glandular tissue is largely replaced with fibrous tissue (courtesy of Dr Jefferiss and Dr J.K. Oates).

physical examination must be performed: the author has seen this symptom in a patient who was found to have a seminoma, and in another who had carcinoma of the prostate. The literature records unusual tumours arising in the seminal vesicles and retrovesical hydatid. It can do no harm to have a prostate-specific antigen measurement done and, when in doubt, a transrectal ultrasound scan — a measure which will reinforce your reassurance to an often somewhat anxious patient [19—22].

References

1 Williams DI, Martin AG (1960) Prostatic abscess in the newborn. *Arch Dis Child* 35: 177.

2 Trapnell J, Roberts JBM (1970) Prostatic abscess. *Br J Surg* 57: 565.

3 Ramirez CT, Ruiz JA, Gomez AZ, Orgaz RE, Del Rio Samper S (1980) A crystallographic study of prostatic calculi. *J Urol* 124: 840.

4 Kirby RS, Lowe D, Bultitude MI, Shuttleworth KED (1982) Intraprostatic urinary reflux: an aetiological factor in abacterial prostatitis. *Br J Urol* 54: 729.

5 Fox M (1963) The natural history and significance of stone formation in the prostate gland. *J Urol* 89: 716.

6 Weidner W, Schiefer HG, Ringert RH (1993) New concepts in the pathogenesis and treatment of prostatitis. *Curr Opinion Urol* 3: 30.

7 de la Rosette JJMCH, Hubregtse MR, Meuleman EJH, Stolk-Engelaar MVM, DeBruyne FMJ (1993) Diagnosis and treatment of 409 patients with prostatitis syndromes. *Urology* 41: 301.

8 Schaeffer AJ, Darras FS (1990) The efficacy of norfloxacin in the treatment of chronic bacterial prostatitis refractory to trimethoprim—sulphamethoxazol and/or carbenicillin. *J Urol* 144: 690.

9 Loup J (1973) Isolated tuberculosis of the prostate. *Ann Urol* 7: 21.

10 Symes JM, Blandy JP (1973) Tuberculosis of the male urethra. *Br J Urol* 45: 432.

11 Sporer A, Auerbach O (1978) Tuberculosis of prostate. *Urology* 11: 362.

12 Teklu B, Ibrahim A (1990) Tuberculosis of prostate. *Saudi Med J* 11: 74.

13 Ibrahim AIA, Awad R, Shetty SD, Saad M, Bilal NE (1988) Genitourinary complications of brucellosis. *Br J Urol* 61: 294.

14 Kirkali Z, Yigitbasi O, Sasmaz R (1990) Urological aspects of Behçet's disease. *Br J Urol* 67: 638.

15 Murty GE, Powell PH (1991) Wegener's granulomatosis presenting as prostatitis. *Br J Urol* 67: 107.

16 Chantelos AE, Parker SH, Sims JE, Horne DW (1990) Malacoplakia of the prostate sonographically mimicking carcinoma. *Radiology* 177: 193.

17 Doble A, Walker MM, Harris JRW, Taylor-Robinson D, Witherow RO'N (1990) Intraprostatic antibody deposition in chronic abacterial prostatitis. *Br J Urol* 65: 599.

18 Fair WR, Sharer W (1986) Prostatitis, in: Blandy JP, Lytton B (eds) *The Prostate*, pp. 33—50. London: Butterworth.

19 Fletcher MS, Herzberg Z, Pryor JP (1981) The aetiology and investigation of haemospermia. *Br J Urol* 53: 669.

20 Whyman MR, Morris DL (1991) Retrovesical hydatid causing haemospermia. *Br J Urol* 68: 100.

21 Ganabathi K, Chadwick D, Feneley RCL, Gingell JC (1992) Haemospermia (review). *Br J Urol* 69: 225.

22 Fain JS, Cosnow I, King BF, Zincke H, Bostwock DG (1993) Cystosarcoma phyllodes of the seminal vesicle. *Cancer* 71: 2055.

Chapter 25: Prostate — benign enlargement

Aetiology

Hormonal factors

The relationship between the prostate and testosterone has been recognised for many years. John Hunter observed that in mammals with a mating season there was a regular swelling and shrinking of the prostate along with the testes [1]. It was noticed that benign enlargement did not develop in eunuchs castrated before puberty, and more recently it has also been observed in men with an inborn deficiency of 5-alpha reductase [2,3]. In practice, castration proved ineffective as therapy for benign enlargement of the prostate [4—8]. No undue incidence of prostatic hypertrophy is seen in acromegaly [9].

Genetic factors

Considerable variations have been reported in the incidence of benign enlargement of the prostate [10]. Comparative rarity in Africans probably reflects want of medical attention rather than a true racial difference [10,11] but elsewhere there is some evidence for genetic differences, e.g. more among those of Welsh [12] and Jewish ancestry [10], and less in natives of Hawaii than Caucasian visitors [13].

Pathology

The precursor of benign prostatic hypertrophy can be detected in the cranial inner prostate as small areas with pale staining and loose texture resembling mesenchyme [14]. Gradually, these areas coalesce and grow into the characteristic nodule of the prostate. It contains varying amounts of fibrous, muscular and acinar tissue (Fig. 25.1). The enlarging nodules squeeze the outer zone tissue into a shell which is left behind after enucleating the prostate, and is often erroneously referred to as the 'capsule' (see p. 370).

Outflow obstruction

In about 10% of males, changes in the prostate lead to outflow obstruction requiring surgical intervention [15]. The cause of obstruction varies among patients.

It may result from compression and elongation of the urethra, but the size of the lump of adenoma has little to do with the severity of the obstruction: the most severe outflow obstruction being often caused by small glands [16—18].

The smooth muscle component of the prostate may fail to relax in synchrony with the contraction of the detrusor, the detrusor may become weaker or there may be a mixture of both.

Response to obstruction

The detrusor responds to outflow resistance by hypertrophy which changes its structure and function. There is an increase in the thickness of its muscle fibres, and infiltration of collagen between them [19,20] (Fig. 25.2). The texture of the wall of the bladder changes from a fine felt to a coarse net, through the gaps of which the urothelium bulges out. The interior of the bladder now resembles the beams (trabeculae) of a vaulted roof. The herniated urothelium forms saccules and diverticula (Fig. 25.3).

These structural changes in the detrusor are accompanied by changes in their function: there is an increase in the voiding pressure within the bladder, while unwanted contractions occur before the bladder is full — detrusor instability — causing frequency and urgency of micturition [18].

Detrusor failure

If the obstruction is not relieved the detrusor will eventually fail. Failure may be gradual or sudden.

In gradual failure, the detrusor begins to be unable to empty the bladder completely and residual urine begins to accumulate. Infection in

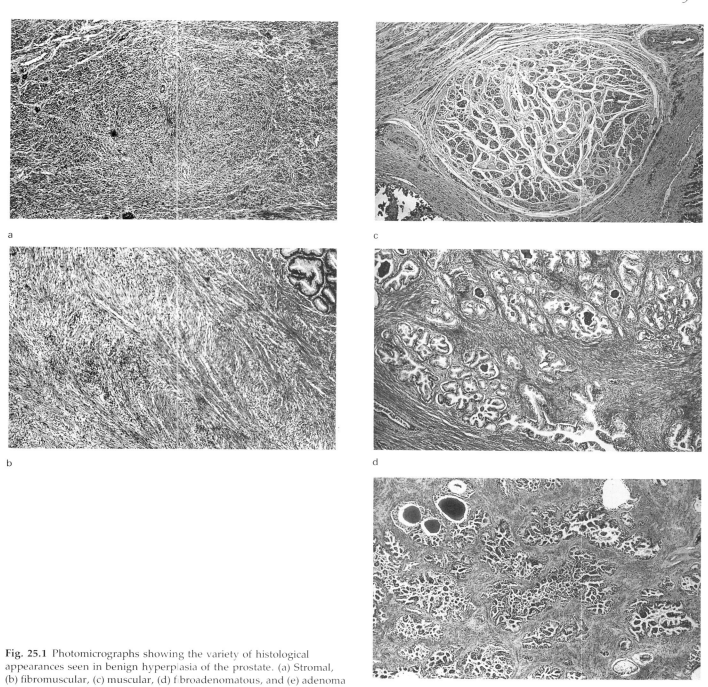

Fig. 25.1 Photomicrographs showing the variety of histological appearances seen in benign hyperplasia of the prostate. (a) Stromal, (b) fibromuscular, (c) muscular, (d) fibroadenomatous, and (e) adenoma (courtesy of Dr E.A. Courtland).

the residual urine may call for treatment. More often the residual urine causes no symptoms. At some stage, the picture is complicated by obstruction to the upper tracts which will occur whenever the voiding pressure in the bladder exceeds about 40 cmH$_2$O [21].

Slowly the detrusor changes from a vigorous pump into an inert bag, weakened by diverticula,

which will never recover its function even when obstruction has been relieved (Fig. 25.4).

Renal function

In practice, it is seldom possible to measure renal tubular function and by the time the serum creatinine is elevated to signify deterioration of

Before voiding

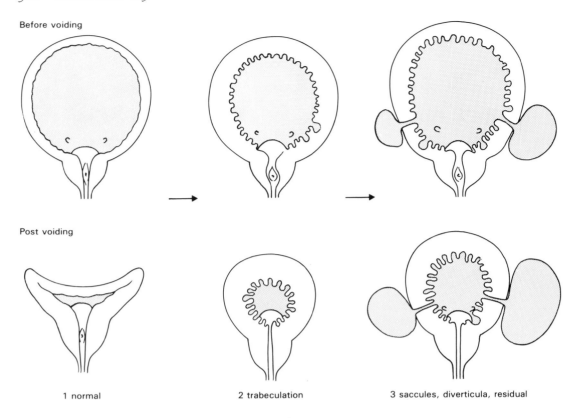

Post voiding

1 normal   2 trabeculation   3 saccules, diverticula, residual

Fig. 25.2 Diagram showing radiographic appearances of the normal and the obstructed bladder.

glomerular filtration, the ability of the tubules to conserve salt and water has become seriously impaired (see p. 58).

Sudden detrusor failure

Sudden failure of the detrusor gives rise to acute retention of urine. Many patients have no warning symptoms. Many others have had increasing frequency and a poor stream and have merely ignored them. Sometimes acute retention is precipitated by some acute local change in the prostate — inflammation or infarct. Occasionally, it is alcohol which has dulled the patient's awareness of the need to empty his bladder until it becomes overdistended.

Complications

Diverticula

Diverticula are herniations of bladder mucosa between hypertrophied bars of muscle. Once the prostatic obstruction has been corrected they can usually be disregarded [22] but they must be removed when they form a stone or cancer, or

when they are so large that they fill up whenever the detrusor is trying to expel urine so that symptoms persist (Figs 25.5 & 25.6).

Diverticulectomy

First cystoscope the patient and catheterize the ureter on the side of the diverticulum — it is much easier to do this through the cystoscope than across the open bladder. Through a Pfannenstiel incision divide the superior vesical pedicle on the side of the diverticulum to allow the bladder to be rolled up towards you (Fig. 25.7). Open the bladder, put a finger inside the diverticulum and cut down on its neck (Fig. 25.8). Trace the neck all round and close the hole in the bladder with catgut. The diverticulum is then dissected out (Fig. 25.9). If the diverticulum is grossly infected it may be safer to leave it alone and drain the cavity (Fig. 25.10).

Calculi

Stones in residual urine either become rounded like pebbles on the beach or assume the characteristic shape of the jack-stone (Fig. 25.11). They

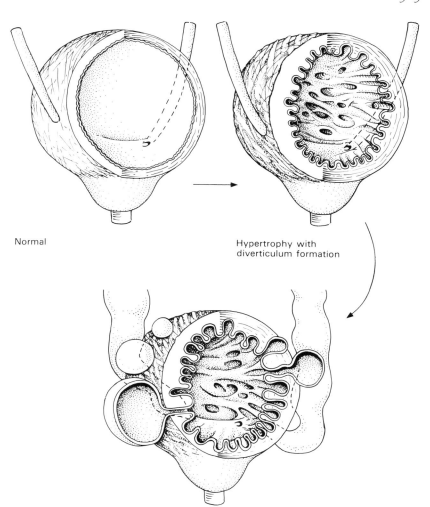

Fig. 25.3 Diagram showing changes in the detrusor secondary to outflow obstruction. The urothelium is herniated between gaps in the trabeculae to form saccules and diverticula. The ureters are hooked up and obstructed.

Normal

Hypertrophy with diverticulum formation

Detrusor failure with chronic retention

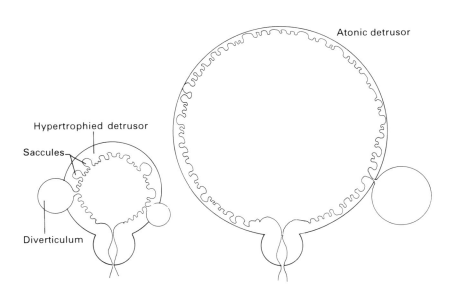

Fig. 25.4 Progressive failure of the detrusor.

Atonic detrusor

Hypertrophied detrusor

Saccules

Diverticulum

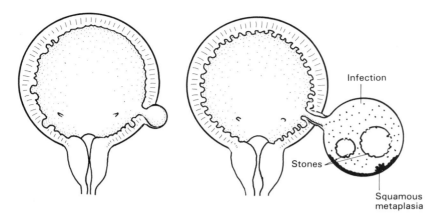

Fig. 25.5 Diagram of the progress of a diverticulum.

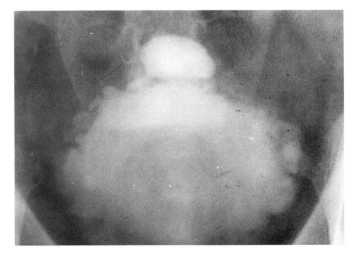

Fig. 25.6 Radiological appearances of the bladder in progressive prostatic obstruction.

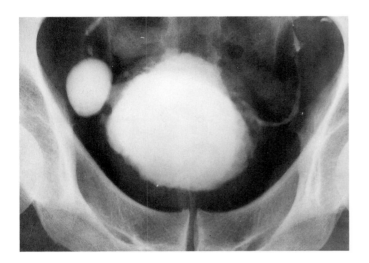

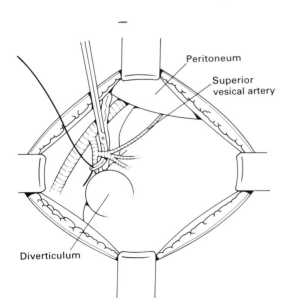

Fig. 25.7 Diverticulectomy. First divide the superior vesical artery between ligatures to mobilize the side of the bladder.

may cause haematuria, and are usually blackened from haemosiderin. They need to be crushed and evacuated — an operation which can be done at the time of transurethral prostatectomy (see p. 232). Stones are rare in men without outflow obstruction.

Infection

Infection in residual urine is seldom cured unless obstruction is relieved but when infection is the presenting feature, a period of drainage and antibiotic treatment is given first. Complications of infection such as epididymitis or septicaemia may be the presenting features of infection in residual urine behind a benign prostate.

Detrusor failure

The end-result of prostatectomy may be disappointing when there is detrusor failure. The

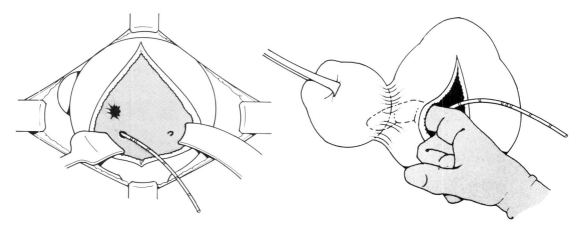

Fig. 25.8 Open the bladder. Protect the ureteric with a catheter. Lift up the diverticulum with a finger and cut down onto its neck.

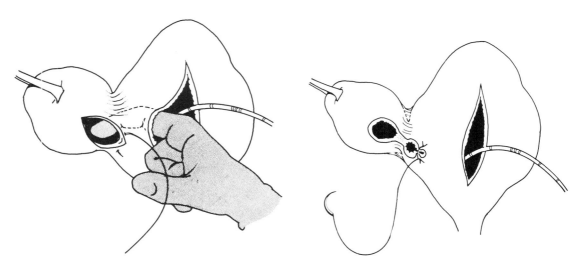

Fig. 25.9 Dissect all round the neck of the diverticulum, and close the hole in the bladder.

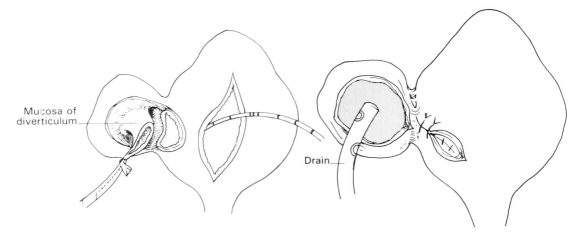

Fig. 25.10 When there has been much inflammation, it is safe to remove the mucosa and leave the tissues around the diverticulum and leave in a drain.

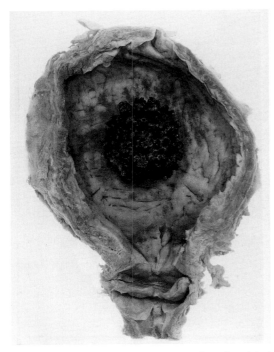

Fig. 25.11 Jack-stone calculus in a grossly trabeculated bladder.

irritability and instability of the detrusor may take several months to resolve after removal of the obstruction [23]. Detrusor instability persisting after prostatectomy may cause incontinence and so the utmost caution is needed before recommending prostatectomy for the patient whose symptoms include urge incontinence.

Instability is not the only change that may be irreversible. Sometimes the detrusor is so infiltrated with collagen that it can no longer empty the bladder under its own power. Even after prolonged catheter drainage the patient may only empty the bladder by abdominal straining and even then, emptying may be incomplete. This is acceptable so long as the residual urine is not infected.

Haematuria

When a patient with a seemingly benign enlargement of the prostate has haematuria, the first concern must be to rule out bladder cancer. At cystoscopy special care must be taken to look right over the top of the middle lobe, and to get a good view inside all the diverticula. If one is not sure that every diverticulum has been examined, check it with a computerized tomographic (CT) scan or pelvic ultrasound. Benign prostates may certainly bleed severely and bleeding may be the principal indication for prostatectomy. These

glands are often very large and require an open operation.

Clinical features

Early symptoms

The earliest symptoms of outflow obstruction are probably due to instability of the hypertrophied detrusor — the so-called 'irritative' symptoms, i.e. increased frequency with urgency of urination and a reduction in the voided volume. The patient may also notice slowing of the stream and difficulty in starting to urinate, most marked in the middle of the night and early morning. These symptoms are often regarded as 'obstructive'.

Much has been made of these early symptoms, and considerable effort has been put into attempting to draw up 'symptom scores' of which there are many versions, those of Boyarsky [24], Madsen [25], Hald [26], the American Urological Association [27] and the International Continence Society [28] being but some of the many schemes that have been proposed — mainly in order to attempt to evaluate new forms of medical or surgical treatment. However, when these symptom scores are compared with objective urodynamic evidence either of detrusor instability or of outflow obstruction there is a disappointing want of correlation [29,30].

The lesson is that these symptoms, which by tradition have been regarded as signifying early prostatic disease, are thoroughly unreliable.

Late symptoms

As obstruction progresses these symptoms may slowly worsen, or they may improve as the detrusor fails and the bladder begins to enlarge. Eventually, the patient may go on to develop retention with overflow, dribbling a little urine whenever he moves. His trousers are constantly wet.

At this stage renal function is often impaired and he is dehydrated, uraemic and anaemic. Confusion adds to his unhappy state. The wise urologist may get more useful information from the wife than the patient. Acute retention may occur without warning at any stage of this progression.

Physical signs

At first there are no physical signs. Rectal exam-

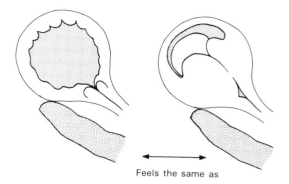

Feels the same as

Fig. 25.12 Digital rectal examination cannot distinguish between a tense bladder and a big benign prostate.

ination will always reveal some enlargement of the prostate, since this is inevitable with age but it gives no information about the state of the bladder.

Later the bladder will become palpable except in a very fat patient. The distended bladder makes the prostate seem larger than it really is on rectal examination: it is impossible to distinguish benign enlargement of the prostate from a full bladder under pressure (Fig. 25.12).

Investigations

In the patient with early outflow obstruction the really crucial measurement needed is the peak voiding pressure in the bladder since it is this which determines whether the kidneys are threatened or not. Full urodynamic studies are too invasive for every patient, but should certainly be performed in those who have frequency and whose flow remains good, to make quite sure that the frequency is not caused by some other lesion, e.g. neuropathy.

For most patients who do not have distressing frequency, the flow rate is easily measured (Fig. 25.13). A peak flow ($Q_{max.}$) of less than 12 ml/s with a voided volume over 150 ml is usually an index of outflow obstruction but the flow rate must be interpreted with common sense. Many patients find it difficult to void on request into a strange machine and it is always sensible to have the test repeated.

Residual urine is easy to measure with ultrasound which also shows the size of the prostate, the presence of a thick and trabeculated bladder and the presence of diverticula or stones (Fig. 25.14). In men who have had haematuria, an IVU is essential but not for those without.

It is prudent to check the prostate-specific antigen in all patients with 'prostatic' symptoms.

Chronic retention of urine

Often the distended bladder is palpable though it may not be in the midline. The ammoniacal reek of wet trousers signifying chronic retention with overflow should make one beware of impaired renal function. Abdominal palpation may fail to detect a very large bladder when it has lost its tone but this will be revealed by ultrasound.

The major problem is not how to correct out-

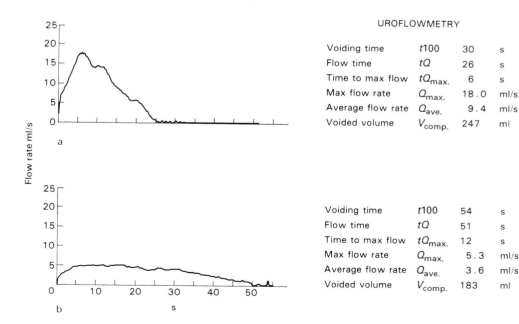

Fig. 25.13 Flow rate (a) normal and in benign enlargement of the prostate (b).

UROFLOWMETRY

Voiding time	$t100$	30	s
Flow time	tQ	26	s
Time to max flow	$tQ_{max.}$	6	s
Max flow rate	$Q_{max.}$	18.0	ml/s
Average flow rate	$Q_{ave.}$	9.4	ml/s
Voided volume	$V_{comp.}$	247	ml

Voiding time	$t100$	54	s
Flow time	tQ	51	s
Time to max flow	$tQ_{max.}$	12	s
Max flow rate	$Q_{max.}$	5.3	ml/s
Average flow rate	$Q_{ave.}$	3.6	ml/s
Voided volume	$V_{comp.}$	183	ml

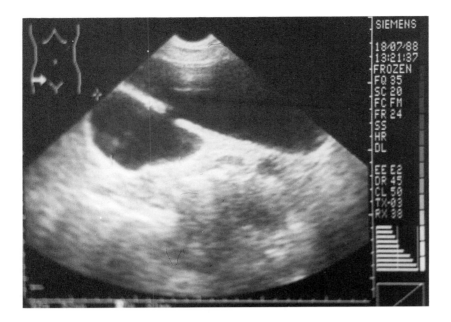

Fig. 25.14 Abdominal ultrasound scan showing a large residual urine and a diverticulum (courtesy of Dr William Hately).

flow obstruction but how to deal with the consequences of obstructive nephropathy. As soon as the bladder is decompressed there may be a tremendous diuresis and these dehydrated men may require intensive intravenous fluid and salt replacement to prevent a decline into hypotension. The correction of salt and water deficiency may take 10 days or more and the anaemia may require transfusion. In the first instance the man should be catheterized. Operation to correct outflow obstruction should be deferred until the patient has reached a steady state.

It is in these patients that the postoperative course is less than perfect. Loss of tubular function may continue the need for water and salt supplement, although in the end it may recover [31]. Irreversible deterioration of the detrusor may mean continuing difficulty in emptying the bladder.

Management

Acute retention

On admission, the patient is in great pain and needs urgent catheterization and pain relieving drugs if this must be delayed. Very occasionally, a warm bath may allow the urine to come away and take the urgency out of the situation. If the patient cannot void then, a narrow (14–16 Charrière) two-way catheter is passed with aseptic precautions. If the catheter does not pass easily, a suprapubic cystostomy cannula is passed (Fig. 25.15).

Percutaneous suprapubic cystostomy

Shave the pubic hair about 5 cm (2 in) all round the chosen site which is a finger's breadth above the symphysis. Infiltrate the skin at the chosen site and for 2.5 cm (1 in) around the area with local anaesthetic and continue to infiltrate down to the bladder until urine is aspirated. This shows how far from the skin the bladder is situated. Using a disposable trocar thrust it firmly into the bladder, withdraw the trocar and advance the catheter until it is well into the bladder. Suture the catheter to the skin.

In the usual patient, an old man in whom acute retention follows on a crescendo of symptoms, there is no doubt that prostatectomy is indicated and it should be done without unnecessary delay. When the patient has no such symptoms, it is reasonable to allow his bladder to rest for a few days and see if he can void again once the catheter is removed or when the suprapubic cystostomy is occluded.

Chronic retention

Chronic retention demands prostatectomy, but only when the patient's general condition has been adequately corrected as outlined above.

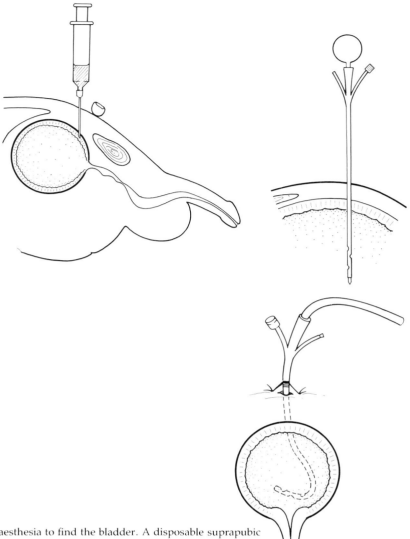

Fig. 25.15 Infiltrating local anaesthesia to find the bladder. A disposable suprapubic cannula is passed down the track.

Prostatism

Patients who fall into neither of these categories, but have suggestive symptoms, require a flow rate and ultrasound measurement of their residual urine and it is wise also to check their prostate-specific antigen whatever the prostate feels like. When there is a large residual urine and a very poor flow rate, treatment should be recommended.

When there is a reasonable flow and negligible residual urine, it is wise to temporize. Nothing is lost by waiting to see how the patient gets on over the next 3–6 months. Many patients go through a stage when their prostate causes symptoms, but they get better spontaneously. All clinical trials for new medications show a 'placebo' effect in about 30% of patients.

Special care is needed in the patient with severe frequency and urge incontinence especially if there is pain or dysuria. Carcinoma *in situ*, and a neuropathic bladder are notorious pitfalls. Make sure the urine has been examined on several occasions for malignant cells. Obtain the advice of a neurologist, who may detect Parkinson's disease or multiple system atrophy. A complete urodynamic assessment is necessary even if it means a suprapubic line.

In summary, refrain from surgical intervention when there is a reasonable flow rate and no residual urine. Have a complete urodynamic investigation and cystoscope the patient to rule out carcinoma *in situ* and rare forms of chronic cystitis.

Treatment

'Medical'

Alpha antagonists

In men with a small prostate and clear evidence of outflow obstruction an alpha blocker may relax the smooth muscle of the bladder neck and prostate [32,33]. At first, phenoxybenzamine was used but blocks both $alpha_1$ and $alpha_2$ components. The prostatic smooth muscle is of the $alpha_1$ type for which prazosin, indoramin or terazosin are specific. They may relax the smooth muscle in the bladder neck and prostate and lead to a useful improvement in flow rate, with disappearance of residual urine and loss of the symptoms of frequency, hesitancy and nocturia.

Since the $alpha_1$ antagonists paralyse the bladder neck most of the semen flows back into the bladder on ejaculation. Men must be warned of this side effect, and also of the risks of fainting when they begin the course of treatment.

$Alpha_1$ antagonists are useful in establishing the diagnosis of bladder neck obstruction in younger patients who may then choose between continuing with the medication or undergoing a bladder neck incision. A good symptomatic result from $alpha_1$ blockers ensures a good result from a bladder neck incision.

In older men, where the obstruction is probably largely due to the bulk of the adenoma, alpha blockers are largely ineffective.

Hormones

Many medications are at present undergoing trials which aim to imitate the effects of castration on the prostate. They include luteinizing hormone-releasing hormone agonists which block the output of testosterone from the testes and adrenals [34,35]; 5-alpha reductase inhibitors which stop testosterone being activated to dihydrotestosterone [36–38]; and drugs which act on the cytosol receptors for dihydrotestosterone [39]. It is claimed that they result in a reduction in the size of the gland by shrinking the acinar component, and that this results in an increase in peak flow rate and diminution in residual urine. It is possible that they might be even more effective if used in combination with $alpha_1$ blockers.

Catheters and stents

From the beginning of time men with prostatic obstruction passed catheters to relieve retention. The results were dreadful: pain, infection, bleeding and false passages were common complications in the best of hands [40]. 'Catheter schooling' was the standard management for prostatic obstruction as late as 1900. Transvesical prostatectomy, for all its dangers and complications, was hailed as a revolution when compared to the horrors of the catheter life [41].

There are still many very old men who are unfit for any operation and who cannot catheterize themselves. A small indwelling catheter may be the only alternative. It is important to make sure the catheter is narrow (less than 16 Charrière) made of a non-irritating substance (e.g. silicone elastomer) and changed at regular intervals.

Several different types of short catheter have been devised which fit inside the prostatic urethra, but leave the external sphincter intact (Fig. 25.16). These are made of various inert metals or plastics. They can be fitted with only local anaesthesia. Their design is constantly being improved. At present they tend to become blocked, embedded in the urethra, and more or less encrusted with stone [42,43].

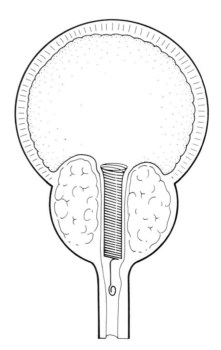

Fig. 25.16 Several different types of short indwelling catheters have been designed to lie in the prostatic urethra.

Endoscopic operations

Bladder neck incision

The bladder neck is divided through a resectoscope, either under general or local anaesthesia. The incision is made with a diathermy electrode or the neodymium-yttrium aluminium garnet (YAG) laser which is said to cause neither pain nor bleeding (Fig. 25.17).

Just where to cut through the bladder neck is a matter of choice. Many choose 5 and 7 o'clock, but this is near the neurovascular bundles supplying the corpora cavernosa and to avoid impotence it is probably better to make the cut almost anywhere else around the circle of the neck of the bladder. Wherever the bladder neck is incised, the patient must be warned of retrograde ejaculation. The long-term results are claimed to be as good as those of transurethral resection [44−47].

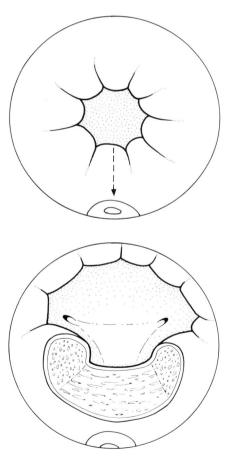

Fig. 25.17 Bladder neck incision. A 6 o'clock incision avoids damage to the penile neurovascular bundles. The incision goes right through the bladder neck which is seen to gape widely.

Transurethral resection of the prostate

This is the standard operation for all but the largest prostates [48]. The purpose of the operation is to remove enough of the obstructing tissue from the cranial inner zone of the prostate to allow the bladder to empty freely.

Transurethral resection of the prostate has two main advantages: (a) it is safer than any open operation and can be offered to men who would be unfit for open surgery; and (b) it has a lower incidence of complications such as deep vein thrombosis, pulmonary embolism and chest infection.

For many years, the main advantage of transurethral resection was its safety [41]. As anaesthesia and postoperative care improved, the mortality for all operations fell to a level where it was difficult to detect any difference.

In recent years, doubts have been cast on the value of transurethral resection. Retrospective studies, which compared those performed some 20 years ago by surgeons who may not all have been adept at transurethral resection with open cases, suggest that more patients operated on transurethrally developed heart disease over the following 15 years [49,50].

Technique

Immediately before prostatectomy the urethra and bladder are examined to rule out strictures, cancers, diverticula and stones.

There are several different styles of transurethral resection and readers should refer to appropriate texts for details [48].

Instruments

Most surgeons use the 30° telescope for resection but beginners may find it easier to keep orientated if they use a 0° telescope with its appropriate sheath (Fig. 25.18). When the gland is very large, a continuous irrigating sheath helps to keep the field clear (Fig. 25.19). The operation has become a great deal more comfortable for the surgeon and instructive for the assistants if closed circuit television is used [51].

Objectives

Transurethral resection removes all the adenoma upstream of the verumontanum and leaves behind a shell of connective tissue and compressed adenoma. Great care is taken to pre-

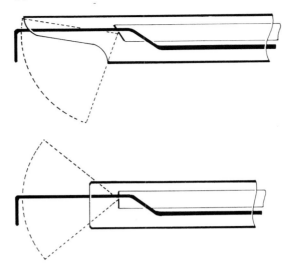

Fig. 25.18 Above, the usual field of view with a 30° telescope and below, the view with a 0° telescope.

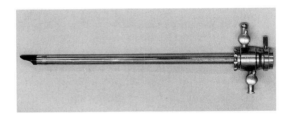

Fig. 25.19 Continuous irrigating sheath.

serve the verumontanum since the intramural sphincter lies so close to it. The neurovascular bundles to the penis are also very close to the membranous urethra and diathermy must be used sparingly in their vicinity. The tissue downstream of the verumontanum is left behind [52] (Fig. 25.20).

Steps of the operation

Begin by identification of the verumontanum and sphincter. Then the circular fibres of the bladder neck are revealed by resecting the overlying middle lobe tissue (Fig. 25.21). Bleeding from the 5 and 7 o'clock arteries of the prostate is controlled by diathermy. The lateral lobe on one side is freed from the bladder neck and capsule by cutting a trench near the midline starting at 1 or 11 o'clock to allow the bulk of the lateral lobe to fall backwards (Fig. 25.22). Bleeding from the anterior prostatic arteries is sealed with coagulation. The remainder of the lateral lobe adenoma is then removed with a series of downwardly directed cuts, exposing the 'capsule', i.e.

the thin layer of remaining adenoma which is right up against periprostatic fat and veins. After one lobe has been resected, the same procedure is applied to the other side (Fig. 25.23). It only remains to clean away any little tags of tissue which have been overlooked, and to obtain perfect haemostasis by coagulation. Throughout the resection the surgeon must continually refer back to the landmarks of the verumontanum, sphincter and bladder neck.

Postoperative management

A three-way irrigating catheter is used by most surgeons, saline being used as the irrigating fluid. The irrigation is stopped when the effluent is reasonably clear and the catheter can usually be removed after 48 h. Others prefer to use a two-way catheter, and rely on intravenous fluids and a diuretic to keep the bladder irrigated. Antibiotics are given when the patient has been catheterized before the operation or if the urine is known to be infected. Patients may go home on the third or fourth day, but are advised not to take vigorous exercise for another 10 days because of the risk of secondary haemorrhage.

Complications

Haemorrhage. Primary haemorrhage on the operating table is the major complication of all forms of prostatectomy, and transurethral resection is no exception. Bleeding can largely be reduced by a preliminary coagulation of the rim of the prostate at the 2, 10, 5 and 7 o'clock positions where the prostatic arteries are found.

Perforation. The capsule is thinner than the loop of the resectoscope [52] so perforations are inevitable. Only when there is a large perforation and the irrigating fluid cannot be recovered is it necessary to insert a drain into the retropubic space.

Perforation into the peritoneal cavity is virtually unknown in transurethral resection, but should it occur, a laparotomy must be done without delay to control bleeding and make sure the intestine has not been damaged by the diathermy.

Perforation into the rectum may occur in cancer of the prostate where normal landmarks are distorted or absent. Small holes will usually heal with a period of catheter drainage. The main risk is that massive faecal contamination of the

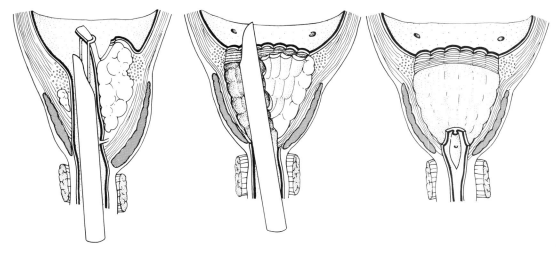

a   Transurethral prostatectomy

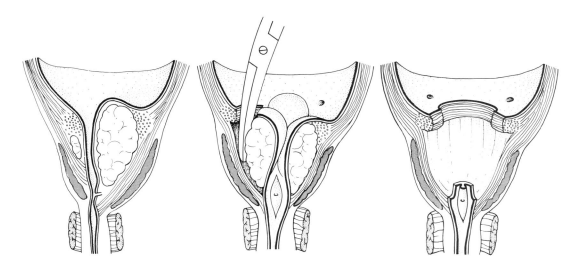

b   Enucleative prostatectomy

Fig. 25.20 The objective of transurethral resection (a) is the same as that of open prostatectomy (b), namely to remove all the tissue from the cranial inner zone.

urinary tract will cause renal infection and septicaemia. If there is any suggestion of urosepsis a loop colostomy is performed and the rectosigmoid irrigated. Later the fistula can be closed (see p. 357).

Haemolysis. If distilled water is used as an irrigant, there is a risk of haemolysis leading to tubular obstruction by haemoglobin and acute renal failure. Non-electrolyte solutions that do not haemolyse the blood should always be used, e.g. glycine, glucose or one of the proprietary sorbitol−mannitol mixtures.

TUR syndrome — dilutional hyponatraemia. Even if solutions are used that cannot cause haemolysis, if a sufficiently large volume enters the vascular space there will be dilution of the plasma electrolytes, especially sodium, and disturbance of muscle and nerve function.

This syndrome is rare, because intravasated fluid is usually rapidly excreted by diuresis but in very frail old men this diuresis may be prevented by an inappropriate secretion of the antidiuretic hormone.

Precautions to avoid intravasation of irrigating fluid include (a) keeping the level of the fluid

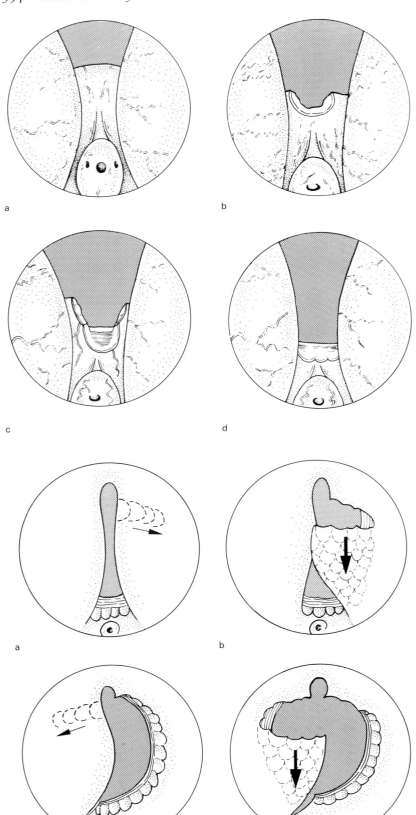

Fig. 25.21 (a) The verumontanum is identified. (b–d) The middle lobe is resected until the bladder neck is visible.

Fig. 25.22 (a) A trench is made between the bladder neck and adenoma at 1 o'clock, allowing the lateral lobe to drop back. (b) The lateral lobe is then resected. (c & d) The same thing is done on the other side.

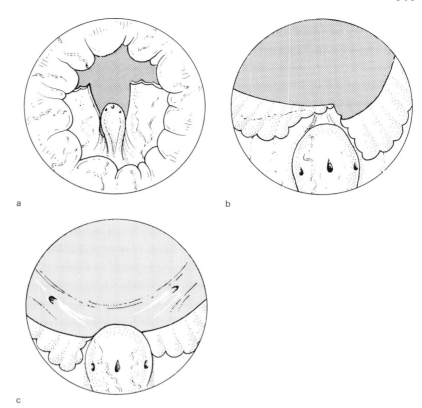

Fig. 25.23 Any little bits of adenoma that have been left behind are removed (a & b) especially around the apices and (c) the verumontanum.

below 20 cm above the operating table; (b) stopping the resection if large veins are opened; (c) using an irrigating resectoscope; and (d) inserting a suprapubic cannula.

The escape of fluid into the patient can be monitored with a scale under the operating table that continually weighs the patient. Other methods include the use of a sodium-sensing electrode into a vein, and measuring the concentration of alcohol in the patient's expired air after adding a minute quantity of ethanol to the irrigating fluid [53,54].

The clinical features include restlessness and hypertension, followed by epileptic fits and transient blindness and hemiparesis. The diagnosis is confirmed by measuring the serum sodium.

No treatment is needed if the patient is well, and is having a good diuresis. When there are uncontrollable epileptic fits, 50 ml of hypertonic solution (29.2% saline) may be given intravenously — preferably through a central venous cannula [55,56].

Incontinence. The risk of incontinence after transurethral resection varies in different series. Its cause is obvious in those cases where endoscopy shows a defect in the intramural sphincter (Fig. 25.24).

In other cases, urodynamic studies may reveal a very unstable detrusor or overt neuropathy. One should certainly reconsider the diagnosis and again think about the possibility of having overlooked carcinoma *in situ* [57,58].

Impotence. The risk of impotence after prostatectomy is about 10% and it increases with the age of the patient and the ill-health of his sexual partner [59,60]. Since the neurovascular bundles to the penis are so close to the verumontanum, coagulation in this region may damage them. The elderly man who is still sexually active should be warned of this risk, as well as the 60% chance of retrograde ejaculation.

Late cardiovascular complications. Retrospective studies of patients treated 20 years ago suggest that those who underwent transurethral resection had a higher incidence of late cardiovascular events than did those who were treated by open prostatectomy [49,50]. These studies have led to a re-evaluation of the strain on the heart during resection. It has been found that if irrigant fluid is used at room temperature some patients show

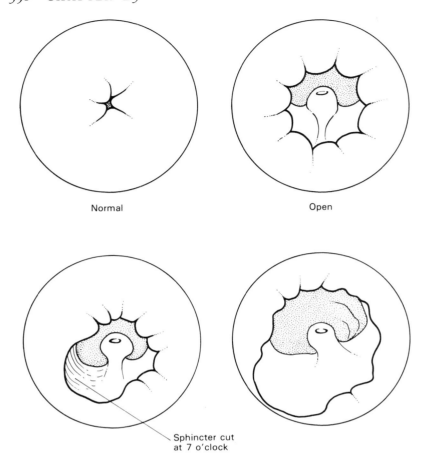

Normal

Open

Sphincter cut
at 7 o'clock

Fig. 25.24 Urethroscopic appearances after the supramembranous intramural sphincter has been cut at 7 o'clock.

significant cardiovascular strain and this can be avoided by keeping the irrigant at normal body temperature [61]. On first principles, it would also seem that all the normal clotting mechanisms are more likely to work best at normal body temperature.

Laser prostatectomy

Recently, the neodymium-YAG laser has been adapted so that it coagulates the tissue of the prostate, and in effect performs a TURP under vision without bleeding. The coagulated tissue is passed by the patient over the next few weeks, during which a suprapubic tube may have to be worn [62]. In later modifications the tissue is completely vapourized by the laser, and a channel created from the beginning. It is too early to evaluate the short-term safety or long-term efficacy of these methods (Fig. 25.25).

Hyperthermia

The prostate can be heated by different types of microwave transmitter put in the urethra or rectum (Fig. 25.26). Optimistic early reports [63–65] were later tempered by more modest claims for subjective improvement and most recently, have been refuted by careful controlled studies which suggest that these techniques are probably valueless [66,67].

Hypothermia

Freezing the prostate was advocated with equal enthusiasm in a former generation [68] but has been given up [69] (Fig. 25.27).

Balloon dilatation

The notion of forcibly dilating the prostate with a balloon occurred to Philip Syng Physick [70], of Philadelphia, one of John Hunter's pupils. It is revived [71] every 50 years or so but always proves a disappointment (Fig. 25.28).

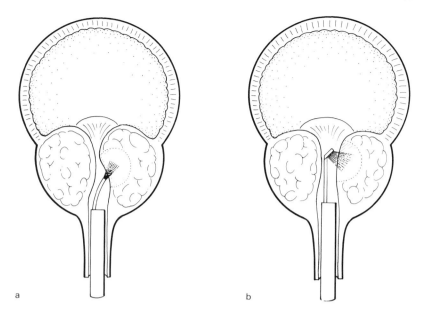

Fig. 25.25 The principle of laser prostatectomy. (a) With a quartz fibre, or (b) a mirror, the laser beam is directed ahead or sideways to coagulate the prostate.

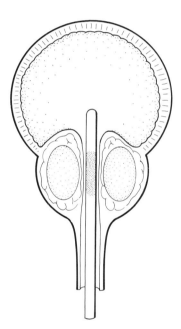

Fig. 25.26 One of many instruments designed to cook the prostate using microwave energy: a coolant is circulated to prevent burning the urethra.

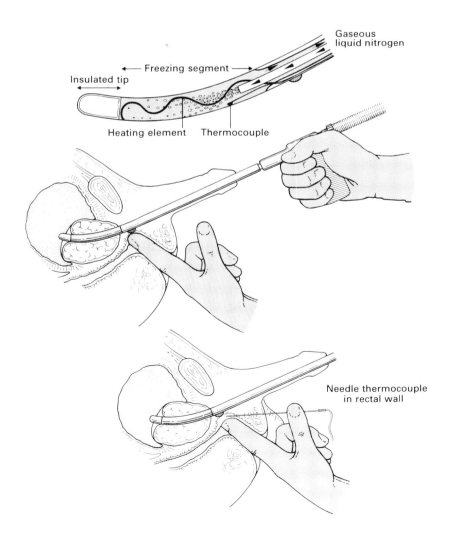

Fig. 25.27 The principle of cryosurgery. The prostate was destroyed by an ice-ball.

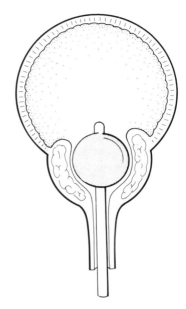

Fig. 25.28 The principle of balloon dilatation of the prostate. A balloon is forcibly expanded inside the prostate.

Open prostatectomy

Transvesical prostatectomy

This is the classic procedure: easy, quick and requiring no special skill. Through a cystostomy the index finger is forced into the internal meatus until it splits to open a plane of cleavage between the adenoma and the so-called 'surgical capsule' (Fig. 25.29). The finger enucleates the adenoma. Once the adenoma is removed there may be a

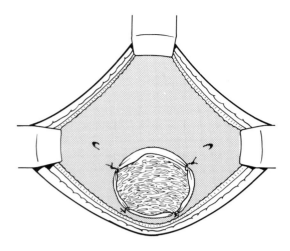

Fig. 25.30 After the adenoma has been enucleated sutures at each quadrant help to control bleeding.

torrent of bleeding from the arteries at the neck of the bladder which are difficult to see or suture. Large stitches are placed with a 'boomerang' needle at the neck of the bladder (Fig. 25.30). The difficulty of securing precise haemostasis is the reason why this operation was replaced by that of Millin [73,74].

Retropubic prostatectomy (Millin's operation)

Make a Pfannenstiel incision. Wipe away the fat around the preprostatic veins and divide them between suture ligatures. The layer of areolar tissue and fat is now carefully wiped laterally with a Lahey pledget in the hope of preserving the neurovascular bundles of the penis (Fig. 25.31).

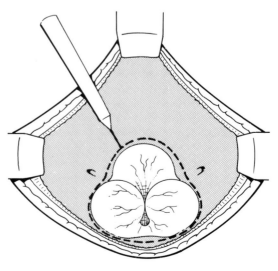

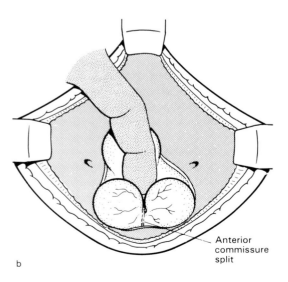

Anterior
commissure
split

Fig. 25.29 (a) Freyer's transvesical prostatectomy. The salient lobes of the prostate are circumcised with the diathermy, and (b) a finger forced into the internal meatus to split the anterior commissure, and then enucleate the adenoma.

a   b

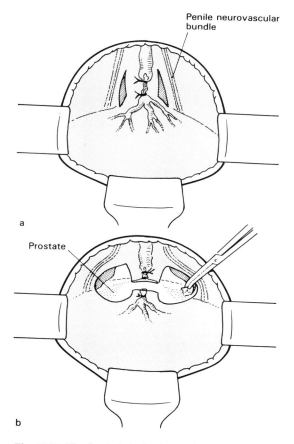

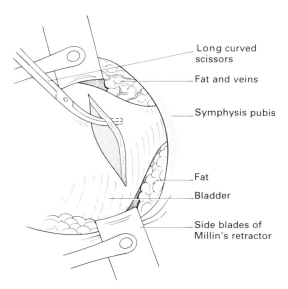

Fig. 25.33 The plane between capsule and adenoma is developed with scissors.

Fig. 25.31 The fascia is incised on either side of the dorsal veins which are then sutured and divided (a) and the penile neurovascular bundle is displaced laterally and backwards (b).

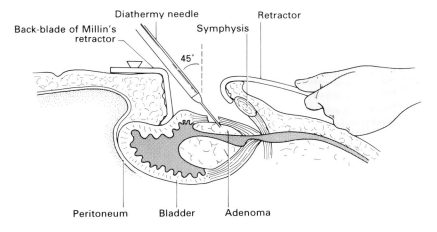

Fig. 25.32 The capsule of the prostate is incised with the diathermy to expose the adenoma.

Make a transverse incision with a diathermy needle at the junction of the bladder and prostate using the coagulating current to control bleeding (Fig. 25.32). As the prostate is thin anteriorly, the incision needs only to be 2 or 3 mm deep before the inner zone adenoma is exposed (Fig. 25.33). The plane of cleavage between 'capsule' and 'adenoma' is opened with scissors on each side.

A finger is firmly thrust into the lumen of the prostatic urethra, breaking through the thin anterior commissure. The nipple of the verumontanum can be felt. Pressure down on either side of the verumontanum breaks into the plane between adenoma and capsule (Fig. 25.34) and leaves a strip of intact urothelium along the midline.

First one lateral lobe and then the other are enucleated with the finger and brought out into the wound (Fig. 25.35). Opening a bladder neck spreader reveals the middle lobe, attached to one or other lateral lobe (Fig. 25.36). This is dissected from the bladder neck with the diathermy needle leaving only the strip of mucosa leading down to the verumontanum which is cut across well proximal to the sphincter.

The retropubic approach permits perfect haemostasis. First a 2-0 absorbable suture is passed through the bladder, bladder neck and capsule at each end of the transverse incision to control bleeding from the main prostatic arteries (Figs 25.37 & 25.38). Smaller vessels along the

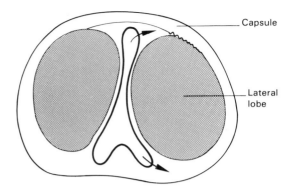

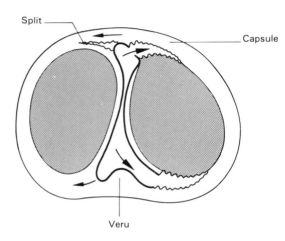

Fig. 25.34 First on one side, then the other, the plane between adenoma and capsule is developed with the finger. Then a second plane is developed between the groove at the side of the verumontanum so as to liberate the lateral lobe completely.

cut edge of the bladder are underrun with fine catgut.

Occasionally an artery continues to spurt from inside the prostatic capsule which is difficult to see. The capsule may be everted by a suture which picks up the lining (Fig. 25.39). Traction on the suture reveals the source of the bleeding which is controlled by suture ligature or diathermy.

A three-way irrigating catheter is put in the bladder; the wound is closed with catgut and a suitable drain. The drain is removed at 48 h and the catheter on the fourth or fifth day when, if generally well, the patient may go home. The skin sutures are usually removed after a week.

Postoperative management

If irrigation is used, it is discontinued when clear. The drain is removed at 24 h and the catheter on the fifth postoperative day. Otherwise the precautions are similar to those for transurethral resection.

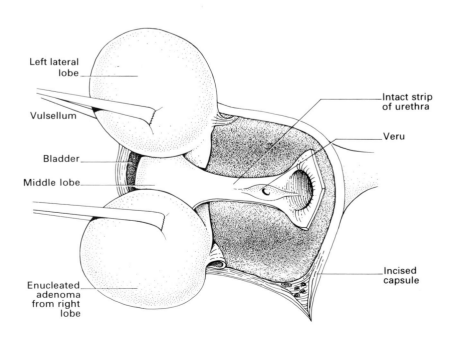

Fig. 25.35 Both lateral lobes are now delivered out of the prostatic shell.

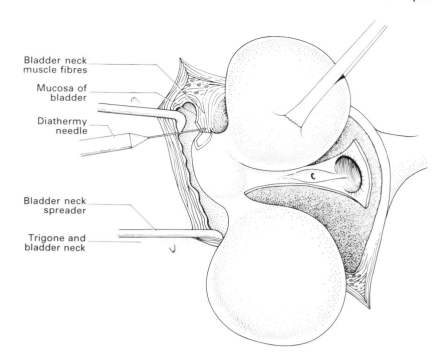

Bladder neck
muscle fibres

Mucosa of
bladder

Diathermy
needle

Bladder neck
spreader

Trigone and
bladder neck

Fig. 25.36 The middle
lobe is dissected from
the bladder neck.

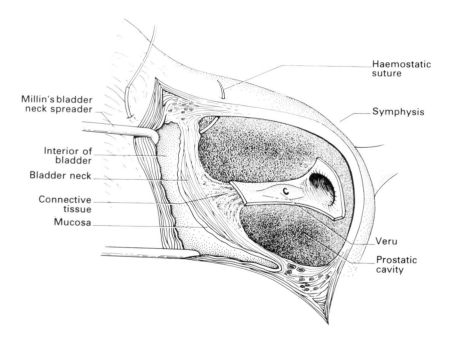

Haemostatic
suture

Symphysis

Millin's bladder
neck spreader

Interior of
bladder

Bladder neck

Connective
tissue

Mucosa

Veru

Prostatic
cavity

Fig. 25.37 Badenoch's
sutures are placed at
each corner to secure the
main arteries of the
prostate.

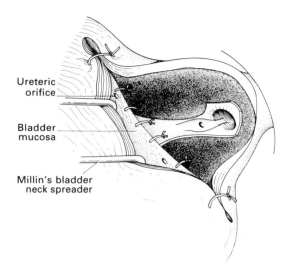

Fig. 25.38 Haemostasis is completed by sutures at the bladder neck.

Ureteric orifice

Bladder mucosa

Millin's bladder neck spreader

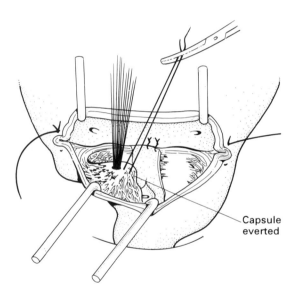

Capsule everted

Fig. 25.39 Bleeding from inside the prostatic capsule can be located by everting the capsule with a suture.

References

1 Palmer JF (1835) (ed.) *The Works of John Hunter*. London: Longman.

2 Harrison R (1893) Castration in enlargement of the prostate. *Br Med J* 2: 798.

3 Walsh PC, Madden JD, Harrod MJ, Goldstein JL, MacDonald PC, Wilson JD (1974) Familial incomplete male pseudohermaphroditism type 2: decreased dihydrotestosterone formation in pseudovaginal perineoscrotal hypospadias. *New Engl J Med* 291: 944.

4 White JW (1893) The present position of the surgery of the hypertrophied prostate. *Ann Surg* 18: 152.

5 Cabot AT (1896) The question of castration for enlarged prostate. *Trans Amer Surg Assoc* 14: 189.

6 Kelsey CB (1896) Failure of castration to cause atrophy of the prostate. *Med Rec* 49: 727.

7 Albarran J, Motz B (1878) Étude experimentale et clinique sur le traitement de l'hypertrophie de la prostate par les operations pratiquées sur les testicules et ses annèxes. *Ann Mal Org Gén Urin* 16: 130.

8 Mansell-Moullin CW (1892) *The Operative Treatment of Enlargement of the Prostate*. London: Bale.

9 Mostofi FK (1970) Benign hyperplasia of the prostate gland, in: Campbell MF, Harrison JH (eds) *Urology*, Vol. 2, p. 1065. Philadelphia: WB Saunders.

10 Lytton B (1989) Demographic factors in benign prostatic hyperplasia, in: Fitzpatrick J, Krane RJ (eds) *The Prostate*, pp. 85–90. Edinburgh: Churchill Livingstone.

11 Lissoos I (1973) Simple prostatic hyperplasia in the Bantu. *S Afr Med J* 47: 389.

12 Ashley DJB (1966) Observations on the epidemiology of prostatic hyperplasia in Wales. *Br J Urol* 38: 567.

13 Conger KB (1947) Racial incidence of prostatism in Hawaii: a report of 172 consecutive cases. *J Urol* 58: 444.

14 Ahluwalia MS, Tandon HD (1965) Nodular hyperplasia of the prostate in North India: an autopsy study. *J Urol* 93: 94.

15 Lytton B, Emery JM, Harvard BM (1968) The incidence of benign prostatic obstruction. *J Urol* 99: 639.

16 Kidd F (1910) *Urinary Surgery: A Review*. London: Longmans & Green.

17 Turner-Warwick RT (1979) A urodynamic view of bladder outlet obstruction in the male and its clinical implications. *Urol Clin N Am* 6: 171.

18 McGuire EJ (1992) The role of urodynamic investigation in assessment of benign prostatic hypertrophy. *J Urol* 148: 1133.

19 Gosling JA, Dixon JS (1980) Structure of trabeculated detrusor smooth muscle in cases of prostatic hypertrophy. *Urol Int* 35: 351.

20 Susset JG (1981) Effect of prostatic obstruction on detrusor function. *Proc A U A* Abstract 347.

21 McGuire EJ, Woodside JR, Bordon TA, Weiss RM (1980) Predictive value of urodynamic testing in myelodysplastic patients. *J Urol* 126: 205.

22 Geridzen RG, Futter NG (1982) Ten year review of vesical diverticula. *Urology* 20: 33.

23 Appell RA (1981) Bladder instability in patients with prostatic hypertrophy. *Postgrad Med J* 57: 640.

24 Boyarsky S, Jones G, Poulsen DF, Prout GR Jr (1977) A new look at bladder neck obstruction by the Food and Drug Administration regulators: guidelines for the investigation of benign prostatic hypertrophy. *Trans Am Ass GU Surg* 68: 29.

25 Madsen PO, Inversen P (1983) A point system for selecting operative candidates, in: Hinman F Jr (ed.) *Benign Prostatic Hyperplasia*, pp. 763–5. New York: Springer.

26 Hald T, Nordling J, Andersen JT, Bilde T, Meyhoff HH, Walter S (1991) A patient-weighted symptom score system in the evaluation of uncomplicated benign prostatic hyperplasia. *Scan J Urol Nephrol Suppl* 138: 59.

27 Barry MJ, Fowler FJ Jr, O'Leary MP *et al.* (1992) American Urological Association index for benign

prostatic hyperplasia. *J Urol* 148: 1549.

28 Abrams PH (1992) Benign prostatic hyperplasia — symptoms and scoring, in: Fitzpatrick JM (ed.) *Non-surgical Treatment of BPH. Société Internationale d'Urologie Reports*, pp. 21–32. London: Churchill Livingstone.

29 Beek C van de, Rollema HJ, Boender H, Wolfs GGMC, Knottnerus JA, Janknegt RA (1993) Relationship between AUA symptom score and objective pressure-flow parameters. *Neurourol Urodyn* 12: 369.

30 Rollema H (1994) Clinical significance of symptoms, signs, and urodynamic parameters in benign prostatic hypertropy, in: Krane RJ, Siroky MB, Fitzpatrick JM (eds) *Clinical Urology*, pp. 847–79. Philadelphia: J B Lippincott.

31 Hill AM, Philpott N, Kay JDS, Smith JC, Fellows GJ, Sacks SH (1993) Prevalence and outcome of renal impairment at prostatectomy. *Br J Urol* 71: 464.

32 Caine M (1995) Reflections on alpha blockade therapy for benign prostatic hyperplasia. *Br J Urol* 75: 265.

33 Lepor H (1992) Alpha-1 adrenergic blockers in the medical management of benign prostatic hyperplasia. *Curr Opinion Urol* 2: 26.

34 Schlegel PN, Brendler CB (1989) Management of urinary retention due to benign prostatic hyperplasia using luteinizing hormone releasing hormone agonist. *Urology* 34: 69.

35 McConnell JD (1990) Androgen ablation and blockade in the treatment of benign prostatic hyperplasia. *Urol Clin N Am* 17: 661.

36 Stoner E (1992) The clinical effects of a 5 alpha reductase inhibitor — Finasteride — on benign prostatic hyperplasia. *J Urol* 147: 1298.

37 Kirby RS, Bryan J, Eardley I *et al.* (1992) Finasteride in the treatment of benign prostatic hyperplasia. A urodynamic evaluation. *Br J Urol* 70: 65.

38 McConnell JD (1992) The role of dihydrotestosterone in benign prostatic hyperplasia. *Curr Opinion Urol* 2: 18.

39 Masai M, Sumiya H, Akimoto S *et al.* (1990) Immunohistochemical study of androgen receptor in benign hyperplastic and cancerous human prostates. *Prostate* 17: 293.

40 Home E (1811) *Practical Observations on the Treatment of the Diseases of the Prostate Gland*, vol. 1. London: Nichol.

41 Blandy JP (1977) Surgery of the benign prostate: the First Sir Peter Freyer Memorial Lecture. *J Irish Med Assoc* 70: 517.

42 Parikh AM, Milroy EJG (1995) Precautions and complications in the use of the Urolume Wallstent. *Eur Urol* 27: 1.

43 Squires B, Gillatt DA (1995) Massive bladder calculus as a complication of a titanium prostatic stent. *Br J Urol* 75: 252.

44 Orandi A (1985) Transurethral incision of prostate (TUIP) — 645 cases in 15 years. A chronological appraisal. *Br J Urol* 57: 703.

45 Nielsen HO (1988) Transurethral prostatotomy versus transurethral prostatectomy in benign prostatic hypertrophy. *Br J Urol* 61: 435.

46 Mobb GE, Moisey CU (1988) Long-term follow-up of unilateral bladder neck incision. *Br J Urol* 62: 160.

47 Costello A, Bowsher WG, Bolton DM, Braslis KG, Burt J (1992) Laser ablation of the prostate in

patients with benign prostatic hypertrophy. *Br J Urol* 69: 603.

48 Blandy JP, Notley RG (1992) *Transurethral Resection*, 3rd edn. London: Butterworth-Heinemann.

49 Roos NP, Wennberg JE, Malenka DJ *et al.* (1989) Mortality and reoperation after open and transurethral resection of the prostate for benign prostatic hyperplasia (special article). *New Engl J Med* 320: 1120.

50 Mebust WK (1992) Increased mortality after transurethral prostatectomy for benign prostatic hyperplasia. *Curr Opinion Urol* 2: 3.

51 O'Boyle PJ (1990) Video-endoscopy: the remote operating technique. *Br J Urol* 65: 557.

52 Page BH (1980) The pathological anatomy of digital enucleation for benign prostatic hyperplasia and its application to endoscopic resection. *Br J Urol* 52: 111.

53 Watkins-Pitchford JM, Payne SR, Rennie CD, Riddle PR (1984) Hyponatraemia during transurethral resection — its practical prevention. *Br J Urol* 56: 676.

54 Hahn RG (1993) Ethanol monitoring of extravascular absorption of irrigating fluid. *Br J Urol* 72: 766.

55 Gale DW, Notley RG (1985) TURP without TURP syndrome. *Br J Urol* 57: 708.

56 Swales JD (1987) Dangers in treating hyponatraemia *Br Med J* 294: 261.

57 Scot FB (1980) Guest editorial: treatment of urinary incontinence. *J Urol* 125: 799.

58 Gundian JC, Barrett DM, Parulkar BG (1993) Mayo clinic experience with the AS800 artificial urinary sphincter for urinary incontinence after transurethral resection of prostate or open prostatectomy. *Urology* 41: 318.

59 Samdal F, Vada K, Lundmo P (1993) Sexual function after transurethral prostatectomy. *Scand J Urol Nephrol* 27: 27.

60 Hanbury DC, Sethia KK (1995) Erectile function following transurethral prostatectomy. *Br J Urol* 75: 12.

61 Evans JWH, Singer M, Chapple CR, Macartney N, Walker JM, Milroy EJG (1992) Haemodynamic evidence for cardiac stress during transurethral prostatectomy. *Br Med J* 304: 666.

62 Marks LS (1993) Serial endoscopy following visual laser ablation of prostate (VLAP). *Urology* 42: 66.

63 Dawkins GPC, Harrison NW, Royle MG, Fletcher MS (1993) Prostate thermotherapy: subjective and objective outcomes correlated in 6 month follow-up study of treatment versus sham groups. *Br J Surg* 80: 105.

64 Strohmaier WL, Bichler KH, Fluchter SH, Wilbert DM (1990) Local microwave hyperthermia of benign prostatic hyperplasia. *J Urol* 144: 913.

65 Zerbib M, Steg A, Conguy S, Debre B (1992) A prospective randomised study of localised hyperthermia vs placebo in obstructive benign hypertrophy of the prostate. *J Urol* 147: 1048.

66 Nawrocki JD, Bell TJ, Lawrence WT, Ward JP (1994) A randomised controlled study of thermotherapy. *British Association of Urological Surgeons Annual Meeting*, July 1994. Abstract 41.

67 Venn SN, Montgomery BS, Sheppard S *et al.* (1994) Microwave hyperthermia in BPH — a placebo controlled clinical trial. *British Association of Uro-*

logical Surgeons Annual Meeting, July 1994, Abstract 42.

68 Soanes WA, Gonder MJ (1971) Cryosurgery in benign and malignant diseases of the prostate. *Int Surg* 51: 104.

69 Kishev SV, Coughlin JD, Dow JA (1970) Late results following cryosurgery of the prostate (a clinical and panendoscopic study of 80 patients). *J Urol* 104: 893.

70 Physick PS (c. 1784) cited by Kuss R, Gregoir V (1989) *Histoire Illustrée de l'Urologie de l'Antiquite à Nos Jours*. Paris: Dacosta.

71 Donatucci CF, Berger N, Kreder KJ, Donohue RE, Raife MJ, Crawford ED (1993) Randomized clinical trial comparing balloon dilatation to transurethral resection of prostate for benign prostatic hyperplasia. *Urology* 42: 42.

72 Harris SH (1933) Prostatectomy with closure. Five years' experience. *Br J Surg* 21: 434.

73 Millin T (1947) *Retropubic Urinary Surgery*. Edinburgh: Churchill Livingstone.

74 Millin T, MacAlister CLO (1970) Retropubic prostatectomy, in: *Urology* Campbell MF, Harrison JH (eds) Philadelphia: WB Saunders.

Chapter 26: Prostate — neoplasms

Aetiology and epidemiology

Carcinoma of the prostate is not linked with any industrial agent, smoking, fertility, socio-economic status, marriage or celibacy [1,2]. It may be more common in blood group A than O [3], and less in men who have been circumcised [4]. There may be a familial susceptibility [5,6]: it was found three times more often in parents or siblings of men who died of it and it may be linked to loss of tumour suppressor genes [7].

Epidemiology

Epidemiological data are obscured by the fact that more histological cancer is found the more it is looked for and differences may reflect the availability of medical care and the method used to make the diagnosis: e.g. clinical screening by rectal examination, macroscopic observations at postmortem or serial sections of autopsy specimens.

In England and Wales there has been a steady increase in the annual number of deaths from cancer of the prostate over the last 30 years (Fig. 26.1), a statistic often cited with alarming implications. In fact, within each age group the incidence has risen hardly at all (Fig. 26.2), and could well be explained by newer methods of detecting the disease. The main factor contributing to the greater number of deaths is the greater number of men who nowadays survive to become old. Far from alarming, it should be reassuring to know that prostate cancer causes death in less than half of 1% of them (Table 26.1).

In the USA, it is estimated that some 96000 new cases of prostate cancer occur per annum in a total male population of over 100 million [9]. The mortality in white men has remained unchanged at about 21 per 100000 over the last 50 years, but has risen in black men from 24 to 36 per 100000. There are curious differences within the same geographical area: the mortality for Japanese men living in California was 12.7 per 100000 compared with 100.2 for black men [10,11].

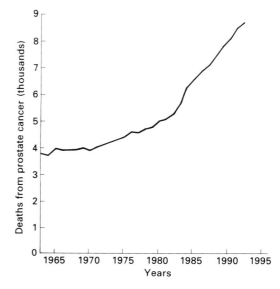

Fig. 26.1 Deaths in England and Wales from prostate cancer (data from the Registrar General, Office of Population Census and Surveys, 1963–1992).

Within the same ethnic groups there are even more curious discrepancies: black men in the USA have 10-fold the incidence of those in West Africa. Japanese men in the USA have four times the incidence of those living in Japan. Chinese living in Singapore or Hong Kong have five or six times more than those in Shanghai [10].

Table 26.1 Deaths from cancer of the prostate: England and Wales 1989. (Office of Population Census and Surveys [8])

Age group (years)	Number of men alive in each age group	Deaths from cancer of prostate	% of men at risk
65–70	1215000	1325	0.11
71–75	784000	2116	0.27
75–80	648300	2365	0.41
81–85	365700	1545	0.42
>85	183900	872	0.47
Total	2203600	8223	0.37

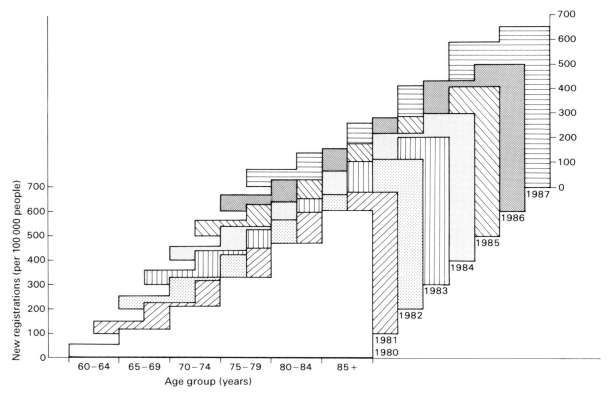

Fig. 26.2 Cancer of the prostate. New registrations per 100 000 population in England and Wales in age groups from 60 to 85+ in 1980–1987 (from the Registrar General, Office of Population Census and Surveys). Note the relatively constant number in each age group.

Speculation as to the possible reasons for these marked differences have included the largely vegetable diet and greater proportion of fish eaten in Japan [11].

Pathology

Classification [12–14]

The majority of cancers of the prostate are adenocarcinomas, but within them a small subgroup has a particularly bad prognosis, namely those which arise from the ducts of the gland [13,14]. There are also rare examples of melanoma, sarcoma and lymphoma (see below).

Macroscopic appearances

The usual advanced case of carcinoma of the prostate forms a large mass which invades the fat and seminal vesicles and spreads around the rectum and the lower third of the ureters, but many years ago Rich pointed out that in up to 14% of postmortems there were multifocal cancers 'so minute that they were neither seen

nor felt even by the pathologist who was able to hold the dissected prostate in his hands and examine the cut surface visually' [15]. This proportion increases the more, and the more thinly, the histological sections are cut and has been found all over the world. By the age of 80 small multifocal cancers are present in almost every prostate [16]. Note the difference between this figure and the clinical incidence of prostatic cancer (Table 26.1).

Microscopic appearances

The same gland may show a wide spectrum of histological appearances (Fig. 26.3) making it difficult to grade prostatic cancer. There are at least four systems [13,17–20]. Most rely on anaplasia, to which has been added the objective measurement of flow cytometry [21].

Quite different is that of Gleason which depends on the low power appearance of the pattern of the tumour [12,17] (Fig. 26.4). It correlates closely with the behaviour of the tumour and its response to treatment, especially when linked to stage [17,20].

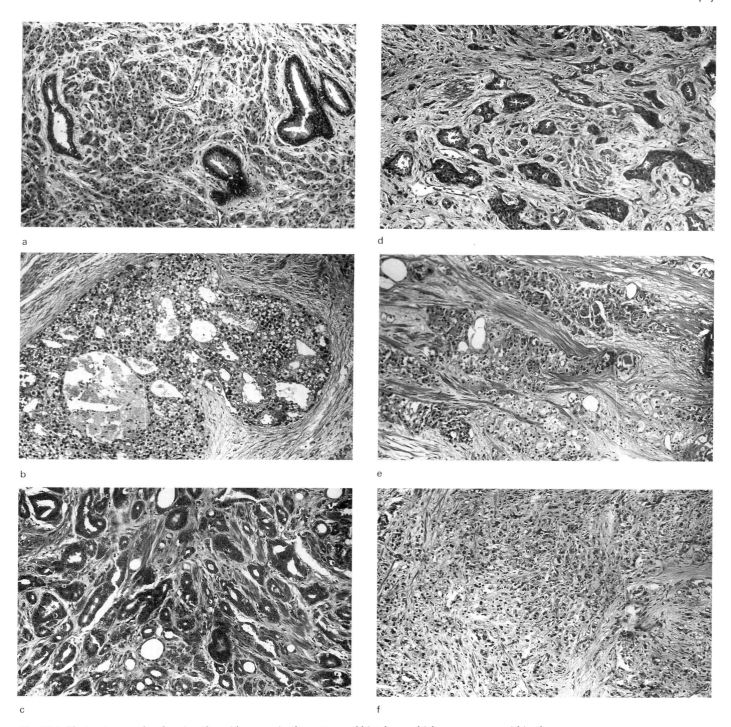

Fig. 26.3 Photomicrographs showing the wide range in the pattern of histology which may appear within the same gland (a). Normal gland with invasive cancer (b), intra-acinar cancer (c), well-differentiated tubular adenocarcinoma (d), moderately differentiated carcinoma (e), and (f) poorly differentiated carcinoma (courtesy of Dr E.A. Courtauld).

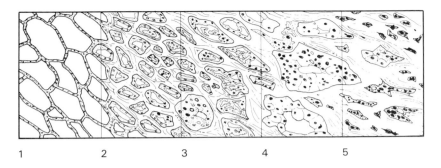

Fig. 26.4 Diagram of the Gleason system of classification of prostate cancer (redrawn from [17]). There are five patterns, based on the low power appearance. For each tumour two fields are chosen, and assigned a pattern 1–5. The sum, e.g. 2 + 3 = 5, is the Gleason score.

1   2   3   4   5

Spread of prostatic cancer

Prostatic cancer spreads by direct invasion, lymphatics, veins and along the perineural spaces.

Direct invasion occurs into seminal vesicles, urethra, base of the bladder and around the rectum. Cancer never penetrates Denonvilliers' fascia unless it has been perforated by a biopsy needle.

Capsule

The notion of the 'capsule' in the context of carcinoma is misleading (see p. 369). The only anatomical capsule is a thin layer of connective tissue continuous with that of the veins and fat around the gland [22,23] (see p. 370). This layer of connective tissue is thinner than the loop of the resectoscope [22] and extends alongside the small nerves, arteries, veins and lymphatics which enter the prostate at many places. In addition to the lymphatics each nerve is surrounded by a perineural space in which cancer readily spreads [24].

Lymph nodes

Lymph nodes may be invaded in many apparently localized cancers — up to 82% of stage 1 and 2 cancers show lymph node invasion [25,26].

Bone invasion

In addition to the involvement of lymph nodes by prostatic cancer, there is a direct route from the prostate through its veins and lymphatics to the marrow of the vertebrae, pelvis and upper third of the femur [27,28].

Pathological staging

The clinical and pathological staging of prostatic cancer has been a matter of controversy. There are several systems [29–31] (Fig. 26.5) which depend on the different methods used to investigate the patient. A clinical staging system — the only one available in cases treated by radiotherapy — cannot be compared with pathological staging based on the examination of the pathological specimen removed by radical prostatectomy with lymphadenectomy.

Carcinoma *in situ*

In the prostate, this is found in acini adjacent to frank carcinoma. Its significance is controversial, and it is variously named atypical dysplasia, atypical hyperplasia and adenosis [32,33] (Fig. 26.6).

Focal carcinoma

Originally, the concept of focal carcinoma of the prostate was cancer that could not be detected at naked eye examination in autopsy material [15,16], or was found by chance on histological examination of tissue removed at transurethral or open prostatectomy for what was considered to be benign disease [34,35].

Transrectal ultrasound renewed interest in the search for focal cancer which might be cured by radical prostatectomy. 'Focal carcinoma' has now come to mean an impalpable tumour detected by transrectal ultrasound and confirmed by needle biopsy.

Whatever staging systems are used, they will be based on the concept that a nodule of cancer starts off very small, and grows in size in an orderly way through the prostate. This is misleadingly simple. Step sections of total prostatectomy specimens show that they are always multifocal and never confined to one lobe [36,37]. Nor is it by any means certain that orderly progression necessarily takes place from stage A, through B, C and D [38] (Fig. 26.7). Small lesions can skip the intervening stages and jump to lymph nodes or bone marrow. The incidence of

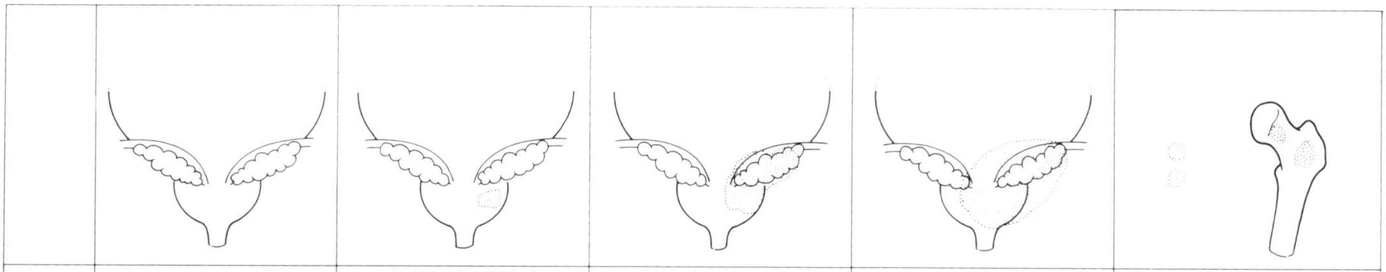

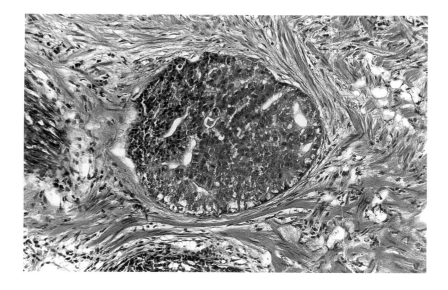

	MICROSCOPIC	CONFINED WITHIN CAPSULE	EXTRACAPSULAR		METASTASES
TNM 1992 [29]	[Tx unassessable T0 no evidence of primary tumour Tis carcinoma *in situ*] T1a Incidental finding in TUR chips <5% tissue T1b Incidental finding in TUR chips >5% tissue T1c Raised PSA: needle bx.	[NB includes invasion of but not through capsule] T2a < half 1 lobe 2b > half 1 lobe 2c both lobes	T3a Unilateral extracapsular T3b Bilateral extracapsular T3c Seminal vesicles invaded	Fixed/invading other organs T4a Bladder neck, external sphincter rectum T4b Levator, pelvic wall.	N0 No regional nodes N1 Single ipsilateral node N2 Bilateral or multiple pelvic nodes N3 Fixed pelvic nodes N4 Extrapelvic nodes M0 No evidence of distant mets. M1 Evidence of distant mets.
JEWETT 1975 [30]	A1 Microscopic focus A2 Diffuse microscopic foci	B1 1 lobe < 1.5 cm B2 both lobes or > 1.5 cm	C1 Localized nodule < 70 g	C2 Fixed to side wall pelvis or > 70 g	D1 Mets confined to pelvis D2 Mets outside pelvis
VACURG 1972 [31]	I Incidental finding in TUR chips. No clinical suspicion of cancer	II Rectal examination nodule. Not clinically outside capsule. Normal PAP	III Rectal examination outside capsule. No metastases. Normal PAP		IV Distant metastases +/or raised PAP

Fig. 26.5 Comparison of staging systems for carcinoma of the prostate. PAP, prostatic acid phosphatase; PSA, prostate specific antigen; TUR, transurethral resection.

Fig. 26.6 Carcinoma *in situ* in prostate. This is a common finding in areas adjacent to cancer (courtesy of Dr Suhail Baithun).

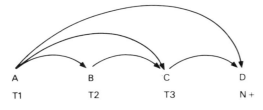

Fig. 26.7 It is by no means necessary that cancer will progress in orderly stages from A to B, etc. It can skip stages (after [38]).

unsuspected lymph node metastases varies from 0 to 23% in stage A and from 0 to 50% in stage B [39].

Cancer in the prostate is by no means straightforward, and in planning the management of the patient it is important not to oversimplify a disease with such a complex and unpredictable natural history.

Melanoma

Melanoma arises from melanin containing cells which are present in up to 4% of prostates [40].

Sarcoma

Sarcomas (usually leiomyosarcoma) occur in younger men, where they present with large tumours [41]. The sarcomatoid carcinoma of the prostate is a particularly malignant version of an anaplastic carcinoma [42].

Lymphoma

Lymphoma and deposits of leukaemia are occasionally found in the prostate.

Clinical features

Today, many symptomless men undergo screening tests and are found to have carcinoma of the prostate. The policy of screening is subject to considerable controversy at present [43]. Nevertheless, the diagnosis is being made with increasing frequency in such patients. Many others have symptoms indistinguishable from those with benign enlargement of the prostate — frequency, a poor stream and perhaps urgency. Many arrive in acute or chronic retention. A relatively short history, and the presence of haematuria, should make one suspicious of cancer [44,45].

In a few patients it is local spread which causes symptoms: bilateral obstruction to the ureters may cause uraemia. Infiltration of the lymphatics in the pelvis may cause oedema of the lower limb, and very occasionally the rectum is encircled by a sheath of cancer leading to intestinal obstruction [46].

In about 10% of patients the first symptoms are those of distant metastases, often causing backache from vertebral involvement — a symptom which may take them to the rheumatologist. Others present with pathological fractures, frequently of the femur. Paraplegia may be a presenting feature. Not uncommonly bone marrow involvement leads to anaemia.

Physical signs

In many patients there are no physical signs. In so-called early cases a hard nodule may be felt in the prostate, but many hard nodules prove to be caused by something other than cancer [47] and often the cancer is present in a part of the prostate other than the palpable nodule.

Investigations

Imaging of the prostate

Transrectal ultrasound

The density of the ultrasonic echo depends on the density of calcification in the prostatic tissue [48] (Fig. 26.8). Depending therefore on the amount of calcium in them, cancers may be hypoechoic, isoechoic or hyperechoic (Fig. 26.9). When the ultrasound pictures are carefully compared with the histological findings after total prostatectomy it becomes clear that the ultrasound has only detected a small number of the many tumours that are actually present [49–53]. Furthermore, the interpretation of ultrasound is open to considerable observer variation [54].

It is especially important to be quite clear what is meant when the report refers to the 'capsule' which, in the case of ultrasound is the interface between the prostatic tissue — whether normal, benign hyperplasia or cancer — and the surrounding fat [48] (Fig. 26.10).

Computerized tomography

Computerized tomography (CT) has, so far, been disappointing in finding small localized carcinomas, but it is useful in demonstrating spread of the cancer into the seminal vesicles and surrounding fat (Fig. 26.11).

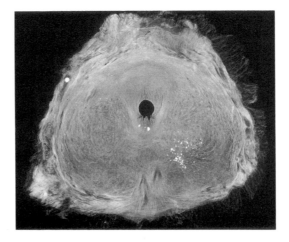

Fig. 26.8 The density of the ultrasound echo in the prostate depends upon the density of calcification in the tissues (courtesy of Mr David R Jones).

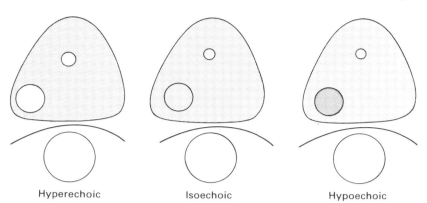

Fig. 26.9 Cancer of the prostate may be more (hyperechoic), less (hypoechoic) or equally dense (isoechoic) on ultrasound as the normal tissue.

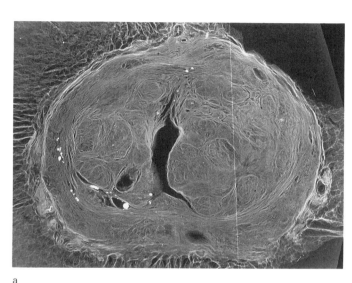

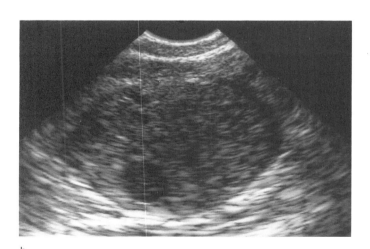

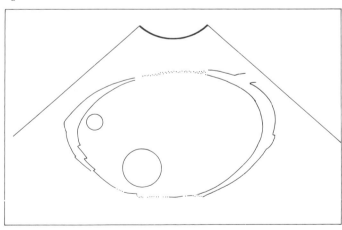

Fig. 26.10 (a) The 'capsule' on ultrasound represents the sonic interface between the prostate and its immediately surrounding vessels and fat (courtesy of Mr David R Jones); (b) ultrasound showing the 'capsule'; (c) note, the bright line of the 'capsule' is the interface: it is not a distinct thick layer of tissue.

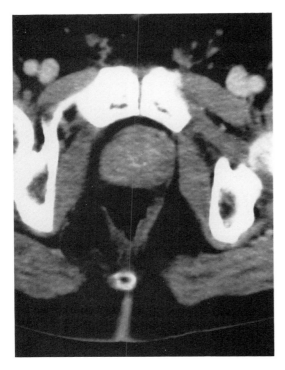

Fig. 26.11 A CT scan showing carcinoma of the prostate gland. Showing some asymmetry on the right posteriorly (courtesy of Dr MJ Kellett).

Magnetic resonance imaging

The continually improving images provided by magnetic resonance imaging (MRI) are still not able to distinguish benign from malignant changes in the prostate but it has advantages over ultrasound in the precision with which it can show invasion of seminal vesicles and the neurovascular bundle to the penis [55–57] (Fig. 26.12).

Tumour markers

In everyday clinical practice, serum acid phosphatase has largely been replaced by prostate-specific antigen (see p. 370). This is a most useful marker, but its interpretation needs care [58–60]. In elderly men, there is a large overlap between the values found with benign enlargement, and those with a small carcinoma (Fig. 26.13). On the other hand, when the value exceeds 30 μg/l there is an 85% chance that there are metastases. As with all these tumour markers, when the cancer cells become very undifferentiated they tend to lose the capacity to elaborate these enzymes, and occasionally one finds a normal result even though there are widespread metastases.

One of its principal uses is to act as a marker with which to monitor response to treatment and detect early relapse.

Biopsy

Cancer is often detected in the chips removed by transurethral resection: the more chips are sectioned, and the more sections the pathologist makes, the more cancers will be discovered. One

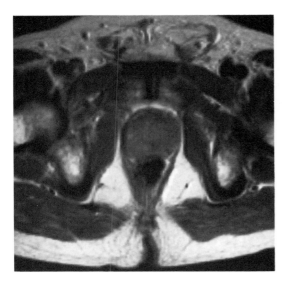

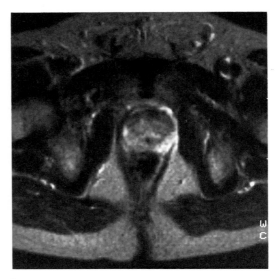

a   b

Fig. 26.12 (a) MRI T1 weighted image showing more clearly asymmetry on the right; (b) T2 weighted MRI image with normal high signal to the peripheral zone on the left and loss of signal due to tumour in the right peripheral zone extending posteriorly (courtesy of Dr Janet Husband).

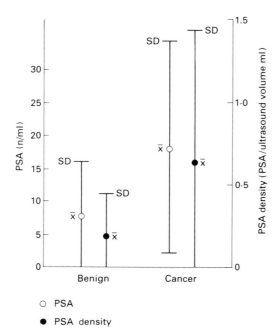

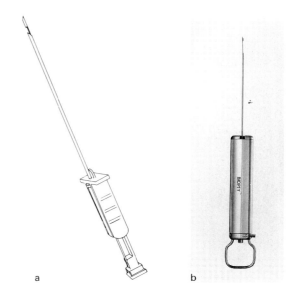

Fig. 26.15 (a) Trucut biopsy needle, (b) Biopty needle.

Fig. 26.13 There is an overlap in the normal values for cancer and benign enlargement. It is better to express prostate-specific antigen (PSA) as a function of volume [60].

important source of error arises because most invasive cancers start in the peripheral outer part of the prostate, and most of the tissue removed during transurethral resection comes from the cranial inner gland (Fig. 26.14). It is thus quite common not to find the carcinoma in the specimen removed by transurethral resection. If there is a clinical suspicion that there might be cancer in the peripheral tissue it is better to take an additional biopsy using a Trucut needle or similar device.

There is now a wide range of modern biopsy needles (Trucut, Monopty or Biopty) (Fig. 26.15) which provide excellent cores of tissue with great ease. More reliable samples are obtained if

the biopsy is obtained with the help of ultrasound [55] (Fig. 26.16).

The biopsy needle may be inserted perineally, or through the rectum. With the transrectal route, it is much more easy to hit the tumour but there is a risk of producing septicaemia. The procedure must always be covered by antibiotics.

These small cores of tissue should be fixed immediately, and the biopsy needle should be thrust straight into formalin.

The search for metastases

If the prostate-specific antigen is over 30 µg/l it is very likely that the patient has metastases. They occur in two main clinical patterns: (a) widespread metastatic deposits in the bones, particularly in the pelvis, femora and vertebrae where the cells are carried in Batson's venous plexus; and (b) glandular metastases, often in

Fig. 26.14 Most invasive cancers arise in the caudal outer zone of the prostate which is not removed by transurethral resection: hence cancer is often found in the tissue left behind.

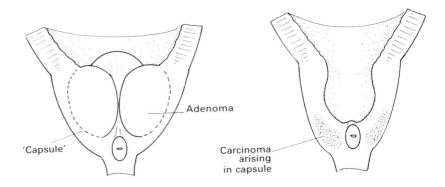

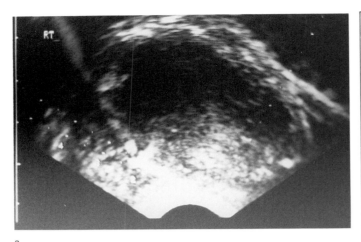

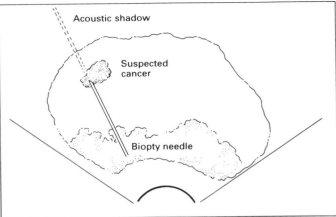

a   b

the para-aortic chain. However, as the disease progresses, metastases may be found in any organ of the body.

Bone scanning

^{99m}Tc-MDP is taken up by bone in proportion to the blood flow, so that where there is increased vascularity (e.g. from a metastasis or a fracture) there will be a 'hot spot' in the scan (Fig. 26.17). When all the bones are uniformly riddled with metastases then there is a diffuse opacity — the so-called 'superscan' (Fig. 26.18).

Management of carcinoma of the prostate

Cancer confined to the prostate: T1–T3, N0 and M0

Nothing in contemporary urology arouses more controversy than the management of this condition. On the one hand, there are many who claim that this is cancer that has been discovered at just the time when surgery has a chance of effecting a cure. Others, more sceptical, point out that small foci of cancer are almost universal in elderly men, and by the time they are found two-thirds of them have been present for more than 10 years, and one-third for more than 20 [61,62].

If the tumour is small, confined to the prostate and well differentiated, the patient's life expectancy is normal, whether treated or not, and by whatever method [63–68].

Small foci arising in the inner zone tend to have a low Gleason number, and although they

Fig. 26.16 Transrectal biopsy of the prostate under ultrasound control. Note the acoustic shadow thrown by the biopty needle (courtesy of Dr Michael Kellett).

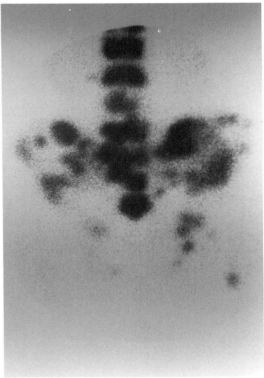

Fig. 26.17 Bone scan showing uptake by metastases (courtesy of Dr Neil Garvie).

may eventually become large they tend not to spread outside the gland. In contrast, those arising in the outer part of the gland tend to be multifocal, have a higher Gleason number and invade the surrounding fat and pelvic lymph nodes [69–71].

The choice of treatment lies between deferred treatment (surveillance), radical prostatectomy, radiotherapy and hormone therapy.

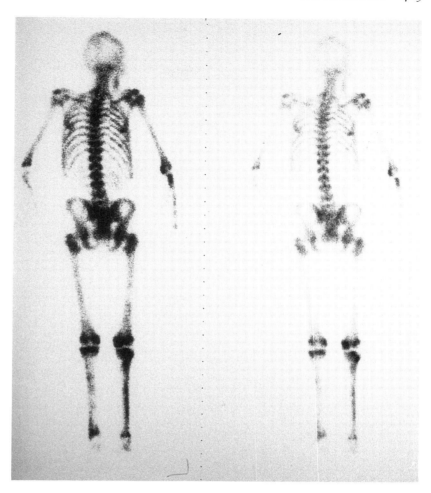

Fig. 26.18 'Superscan' — almost all the bones are invaded and take up the isotope (courtesy Dr Neil Garvie).

Deferred treatment — surveillance

This can be difficult for the patient who is told he has cancer and anxiously faces repeated follow-up visits and investigations. Although the results of such deferred treatment are no worse than those of active intervention [72–74], it is always more difficult for surgeon and patient *not* to do anything. The symptomless patient whose cancer has been detected by screening may well ask why bother to undergo screening if the lesion does not need to be treated anyway?

Radical prostatectomy

Radical prostatectomy was first performed by the perineal route [63] which could take no account of the state of the pelvic lymph nodes. The long survival advantage claimed for radical prostatectomy still rests largely on the data obtained with the perineal operation [63,64]. For a time in the UK, the perineal operation was superseded by the retropubic total prostatectomy of Millin [75] and in turn this was largely given up with the advent of stilboestrol.

It has been revived in recent years, thanks to the radical improvements introduced by Walsh who has shown how, by attention to technique, it is possible to preserve the neurovascular bundles of the penis as well as the intramural sphincter [76,77].

Preliminary laparoscopic node dissection

Before embarking on radical retropubic prostatectomy it is usual to dissect the lymph nodes on both sides from the internal iliac and obturator group. This can be done at a preliminary session using a minimally invasive technique either with an extra- or a transperitoneal approach [78]. This has the advantage that paraffin sections can be studied before making the decision to proceed to radical prostatectomy (Figs 26.19 & 26.20)

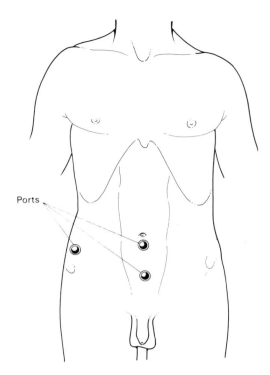

Fig. 26.19 Laparoscopic dissection of the internal iliac nodes. After inducing a pneumoperitoneum and placing the ports, the peritoneum is incised medial to the vas deferens.

Laparoscopic pelvic lymph node dissection

The patient is placed head-down, and rolled a little towards the opposite side to allow the bowel to fall away from the operative field. The peritoneum is incised along and just lateral to the obliterated hypogastric artery, up to the ureter — which should always be identified for safety — and down to the pubis, dividing the vas

deferens *en route*. All the fibrofatty tissue with its content of lymph nodes is then separated by blunt dissection within a triangle formed by the external iliac artery, the pubis and the obliterated hypogastric artery. The apex of the triangle is the bifurcation of the common iliac artery. At the conclusion of the dissection the external iliac vessels, obturator vessels and nerve have been completely cleaned.

Technique of radical prostatectomy

With the patient head-down the bladder is catheterized. A long lower midline incision is made and, if not done already at laparoscopy, a node dissection is now performed, and the results of frozen section are awaited.

The bladder is retracted upwards and the fat cleaned from the retropubic veins. The pelvic fascia is incised on either side of the puboprostatic ligament which contains the dorsal vein (Fig. 26.21). The leash of veins is carefully suture ligated, and the layer of pelvic fascia containing the neurovascular bundles are displaced laterally (Fig. 26.22). A silicone sling is passed around the urethra and pulled up. The urethra is opened just distal to the apex of the prostate and just cephalad to the membranous urethra and its intramural sphincter (Fig. 26.23). The catheter is now used to pull up the prostate, and the tissue behind the prostate — the rectourethralis muscle — is divided in the midline and again displaced laterally and backwards away from the prostate on either side to preserve the penile neurovascular bundles (Fig. 26.24). Medial to this bundle there is a stout leash of inferior vesical vessels which must be suture ligated (Fig. 26.25).

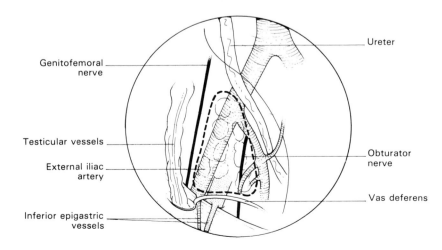

Fig. 26.20 The sleeve of nodes is teased off the internal iliac vessels. Haemostasis is obtained by diathermy.

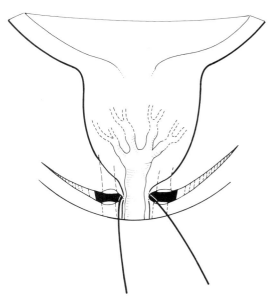

Fig. 26.21 Walsh's technique of nerve sparing radical prostatectomy. First the pelvic fascia is incised on either side of the dorsal veins which are carefully suture ligated and divided.

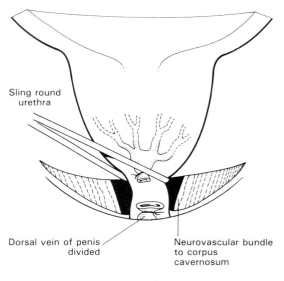

Sling round
urethra

Dorsal vein of penis
divided

Neurovascular bundle
to corpus
cavernosum

Fig. 26.22 The neurovascular bundles are displaced laterally and posteriorly.

Now open the bladder at the bladder neck (Fig. 26.26). Deflating the balloon of the catheter, and using the catheter as a sling, the prostate is lifted up and the bladder is dissected away from the prostate. When the bladder is finally cut across, its calibre is similar to that of the cut edge of the urethra. As the back of the trigone is dissected from the prostate the seminal vesicles and vasa deferentia are displayed (Fig. 26.27). Their arterial bundles are ligated and divided

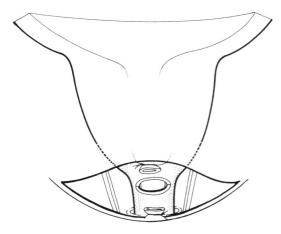

Fig. 26.23 The urethra is opened just cephalad to the membranous urethra and its intramural sphincter.

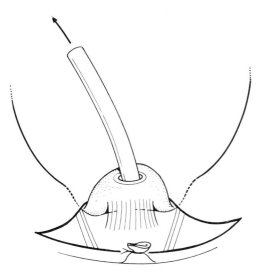

Fig. 26.24 The catheter pulls up the prostate, and the rectourethralis muscle is divided in the midline, so that the neurovascular bundles can be again displaced laterally.

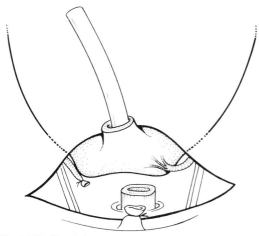

Fig. 26.25 The inferior vesical vessels are suture ligated.

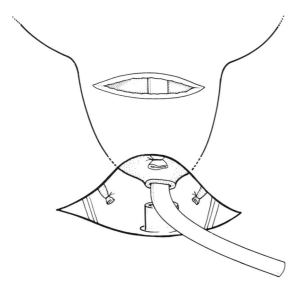

Fig. 26.26 The bladder is opened at the bladder neck. The prostate is now slung up with the catheter.

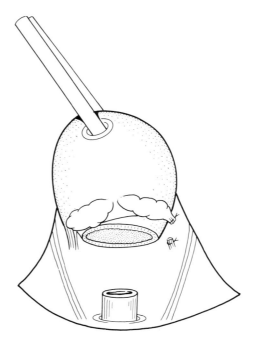

Fig. 26.28 The vascular leash of the seminal vesicles is divided well medial to the penile neurovascular bundles.

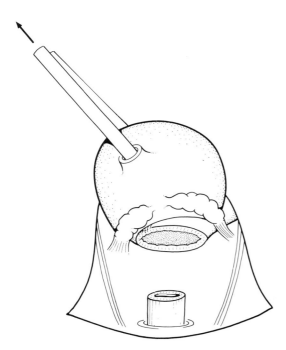

Fig. 26.27 The bladder is dissected away from the prostate, displaying the seminal vesicles and vasa.

well medial to the penile neurovascular bundles (Fig. 26.28).

The bladder neck may have to be narrowed with one or two sutures before it is anastomosed over a 20 Charrière silicone catheter to the stump of the urethra. Great care is taken in making this anastomosis to get a precise urothelial junction, and not to injure the intramural sphincter

mechanism immediately distal to the site of division (Fig. 26.29). It helps to place all the sutures before tying them.

The catheter remains for 3 weeks. Slight stress incontinence is normal for the first few weeks and urinary frequency persists for another month or so. A stricture often occurs at the anastomosis and may require dilatation from time to time.

Radiotherapy

The history of radiation treatment for cancer of the prostate goes back for nearly a century. Two types of radiotherapy are used for carcinoma of the prostate: (a) external beam therapy; or (b) interstitial irradiation.

External beam therapy

External beam therapy from a linear accelerator is directed by a computerized tomographic scanning simulator so as to include the lymph nodes of the pelvis and avoid the rectum and small bowel [79]. Common sequelae include radiation proctitis which can be controlled by hydrocortisone enemas, and impotence which occurs in about 10% and is unpredictable.

The results of radiation therapy for cancer are comparable to those obtained by radical surgery

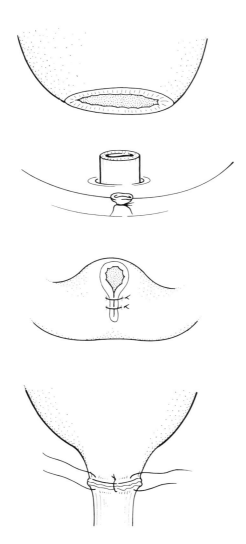

Fig. 26.29 After narrowing the bladder neck, a precise mucosa-to-mucosa anastomosis is made between the bladder neck and the urethra over a 20 Charrière catheter. Place all the sutures before tying them.

even when no account is taken of the errors which necessarily arise when comparing cases staged clinically with those staged pathologically [80–84].

Attempts have been made to improve the results of radiation treatment by radical transurethral 'debulking' surgery or hormone therapy [85,86].

Interstitial radiation

A number of radioactive sources have been used, including ^{125}iodine seeds, ^{198}Au gold grains and iridium wires. These are implanted at open operation, after the lymph nodes have been

staged or through a series of perineal cannulae, placed under ultrasound control, using an after-loading method. The results more or less reflect the tumour grade. Impotence occurs, probably from endarteritis (as with teletherapy) in 5–10% [87,88].

Although survival statistics seem to show little difference between the results of radiotherapy and those of radical surgery, when the irradiated prostate is biopsied, a large number are still found to show cancer cells. Whether these are 'viable' or not is uncertain but the fact that the patient still has cancer causes anxiety for him and his doctor [89,90].

Adjuvant orchiectomy

A multicentre combined clinical trial set out to see if there was any advantage in adding orchiectomy to radiotherapy for localized cancer of the prostate. There was no prolongation of survival or lessening of local symptoms, but orchiectomy postponed the appearance of metastases [91].

Hormone therapy in confined disease

This is another area where there is intense controversy. In some centres, hormone therapy such as orchiectomy is routinely added to a radical prostatectomy, and remarkable results are claimed even in cases where the lymph nodes are involved [92]. Most urologists feel that the side effects of hormone treatment are not justified in localized disease, and keep them in reserve until there is definite evidence of symptomatic metastases.

Urinary obstruction — the role of transurethral resection

Most patients come to the urologist with symptoms of urinary obstruction. Often the diagnosis of cancer is not made until the chips are examined histologically. There is always a fear that opening up the veins in the periphery of the gland, which is inevitable during this procedure, will allow cancer cells to escape into the circulation and give rise to metastases. Many careful studies have looked into this question and there is as yet no clear answer [93].

Many patients have severe outflow obstruction, and even though there is evidence of widespread metastases, transurethral resection is needed to give symptomatic relief. In such cases, the technique is somewhat different from that used in benign hyperplasia. When there are widespread metastases, there may be abnormal circulating fibrinolysins, and if there is any suggestion of spontaneous bruising it is wise to obtain expert haematological advice. Amino-caproic acid may be required.

The prostatic urethra may be so stiff and rigid that passing the resectoscope risks creating a false passage. A useful trick is to pass a filiform guide first (Fig. 26.30), and then use an angled Timberlake obturator (Fig. 26.31) with a screw attachment or a flexible Phillips follower which snugly fits the resectoscope sheath and guides the resectoscope sheath through the rigid cancer. Once the first few chips have been removed the resectoscope becomes mobile.

The aim of the operation is not to take out all the tumour down to the capsule: since most cancers originate in the peripheral part of the prostate, this is futile. The aim is to cut out a generous cone of tissue with its apex at the verumontanum (Fig. 26.32). Keep well away from the region of the sphincter which may already be invaded by cancer. Resecting in its vicinity may bring on incontinence. (It is a wise precaution to warn the patient of the risk of incontinence when you know he has cancer.)

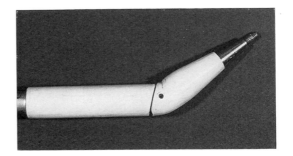

Fig. 26.31 An angled Timberlake obturator, which snugly fits the resectoscope, is screwed on to the filiform and guides it through the rigid cancer.

Laser treatment

After the bulk of the tumour has been removed, it has been suggested that the cancer might be got rid of by coagulating the shell that is left behind with the neodymium-yttrium aluminium garnet (YAG) laser [94]. The method is still under trial.

Cryosurgery for cancer

It was hoped that freezing cancer of the prostate would liberate modified antigens that would provoke an immunological attack against the cancer. It was an ingenious idea but it did not work [95].

Cancer of the prostate with metastases

Huggins [96] applied John Hunter's observations on the relationship of the prostate to the testicles and showed that castration, while it might have made little difference to benign disease, certainly made metastases disappear. He followed this by showing that the synthetic oestrogen diethylstil-boestrol would have the same effect. This opened the door to the hormone treatment of prostatic cancer which gave relief to countless patients, and won Huggins a Nobel prize.

The timing of hormone treatment

If the patient has pain or the bone scan reveals a metastasis that threatens to cause serious illness, it is universally agreed that treatment is needed. Examples are metastases in the neck or shaft of the femur which might cause a crippling patho-logical fracture, or those in the vertebrae which might lead to paraplegia.

Otherwise many favour a policy of surveillance [73,74]. The patient is kept under regular review

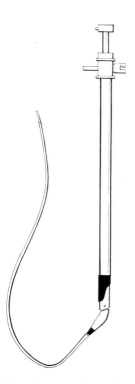

Fig. 26.30 When the prostatic urethra is very rigid a filiform guide is passed first.

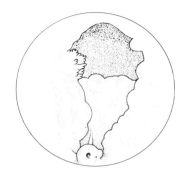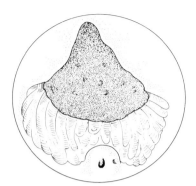

Fig. 26.32 The aim of transurethral resection in prostatic cancer is to cut out an even cone.

by means of prostate-specific antigen estimations and a bone scan if this is seen to rise alarmingly or if the patient complains of pain. Others prescribe hormone treatment at once. There is no clear advantage of one policy over the other. All forms of hormone treatment have their disadvantages. There are many to choose from.

Hormone treatment — the options

The background has been described above (see p. 363). In summary, many cancers of the prostate depend on dihydrotestosterone, the active form of testosterone. Testosterone is nearly all made in the Leydig cells of the testicles, but the adrenals secrete an unknown additional amount of

steroid precursors which are converted to testosterone in the prostate cells (see below).

Testosterone is converted to dihydrotestosterone by the enzyme 5-alpha reductase which is present in the prostate cells. The active dihydrotestosterone interacts with a cytosol receptor in prostate cells and sets off a train of events which make the cell thrive and divide (Fig. 26.33).

Orchiectomy is irreversible and, compared with the other options, cheap. Through a transverse scrotal incision one testis is delivered, the tunicae are incised, the testicular tubules are wiped away, and haemostasis is obtained by suture and diathermy (Fig. 26.34). The same is done on the other side. Great care must be taken over

Dehydroepiandrosterone

Testosterone

Androstenedione

Aromatase

5α-reductase

Dihydrotestosterone

Fig. 26.33 Testosterone is converted to dihydrotestosterone by 5-alpha reductase.

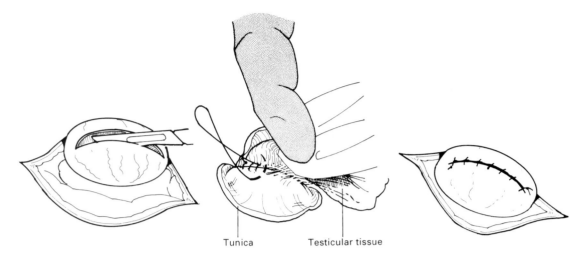

Tunica   Testicular tissue

Fig. 26.34 Subcapsular orchiectomy.

haemostasis to prevent a haematoma. It can be done under local anaesthesia using bilateral inguinal blocks and infiltration of the scrotal skin.

Stilboestrol. The action of testosterone may be blocked by the synthetic oestrogen diethylstilboestrol. This is cheap; the dose is only 1 mg/ day. Higher doses led to an unacceptable incidence of cardiovascular side effects [97] and although the cure rate is the same as orchiectomy this risk has made most surgeons give it up [98]. With minimal precautions against cardiovascular side effects such as an aspirin a day, it is probably as safe and a great deal cheaper than the alternatives.

LHRH agonists. Although orchiectomy lowers the plasma testosterone by over 90%, it only reduces the level of testosterone in the prostate by about 75% [99]. The residual testosterone is derived from adrenal precursors dehydroepiandrosterone and androstenedione which are converted in the cell to testosterone. (For a time in the 1960s, adrenalectomy was widely used for clinical relapse after orchiectomy, but the results did not justify the morbidity of the operation.)

The secretions of both testicle and adrenal are governed by the luteinizing hormone which is released by the anterior pituitary. This in turn is released by a luteinizing hormone-releasing hormone (Fig. 26.35). Compounds which imitate the action of LHRH — the LHRH agonists — boost the output of LH by the pituitary until it is exhausted. For about a week the testicles and adrenals are in overdrive and there is a surge in the level of testosterone in the blood which produces a flare of symptoms which can sometimes

be serious, e.g. paraplegia. The results of treatment with LHRH agonists are equivalent to orchiectomy or stilboestrol, without the cardiovascular side effects of the latter [100,101].

During the first week of treatment with LHRH agonists, the side effects of the surge in testosterone level may be prevented by drugs which act on the next steps in the process — the conversion of testosterone to dihydrotestosterone — or the reaction of dihydrotestosterone with the cytosol receptor.

Drugs which block the cytosol receptor. These compounds are known as antiandrogens. There are two main types. The first are the steroids cyproterone acetate and megestrol acetate. These prevent flare in the first couple of weeks of treatment with LHRH agonists and also subsequently prevent the tiresome side-effect of 'hot flushes' seen either with orchiectomy or LHRH treatment – though far more expensive than a low dose of diethylstilboestrol. The second are non-steriodal compounds such as flutamide, nilutamide and bicalutamide [102, 103].

Used on their own, the antiandrogens can have a therapeutic benefit that compares reasonably with orchiectomy [104], but when given to the patient whose metastases have escaped from the effect of orchiectomy or LHRH agonists, they have little effect.

It was reasonable therefore to give the antiandrogens at an earlier stage — the so-called 'total androgen blockade'. Extravagant claims were made that this would improve and delay the onset of relapse. Careful controlled trials do indeed show that there is a detectable benefit: but it is very small and short-lived, and the expense prodigious [105−108]. The probable

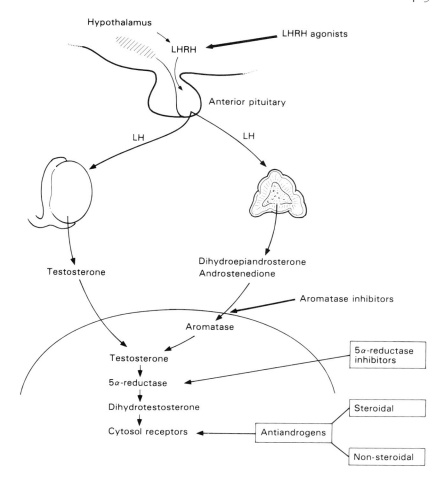

Fig. 26.35 The pituitary secretes luteinizing hormone-releasing factor (LHRH), which governs the secretions of the testes and adrenal.

explanation is that clones of cells have grown out which no longer need testosterone.

Localized metastases

Frequently a single metastasis is seen that causes disproportionate pain. A short course of radiotherapy directed to the site will often stop the pain at once, and give relief which will last until the end of the patient's life.

Generalized metastases

If the whole body is irradiated all at once, the marrow will be destroyed and the patient will have a fatal anaemia. This can be avoided by the ingenious technique of half-body irradiation [109]. One half is irradiated first. Then an interval is allowed, during which marrow cells migrate from the unirradiated bone marrow, and repopulate the irradiated marrow. Then the other half is treated similarly. This method can give profound and lasting relief of pain, although it does not prolong life.

Radioactive strontium and phosphorus

^{32}Phosphorus is taken up by bony metastases and can give immediate pain relief [110]. In the near future it may be replaced by radioactive ^{89}strontium, currently the subject of clinical trials [111].

Diphosphonate

Comparable pain relief can be obtained by giving patients diphosphonate [112].

Corticosteroids

It is worth bearing in mind that useful pain relief is provided with corticosteroids and, for the dying patient, they may bring a measure of welcome euphoria [113].

References

1 Majeed FA, Burgess NA (1994) Trends in death rates and registration rates for prostate cancer in

England and Wales. *Br J Urol* 73: 377.

2 Ross RK, Deapen D, Casagrande J, Paganini-Hill A, Henderson BE (1981) A cohort study of mortality from cancer of the prostate in Catholic priests. *Br J Cancer* 43: 223.

3 Bourke JB, Griffin JP (1962) Blood groups in benign and malignant prostatic hypertrophy. *Lancet* ii: 1279.

4 Apt A (1968) Circumcision and prostatic cancer. *Acta Med Scand* 178: 493.

5 Carter BS, Bova GS, Beaty TH *et al.* (1993) Hereditary prostate cancer: epidemiologic and clinical features. *J Urol* 150: 797.

6 Bastacky SI, Wojno KJ, Walsh PC, Carmichael MJ, Epstein JI (1995) Pathological features of hereditary prostate cancer. *J Urol* 153: 987.

7 Paulson DF (1993) Clinically localized prostatic carcinoma (editorial). *Cancer* 71: 3797.

8 *Office of Population Censuses and Surveys*. London: HMSO.

9 U.S. National Cancer Institute (1982) Monograph 59. *Cancer Mortality in the United States 1950–1977.* National Cancer Institute, Bethesda, Maryland. pp 190–5.

10 Lytton B (1989) Demography of prostatic carcinoma, in: Fitzpatrick JM, Krane RJ (eds) *The Prostate*, pp. 253–9. Edinburgh: Churchill Livingstone.

11 Mettlin C, Natarajan N (1983) Epidemiological observations from the American College of Surgeons' survey on prostate cancer. *Prostate* 4: 323.

12 Gleason DF (1966) Classification of prostatic carcinoma. *Cancer Chemother Rep* 50: 125.

13 Mostofi FK (1975) Grading of prostatic carcinoma. *Cancer Chemother Rep* 59: 111.

14 Christensen WN, Steinberg G, Walsh PC, Epstein JI (1991) Prostatic duct adenocarcinoma: findings at radical prostatectomy. *Cancer* 67: 2118.

15 Rich AR (1935) On the frequency of occurrence of occult carcinoma of the prostate. *J Urol* 33: 215.

16 Breslow N, Chan CW, Dhom G *et al.* (1977) Latent carcinoma of prostate at autopsy in seven areas. *Int J Canc* 20: 680.

17 Gleason DF (1987) *Histologic Grade, Clinical Stage and Patient Age in Prostate Cancer*, pp. 15–18. National Cancer Institute Monograph 7.

18 Utz DC, Farrow GM (1969) Pathologic differentiation and prognosis of prostatic carcinoma. *J Am Med Assoc* 209: 1701.

19 Gaeta JF, Asirwatham JE, Miller G, Murphy GP (1980) Histologic grading of primary prostatic cancer: a new approach to an old problem. *J Urol* 123: 689.

20 Benson MC, Olsson CA (1989) The staging and grading of prostatic cancer, in: Fitzpatrick JM, Krane RJ (eds) *The Prostate*, pp. 261–72. Edinburgh: Churchill Livingstone.

21 Winkler HZ, Rainwater LM, Myers RP *et al.* (1988) Stage D1 prostatic adenocarcinoma: significance of nuclear DNA ploidy patterns studied by flow cytometry. *Mayo Clin Proc* 63: 103.

22 Page BH (1980) The pathological anatomy of digital enucleation for benign prostatic hyperplasia and its application to endoscopic resection. *Br J Urol* 52: 111.

23 Jones DR, Griffiths GJ, Parkinson MC *et al.* (1989)

Comparative histopathology, microradiography and per-rectal ultrasonography of the prostate using cadaver specimens. *Br J Urol* 63: 508.

24 Villers A, McNeal JE, Redwine EA, Freiha FS, Stamey TA (1989) The role of perineural space invasion in the local spread of prostatic adenocarcinoma. *J Urol* 142: 763.

25 Arduino LJ, Gluckman MA (1962) Lymph node metastases in early carcinoma of the prostate. *J Urol* 88: 91.

26 Doublet JD, Gattegno B, Thibault P (1994) Laparoscopic pelvic lymph node dissection for staging of prostatic cancer. *Eur Urol* 25: 194.

27 Batson O (1940) The function of the vertebral veins and their role in the spread of metastases. *Ann Surg* 112: 138.

28 Kahler JE (1939) Carcinoma of the prostate gland: a pathological study. *J Urol* 41: 557.

29 Hermanek P, Sobin LH (eds) (1992) *UICC International Union against Cancer TNM Classification of Malignant Tumours*, 4th edn, 2nd revision. Berlin: Springer.

30 Jewett HJ (1975) The present status of radical prostatectomy for stage A and B prostatic cancer. *Urol Clin N Am* 2: 105.

31 Byar DP, Mostofi FK and the Veterans Administration Cooperative Urological Research Group (1972) Carcinoma of the prostate: prognostic evaluation of certain pathologic features in 208 radical prostatectomies. *Cancer* 30: 5.

32 Cantrell BB, de Klerk DP, Eggleston JC *et al.* (1981) Pathological factors that influence prognosis in stage A prostatic cancer: the influence of extent versus grade. *J Urol* 125: 516.

33 Waisman J (1988) Pathology of neoplasms of the prostate gland, in: Skinner DG, Lieskovsky G (eds) *Diagnosis and Management of Genitourinary Cancer*, pp. 161–2. Philadelphia: WB Saunders.

34 Franks LM (1954) Benign nodular hyperplasia of the prostate (review). *Ann Roy Coll Surg Engl* 14: 92.

35 McNeal JE (1970) Age related changes in prostatic epithelium associated with carcinoma, in: Griffiths K, Pierrepoint CG (eds) *Third Tenovus Workshop, Cardiff, Wales*. Alpha Omega Alpha 23–32.

36 Aihara M, Wheeler TM, Ohori M, Scardino PT (1994) Heterogeneity of prostate cancer in radical prostatectomy specimens. *Urology* 43: 60.

37 Haggman M, Norberg M, de la Torre M, Fritjofsson A, Busch C (1993) Characterization of localized prostatic cancer: distribution, grading and pT-staging in radical prostatectomy specimens. *Scand J Urol Nephrol* 27: 7.

38 Whitmore WF (1989) *Overview: Historical and Contemporary*, p. 7. National Cancer Institute Monograph.

39 Donohue RE, Fauver HE, Whitesel JA *et al.* (1981) Prostatic carcinoma. *Urology* 20: 559.

40 Block NL, Weber D, Schinella R (1972) Blue nevi and other melanotic lesions of the prostate: report of three cases and review of the literature. *J Urol* 107: 85.

41 Stenram U, Holby L (1969) A case of circumscribed myosarcoma of the prostate. *Cancer* 24: 803.

42 Shannon RL, Ro JY, Grignon DJ *et al.* (1992) Sarcomatoid carcinoma of the prostate. *Cancer* 69: 2676.

43 Chodak GW (1993) Questioning the value of screening for prostate cancer in asymptomatic men. *Urology* 42: 116.

44 Chodak GW, Thisted RA, Gerber GS *et al.* (1994) Results of conservative management of clinically localized prostate cancer. *New Engl J Med* 330: 242.

45 Barnes RW (1940) Carcinoma of the prostate: a comparative study of modes of treatment. *J Urol* 44: 169.

46 Barry J, Wild SR (1991) Radiological appearances in prostatic cancer with rectal spread. *Br J Urol* 67: 441.

47 Howard GCW (1993) The management of carcinoma of the prostate after failed primary therapy. *Br J Urol* 72: 269.

48 Jones DR, Griffiths GJ, Parkinson C *et al.* (1989) Comparative histopathology, microradiography and per-rectal ultrasonography of the prostate using cadaver specimens. *Br J Urol* 63: 508.

49 Palken M, Cobb OE, Simons CE, Warren BH, Aldape HC (1991) Prostate cancer: comparison of digital rectal examination and transrectal ultrasound for screening. *J Urol* 145: 86.

50 Weaver RP, Noble MJ, Weigel JW (1991) Correlation of ultrasound guided and digitally directed biopsies of palpable prostatic abnormalities. *J Urol* 145: 516.

51 Lee F, Torp-Pedersen ST, Siders DB, Littrub PJ, McLeary RD (1989) Transrectal ultrasound in the diagnosis and staging of prostatic carcinoma. *Radiology* 170: 609.

52 Shinohara K, Wheeler TM, Scardino PT (1989) The appearance of prostate cancer on transrectal ultrasonography: correlation of imaging and pathological examinations. *J Urol* 142: 76.

53 Worischek JH, Kutrz ME, Parra RA (1991) Evaluation of digital rectal examination, transrectal ultrasound and prostatic specific antigen in the diagnosis and staging of prostatic carcinoma. *J Urol* 145: 351A.

54 Rorbik J, Halvorsen OJ, Servoll E, Haukaas S (1994) Transrectal ultrasonography to assess local extent of prostatic cancer before radical prostatectomy. *Br J Urol* 73: 65.

55 Chadwick DJ, Cobby M, Goddard P, Gingell JC (1991) Comparison of transrectal ultrasound and magnetic resonance imaging in the staging of prostatic cancer. *Br J Urol* 67: 616.

56 Vapneck JM, Shinohara K, Carroll PR, (1991) Staging accuracy of magnetic resonance imaging versus transrectal ultrasound in stages A and B prostatic cancer. *J Urol* 145: 352A.

57 Tempany CMC, Rahmouni AD, Epstein JI, Walsh PC, Zerhouni EA (1991) Invasion of the neurovascular bundle by prostate cancer: evaluation with MR imaging. *Radiology* 181: 107.

58 Babaian RJ, Camps JL, Frangos DN *et al.* (1991) Monoclonal prostatic-specific antigen in untreated prostate cancer. *Cancer* 67: 2220.

59 Brawer MJ (1994) Prostate specific antigen: critical issues (review). *Urology* 44: Symposium No 6A. p9.

60 Bare R, Hart L, McCullough DL (1994) Correlation of prostatic specific antigen density with outcome of prostate biopsy. *Urology* 43: 191.

61 Gleason DF (1988) *Histologic Grade, Clinical Stage and Patient Age in Prostate Cancer*, pp. 15—18. National Cancer Institute Monograph 7.

62 Franks LM (1954) Latent carcinoma of prostate. *J Pathol* 68: 617.

63 Belt E, Schröder FH (1972) Total perineal prostatectomy for carcinoma of the prostate. *J Urol* 107: 91.

64 Jewett HJ, Bridge RQ, Gray GF Jr, Shelley WM (1968) The palpable nodule of prostatic cancer: results 15 years after radical excision. *J Am Med Assoc* 203: 403.

65 Byar DP, Corle DK and the Veterans Administration Cooperative Urological Research Group (1981) VACURG randomized trial of radical prostatectomy for stages I and II prostate cancer. *Urology* 17 (Suppl 4): 7.

66 Matzkin H, Patel JP, Altwein JE, Soloway MS (1994) Stage T1a carcinoma of prostate. *Urology* 43: 11.

67 Rana A, Chisholm GD, Christodoulou S, McIntyre MA, Elton RA (1993) Audit and its impact in the management of early prostatic cancer. *Br J Urol* 71: 721.

68 Zhang G, Wasserman NF, Sidi AA, Reinberg Y, Reddy PK (1991) Long-term follow up results after expectant management of stage A1 prostatic cancer. *J Urol* 146: 99.

69 McNeal JE (1993) Prostatic microcarcinomas in relation to cancer origin and the evolution to clinical cancer. *Cancer* 71: 984.

70 Mostofi FK, Sesterhenn IA, Davis CJ (1993) A pathologist's view of prostatic carcinoma. *Cancer* 71: 933.

71 Franks LM (1989) Pathology and biological activity of prostate tumours, in: Oliver RTD, Blandy JP, Hope-Stone HF (eds) *Urological and Genital Cancer*, pp. 195—202. Oxford: Blackwell Scientific Publications.

72 Adolfsson J, Carstensen J, Lowhagen T (1992) Deferred treatment in clinically localised prostatic carcinoma. *Br J Urol* 69: 183.

73 Parker MC, Cook A, Riddle PR, Fryatt I, O'Sullivan J, Shearer RJ (1985) Is delayed treatment justified in carcinoma of the prostate? *Br J Urol* 57: 724.

74 Handley R, Carr TW, Travis D, Powell PH, Hall RR (1988) Deferred treatment for prostate cancer. *Br J Urol* 249.

75 Millin T (1947) *Retropubic Urinary Surgery.* Edinburgh: Churchill Livingstone.

76 Catalona WJ, Basler JW (1993) Return of erections and urinary continence following nerve-sparing radical retropubic prostatectomy. *J Urol* 150: 905.

77 Fowler FJ, Roman A, Barry MJ, Wasson J, Grace L-Y, Wennberg JE (1993) Patient reported complications and follow-up treatment after radical prostatectomy. *Urology* 42: 622.

78 Prasad BR, Parr NJ, Fowler JW (1994) Laparoscopic pelvic lymphadenectomy — early results. *Br J Urol* 73: 271.

79 Ennis RD, Peschel RE (1993) Radiation therapy for prostate cancer. *Cancer* 72: 2644.

80 Lannon SG, El-Araby AA, Joseph PK, Eastwood BJ, Awad SA (1993) Long-term results of combined interstitial gold seed implantation plus external beam irradiation in localised carcinoma of the prostate. *Br J Urol* 72: 782.

81 Bagshaw MA, Kaplan ID, Cox RC (1993) Radiation therapy for localized disease. *Cancer* 71: 939.

82 Lawton CA, Cox JD, Glisch C, Murray KJ, Byhardt RW, Wilson JF (1992) Is long-term survival possible with external beam irradiation for stage D1 adenocarcinoma of the prostate? *Cancer* 69: 2761.

83 Fowler JE, Braswell NT, Pandey P, Seaver L (1995) Experience with radical prostatectomy and radiation therapy for localized prostate cancer at a veterans affairs medical center. *J Urol* 153: 1026.

84 Zagars GK, von Eschenbach AC, Johnson DE, Oswald MJ (1988) The role of radiation therapy in stage A2 and B adenocarcinoma of the prostate. *Int J Radiat Oncol Biol Phys* 14: 701.

85 Shearer RJ, Davies JH, Gelister JSK, Dearnley DP (1992) Hormonal cytoreduction and radiotherapy for carcinoma of the prostate. *Br J Urol* 69: 521.

86 Zelefsky MJ, Whitmore WF, Leibel SA, Wallner KE, Fuks Z (1993) Impact of transurethral resection on the long-term outcome of patients with prostatic carcinoma. *J Urol* 150: 1860.

87 Gomella LG, Steinberg SM, Ellison MF, Reeves WW, Flanigan RC, McRoberts JW (1991) Analysis of iodine[125] interstitial therapy in the treatment of localised carcinoma of the prostate. *J Surg Oncol* 46: 235.

88 Grossman HB, Batata M, Hilaris B (1982) [125]I implantation for carcinoma of the prostate: further follow up of first 100 cases. *Urology* 20: 591.

89 Scardino PT, Wheeler TM (1988) *Local Control of Prostate Cancer with Radiotherapy: Frequency and Prognostic Significance of Positive Results of Postirradiation Prostatic Biopsy*, p. 95. National Cancer Institute Monograph 7.

90 Kuban DG, El-Mahdi AM, Schellhammer PF (1988) I[125] interstitial implantation for prostate cancer. *Cancer* 63: 2415.

91 Fellows GJ, Clark PB, Beynon LL et al. (1992) Treatment of advanced localised prostatic cancer by orchiectomy, radiotherapy, or combined treatment. Medical Research Council study. *Br J Urol* 70: 304.

92 Winckler HZ, Rainwater LM, Myers RP et al. (1988) Stage D1 prostatic adenocarcinoma: significance of nuclear DNA ploidy patterns studied by flow cytometry. *Mayo Clin Proc* 63: 103.

93 Meacham RB, Scardino PT, Hoffman GS, Easley JD, Wilbanks JH, Carlton CE (1989) The risk of distant metastases after transurethral resection of the prostate versus needle biopsy in patients with localized prostate cancer. *J Urol* 142: 320.

94 Sander S, Bresland HO (1984) Laser in the treatment of localised prostatic carcinoma. *J Urol* 132: 280.

95 Soanes WA, Gonder MJ (1971) Cryosurgery in benign and malignant diseases of the prostate. *Int Surg* 51: 104.

96 Huggins C, Hodges CV (1941) Studies on prostatic cancer I. The effect of castration, of estrogen and of androgen injection on serum phosphatases in metastatic carcinoma of the prostate. *Cancer Res* 1: 293.

97 Blackard CE, Mellinger GT (1972) Current status of estrogen therapy for prostatic carcinoma. *Postgrad Med* 51: 140.

98 Johansson J-E, Andersson S-O, Holmberg L, Bergstrom R (1991) Primary orchiectomy versus estrogen therapy in advanced prostatic cancer — a randomised study: results after 7—10 years of follow-up. *J Urol* 145: 519.

99 Geller J (1993) Basis for hormonal management of advanced prostate cancer. *Cancer* 71: 1039.

100 Waymont B, Lynch TH, Dunn JA et al. (1992) Phase III randomised study of Zoladex versus stilboestrol in the treatment of advanced prostate cancer. *Br J Urol* 69: 614.

101 Kaisary AV, Tyrrell CJ, Peeling WB, Griffiths K (1991) Comparison of LHRH analogue (Zoladex) with orchiectomy in patients with metastatic prostatic carcinoma. *Br J Urol* 67: 502.

102 McLeod DG (1993) Antiandrogenic drugs. *Cancer* 71: 1046.

103 Buchholz N-P, Mattarelli G, Huber Buchholz M-M (1994) Post-orchiectomy hot flushes. *European Journal of Urology* 26: 120.

104 Ostri P, Bonnesen T, Nilsson T, Frimodtmoller C (1991) Treatment of symptomatic metastatic prostatic cancer with Cyproterone acetate versus orchiectomy — a prospective randomised trial. *Urol Int* 46: 167.

105 Crawford ED, Eisenberger MA, McLeod DG et al. (1989) A controlled trial of leuprolide with and without flutamide in prostatic carcinoma. *New Engl J Med* 321: 419.

106 Schroder FH (1993) Endocrine therapy for prostate cancer: recent developments and current status. *Br J Urol* 71: 633.

107 Denis LJ, Carneiro de Moura JL, Bono A et al. (1993) Goserelin acetate and flutamide versus bilateral orchiectomy: a phase III EORTC trial (30853). *Urology* 42: 119.

108 Janknegt RA, Abbou CC, Bartoletti R et al. (1993) Orchiectomy and Nilutamide or placebo as treatment of metastatic prostatic cancer in a multinational double-blind randomized trial. *J Urol* 149: 77.

109 Keen CW (1991) Second-line treatment of advanced prostate cancer: hemi-body radiation, in: Alderson AR, Oliver RTD, Hanham IW, Bloom HJG (eds) *Urological Oncology: Dilemmas and Developments*, p. 253. Chichester: Wiley.

110 Johnson DE, Haynie TP (1977) Phosphorus[32] for intractable pain in carcinoma of prostate. *Urology* 9: 137.

111 Laing AH, Ackery DM, Bayly RJ et al. (1991) Strontium[89] chloride for pain palliation in prostatic skeletal malignancy. *Br J Radiol* 64: 816.

112 Elomaa I, Blomqvist C, Grohn P et al. (1983) Long-term controlled trial with diphosphonate in patients with osteolytic bone metastases. *Lancet* i: 146.

113 Tannock I (1989) Treatment of metastatic prostatic cancer with low-dose predisone: evaluation of pain and quality of life as pragmatic indices of response. *J Clin Oncol* 17: 590.

PART 5
URETHRA
AND PENIS

Chapter 27: Urethra and penis — structure and function

Anatomy and physiology

Comparative anatomy

There is a wide variation in the anatomy of the penis and scrotum in mammals. In elephants, whales and hedgehogs the testes are abdominal — respectively just caudal to the kidneys, in the pelvis or at the internal ring. In pigs, they are in the superficial inguinal pouch; in sheep and man they lie at the bottom of a pendulous scrotum.

The rich blood supply of the testicle and the scrotum has been seen both as a heat-exchanging mechanism and a sexual signal. In many monkeys the brightly coloured scrotum is important in the mating season. The penis varies considerably in size and shape among mammals. In some monkeys it is equipped with sharp recurved spines of unknown function [1].

Embryology

Two crucial events occur in the male embryo, between the fifth and seventh week — the disappearance of the Müllerian ducts and the transformation of the phallic tubercles — events both orchestrated by the two sex chromosomes (see p. 537).

On the Y chromosome the HY gene produces the HY enzyme which makes the germ cells differentiate, first into Sertoli cells (whose Müllerian duct inhibiting factor causes the Müllerian ducts to disappear); and second, a week later, the germ cells differentiate to Leydig cells which secrete testosterone which enters the Wolffian ducts and the phallic and genital tubercles. These tissues have 5-alpha reductase which activates the testosterone to dihydrotestosterone. This binds to a cytosol receptor protein and sets off the changes in growth which make the Wolffian ducts turn into the vasa deferentia, seminal vesicles and epididymis, and the phallic and genital tubercles become the penis, scrotum and urethra (Fig. 27.1). The cytosol receptor protein is coded by a gene on the X chromosome. Each step on this ladder of events is carried out by a certain enzyme coded by a single gene. Each step may go wrong and result in one of the variations of intersex (see p. 440).

By 7 weeks the cloacal membrane dissolves and the primitive bladder opens on the ventral aspect of the genital tubercle (Fig. 27.2). This elongates to form the penis under which a groove is folded in from either side to form the urethra (Fig. 27.3). Rods of mesenchyme in each fold differentiate into the corpora cavernosa and spongiosum. At the tip of the penis a groove demarcates the glans through which a solid cord extends and then becomes canalized as the terminal urethra (Fig. 27.4). Skin grows forwards from the coronal sulcus to enclose the glans in the prepuce, and then becomes adherent.

The scrotum is formed by the meeting together in the midline of the two genital tubercles over the urethra (Fig. 27.5).

All these processes must be complete within a critical window of time: if the genital folds and penis are not completed by 12 weeks they never will be: however much androgen is given later on, all it can do is slightly enlarge the penis [2,3].

Neuter state

Without a Y chromosome or its HY enzyme the fetus stays neuter. The neuter state seems at first glance to be female: there is no phallus; the Müllerian ducts persist; the Wolffian ducts fail to turn into the vas deferens.

Topographical anatomy

Penis

The penis has three elements — the two corpora cavernosa, and the corpus spongiosum which expands distally to form the glans penis (Fig. 27.6). Each corpus consists of a sponge of intercommunicating venous sinuses. Each corpus cavernosum is attached to the medial aspect of

Y chromosome

HY gene

Germ cells

Sertoli cell

Leydig cells

Müllerian duct inhibiting factor

Testosterone
↓
Dihydrotestosterone

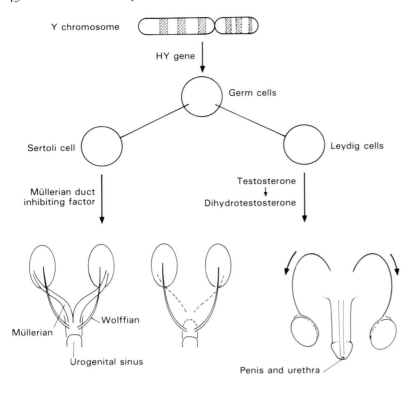

Müllerian

Wolffian

Urogenital sinus

Penis and urethra

Fig. 27.1 The Y chromosome produces the HY gene which turns germ cells either into Sertoli cells which secrete the Müllerian duct inhibiting factor; or turns germ cells into Leydig cells. The Leydig cells secrete testosterone, which is hydrogenated to dihydro-testosterone, and binds to receptors in the Wolffian ducts and phallic tubercles.

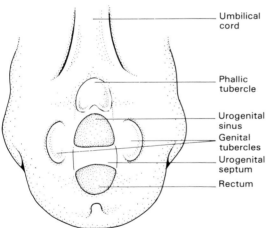

Umbilical cord

Phallic tubercle

Urogenital sinus

Genital tubercles

Urogenital septum

Rectum

Fig. 27.2 When the cloacal membrane dissolves the bladder opens behind the genital tubercle.

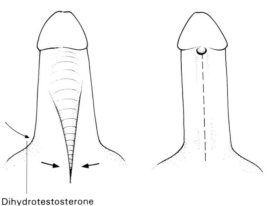

Dihydrotestosterone

Fig. 27.3 Under the influence of dihydrotestosterone the genital tubercle elongates, and a groove folds in on either side to form the urethra, up to the groove behind the solid glans penis.

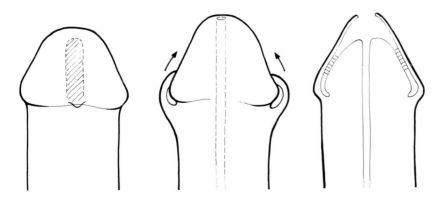

Fig. 27.4 A cord extends through the solid glans, and then becomes canalized to form the terminal urethra. Skin grows forwards from the coronal sulcus to enclose and adhere to the glans.

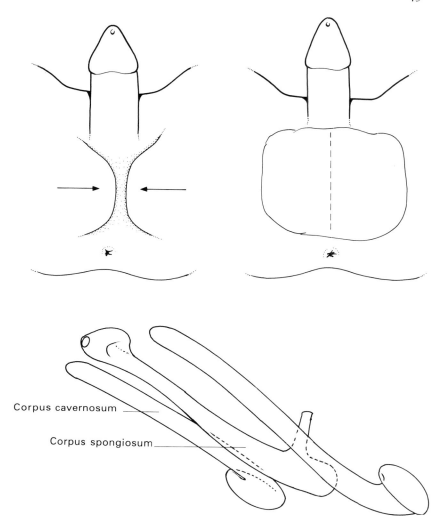

Fig. 27.5 The scrotum is formed by the inrolling of the two genital tubercles over the urethra.

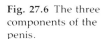

Corpus cavernosum

Corpus spongiosum

Fig. 27.6 The three components of the penis.

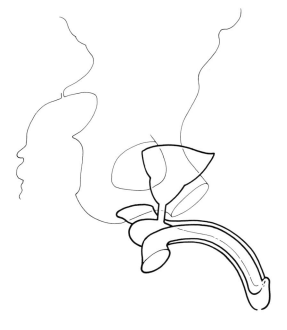

Fig. 27.7 Bony attachments of the urethra: the corpora cavernosa are fixed to the ischia, the prostate to the back of the symphysis pubis. The hilum of the penis is attached to the front of the symphysis by the suspensory ligament.

the ischiopubic ramus (Fig. 27.7). They join under the symphysis pubis to form the hilum of the penis, which is attached by the suspensory ligament.

Each corpus is enclosed in the specialized tunica albuginea made of strong fibroelastic tissue (Fig. 27.8). Between the corpora, the tunicae fuse to form the pectinate septum which is perforated by many small veins so that contrast injected into one corpus instantly fills the other.

The three corpora are enclosed in Buck's fascia in which run the deep dorsal vein and the sensory nerves supplying the glans penis. Between Buck's fascia and the skin is a loose layer of vascular connective tissue. The skin continues over the glans as the prepuce [4].

Arteries

The arteries of the penis are terminal branches of the internal pudendal artery — last branch of

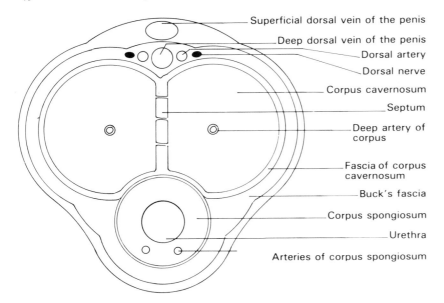

Superficial dorsal vein of the penis

Deep dorsal vein of the penis

Dorsal artery

Dorsal nerve

Corpus cavernosum

Septum

Deep artery of corpus

Fascia of corpus cavernosum

Buck's fascia

Corpus spongiosum

Urethra

Arteries of corpus spongiosum

Fig. 27.8 Transverse section through the penis.

the internal iliac artery. Each internal pudendal artery splits into three (Fig. 27.9):

1 A dorsal artery runs in Buck's fascia either side of the deep dorsal vein of the penis.

2 A second larger cavernous artery runs in the middle of each corpus cavernosum and is the main artery responsible for erection.

3 A pair of bulbar arteries run in the corpus spongiosum either side of the urethra [5,6].

The cavernous arteries supply blood for tumescence of the corpora cavernosa in the first and second stages of erection (see p. 436): the dorsal and bulbar arteries are responsible for

distension of the glans penis in the third stage.

The arteries of the corpora cavernosa and spongiosum give off short branches which open directly into the venous sinuses. In the flaccid state these arteries are constricted: in the first and second phases of erection they dilate (Fig. 27.10).

Veins

The venous sinuses of the spongy tissue drain into efferent veins. Those of the glans enter a coronal plexus which flows into the deep dorsal

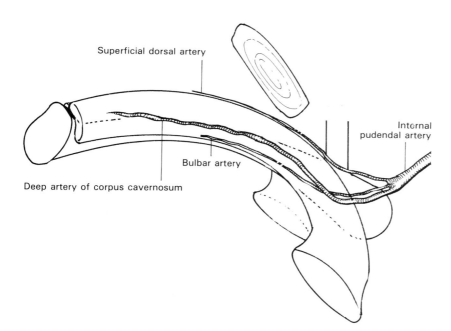

Superficial dorsal artery

Internal pudendal artery

Bulbar artery

Deep artery of corpus cavernosum

Fig. 27.9 Arterial supply to the penis.

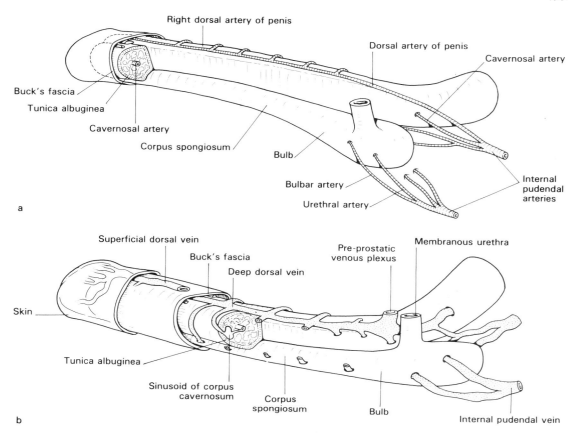

Fig. 27.10 Blood supply to the penis (a) arterial, (b) venous.

vein. Those of the middle part of the penis run obliquely through the tunica albuginea into the deep dorsal vein directly or via circumflex veins (Fig. 27.11).

The veins of the bulb and proximal corpora cavernosa join up to form large cavernosal veins which flow into the deep dorsal vein which itself runs under the symphysis into the pre-prostatic plexus of Santorini.

A superficial venous system drains the subcutaneous tissues of the penis via the superficial dorsal vein of the penis into the saphenous vein.

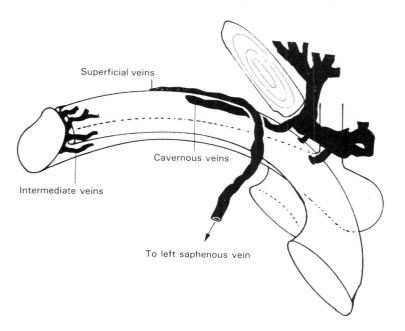

Fig. 27.11 Venous drainage of the penis.

There are many communications between these two venous systems [5,6].

Lymphatics

Most of the lymphatics of the penis drain into the medial group of superficial inguinal lymph nodes: some flow through the 'sentinel' node lying over the fossa ovalis while others accompany the deep dorsal vein under the pubis into the lymphatics of the pelvis [7].

Nerve supply

Autonomic

A rich autonomic plexus forms a sleeve around the cavernous and bulbar arteries. This is linked to ancient centres in the brain — the hippocampus, cingulate gyrus and thalamus [8,9]. There are two spinal centres concerned with erection, one at T12−L3, the other at S2−S4 [10].

The main neurovascular bundle lies posterolateral to the prostate gland, and can sometimes be preserved during prostatectomy or cystectomy by displacing the bundle laterally in its layer of pelvic fascia [11].

Somatic afferent and efferent nerves

Sensory branches of the pudendal nerve (S2, S3) run with the two dorsal nerves of the penis in Buck's fascia to the skin and glans penis. Care must be taken to safeguard these nerves when operating for Peyronie's disease.

Efferent fibres in the pudendal nerve supply the bulbospongiosus and ischiocavernosus muscles to raise the blood pressure within the corpora above the systolic pressure during the third phase of erection.

Scrotum

The skin of the scrotum is hairy and rich in sebaceous glands. There is a distinct plane of cleavage between the scrotal skin and the dartos which has a rich vascular supply and is innervated by sympathetic fibres of S4. The dartos is part of the panniculus carnosus of the body, and continues as a distinct layer over the penis. It has a profuse blood supply, and is sensitive to temperature: when cold it contracts, converting the scrotum into a compact lump. When warm, the scrotum becomes a loose dependent bag.

Fascia

The fascia of Colles is attached behind to the perineal membrane, each side to the pubis, and continues upwards as the fascia of Scarpa onto the abdominal wall. Blood and extravasated urine will collect in this space and sharply define its limits (Fig. 27.12).

Arteries

The scrotum derives its arterial supply from the superficial and deep external pudendal branches of the femoral artery, and the internal pudendal artery.

Veins

The venous drainage of the scrotum is via the saphenous to the femoral vein. The scrotal veins anastomose freely with those of the penis.

Lymphatics

The scrotal lymphatics drain into the medial group of the inguinal lymph nodes, and from there along the course of the external iliac artery.

Nerves

The anterior third of the scrotum is innervated by the ilio-inguinal nerve (L1): the posterior two-thirds by the scrotal branches of the perineal (S3) and posterior cutaneous nerve of the thigh (S2) (Fig. 27.13) [12].

Urethra

Male

The male urethra is an elastic tube capable of doubling in length during erection. It is lined with transitional epithelium as far as the bulb where it is squamous for the next 5 cm and cuboidal for the remainder of its length. Para-urethral glands enter the urethra along its length, being most numerous in the bulb and near the external meatus (Fig. 27.14). Cowper's glands lie within the levator ani muscle and send their ducts down beside the bulbar urethra to open into it. Paired glands of Littré open on either side of the external urinary meatus.

A sleeve of spongy tissue — the corpus spongiosum — with a structure similar to that of the corpora cavernosa, surrounds the urethra and is

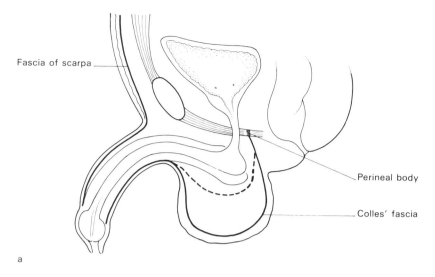

Fascia of scarpa

Perineal body

Colles' fascia

a

Fig. 27.12 Attachments of the fasciae of Colles and Scarpa which (a) limit the spread of extravasated blood and urine in the perineum, but (b) allow it to diffuse up in the fat of the abdominal wall.

b

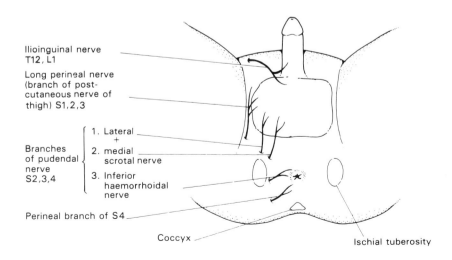

Fig. 27.13 Cutaneous nerves of the scrotum.

Ilioinguinal nerve T12, L1

Long perineal nerve (branch of post-cutaneous nerve of thigh) S1,2,3

Branches of pudendal nerve S2,3,4

1. Lateral +
2. medial scrotal nerve
3. Inferior haemorrhoidal nerve

Perineal branch of S4

Coccyx

Ischial tuberosity

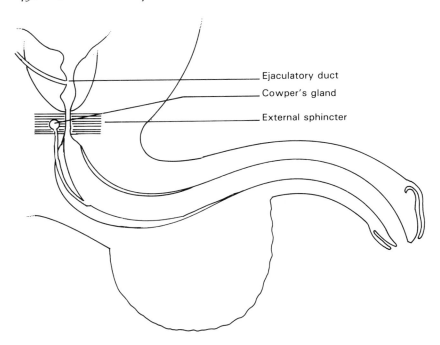

Ejaculatory duct
Cowper's gland
External sphincter

Fig. 27.14 Topographical anatomy of the male urethra.

continuous with the glans penis. Like the corpora cavernosa the nerves of the corpus spongiosum and urethra come from the neurovascular bundles just posterolateral to the prostate.

In small boys, the urethra is extremely narrow and does not enlarge until puberty. The calibre of the adult male urethra is very variable, but at its most narrow is about 8 mm in diameter (24 Charrière).

Female

The female urethra is lined with transitional epithelium above and squamous epithelium below: the junction between the two types of epithelia is variable, and it is normal for the squamous epithelium to extend up onto the trigone [13] (Fig. 27.15).

The urethra is surrounded by erectile spongy tissue which is anatomically continuous with the glans of the clitoris (Fig. 27.16).

Surrounding the spongy tissue is a sleeve of smooth and striated muscle fibres, entirely distinct from the levator ani sheet. These muscles contain fast- and slow-twitch fibres, very similar to those of the intramural sphincter of the male membranous urethra (see p. 371).

The lumen of the female urethra forms a crescent, with a marked crest on the posterior wall (Fig. 27.17). Numerous paraurethral glands of unknown function open into the urethra.

Erection

When the penis is flaccid its arterioles are constricted and there is a very low blood flow. Parasympathetic activity from conscious erotic stimulation or local contact, releases neurotransmitter substances which relax the branches of the deep artery of the corpora cavernosa.

The action of these neurotransmitter substances is complex. Acetylcholine may release a factor

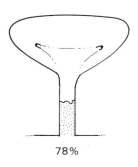
78%

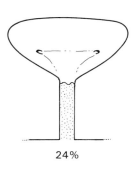
24%

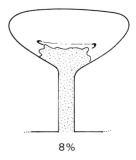
8%

Fig. 27.15 The level at which squamous epithelium extends up the lining of the female urethra is very variable.

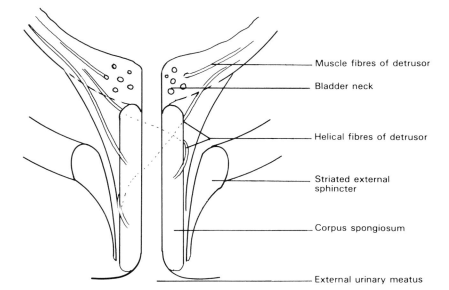

Fig. 27.16 Surrounding the corpus spongiosum of the female urethra is a sleeve of smooth and striated muscle, similar to the supramembranous intramural sphincter of the male. Outside this is the striated external sphincter, part of the levator ani sheet.

- Muscle fibres of detrusor
- Bladder neck
- Helical fibres of detrusor
- Striated external sphincter
- Corpus spongiosum
- External urinary meatus

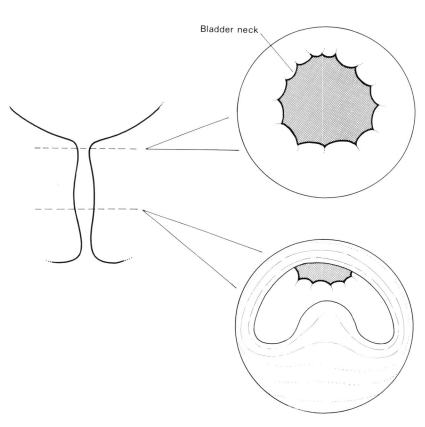

Bladder neck

Fig. 27.17 The lumen of the female urethra is crescentic in shape. The bladder neck is seen in the distance.

from endothelium causing the smooth muscle to relax, or may act with vasoactive intestinal polypeptide (VIP) [4]. There are alpha and beta adrenergic receptors in the muscle of the penile blood vessels. Injections of alpha-blocking agents produce erection.

There are five phases in erection:

1 Tumescence. As the first stimuli reach the penis there is an increased blood flow. The spaces of the corpora fill with blood. At first there is no increase in pressure, and the penis remains soft though it may increase in length and girth.

2 Erection. When the vascular sinusoids are filled there is an increase in pressure inside the corpora which makes the penis stiff. At the end of this phase the blood flow into the penis slows down.

3 Full erection. In this phase the penis is fully erect but the pressure inside the corpora is still only 10 mmHg below the systolic pressure. The inflow of blood has almost stopped.

4 Rigid erection. Full erection is followed by the phase of rigid erection, when the intracavernous pressure rises to several times that of the systolic blood pressure. The change from 'full' to 'rigid' erection requires closure of the efferent veins which are kinked where they exit through the tunica albuginea (Fig. 27.18). In addition, the bulbospongiosus muscles contract and blood ceases to flow in or out of the penis.

5 Detumescence. Here, the venous outflow starts again, the arterial inflow remaining very small: the penis shrinks and gradually returns to its flaccid state [4].

Function of the scrotum

The marked alterations in the size and shape of the scrotum with temperature, and the pampiniform plexus of the spermatic cord, have been interpreted as a temperature regulating system designed to keep the testicles cool — a concept which has been disputed in view of the intra-abdominal position of the testes in so many other mammals [12].

Physiology of the urethra

The urethra is a most important element in the sphincter mechanism in both sexes. The role of the intramural or supramembranous sphincter in preserving continence after prostatectomy is

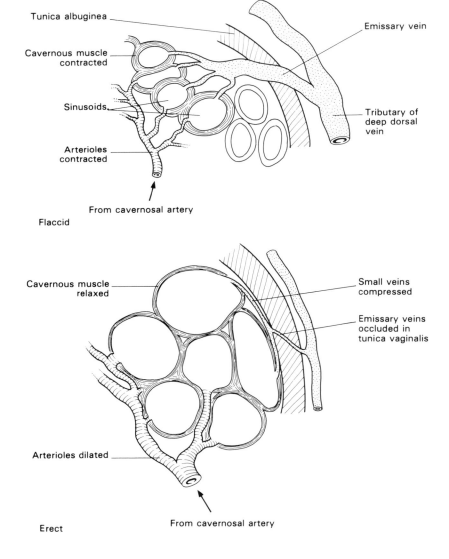

Fig. 27.18 The efferent veins from the corpora cavernosa are closed by being kinked where they pass through the tunica albuginea.

described on p. 249. The role of the muscles of the urethra in females is essential for continence at all times, for in women the bladder neck appears to be open at rest (see p. 251). The function of the paraurethral glands in either sex is not known.

References

1 Hill WCO (1956–1966) *Primates: Comparative Anatomy and Taxonomy*, 6 vols. Edinburgh: Edinburgh University Press.

2 Marshall FF (1978) Embryology of the lower genitourinary tract. *Urol Clin N Am* 5: 3.

3 Vaughan ED, Middleton GW (1975) Pertinent genitourinary embryology: review for the practising urologist. *Urology* 6: 139.

4 Gosling JA, Dixon JS, Humpherson JR (1983) *Functional Anatomy of the Urinary Tract*. London: Gower.

5 Tanagho EA, Lue TF (1990) Physiology of penile erection, in: Chisholm GD, Fair WR (eds) *Scientific Foundations of Urology*, 3rd edn, pp. 420–6. Oxford: Heinemann.

6 Fugleholm K, Schmalbruch H, Wagner G (1989) The vascular anatomy of the cavernous body of green monkeys. *J Urol* 142: 181.

7 Riveros M, Garcia R, Cabanas R (1967) Lymphangiography of the dorsal lymphatics of the penis. *Cancer* 20: 2026.

8 MacLean PD, Denniston RH, Dua S (1963) Further studies on cerebral representation of penile erection: caudal thalamus, midbrain and pons. *J Neurophysiol* 26: 274.

9 Slimp JC, Hart BL, Goy RW (1978) Heterosexual, autosexual and social behavior of adult male rhesus monkeys with medial preoptic-anterior hypothalamic lesions. *Brain Res* 142: 105.

10 Lue TF, Zeineh SJ, Schmidt RA, Tanagho EA (1984) Neuroanatomy of penile erection: its relevance to iatrogenic impotence. *J Urol* 131: 273.

11 Walsh PC, Donker PJ (1992) Impotence following radical prostatectomy: insight into etiology and prevention. *J Urol* 130: 1237.

12 Setchell BP (1978) *The Mammalian Testis*. London: Elek.

13 Smith P (1972) Age changes in the female urethra. *Br J Urol* 44: 667.

Chapter 28: Urethra and penis — congenital abnormalities

Ambiguous genitalia — intersex

The neuter pattern of human genitalia seems at first glance to be female. A child with genitalia of ambiguous appearance may either be a genetic female subjected to masculinization or a genetic male in whom the process of masculinization has been impaired [1–3].

Female subject to masculinization

1 There may be no synthesis of cortisol from a genetic lack of one of a group of enzymes — of which 17-hydroxylase and 11-hydroxylase are the most common (Fig. 28.1). Want of cortisol leads to an increased secretion of adrenocortico-trophic hormone (ACTH) and hence to adrenal

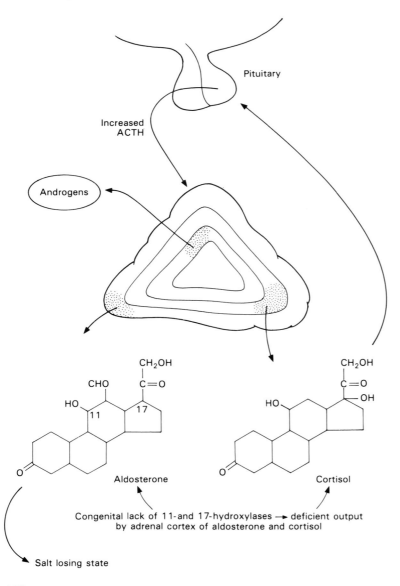

Pituitary

Increased ACTH

Androgens

CH₂OH
CHO   C=O
HO   11   17

O
Aldosterone

CH₂OH
C=O
OH
HO

O
Cortisol

Congenital lack of 11-and 17-hydroxylases → deficient output by adrenal cortex of aldosterone and cortisol

Salt losing state

Fig. 28.1 Females subject to masculinization. Mechanisms causing an excess of androgens.

hyperplasia and the overproduction of androgens. But at the same time there may be an inability to synthesize aldosterone, leading to excessive loss of salt in the urine.

2 The genetic XX female may be poisoned with androgens because her mother has an adrenal tumour, or has been given androgens during pregnancy.

Male with imperfect masculinization

The neuter pattern may fail to become masculine for three main reasons (Fig. 28.2):

1 Testosterone may not be being formed, because of a congenital deficiency of 17-ketosteroid reductase.

2 Testosterone is not converted to dihydro-testosterone because of a genetic lack of 5-alpha reductase.

3 There is an error on the X chromosome leading to a lack of the cytosol receptor for dihydrotestosterone.

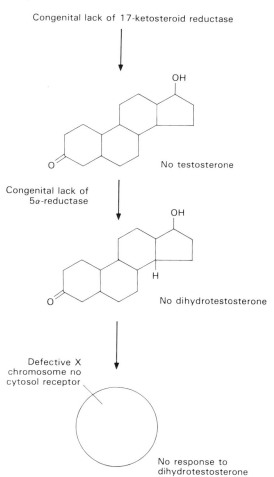

Fig. 28.2 Mechanism causing imperfect masculinization in males.

Females subjected to masculinization

Adrenogenital syndrome

In this, the most common and serious type of intersex there is some urgency about making the diagnosis because of the risk of a lethal salt losing state. The diagnosis is confirmed by showing a positive buccal smear and a raised urinary secretion of 17-ketosteroids. The treatment is by giving steroids. This halts the process of virilization, but it leaves the problem of the enlarged clitoris and the covered-up urogenital sinus (Figs 28.3 & 28.4).

Later on in childhood, the clitoris can be mobilized and part of its shaft removed with careful preservation of the nerve supply (Fig. 28.5). The covered urogenital sinus is laid open, sometimes with the aid of a flap of skin. When the child reaches puberty it is necessary to check, and if necessary correct, any remaining stenosis of the vaginal introitus.

In those genetic females that have been masculinized by androgens given to the mother in pregnancy, the process ceases at birth, but the problems of the clitoris and covered vagina remain.

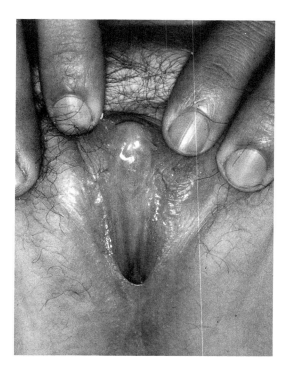

Fig. 28.3 Mild virilization: girl with genetic lack of 21-hydroxylase. Hypertrophied clitoris and fusion of posterior parts of labia (courtesy of Mr J.H. Johnston).

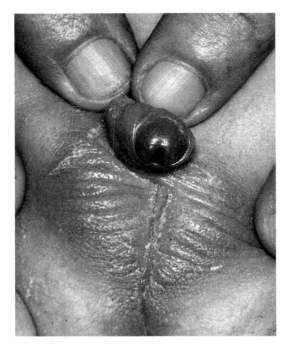

Fig. 28.4 Severe virilization: girl with more severe genetic enzyme defects: complete fusion of labia and urogenital sinus opens at tip of phallus (courtesy of Mr J.H. Johnston).

Males with imperfect masculinization

Male pseudohermaphroditism

The most common and severe disorder occurs in testicular feminization which is a sex-linked inherited condition. The appearance is female, but the vagina is short. Inguinal herniae are common, and the testicles show Leydig cells but no spermatogenesis, and have a considerable risk of forming malignant tumours (Fig. 28.6). The various biochemical investigations may be able to discover whether there is a deficiency of the production of testosterone (from want of 17-ketosteroid reductase), failure of activation to dihydrotestosterone, or want of the cytosol receptor protein. None of these can be corrected. The child should be reared as a girl until puberty when the testicles should be removed to prevent cancer and oestrogen replacement therapy is given.

When the syndrome is incomplete the clitoris may be very large. With the onset of puberty these children may rapidly virilize and it is necessary to remove the gonads in childhood.

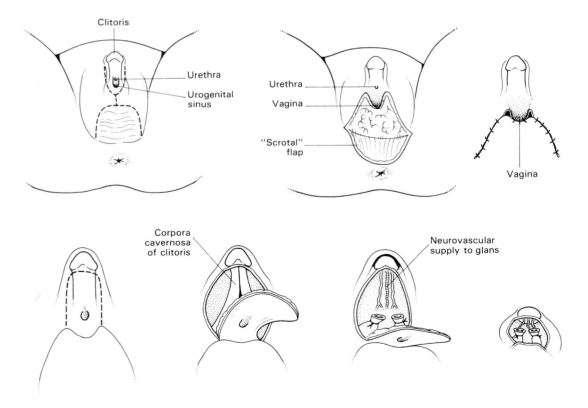

Fig. 28.5 Correction of virilization: the covered urogenital sinus is laid open and the clitoris is reduced with careful preservation of its nerve supply.

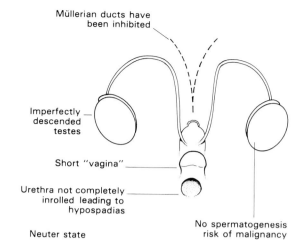

Müllerian ducts have been inhibited

Imperfectly descended testes

Short "vagina"

Urethra not completely inrolled leading to hypospadias

Neuter state

No spermatogenesis risk of malignancy

a

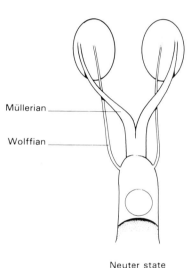

Müllerian

Wolffian

Neuter state

b

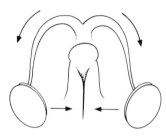

Descent of gonads hypertrophy of clitoris no inhibition of Müllerian ducts inrolling of urethra

Fig. 28.6 Male pseudo-hermaphroditism (a) with and (b) without inhibition of Müllerian ducts.

There are a large number of genetic males who are only slightly imperfectly masculinized. Some merely have hypospadias and need no other treatment. Others may have persistent Müllerian structures and more or less maldescent of the testicles [4]. These children may be reared as boys, and any minor deformity of the genitalia can be corrected appropriately.

Mosaicism (XO/XY)

In these rare chromosomal abnormalities one gonad may be a testis, the other a 'streak' gonad — an ovary without any follicles. Their management calls for great care, and the child should only be reared as a boy if there is a well-developed phallus.

Klinefelter's syndrome (XXY)

Many of these children grow up to be physically quite normal, but their testicles are small, and they are referred because of infertility (Fig. 28.7). More severe cases may be deficient in masculine body hair, and require treatment with androgens. The diagnosis is easily made with a buccal smear [5].

Turner's syndrome (XO)

Here the child remains in the neuter–female state. The gonads are streaks of connective tissue in the broad ligaments. There are often associated cardiac defects. The patient is short, with a broad chest and webbed neck [6] (Fig. 28.8).

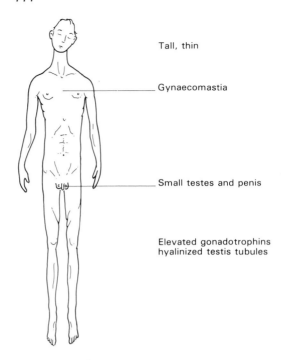

Fig. 28.7 Klinefelter's syndrome (XXY).

Investigation of intersex

The buccal smear will detect the presence of a second X chromosome. The collection of a 24-h specimen of urine for 17-ketosteroids is urgently needed, but one must be aware of a source of error here, since in the first few days of life the levels in the healthy infant may be above normal. In the salt losing state the serum electrolytes will usually reveal a high potassium and a low sodium.

As soon as possible the child should be referred to a paediatric centre with experience of these conditions. Subsequent investigations will include examination of the genitalia with contrast media and endoscopy, and perhaps laparotomy and biopsy of the gonads.

Absence of the penis

The urethra opens in front of or behind the scrotum. Although a sort of penis may be constructed in a series of staged plastic surgical procedures, it never functions and the best advice is to raise the child as a girl [2].

Micropenis and microphallus

Micropenis is a small penis without hypospadias; microphallus signifies an ambiguous organ associated with hypospadias [1]. Do not jump to either of these diagnoses in fat little boys whose penis seems to be hidden: gentle retraction of the fat often discloses a normal penis.

Micropenis may occur with incomplete androgen resistance. Chorionic gonadotrophin will make the penis develop enough for adequate sexual function [7,8].

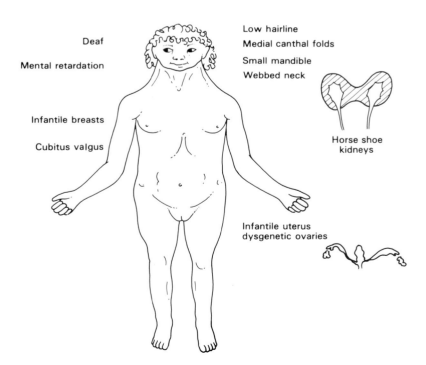

Fig. 28.8 Turner's syndrome (XO).

Duplex phallus

If the paired phallic tubercles fail to fuse there will be a double penis: it is sometimes associated with exstrophy, diastasis of the pubis and duplication of the bladder [9] (Fig. 28.9).

Torsion of the penis

The penis may be twisted on its long axis (Fig. 28.10). There may be hypospadias. It can be remedied by sleeving the penile skin back through a circumferential incision, untwisting the penis, and sewing the skin back straight.

Phimosis

The fold of skin which grows forwards to enclose the embryo glans soon becomes adherent. The cleft between the two layers of skin does not reappear in many boys until 4 or 5 years of age [10]. Efforts to force back the prepuce before the plane of cleavage has reappeared may lead to fibrosis which makes it even less easy to reduce. The irretractible prepuce may cause recurrent balanitis and secondary adhesions, and the prepuce often becomes inflamed from ammoniacal dermatitis in infancy. The scarred, irretractible prepuce may become so tight that it causes urinary obstruction.

Circumcision

History and background

Cave paintings show that ritual circumcision was practised from the most ancient times along with amputations of fingers and other ritual mutilations which persist in some Stone Age

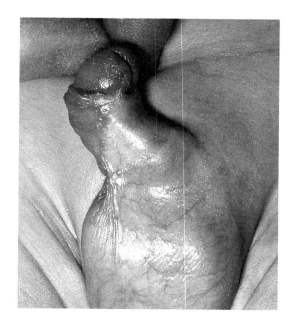

Fig. 28.10 Torsion of the penis associated with hypospadias (courtesy of Mr J.H. Johnston).

cultures even today where it is a pubertal rite of passage [11−14].

It is customary for surgeons to distance themselves from ritual mutilations, whether done in the name of justice or religion [15−18]. There are some therapeutic arguments in favour of circumcision.

Urinary infections in infant boys are very slightly more common (0.24%) in uncircumcised than circumcised boys (0.19%) [16].

Virus infections in adults are more likely to attack the moist, easily abraded skin of the prepuce and uncircumcised glans. Condylomata acuminata and recurrent herpes are comparatively rare in circumcised men [19]. Transmission of the hepatitis virus may be prevented by circumcision. Circumcision has been recommended for homosexual males to protect them against the human immunodeficiency virus (HIV) [20].

Prevention of cancer. Circumcision prevents cancer of the penis. Partly this may be because so many cancers arise in the prepuce, but cancer is associated with balanitis and infection with *Haemophilus ducreyi* which are prevented by circumcision. It has also been shown that extracts of smegma are carcinogenic in animals.

The ritual circumcision of Jewish boys on the eighth day confers almost absolute protection

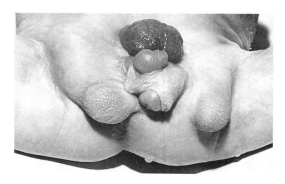

Fig. 28.9 Double penis — associated with exstrophy (courtesy of Mr J.H. Johnston).

against cancer: circumcision of Muslim boys in later childhood affords somewhat less protection, and for adolescents even less [21]. Regular washing under the prepuce and glans penis probably offers protection equal to that of circumcision [22].

Carcinoma of the cervix. The rarity of cancer of the female cervix among Jewish women has been interpreted to mean that circumcision protects perhaps by lessening the transmission of papillomavirus. Other factors may be equally important [23,24].

The morbidity of the operation is by no means negligible [25,26]. Jewish communities have a cadre of officers (Mohelim) who are trained in the technique of ritual circumcision. Even so, there is morbidity, including injuries to the glans penis and urethra, removal of too much penile skin and severe haemorrhage.

In gentile communities circumcision is often left to less adept operators. In communities which demand male circumcision, but make no provision for it, accidental amputation of the penis, sloughing of the glans and life-threatening haemorrhage are commonplace. It is a matter for ethical debate whether surgeons should try to prevent these disasters by offering to perform this ritual mutilation correctly, thus becoming an accomplice to an assault for which there is no therapeutic reason and no informed consent [27].

Alternatives to circumcision

1 Retraction of the prepuce. Many circumcisions can be avoided by counselling the mother. Retraction of the prepuce may be performed if the penis is first steeped in local anaesthetic cream for 10 min or so [28,29]. Once the prepuce has been retracted, the mother may repeat the process each day in the bath. This will avoid circumcision in about 80% of little boys.
2 Dorsal slit. A short vertical incision in the prepuce — the dorsal slit — just enough to allow the prepuce to be retracted fully, serves the same purpose but the result is somewhat unsightly. Closing the incision transversely may be the answer (Fig. 28.11).

Technique of therapeutic circumcision

Circumcision may be performed with local or general anaesthesia: if local anaesthetic is used it must not contain adrenaline because arterial spasm caused by adrenaline may lead to necrosis

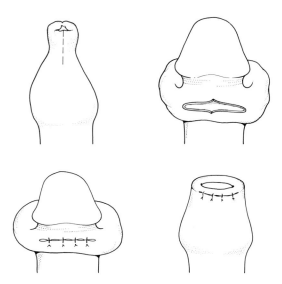

Fig. 28.11 Preputioplasty. Only the tight band need be incised. Afterwards the parent must keep the prepuce regularly reduced.

of the penis. Care must be taken in using the diathermy to avoid coagulation of the vessels of the penis. The bipolar diathermy is safe, but if this is not available the penis should be surrounded by swabs soaked in saline to provide a wide pathway for the current to return to earth (Fig. 28.12).

Draw the foreskin forwards. Make a clean incision with a knife level with the corona of the glans (Fig. 28.13). Then draw the foreskin backwards, if necessary making a small slit in the prepuce. Make a second clean incision with the knife 3 mm proximal to the sulcus of the glans. Join the two incisions and dissect the sleeve of skin off the shaft of the penis. Seal every small vessel with the bipolar diathermy or very fine catgut.

If the frenulum is so short that it causes pain on intercourse [30] take the opportunity to elongate the frenulum by closing the transverse incision in the midline (Fig. 28.14).

Use only very fine absorbable sutures. Perfect haemostasis must be achieved: avoid 'haemostatic' dressings which may cause pressure necrosis of the underlying skin. As soon as the blood has dried no dressing is needed other than a fold of sterile Vaseline gauze to prevent bedclothes or pants from sticking.

Hypospadias

Most of the urethra is formed by inrolling of the urethral folds either side of the developing

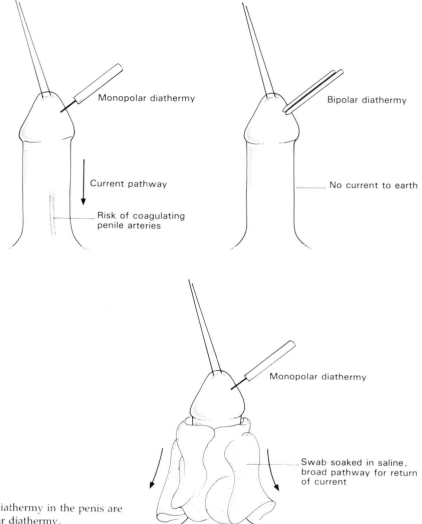

Monopolar diathermy

Bipolar diathermy

Current pathway

No current to earth

Risk of coagulating
penile arteries

Monopolar diathermy

Swab soaked in saline,
broad pathway for return
of current

Fig. 28.12 The hazards of diathermy in the penis are
avoided by using the bipolar diathermy.

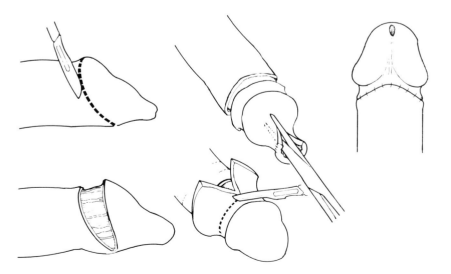

Fig. 28.13 Technique of
circumcision.

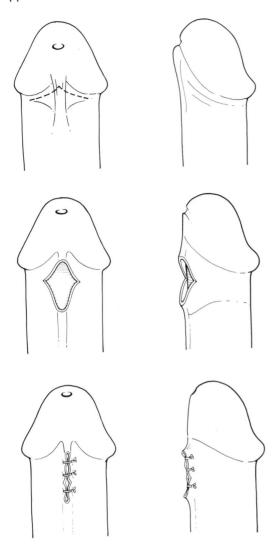

Fig. 28.14 Technique for elongating the frenulum.

phallus, but the last part — the channel through the glans — starts as a solid rod and then canalizes. Any part of this complex process may go wrong. Its most severe forms are often associated with undescended testes and should raise the suspicion of intersex (see p. 442).

If the solid cord that burrows through the glans fails to canalize, the urethra opens on its ventral aspect — glandular hypospadias. This is common, and apart from looking slightly unusual, never causes any trouble (Fig. 28.15).

Failure of inrolling of the urethral folds is accompanied by errors in development of the corpora cavernosa and spongiosum. The distal part of the corpus spongiosum may be a thin strand of fibrous tissue which acts like the cord of a bow causing the penis to bend over during erection — chordee.

Glandular hypospadias

In this common minimal form of hypospadias the only abnormality is a prepuce which opens in front and a meatus that is level with the corona glandis. These boys grow to manhood without disability: rarely a meatal hood makes them spray when they void. Few little boys worry about this. Most learn to aim, marry, have children and in the evening of their lives come to prostatectomy without ever realizing that they had an abnormality.

Today, it is the fashion to subject these boys to an operation — 'meatus advancement glanuloplasty' (MAGPI) — which alters the appearance of the penis to that of a boy who has been circumcised [31,32]. The child has no say in this procedure which is done to please the parents.

MAGPI operation

Cut the little fold at the distal end of the pit which represents the true meatus in the midline and close it transversely (Fig. 28.16). Make a second transverse incision just proximal to the urethra. Draw it up with a skin hook. Mobilize the prepuce on either side and swing it down beneath the glans to cover the raw area. The penis now looks as if circumcision has been performed. No catheter is needed. The little operation can be done as a day-case. The long-term results are disappointing, as there is a tendency for the appearance of the glans to revert to its original one.

Penile hypospadias

Usually the urethra opens half-way along the urethra and there is a pronounced chordee when the child has an erection. The two objectives of operation are (a) to correct the chordee; and (b) bring the urethra to the end of the penis. The innumerable techniques mean that this is an operation which is not easy or always successful. Good results are obtained only by teams that deal with many cases. Hypospadias is not for the occasional operator.

The most experienced paediatric urological units offer a one-stage operation, using a myo-cutaneous skin flap [33–37] of which there are several variants (Fig. 28.17). They all begin with a circumferential incision behind the corona just distal to the opening of the urethra. The skin is sleeved back together with the urethra. The fibrous strand is dissected away until the chordee

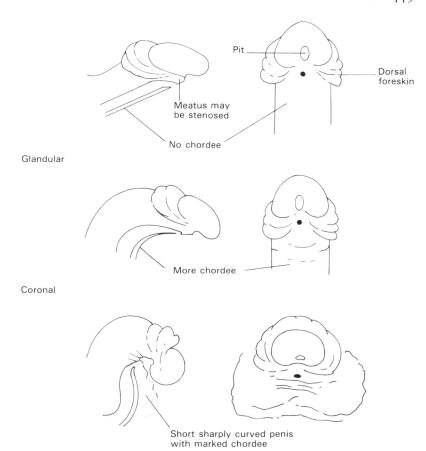

Glandular

Pit

Dorsal foreskin

Meatus may be stenosed

No chordee

More chordee

Coronal

Short sharply curved penis with marked chordee

Penoscrotal and perineal

Fig. 28.15 Degrees of hypospadias.

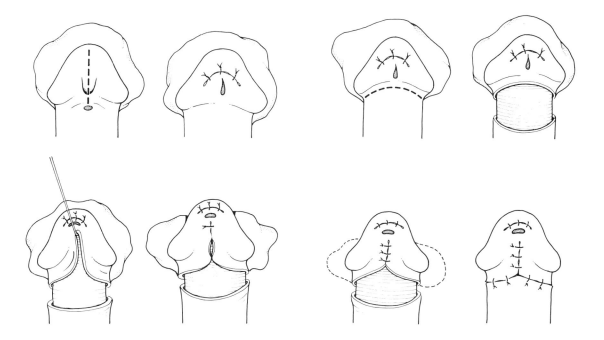

Fig. 28.16 MAGPI operation.

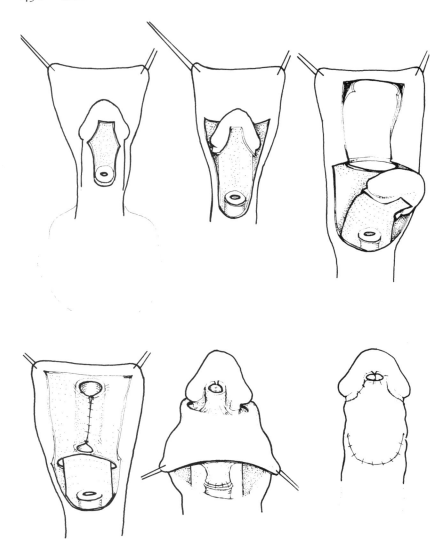

Fig. 28.17 One variant of one-stage hypospadias repair.

is corrected. When the penis is straight the urethra may have dropped back right down the shaft of the penis.

A new urethra is formed of a tube of foreskin which is provided with a vascular pedicle of dartos muscle. Variations in the way of making this skin tube have given rise to many different eponyms for what is essentially the same operation. During the period of healing, the urine is diverted with a suprapubic or a very narrow urethral catheter.

The main complication of this type of hypospadias repair is breakdown of part of the suture line, resulting in a fistula. Several months should be allowed to pass before attempting to repair it. This is a common complication. Always warn the parents that it might happen, and that all is not lost if it does.

A more reliable alternative to these one-stage operations are the two-stage procedures which are usually performed for the more severe degrees of hypospadias.

Complete hypospadias

It may help to give androgens in the form of local cream or systemic injection to enlarge the phallus before the first stage when the chordee is corrected. Skin is brought round from the prepuce to the ventral side of the penis. One reliable method starts by dividing the prepuce in the dorsal midline (Fig. 28.18). Two large flaps are brought down on each side to cover the gap on the underside of the penis. At a second stage the urethra is formed by forming a skin tube [38] (Fig. 28.19).

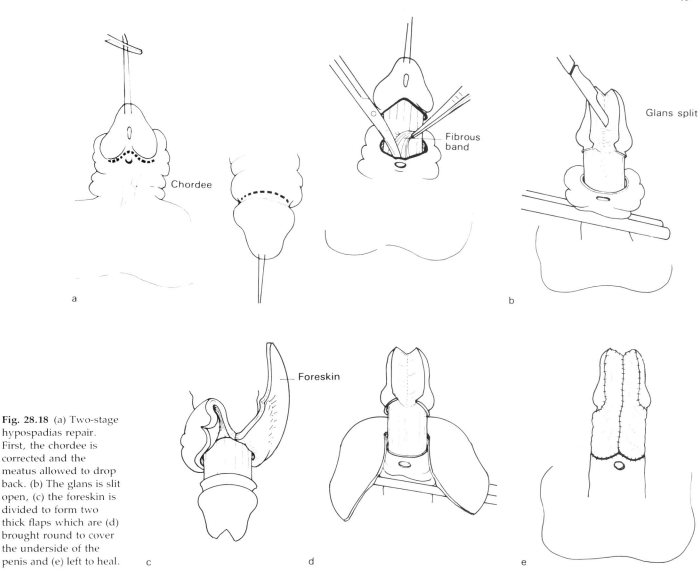

Fig. 28.18 (a) Two-stage hypospadias repair. First, the chordee is corrected and the meatus allowed to drop back. (b) The glans is slit open, (c) the foreskin is divided to form two thick flaps which are (d) brought round to cover the underside of the penis and (e) left to heal.

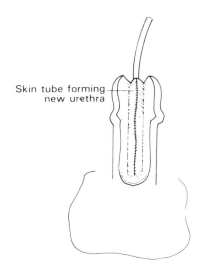

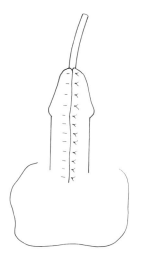

Fig. 28.19 At a second stage a full thickness skin tube is outlined and the skin closed over it to form a new urethra.

Late repair of hypospadias

It is deplorable that so many children suffer several unsuccessful attempts at repair of hypospadias before they are referred to a surgeon who specializes in the procedure by which time the foreskin has been used up. It is then necessary to resort to free grafts of skin, bladder mucosa or the lining of the mouth [39,40].

Hypoplasia of corpus cavernosum

Young adults notice that the erect penis bends to one side, or has a ventral chordee. It is painless and usually only needs reassurance. Cavernosography shows a difference in the length and diameter of the two corpora. If treatment is really needed use Nesbit's procedure (see p. 532).

Congenital anomalies of the urethra

There are two main groups of congenital anomalies of the urethra: (a) where there has been an error in the development of the cloacal membrane, leading to exstrophy and epispadias (see p. 256); and (b) where there has been an error in the inrolling of the genital folds to form the urethra.

Atresia of the urethra

Formerly regarded as incompatible with life, this rare condition is now diagnosed by ultrasound during pregnancy. A vesicoamniotic shunt is inserted percutaneously, allowing the urine to escape into the amniotic cavity. Then it has been possible to dialyse the baby until such time that a maternal transplant was accomplished at 1 year of age [41].

Congenital urethral valves

This anomaly is frequently detected by antenatal ultrasound scanning in the last trimester of pregnancy. Its cause is unknown. A membrane like a parachute lies across the prostatic urethra, exaggerating the folds that normally lead down from the verumontanum (Fig. 28.20) and obstructing the outflow from the bladder (Figs 28.21 & 28.22).

Urine is continually secreted *in utero* to make the amniotic fluid. The boy with urethral valves develops chronic retention, hydroureters and hydronephrosis. The distended bladder prevents proper development of the abdominal wall (Fig. 28.23).

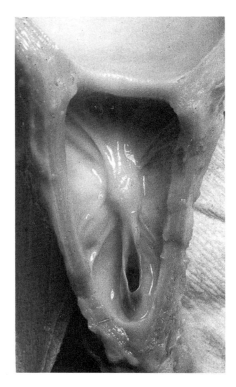

Fig. 28.20 Autopsy specimen showing posterior urethral valve (courtesy of Mr J.H. Johnston).

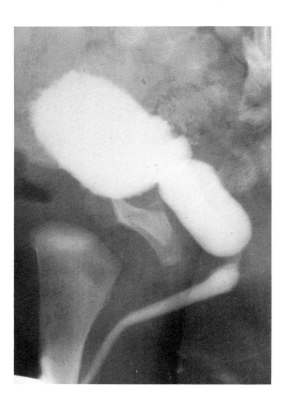

Fig. 28.21 Micturating cystogram in a boy with congenital posterior urethral valves (courtesy of Mr J.H. Johnston).

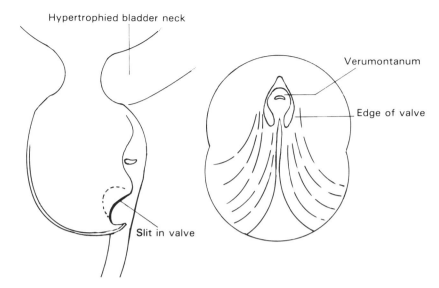

Fig. 28.22 Congenital posterior urethral valves.

Sometimes the dilatation of the upper urinary tract, detected *in utero* by ultrasound, is found to resolve spontaneously but the damage has been done, and when the child is born he is found

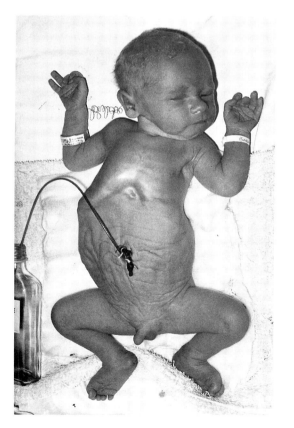

Fig. 28.23 Prune belly deformity associated with congenital posterior urethral valves and gross dilatation of the urinary tract (courtesy of Mr J.H. Johnston).

to have a trabeculated bladder, thinned out kidneys, and a thin, wrinkled abdominal wall. All evidence of obstruction has disappeared, suggesting that the valves have ruptured spontaneously [42].

It is possible to overcome the obstruction by inserting a vesicoamniotic shunt (Fig. 28.24) and then, after the child has been delivered, the diagnosis is confirmed with ultrasound. A thin hook, insulated except for a segment on its concavity, is passed into the urethra (Fig. 28.25). When the valve is engaged — and confirmed with ultrasound — a touch of diathermy destroys the valve and obstruction is relieved [43]. The boy is left with permanently dilated upper tracts. The long-term outlook is guarded — about 30% persist with incontinence and continued bladder dysfunction [44].

Urethral duplication

The usual type of urethral duplication is incomplete — a double-barrelled urethra with its second channel inferior to the normal one (Fig. 28.26). At operation the second urethra is found to be surrounded by spongy tissue and there are one or more openings into the normal urethra (Fig. 28.27). When the boy passes urine the second channel fills out and compresses the normal one — hence the term 'anterior urethral valve' [45,46].

The clinical history is typical. The child has a poor stream. He strains so hard that 'he dirties when he wets'. The ballooned second urethra slowly empties and so the boy seems to be continually incontinent. There is a translucent

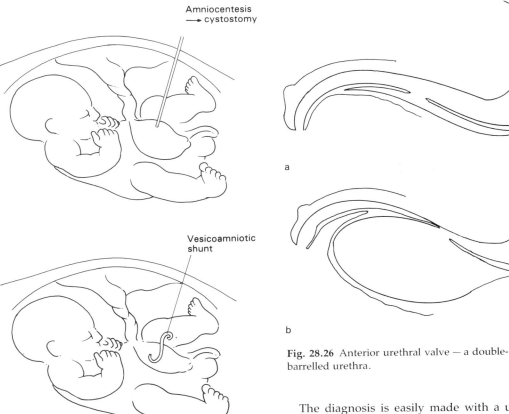

Amniocentesis
→ cystostomy

Vesicoamniotic
shunt

Fig. 28.24 Principle of intrauterine shunt for urinary obstruction caused by congenital valves.

Fig. 28.26 Anterior urethral valve — a double-barrelled urethra.

swelling in the midline. Often this collection of urine becomes infected and the child presents with an abscess which is incised and leaves a permanent fistula. There may be severe upper tract obstruction. They may present in adult life with a stone in the sac (Fig. 28.28).

The diagnosis is easily made with a urethrogram or ultrasound examination of the perineum. Endoscopy shows an opening in the floor of the urethra.

If the anterior leaf of the 'valve' is incised (Fig. 28.29) the obstruction is relieved. The child may be left with a baggy urethra, and if this causes trouble, it is easy to remodel it at a later stage. In severe cases the sac can be excised and the hole in the urethra repaired as in urethroplasty (see p. 489).

Urethral duplications also occur dorsal to

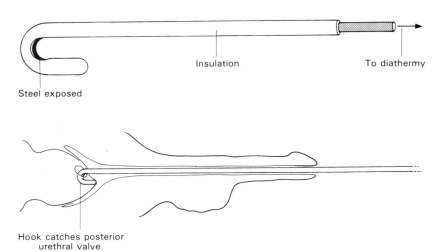

Insulation

To diathermy

Steel exposed

Hook catches posterior
urethral valve

Fig. 28.25 Insulated urethral hook for destroying congenital valves.

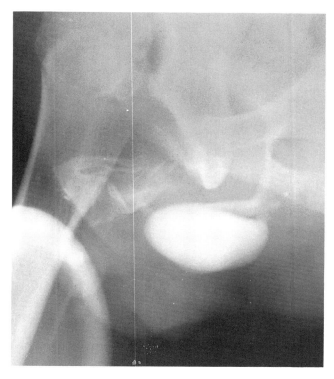

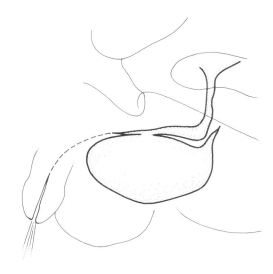

Fig. 28.27 Anterior urethral valve. Radiograph during an attempt at voiding.

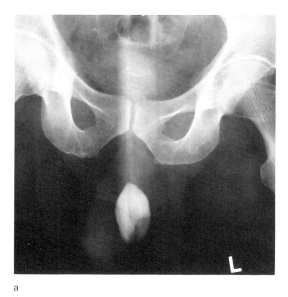

a

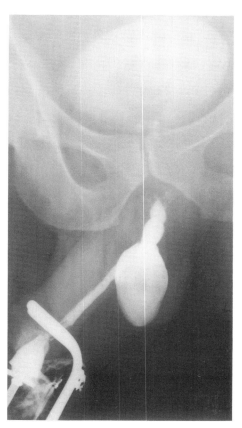

b

Fig. 28.28 (a) Plain X-ray and (b) urethrogram of a postman who complained of perineal discomfort after cycling. The stone had formed in the diverticulum.

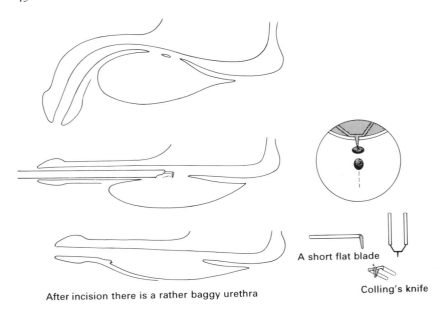

After incision there is a rather baggy urethra

A short flat blade

Colling's knife

Fig. 28.29 The anterior leaf of the 'valve' may be incised endoscopically, but the very large urethra may need repairing later on.

the normal channel (Fig. 28.30). They may be complete or incomplete. They are very rare and do not need any treatment. They can be a site for persistent infection with *Neisseria gonorrhoeae*.

Congenital midbulbar strictures

It is common to notice helical rings in the normal bulbar urethra, resembling the rifling of a gun-barrel. An exaggeration of this may occasionally cause a midbulbar stricture which can be a cause of obstruction in adolescents [47–48] (Fig. 28.31).

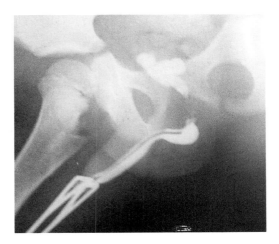

Fig. 28.30 Urethral duplication dorsal to the normal urethra (courtesy of Mr J.H. Johnston).

Dilated Cowper's ducts

Cowper's glands lie within the levator ani shelf. Their ducts pass down to open in the bulbar urethra. Sometimes these ducts become dilated and infected. The urethrographic appearances then resemble an anterior urethral valve (Fig. 28.32). The difference is that these are always double — one beside the other. Attempts to remove them are seldom successful or worthwhile; unless the glands are also removed the ducts will regenerate.

Cowper's glands are rarely the site of persistent infection with *Neisseria* or other organisms. Clinical examination shows a pea-sized swelling, exquisitely tender, between the layers of the pelvic fascia just anterior to the rectum (Fig. 28.33).

Urethral diverticula in the female

Two kinds of urethral diverticula occur in females [49]. The most common is a single pouch opening in the midline in the floor of the urethra (Fig. 28.34). It presents as a tender swelling along the urethra. Pus emerges on gentle pressure. Sometimes stones form and, very rarely, carcinoma.

The second type is double, one on either side of the midline, and they each have a long process leading back up and behind the bladder (Fig. 28.35). They probably represent an ectopic ureterocele without a kidney component. They are rare. They have twin openings in the urethra. In the author's experience attempts to excise

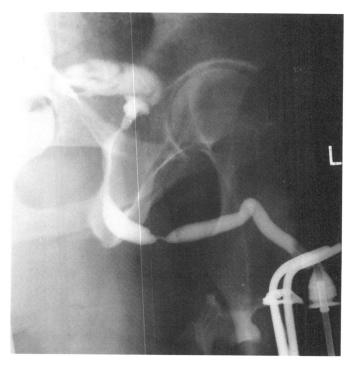

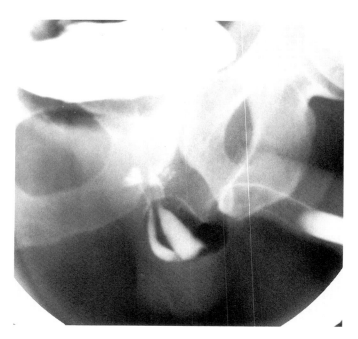

Fig. 28.32 Dilated Cowper's ducts resemble congenital anterior valves but they are usually double.

Fig. 28.31 Midbulbar stricture thought to have been of congenital origin.

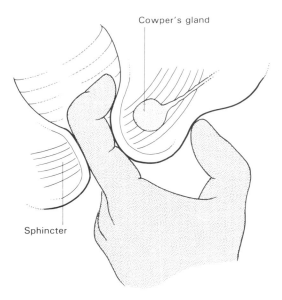

Fig. 28.33 An abscess of Cowper's gland presents as a very tender swelling in the pelvic floor felt anterior to the anal canal.

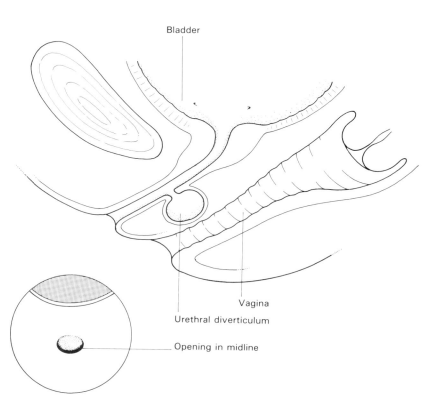

Fig. 28.34 (*Right*) Urethral diverticulum in a female patient.

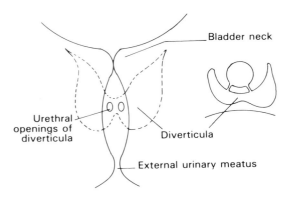

Fig. 28.35 Diagram of bilateral 'saddle-bag' urethral diverticula in females. They may represent a form of ureterocele.

them have usually been followed by recurrence [49].

The approach to urethral diverticula in the female is via a laterally based trapdoor incision (Fig. 28.36). This avoids having a suture line in front of the urethra and prevents fistula. Marsupializing the sac may lead to incontinence [50]. Care is taken to repair all the layers of the wall of the urethra, for these contain the sleeve of smooth and striated muscle upon which continence depends.

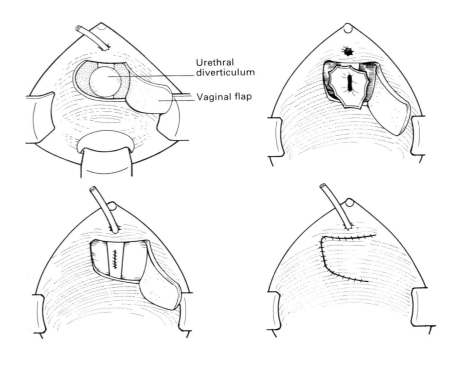

Fig. 28.36 Operative approach to urethral diverticulum in a female. A trapdoor vaginal flap prevents formation of a fistula afterwards.

References

1 Whitaker RH, Barnes ND (1987) *Intersex: Cambridge Guide to Diagnosis and Management in Neonates.* Cambridge: Cambridge Childrens Kidney Care Fund.

2 Allen TD (1976) Disorders of sexual differentiation. *Urology* 7 (Suppl): 1.

3 Izquierdo G, Glassberg K (1993) Gender assignment and gender identity in patients with ambiguous genitalia. *Urology* 42: 232.

4 Gustafson ML, Lee MM, Asmundson L, Maclaughlin DT, Donahoe PK (1993) Müllerian inhibiting substance in the diagnosis and management of intersex and gonadal abnormalities. *J Ped Surg* 28: 439.

5 Klinefelter HF Jr, Reifenstein CE Jr, Albright F (1942) Syndrome characterised by gynecomastia, aspermatogenesis without A-Leydigism and

increased excretion of follicle stimulating hormone. *J Clin Endocrinol* 2: 615.

6 Turner HH (1938) A syndrome of infantilism, congenital webbed neck, and cubitus valgus. *Endocrinology* 23: 566.

7 Reilly JM, Woodhouse CRJ (1989) Small penis and the male sexual role. *J Urol* 142 (part 2): 569.

8 Young HH, Cockett ATK, Stoller R, Ashley FL, Goodwin WE (1971) The management of agenesis of the phallus. *Pediatrics* 47: 81.

9 Savir A, Lurie A, Lazenbik J (1970) Diphallia: report of a case. *Br J Urol* 42: 498.

10 Gairdner D (1949) The fate of the foreskin. *Br Med J* 2: 1433.

11 Remondino PC (1891) *History of Circumcision.* Philadelphia: Davis.

12 Murphy LJT (1974) Subincision of the urethra. *Br J Urol* 46: 123.

13 Genesis 17: 10–23.

14 Ghalioungui P (1963) *Magic and Medical Science in Ancient Egypt*. London: Hodder & Stoughton.

15 Cetinkaya M, Saglam HS, Beyribey S (1993) Two serious complications of circumcision. *Scand J Urol Nephrol* 27: 121.

16 Wiswell TE, Hahey WE (1993) Urinary tract infections and the uncircumcised state: an update. *Clin Ped* 32: 130.

17 Editorial (1979) The case against neonatal circumcision. *Br Med J* 1: 1163.

18 Rickwood AMK, Hemalatha V, Batcup G, Spitz L (1980) Phimosis in boys. *Br J Urol* 52: 147.

19 Oates JK (1983) Venereal disease: genital herpes. *Br J Hosp Med* 29: 13.

20 Marx JL (1989) Circumcision may protect against the AIDS virus. *Science* 245: 470.

21 Blandy JP (1977) Circumcision, in: Chamberlain G (ed.) *Contemporary Obstetrics and Gynaecology*, pp. 240–2. London: Northwood.

22 Reddy DJ, Indira C (1963) Some aspects of the pathology of carcinoma penis. *J Indian Med Ass* 41: 277.

23 Aitken-Swan J, Baird D (1965) Circumcision and cancer of the cervix. *Br J Cancer* 19: 217.

24 Terris M, Wilson F, Nelson JH (1973) Relation of circumcision to cancer of the cervix. *Am J Obstet Gynecol* 117: 1056.

25 Talarico RD, Jasaitis JE (1973) Concealed penis: a complication of neonatal circumcision. *J Urol* 110: 732.

26 Shulman J, Ben-Hur N, Neuman Z (1964) Surgical complications of circumcision. *Am J Dis Child* 107: 149.

27 Gordon A, Collin J (1993) Save the normal foreskin. *Br Med J* 306: 1.

28 Cooper GG, Thomson GJL, Raine PAM (1983) Therapeutic retraction of the foreskin in childhood. *Br Med J* 286: 186.

29 MacKinlay GA (1988) Save the prepuce. Painless separation of preputial adhesions in the outpatient clinic. *Br Med J* 297: 590.

30 Whelan P (1977) Male dyspareunia due to short frenulum: an indication for adult circumcision. *Br Med J* 2: 1633.

31 Duckett JW (1981) MAGPI (meatoplasty and glanuloplasty): a procedure for subcoronal hypospadias. *Urol Clin N Am* 8: 513.

32 Scherz HC, Kaplan GW, Packer MG (1989) Modified meatal advancement and glanuloplasty (Arap hypospadias repair): experience in 31 patients. *J Urol* 142 (part 2): 620.

33 Devine CJ, Horton CE (1961) A one-stage hypospadias repair. *J Urol* 85: 166.

34 Harris DL, Jeffery RS (1989) One-stage repair of hypospadias using split preputial flaps (Harris): the first 100 patients treated. *Br J Urol* 63: 401.

35 Dewan PA, Dinneen MD, Duffy PG, Winkle D, Ransley PG (1991) Pedicle patch urethroplasty. *Br J Urol* 67: 420.

36 Hodgson NB (1970) A one-stage hypospadias repair. *J Urol* 104: 281.

37 Rober PE, Perlmutter AD, Reitelman C (1990) Experience with 81 one-stage hypospadias chordee repairs with free graft urethroplasties. *J Urol* 144 (part 2): 526.

38 Byars LT (1955) A technique for consistently satisfactory repair of hypospadias. *Surg Gynecol Obstet* 100: 184.

39 Scherz HC, Kaplan GW, Packer MG, Brock WA (1988) Post-hypospadias repair urethral strictures: a review of 30 cases. *J Urol* 140 (part 2): 1253.

40 El-Kasaby AW, Fath-Alla M, Noweir AM, El-Halaby MR, Sakaria W, El-Beialy MH (1993) The use of buccal mucosa path graft in the management of anterior urethral strictures. *J Urol* 149: 276.

41 Steinhardt G, Hogan W, Wood E, Weber T, Lynch R (1990) Long-term survival in an infant with urethral atresia. *J Urol* 143: 336.

42 Grieg JD, Raine PAM, Young DG *et al.* (1989) Value of antenatal diagnosis of abnormalities of the urinary tract. *Br Med J* 298: 1417.

43 Whitaker RH, Sherwood T (1986) An improved hook for destroying posterior urethral valves. *J Urol* 135: 531.

44 Parkhouse HF, Barratt TM, Dillon MJ *et al.* (1988) Long-term outcome of boys with posterior urethral valves. *Br J Urol* 62: 59.

45 Gingell JC, Mitchell JP, Roberts JBM (1972) Anterior urethral diverticulum. *Proc Roy Soc Med* 65: 304.

46 Abeshouse BS (1951) Diverticula of the anterior urethra in the male: a report of four cases and a review of the literature. *Urol Cutan Rev* 55: 690.

47 Cobb BG, Wolf JA, Ansell JS (1968) Congenital stricture of the proximal urethral bulb. *J Urol* 99: 629.

48 English PJ, Pryor JP (1986) Congenital bulbar urethral stricture occurring in a father and son. *Br J Urol* 58: 732.

49 Woodhouse CRJ, Flynn JT, Blandy JP (1980) Urethral diverticulum in females. *Br J Urol* 52: 305.

50 Spence H, Duckett J (1970) Diverticulum of the female urethra, clinical aspects and presentation of a simple operative technique for cure. *J Urol* 104: 432.

Chapter 29: Urethra and penis — trauma

Penis and scrotum

The foreskin may be injured during minor trauma, e.g. by being jammed in a zip-fastener, or may suffer major degloving injuries, e.g. when a vacuum cleaner is used for masturbation [1]. Industrial or criminal assaults, and bites from *Homo sapiens* or other domestic animals are also seen [2].

All but the most trivial injuries should be taken very seriously as mixed infection is apt to lead to cellulitis with more loss of skin. All crushed tissue should be excised. No attempt is made at primary closure. Delayed primary or secondary suture is effected after 3–4 days, in which intensive combination chemotherapy is given including metronidazole for anaerobic infection. With human bites mixed infection is especially common together with the risk of fasciitis [2].

When there is extensive loss of shaft skin, as a temporary measure the penis may be placed in a tunnel of scrotum (Fig. 29.1). This preserves the penis, and keeps the option of applying split skin to the penis at a later stage, or of providing it with a new covering of scrotal skin.

Fracture of the penis

The penis may be 'fractured' during strenuous coitus. The tunica albuginea bursts, often with an audible crack. There is extravasation of blood. Usually a corpus cavernosum has ruptured, but the corpus spongiosum may also be torn (Fig. 29.2). The best results follow early exploration, evacuation of the haematoma, and repair of the tunica albuginea [3–4]. If this is not done the haematoma may organize leaving a fibrous plaque in the corpus with the features of Peyronie's disease.

Amputation of the penis

This may occur in an industrial accident, but more often follows a domestic or criminal assault.

It is occasionally seen after unskilful attempts at circumcision. If the penis can be found an attempt should be made to suture it back using microvascular anastomosis of at least one of the penile arteries. There is no need to suture any of the veins — the corpora cavernosa will provide adequate venous return. The urethra is sutured with absorbable sutures over a suitable catheter, and the urine is diverted suprapubically [5].

Battery burn

Severe burns have been caused when an electric battery gets into a baby's wet napkin [6].

Trauma causing priapism or impotence

Cycling may give rise to temporary impotence which recovers spontaneously. Blunt injury has also been reported to cause high flow priapism [7,8].

Lacerations and avulsions of the scrotum

As with injuries to the penis, all scrotal injuries require thorough debridement because of the risk of infection. When in doubt, it is wise to delay primary suture for 3–4 days. This is particularly so in gun-shot wounds [9]. If there is any suspicion of urethral injury, a suprapubic cystostomy is inserted. It is astonishing to see how well the scrotum will regenerate even though the major part has been avulsed. In the management of these injuries one can afford to be very conservative, and postpone skin grafting. If the testes have been exposed by the original injury, they should be temporarily placed in the suprapubic fat pad.

Urethral trauma

Iatrogenic

A clean incision in the urethra made with a

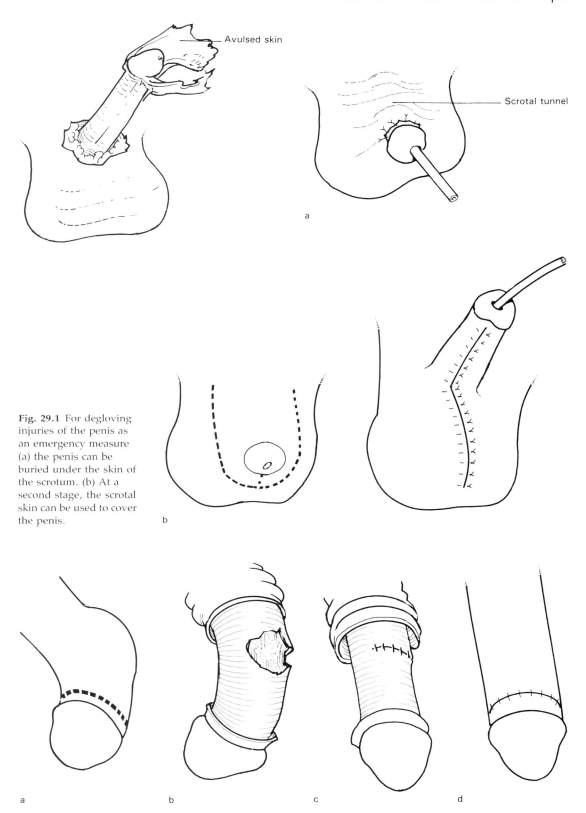

Fig. 29.1 For degloving injuries of the penis as an emergency measure (a) the penis can be buried under the skin of the scrotum. (b) At a second stage, the scrotal skin can be used to cover the penis.

Fig. 29.2 Fracture of the penis. (a) The penile skin is pulled back, (b) the tear in the tunica albuginea is repaired, and (c) the skin is replaced (d).

urethrotome, heals with a linear white scar without stenosis [10] (Fig. 29.3). Passing a urethral instrument is often difficult and followed by bleeding, but strictures are very rare unless infection is present. When in doubt a suprapubic cystostomy tube should be inserted and the urethra re-examined 10–14 days later by which time most iatrogenic lacerations will be found to have healed perfectly.

A more important cause of iatrogenic urethral damage is ischaemic necrosis of the urethra caused by a catheter, as in a bedsore (Fig. 29.4). Urethroscopy in a man catheterized for chronic retention of urine often shows a white ischaemic patch either at the penoscrotal junction or near the external sphincter. These are common sites for 'post-prostatectomy' strictures and they are not caused by the prostatectomy but pressure necrosis from the catheter [11] (Fig. 29.5).

One very important variety of this iatrogenic damage is seen after surgery on the heart or aorta. For a time a toxic component of the latex rubber or plastic of the catheter was blamed: but it is more likely that the cause is pressure of the catheter, whatever it is made of, on a urethra that has become relatively ischaemic during aortic obstruction or cardiac standstill. These 'catheter strictures' may involve the whole length of the urethra and are difficult to treat [12–14] (Fig. 29.6).

From perineal injury

A fall-astride injury or a blow on the perineum forces the urethra up against the inferior edge of

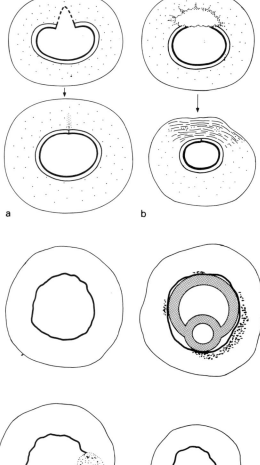

Fig. 29.3 (a) A linear incision in the urethra heals without stenosis. (b) In contrast, a lesion which results in an area of necrosis, especially one involving the corpus spongiosum, heals with a scar that undergoes contraction.

Fig. 29.4 Ischaemic necrosis caused by the pressure of a catheter leads to a scar which heals by contraction — a catheter stricture.

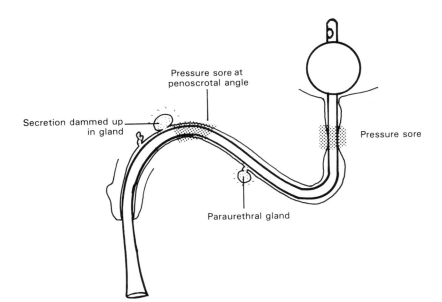

Fig. 29.5 Common sites for catheter strictures are at the penoscrotal junction and the external sphincter.

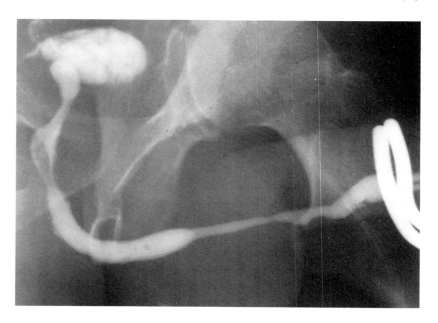

Fig. 29.6 Catheter strictures following open heart surgery often extend the whole length of the urethra.

the symphysis pubis (Fig. 29.7). There is a more or less complete rupture of the corpus spongiosum and urethral wall. Usually, the corpora cavernosa are not injured and they hold the ends of the corpus spongiosum together (Fig. 29.8) so that even if the injury heals with a stenosis, it is always short and easily treated [15] (Fig. 29.9).

Management

If seen early the diagnosis can easily be confirmed by injecting 10−20 ml of water-soluble contrast medium. If there is any extravasation one must assume that the urethra has been lacerated. The

patient should be advised not to void, in the hope of preventing extravasation of urine into the tissues of the scrotum. A suprapubic cystostomy is placed at once.

If seen later on, the patient will have passed urine into the soft tissues of the scrotum (Fig. 29.10) and, unless this is drained, the combination of hypertonic urine and infection will lead to necrosis of the fat and connective tissue, which will in turn lead to necrosis of the overlying skin. The sloughing of the skin caused by the extravasated urine is demarcated by the limits of Colles' fascia, i.e. it is limited posteriorly to the perineal body, and laterally by the crease of

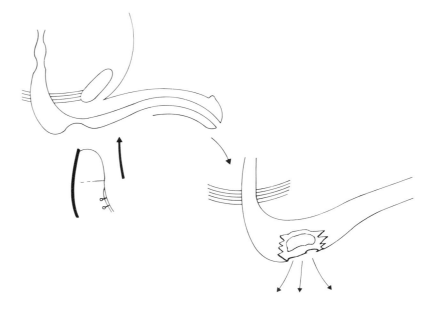

Fig. 29.7 A fall-astride injury forces the urethra up against the edge of the symphysis.

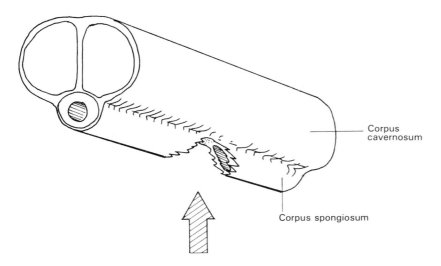

Fig. 29.8 The urethra and its corpus spongiosum are splinted by the corpora cavernosa, and the torn ends cannot retract.

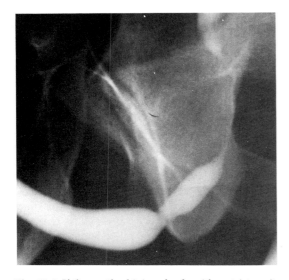

Fig. 29.9 If the urethral injury heals with a stricture it is a short one.

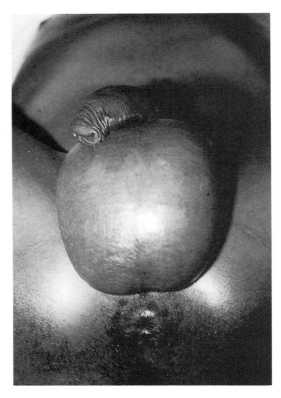

Fig. 29.10 Urine and blood extravasate into the space confined by the fasciae of Scarpa and Colles.

the groin, but involves the entire skin of the scrotum and penis, and a variable amount in front of the symphysis. To prevent this sloughing, the perineum must be adequately drained and, in doing this, one must make sure that both compartments of the scrotum are opened [16] (Fig. 29.11).

In most cases that are diagnosed reasonably early the urethra will be healed within 10−14 days without any stricture. The patient should be carefully followed up and a urethrogram or flexible urethroscopy performed after 2−3 months. If at this stage a stricture is found, since the ruptured ends of the urethra are held in apposition by their attachment to the corpora cavernosa, the stricture is always short and easily treated by dilatation or urethrotomy. If, as is

unusual, urethroplasty is needed, an end-to-end anastomosis can often be performed (see p. 486).

Ruptured membranous urethra associated with fractures of the pelvis

Two main types of fracture of the pelvis lead to membranous urethral injury — they are quite different and require different management [17].

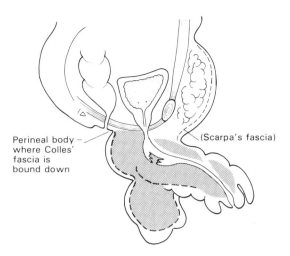

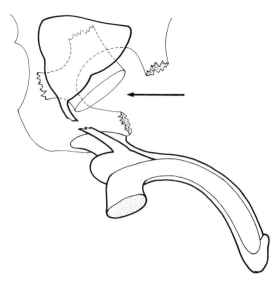

Perineal body – where Colles' fascia is bound down

(Scarpa's fascia)

Fig. 29.11 To prevent sloughing both fascial compartments of the scrotum must be drained.

Fig. 29.12 The symphysis is forced backwards carrying the prostate with it, stretching and then tearing the membranous urethra.

Type I

This is the usual injury. The pelvis is compressed front to back: the weakest parts of the ring — the rami of the pubis and ischium — give way, and the symphysis is forced backwards, carrying the bladder with it (Fig. 29.12). The corpora cavernosa are densely attached to the inner edge of the ischial rami and the urethral bulb. The prostate, firmly attached to the symphysis, is wrenched away from the corpora cavernosa which remain joined to the ischial rami. The urethra stretches until it tears, more or less completely. When the compressing force of the injury is relieved, the displaced symphysis springs back towards its former position. The ends of the urethra return to nearly, but not quite, their original position (Fig. 29.13). Usually, the prostatic urethra ends up just behind and to one or other side of the lower end — the bulbar urethra.

The diagnosis is suspected by the nature of the injury and the appearance of blood from the urethral meatus. It is confirmed by the injection of 10–20 ml of water-soluble contrast medium up the urethra: any extravasation signifies a laceration of the urethra and, whatever its extent, this calls for a suprapubic cystostomy.

Many of these patients have other more serious injuries which take priority, but if the patient is otherwise well, then as soon as possible a urethroscopy should be performed to see whether the lumen of the urethra is still patent. A flexible cystoscope is an ideal instrument with which to make this examination since only a little local anaesthetic is necessary. If the way can be seen clear up to the bladder one can be confident that the laceration will heal (Fig. 29.14). Progress of healing is checked from time to time.

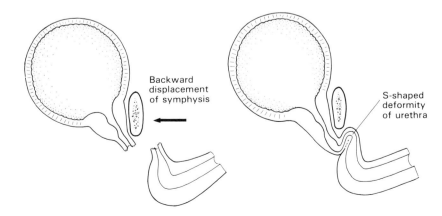

Fig. 29.13 The symphysis springs back but not quite completely and the prostate comes to lie just behind its original position.

Backward displacement of symphysis

S-shaped deformity of urethra

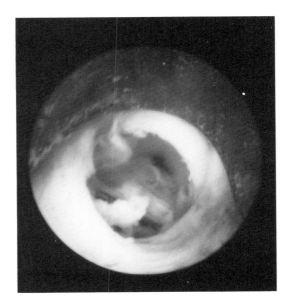

Fig. 29.14 Endoscopic view of an incomplete tear of the membranous urethra.

If the prostatic urethra heals just behind the bulbar urethra, the lumen of the urethra will form an S-shaped bend, leaving two shelves which may need to be incised with a urethrotome (Fig. 29.15). Occasionally, it helps to introduce the flexible cystoscope through the cystostomy track and use its light as a guide for the incision of the obstructing shelves or as a means of introducing a guide-wire for subsequent dilatation [18].

If the lumen is completely blocked, then as soon as reasonably possible — i.e. within the next 10 days — the bulbar urethra should be ex-

plored and anastomosed directly to the torn prostatic urethra (Fig. 29.16). If this exploration is done at this time, the dissection is made easy by the presence of haematoma. Thereafter it becomes progressively more difficult as the scar tissue becomes more dense. The patient must be carefully followed so that any stricture at the anastomosis can be corrected — but the results are excellent [17,19] (Fig. 29.17).

Type II

In the second type of pelvic fracture, the force is (usually) transmitted up the lower limb (Figs 29.18 & 29.19) to wrench the hemi-pelvis out of alignment and dislocate the sacroiliac joint. The bladder and prostate are carried up with the dislocated hemi-pelvis while the bulbar urethra remains attached to the ischial ramus on the other side. Between the severed ends of the urethra there is a gap which is equal to the distance between the bony fragments. If the dislocation cannot be reduced this gap will remain and becomes increasingly difficult to bridge [17].

Most of these patients have other more serious injuries whose treatment takes priority, but as soon as possible the suspected diagnosis should be confirmed by means of a urethrogram using water-soluble contrast medium. Any extravasation signifies some degree of urethral laceration, and demands a suprapubic cystostomy. The pelvic haematoma may make this procedure difficult and it is wise to make sure that the suprapubic tube is really in the bladder by injecting some contrast medium at this time.

To reduce the gap between the severed ends of

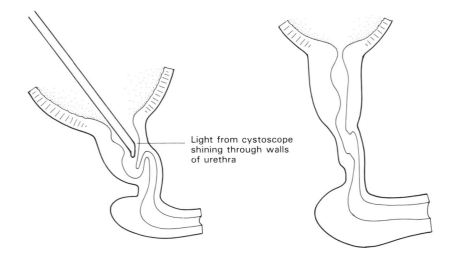

Light from cystoscope shining through walls of urethra

Fig. 29.15 The urethra takes an S-shaped bend whose two leaves can be incised with the urethrotome. It may help to introduce a cystoscope from above and cut down on the light.

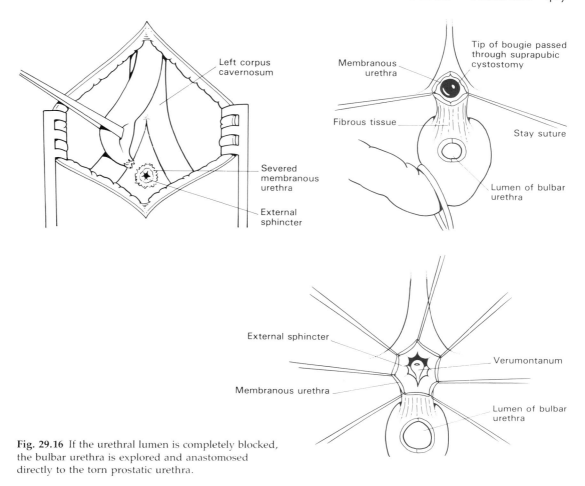

Left corpus cavernosum

Severed membranous urethra

External sphincter

Membranous urethra

Fibrous tissue

Tip of bougie passed through suprapubic cystostomy

Stay suture

Lumen of bulbar urethra

External sphincter

Membranous urethra

Verumontanum

Lumen of bulbar urethra

Fig. 29.16 If the urethral lumen is completely blocked, the bulbar urethra is explored and anastomosed directly to the torn prostatic urethra.

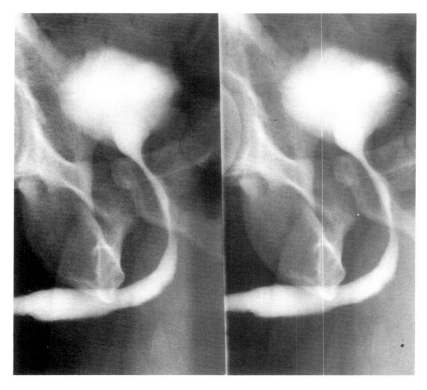

Fig. 29.17 Result of anastomotic repair of type I injury.

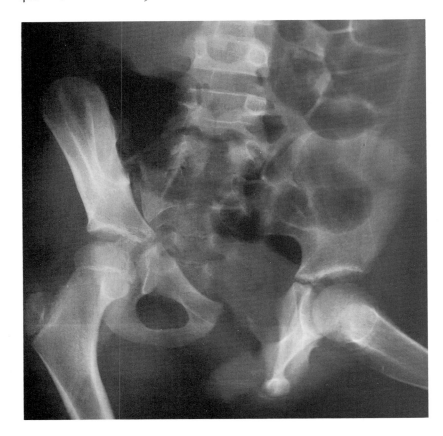

Fig. 29.18 X-ray in type II injury with gross displacement of hemi-pelvis.

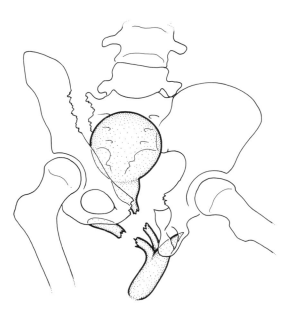

Fig. 29.19 Diagram of type II injury: the right hemi-pelvis is forced upwards, carrying the prostate with it. The left hemi-pelvis stays put, together with the corpus cavernosum and urethra.

the prostate and bulbar urethra, it is necessary to reduce the dislocation of the pelvis. Recently, it has been reported that magnetic resonance imaging (MRI) gives a helpful picture of the damage done to the corpora cavernosa [20].

If the patient is generally well, this reduction is achieved and maintained by a system of external fixation (Fig. 29.20). Later, when the condition of the patient permits, the urethra can be examined with a flexible cystoscope, and sometimes the way through into the bladder can be seen, a guide-wire introduced and the inevitable subsequent stricture dealt with by dilatation or urethrotomy.

Reducing the dislocation of the bones of the pelvis reduces the gap between the ends of the urethra, and makes it relatively easy to perform an end-to-end anastomosis through a suprapubic Pfannenstiel or a perineal incision, according to the general condition of the patient and the presence of his other injuries (Figs 29.21 & 29.22).

Where it is not possible to reduce the bony dislocation, the suprapubic tube is left in position, but this leaves a long defect which has to be bridged. There are several techniques for this

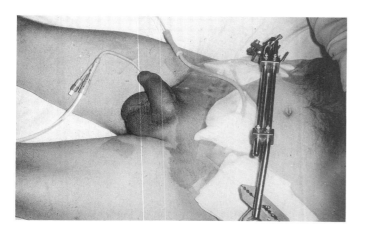

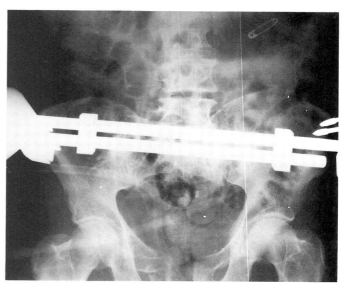

Fig. 29.20 External fixation maintains reduction of the dislocated pelvis.

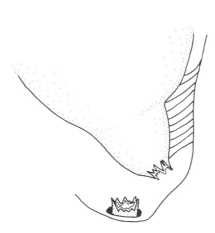

Fig. 29.21 Once the fracture has been reduced, the retropubic space is explored and the prostate mobilized.

(see p. 485). None of them are minor operations and the long-term follow-up is fraught with complications [17,21].

Urethral combined with rectal injury

A massive crushing injury may lacerate the urethra and rectum [22] (Fig. 29.23). The external urethral sphincter may be destroyed, but the bladder neck is usually intact except in young boys where the prostate is often torn across. The laceration may also rupture the anal sphincter. These patients always have many other injuries and although some of these may take priority it is urgent that the perineal wound is thoroughly

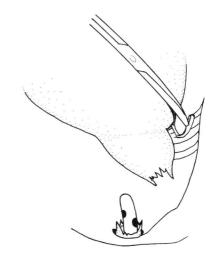

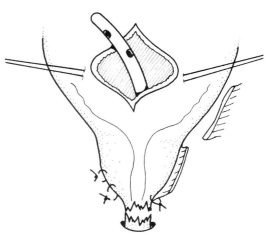

Fig. 29.22 The mobilized prostate is brought down to the torn urethra without any tension and secured over a catheter.

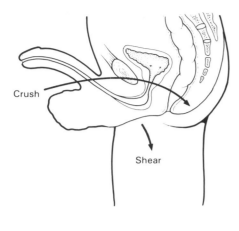
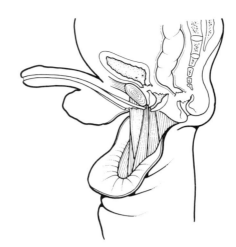

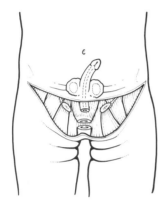

Fig. 29.23 Severe crushing injuries may lacerate urethra and rectum, avulse the adductors and partially deglove the lower limb.

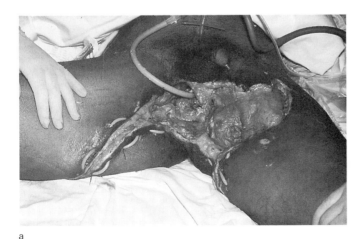

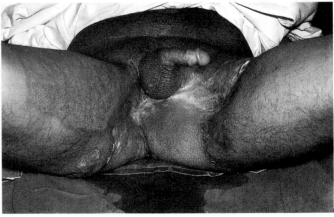

a   b

debrided and the urinary and faecal streams are diverted to avoid gas gangrene, which is a common complication and leads to loss of soft tissue that could be useful in the subsequent repair. No attempt is made at primary suture [22,23] (Fig. 29.24).

Gun-shot injuries

In gun-shot injuries, the damage to the urethra is only one part of multiple injuries involving bone, major blood vessels and bowel. Again, the first priority is adequate debridement with urinary and faecal diversion, and no attempt should be made at primary suture [23].

Fig. 29.24 Severe crushing injury involving urethra and rectum (a) 2 weeks after the accident, and (b) 2 years later.

In both these types of injury, a suprapubic catheter may not divert the urinary stream especially if the prostate and internal sphincter have been torn. It may be necessary to make a temporary ileal conduit diversion to allow the perineal wounds to heal (see p. 324).

The urethra and rectum can be reconstructed months later on.

In children

The urethral injury following pelvic fractures that is seen in boys often differs from that seen in adults. The prostate is so small that it tends to be torn rather than the membranous urethra alone. Repair is made more difficult by the narrow urethra of the child and the risk of creating a catheter stricture. Wherever possible a primary repair should be performed, but there is always a risk that the damage to the bladder neck may be followed by incontinence [24,25].

References

1 Citron ND, Wade PJ (1980) Penile injuries from vacuum cleaners. *Br Med J* 2: 26.
2 Wolf JS, Gomez R, McAninch JW (1992) Human bites to the penis. *J Urol* 147: 1265.
3 Hamarneh SA, Sikafi ZH, Salih AJM (1993) Fracture of the penis. *Emirates Med J* 11: 25.
4 Nymark J, Kristensen JK (1983) Fracture of the penis with urethral rupture. *J Urol* 129: 147.
5 Aboseif S, Gomez R, McAninch JW (1993) Genital self-mutilation. *J Urol* 150: 1143.
6 Witt MA, Goldstein I, Saenz de Tejada I, Greenfield A, Krane RJ (1990) Traumatic laceration of intracavernosal arteries: the pathophysiology of nonischemic, high flow, arterial priapism. *J Urol* 143: 129.
7 Desai KM, Gingell JC (1989) Hazards of long distance cycling. *Br Med J* 298: 1072.
8 Mecrow IK (1988) Burn to toddler's penis from an electrochemical battery. *Br Med J* 297: 1315.
9 Gomez RG, Castenheira ACC, McAninch JW (1993) Gun-shot wounds to the male external genitalia. *J Urol* 150: 1147.
10 Singh M, Blandy JP (1976) The pathology of urethral stricture. *J Urol* 115: 673.
11 Blandy JP (1980) Urethral stricture. *Postgrad Med J* 56: 383.
12 McEntee G, Smith J, Neligan MC, O'Connell D (1984) Urethral strictures following cardiac surgery. *Br J Urol* 56: 506.
13 Prabhu S, Cochran W, Raine PAM, Azmy AF (1985) Postcatheterization urethral strictures following cardiac surgery in children. *J Ped Surg* 20: 69.
14 Walsh A (1982) Urethral strictures after open heart surgery. *Lancet* i: 392.
15 Blandy JP (1990) Posterior urethroplasty after trauma Part II. *AUA Update Series* 9(28): 218.
16 Singh M (1967) Emergency treatment of impassable urethral strictures in the tropics. *Proc Roy Soc Med* 60: 871.
17 Jenkins BJ, Badenoch DF, Fowler CG, Blandy JP (1992) Long-term results of treatment of urethral injuries in males caused by external trauma. *Br J Urol* 70: 73.
18 Towler JM, Eisen SM (1987) A new technique for the management of urethral injuries. *Br J Urol* 60: 162.
19 Webster GD, Ramon J (1991) Repair of pelvic fracture posterior urethral defects using an elaborated perineal approach. Experience with 74 cases. *J Urol* 145: 744.
20 Dixon CM, Hricak H, McAninch JW (1992) Magnetic resonance imaging of traumatic posterior urethral defects and pelvic crush injuries. *J Urol* 148: 1162.
21 McAninch JW (1990) Urethral injuries. *World J Urol* 7: 184.
22 Blandy JP, Singh M (1972) Fistulae involving the adult make urethra. *Br J Urol* 44: 632.
23 Kudsk KA, McQueen MA, Woeller GR, Fox MA, Mangiante EC, Fabian TC (1990) Management of complex perineal soft-tissue injuries. *J Trauma* 30: 1155.
24 Baskin LS, McAninch JW (1993) Childhood urethral injuries: perspectives on outcome and treatment. *Br J Urol* 72: 241.
25 Pritchett TR, Shapiro RA, Hardy BE (1993) Surgical management of traumatic posterior urethral strictures in children. *Urology* 42: 59.

Chapter 30: Urethra and penis — inflammation

Acute inflammation of the penis and scrotum

Acute balanoposthitis

This is a very common finding in boys and men who are uncircumcised, and cannot clean under the prepuce. In diabetics it can be very serious and lead to cellulitis. Most cases respond to saline irrigations under the prepuce combined with systemic antibiotics, but in severe examples it is necessary to drain the preputial space. A dorsal slit may be the least invasive means of doing this but it leaves a grossly oedematous foreskin which takes weeks to heal and it is usually better to proceed to a complete circumcision, even in the presence of infection.

Herpes of the penis

Patients seldom notice the first vesicular eruption on the penis and become aware only when the vesicles rupture leaving raw and painful patches on the prepuce and glans. Of the two common types of herpesvirus, herpes simplex virus type 1 (HSV-1) usually causes infections elsewhere and it is HSV-2 which involves the genitalia (Fig. 30.1). Both are DNA viruses like

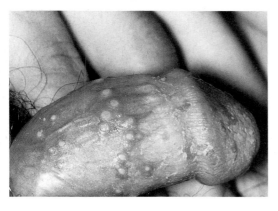

Fig. 30.1 Multiple herpesvirus erosions of the shaft of the penis (courtesy of Dr J.K. Oates).

varicella zoster, cytomegalovirus and Epstein–Barr virus which linger in their hosts, remaining latent indefinitely. The virus enters a cell, its DNA core enters the nucleus, is there transcribed and forms capsids which contain DNA and are infectious.

The virus is identified by electron microscopy of vesicle fluid, by immunofluorescent staining of scrapings from the lesions or by tissue culture — for which the specimens must be sent fresh or in Stuart's transport medium.

The infection is transmitted by sexual intercourse, especially orogenital contact. It gives rise to little or no illness in half the patients who are infected. The other half — after a week's incubation period —develop local burning, itching and pain, sometimes with systemic fever and muscle aches resembling influenza. Small groups of 2 mm red papules appear, form vesicles and burst, leaving painful ulcers, which scab over and heal but are succeeded by further waves of fresh infection. Headache, neck stiffness and photophobia signify meningeal infection from which patients recover spontaneously. Infection of the sacral nerve roots may give pain in the thighs and difficulty in voiding.

In immunosuppressed patients, these symptoms may be much more severe. Female partners of men with herpes genitalis incur an increased risk of carcinoma of the cervix.

Local discomfort may be relieved by 1% lignocaine gel, a weak solution of potassium permanganate or an ice bag. Secondary infection with *Candida* should be treated. Acyclovir cream 5% or idoxuridine 5% in dimethyl sulphoxide give rapid relief of symptoms but do not prevent recurrence. Interferon accelerates response though its cost can seldom be justified [1]. Repeated attacks call for circumcision.

Recently, it has been pointed out that skin damaged by herpesvirus infection, or other forms of genital ulceration, may facilitate infection with the human immunodeficiency virus (HIV) virus [2,3].

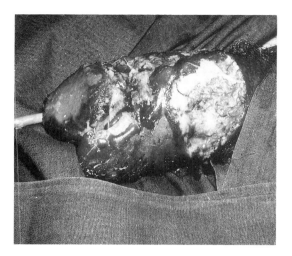

Fig. 30.2 Fournier's gangrene — necrotizing fasciitis of the penis.

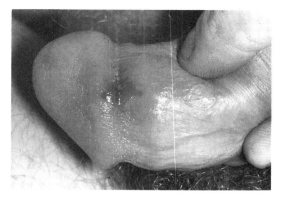

Fig. 30.3 Single early primary chancre of syphilis: no ulceration or induration: dark field positive for *Treponema pallidum* (courtesy of Dr J.K. Oates).

Fournier's gangrene

This is a potentially lethal cellulitis caused by a mixed infection in the skin and deep fascia of the penis and scrotum [4,5]. It is seen in debilitated patients, diabetics and arterial diseases such as periarteritis nodosa and temporal arteritis [6].

It begins with a painful cellulitis of the penis and scrotum making the oedematous skin copper coloured. There may be bacteraemic shock. If there is any suspicion of extravasation of urine, a suprapubic cystostomy should be performed without delay. All necrotic tissue must be excised as soon as possible. The superficial and deep spaces of the scrotum must both be drained. The necrosis involves deep fascia and is always more extensive than it first seems. Intensive combination antimicrobial chemotherapy is given. If there is any evidence of further spread of subcutaneous necrosis, the affected tissue should be re-explored and excised widely (Fig. 30.2). This is one condition where hyperbaric oxygen therapy may be of value.

Chronic infections of the penis and scrotum

Syphilis

The classical Hunterian chancre of primary syphilis starts as a dull red papule of variable size, on the prepuce, glans or coronal sulcus (Fig. 30.3). There may be more than one papule, mimicking herpes. The papule becomes an ulcer, which may become secondarily infected. Typically, there is an enlarged lymph node in the inguinal region. The diagnosis is confirmed by dark-ground examination of the fluid expressed from the chancre if necessary abrading it first with a rough swab or a needle. The fluid teems with *Treponema pallidum* (Fig. 30.4). Serological tests for syphilis are seldom positive at this stage. If no spirochaetes can be found, the patient must be followed up with regular serological testing. Contact tracing and the investigation and treatment of syphilis requires the expertise of a specialist in venereology.

Chancroid

The organism *Haemophilus ducreyi* causes a large, sloughing ulcer of the penis and prepuce with secondary infection and inflammation of the regional inguinal lymph nodes which often sup-

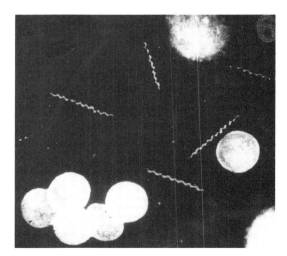

Fig. 30.4 Dark field preparation showing *Treponema pallidum* (courtesy of Professor J.D. Williams).

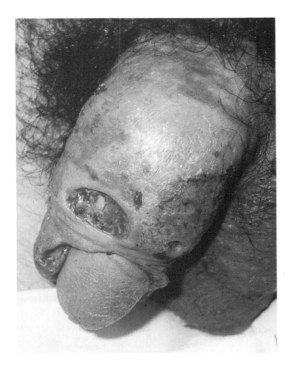

Fig. 30.5 Healing chancroidal ulcers of prepuce (courtesy of Dr J.K. Oates).

purate (Fig. 30.5). *H. ducreyi* is cultured from the exudate. It responds to antibiotics, but the follow-up must include tests for unsuspected syphilis [7].

Granuloma inguinale

The lesion of granuloma inguinale on the penis produces a shallow painful ulcer with a bright red granulating base from which the typical 'Donovan bodies' — hordes of *Donovania granulomatis* in mononuclear cells (Fig. 30.6) — can be found in scrapings stained with Giemsa. The urologist is likely to make the diagnosis only in a biopsy. It responds rapidly to tetracyclines [7].

Balanitis of Zoon

This occurs on the glans penis of uncircumcised adults. The painless inflamed copper coloured flat lesion (Fig. 30.7) cannot be distinguished from the precancerous erythroplasia of Queyrat (see p. 177) and demands a biopsy which shows a chronic inflammation with many plasma cells. No allergic cause has been found for this condition. Neither steroid cream nor antibiotics improve it. It is not premalignant. It always gets better once the patient has been circumcised. Its aetiology remains a mystery [8].

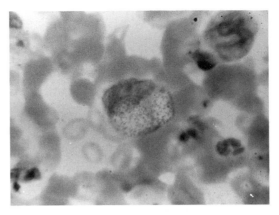

Fig. 30.6 Donovan bodies in a large mononuclear cell: scrape from penile lesion of granuloma inguinale (courtesy of Dr J.K. Oates).

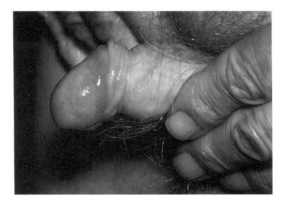

Fig. 30.7 Balanitis of Zoon.

Balanitis xerotica obliterans (BXO)

This equally mysterious condition is potentially more dangerous (Fig. 30.8). It is identical with the change seen in the vulva and on the elbows known to dermatologists as lichen sclerosus et obliterans. Histologically, there is a loss of the rete pegs that nail the epidermis to the dermis so the dermis tends to flake off (Fig. 30.9). There is a thickening of the collagen layer of the dermis into which lymphocytes invade, and this collagen tends to contract so that the skin shrinks.

BXO is seen at any age, though relatively rare in children. Its cause is unknown. At first, it affects the prepuce which becomes itchy, whitened and then stiff so that retracting the prepuce becomes more difficult and the skin may split and cause discomfort on intercourse. After erection the prepuce may not go back, resulting in a painful paraphimosis.

Treatment is circumcision: but the patient must be carefully followed up for two reasons: (a)

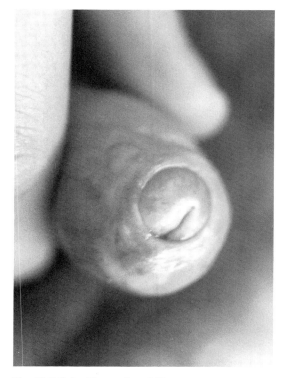

Fig. 30.8 Balanitis xerotica obliterans.

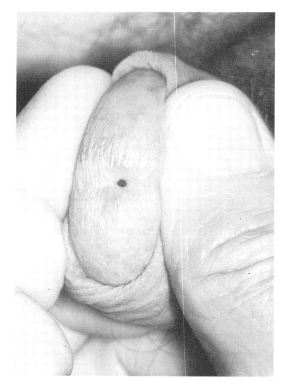

Fig. 30.10 Meatal stenosis following balanitis xerotica obliterans: this had caused uraemia and hypertension.

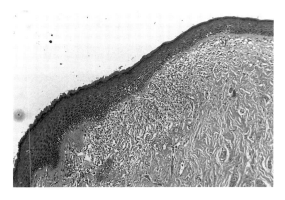

Fig. 30.9 Histological section of balanitis xerotica obliterans (courtesy of Dr Suhail Baithun).

because BXO inevitably recurs, and when it involves the meatus it may produce meatal stenosis which may occasionally lead to hydronephrosis, hypertension and uraemia (Fig. 30.10). (b) BXO is precancerous. In the vulva, it is followed by squamous cell carcinoma in 6% of patients [9]. The risk is probably much smaller in males, but is still high enough to require follow-up [10,11].

Candidiasis

Infection under the prepuce with *Candida* is com-

mon in diabetics and may be transmitted by sexual intercourse. It usually responds readily to fungicidal cream but circumcision may be advisable for frequent relapses [7].

Lymphoedema

In the West, the most common cause of oedema of the penis is undiagnosed cardiac failure with dependent oedema. In the tropics, lymphoedema of the penis often has an inflammatory origin in parts where microfilarial infestation with *Wuchereria bancrofti* is endemic. Elsewhere the cause is unknown. The penis is enlarged: at first the swelling is intermittent, but eventually becomes permanent. Investigations for filariasis are usually negative. Lymphangiography is seldom helpful and not worth doing.

This condition is profoundly distressing to the unhappy patient: intercourse is impossible, and micturition messy because of spraying of the stream.

Because the cause is unknown treatment has to be empirical and consists of excision of the oedematous subcutaneous tissues of the penis.

Through a circumferential incision in the coronal sulcus, the skin is sleeved back, down to Buck's fascia. The dorsal neurovascular bundle is preserved. All the subcutaneous tissue is dissected away, leaving only enough skin to cover the penis. The condition seldom recurs.

Inflammation and stricture of the urethra

The commonest cause of stricture has always been urethritis. Originally, the usual cause was gonorrhoea, but today more strictures are caused by *Chlamydia* [12].

The pathogenesis of gonococcal stricture was worked out a century ago. Abscesses would form in paraurethral glands and burst out into the surrounding corpus spongiosum (Fig. 30.11). Healing by fibrous tissue led to stricture [13].

The sites affected by gonococcal stricture are those with the largest number of paraurethral glands (Fig. 30.12). They are most profuse in the bulb and it is here that gonococcal strictures are most common.

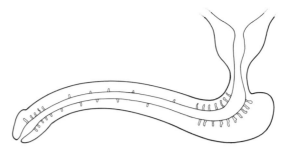

Fig. 30.12 Paraurethral glands are most numerous in the terminal centimetre and in the bulb of the urethra.

Once stenosis occurs, infected urine accumulates under pressure upstream of the stenosis and extravasates into the corpus spongiosum. As a result there is a tendency for the process of scarring and stricture to creep spread slowly up towards the prostate [14] (Fig. 30.13).

Chronic inflammation

Tuberculosis of the urethra is rare in the West [15] and nearly always associated with tuberculous

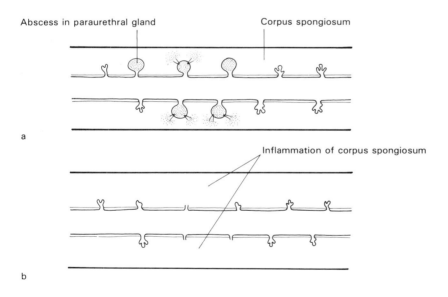

Abscess in paraurethral gland   Corpus spongiosum

a

Inflammation of corpus spongiosum

b

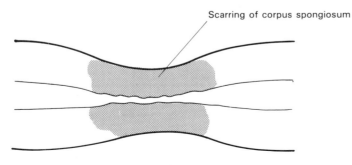

Scarring of corpus spongiosum

c

Fig. 30.11 (a) Acute gonococcal inflammation of the paraurethral glands bursts out into the corpus spongiosum to produce inflammation (b) which heals by scarring — hence (c) the stricture.

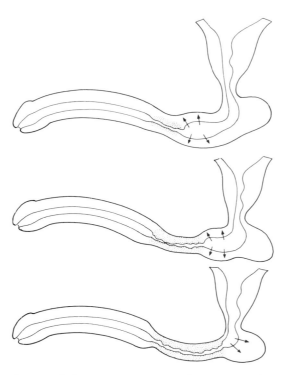

Fig. 30.13 Inflammatory stricture tends to creep up the urethra as infected urine is forced into the corpus spongiosum upstream of a stricture.

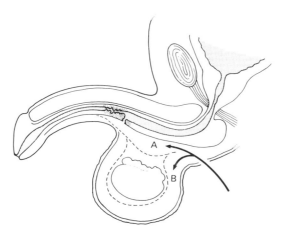

Fig. 30.14 In extravasation of urine it is important to make sure that both compartments A and B of Colles' fascia are drained.

prostatitis. It should be suspected in any long or tortuous stricture, especially when there are fistulae and abscesses.

Bilharziasis can affect any organ in the body, and *Schistosoma* ova may be found anywhere in the urethra and corpus spongiosum giving rise to fibrosis and stenosis [16].

Complications of urethral stricture

Extravasation of urine. The most dangerous complication of stricture is extravasation of urine into the scrotum and perineum. Unless both compartments are promptly drained (Fig. 30.14) infected hypertonic urine causes necrosis of fat and fascia of the perineum, scrotum, penis and the lower part of the abdominal wall: only the testicles survive thanks to their separate blood supply (Fig. 30.15). The patient who survives this life-threatening complication, will often end up with several fistulae.

Periurethral abscess. An infected paraurethral gland may burst outside the corpus spongiosum to form a paraurethral abscess which may discharge spontaneously (Fig. 30.16).

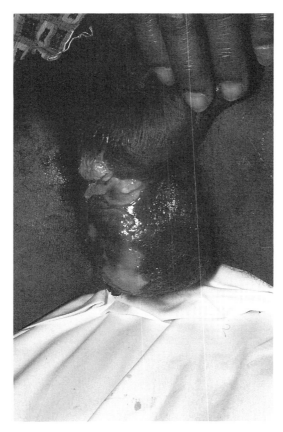

Fig. 30.15 Sloughing of the skin of the scrotum following extravasation of urine.

Fistula. Whether such a paraurethral abscess discharges or is incised, urine will continue to leak so long as there is a stenosis downstream [17]. A maze of channels may link one fistula with another — the watering-can perineum (Fig. 30.17).

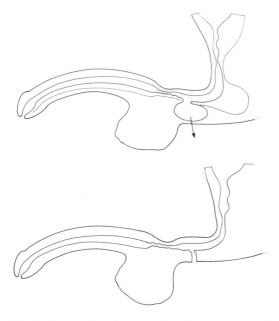

Fig. 30.16 An infected paraurethral gland upstream of a stricture may cause an abscess which will discharge, giving rise to a urinary fistula which will persist so long as the stricture persists.

Diverticulum. An abscess may fail to burst through the overlying skin, and so form a diverticulum where a stone may form.

Cancer. Every patient with a long-standing stricture, who has a swelling upstream of a stricture, should be suspected of having cancer (see p. 500).

Urinary infection is a common sequel of urethral stricture. Stones, epididymitis and prostatitis are common complications [18,19].

Clinical features of urethral stricture

The symptoms of urethral stricture are the same as those of other types of outflow obstruction — slow stream, frequency and dribbling of urine after voiding. Obstructed ejaculation suggests stricture and indeed may be an important cause of infertility, often noted in retrospect when the stricture has been cured. A stricture is often found only when one of its complications has developed.

Physical signs

Induration may be felt along the urethra and a distended bladder will be found when there is acute or chronic retention.

Investigations

The flow rate confirms the history of a restricted stream (Fig. 30.18). It is useful in monitoring the progress of the patient. It may give a false sense of security because flow is proportional to the square of the diameter of the urethra, and the urethral calibre can be reduced to only a millimetre before the patient is aware of a lessened stream [20]. The flow–rate curve is said to have a characteristic 'box shape'.

An ascending urethrogram is the standard investigation. It is performed with water-soluble contrast. It should be combined with a descending study to give a complete picture of the urethra (Fig. 30.19). This is beginning to be replaced by ultrasound which gives a good image of the urethra and has the additional advantage of revealing the extent of fibrosis in the corpus spongiosum [21,22] (Fig. 30.20).

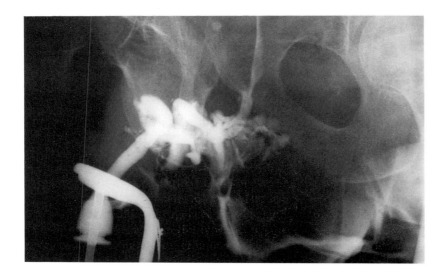

Fig. 30.17 Multiple fistulae and paraurethral abscesses associated with a stricture — the watering-can perineum.

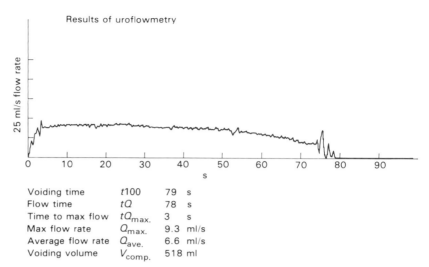

Results of uroflowmetry

Voiding time	$t100$	79	s
Flow time	tQ	78	s
Time to max flow	$tQ_{max.}$	3	s
Max flow rate	$Q_{max.}$	9.3	ml/s
Average flow rate	$Q_{ave.}$	6.6	ml/s
Voiding volume	$V_{comp.}$	518	ml

Fig. 30.18 Flat 'box-shaped' flow—rate curve in urethral stricture.

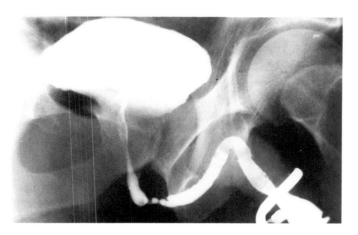

Fig. 30.19 'Up-and-down-a-gram' — descending and ascending urethrogram combined to show entire extent of the stricture.

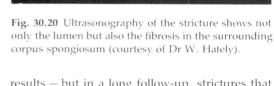

Fig. 30.20 Ultrasonography of the stricture shows not only the lumen but also the fibrosis in the surrounding corpus spongiosum (courtesy of Dr W. Hately).

Urethroscopy with the 0° telescope is now always performed as part of the procedure of optical urethrotomy, but for outpatient diagnostic purposes the flexible cystoscope has largely replaced the urethroscope.

Management of urethral stricture

Dilatation

'The skill of the urologist is measured by his gentleness' [23]. Many strictures are still well managed by dilatation. The classical practice was to double the interval between dilatations, so long as they were painless and easy, until the patient returned once a year. He was never discharged. The doctrine was 'once a stricture always a stricture'. With an easy stricture and a skilled surgeon this method gave excellent results — but in a long follow-up, strictures that were not always easy and were often delegated to junior urologists of varying skill, had a considerable morbidity [18].

For centuries bougies and sounds (today the terms are interchangeable) were made of different materials. The names are of historical interest: *bougie*, comes from Bujiyah (Fig. 30.21) — the Algerian port whence came the best French wax candles — and thin wax tapers were found to make excellent dilators. Curved metal instruments were used for dilating strictures as well as for 'sounding' for stone — hence 'sound' (Fig. 30.22). The very thin pliable bougie — 'filiform' — is named after the thread it resembles and it was an ingenious Dutch urologist named Phillips who invented the screw-on flexible followers [24] (Fig. 30.23).

The fully equipped urologist needs a complete

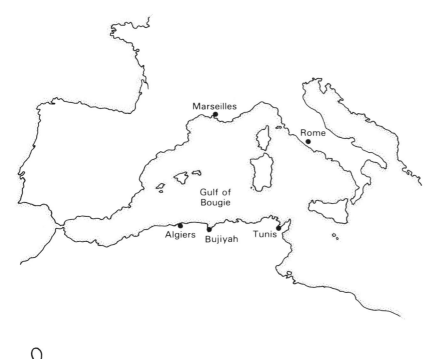

Fig. 30.21 Bougie — French for candle. The best wax candles came from Bujiyah in Algiers.

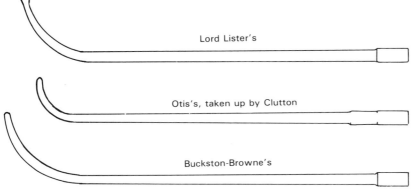

Lord Lister's

Otis's, taken up by Clutton

Buckston-Browne's

Fig. 30.22 Classical designs of sounds used for dilating strictures.

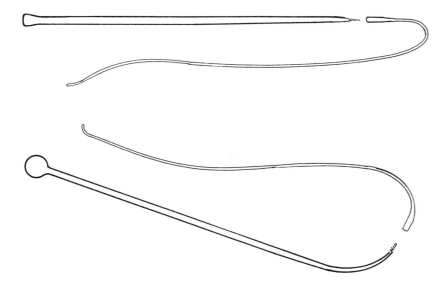

Fig. 30.23 Filiform bougies, with flexible or rigid followers.

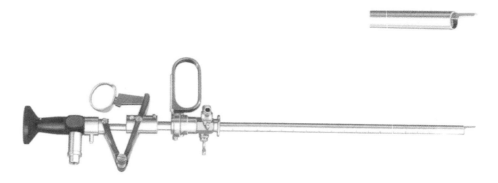

Fig. 30.24 Sachse optical urethrotome.

set of filiforms with Phillips' followers, flexible bougies, steel sounds, as well as an optical Sachse urethrotome (Fig. 30.24).

Dilatation of a new stricture

Fill the urethra with local anaesthetic gel, and begin with a filiform. Since the opening of the stricture is often eccentric, give the end of the filiform a dog-leg bend (Fig. 30.25) and feel for the way through the stricture by gently rotating the filiform. This is more easy and reliable than the 'faggot' technique of filling the urethra up with a series of filiforms (Fig. 30.26). Better still, pass the filiform or a guide-wire under vision with a flexible cystoscope.

Once the filiform passes the stricture, screw on flexible Phillips' followers of increasing size and dilate the stricture, aiming not to tear the urethra by too rapid dilatation the first time.

On subsequent visits dilatation using polished steel sounds is usually more satisfactory. They come in different shapes but the short curve designed by Otis (and adopted by Clutton) is best.

In passing any instrument, the utmost gentleness should be exercised: 'the urethra should swallow the bougie'. There should be no pain, no blood and no fever.

Autodilatation

For millenia patients have dilated their own strictures with excellent results. In recent years, self-lubricating catheters have made the task easier [25]. When complications develop, or when either the patient or the surgeon finds the operation difficult, alternatives should be considered [26].

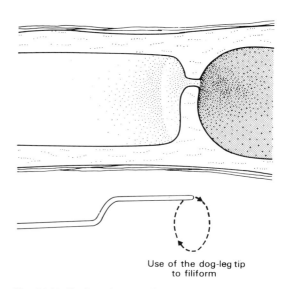

Use of the dog-leg tip to filiform

Fig. 30.25 Finding the way through the eccentric opening of a urethral stricture with a filiform bougie which is given a dog-leg bend.

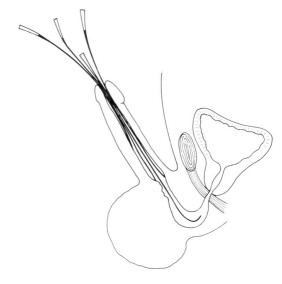

Fig. 30.26 The faggot technique of using multiple filiforms.

Internal urethrotomy

This is another ancient operation: knives for slitting the stricture from within have been used for centuries [27]. Today, the optical urethrotome of Sachse [28] has superseded them all. The operation is easy and may be performed under local or general anaesthetic.

Having introduced the sheath, using normal saline rather than water (in view of the risk of haemolysis if water is extravasated), the stricture is slit under vision with one of the knives supplied with the instrument (Fig. 30.27). When it is difficult to see beyond the stricture, a flexible guide-wire is passed before cutting. Once the stricture has been divided, a catheter is left in the urethra for 24 h. Thereafter the stricture must be followed by regular dilatation or auto-dilatation. Several urethrotomies are often needed and every case must be carefully followed [29].

Balloon dilatation

Urethral strictures can be dilated with the type of balloon provided for angioplasty. Its proponents claim a theoretical advantage for it since the force of the balloon is exerted radially rather than shearing the scar tissue in the urethra (Fig. 30.28). So far only early results are available. These balloons will always be much more expensive than classical sounds or bougies and it remains to be seen whether they will have any long-term advantage [30, 31].

Laser urethrotomy

With an appropriate laser the scar tissue may be vapourized or incised. It is claimed that this type of thermal injury is followed by less scarring than conventional incision. There are no controlled trials and so far no long-term follow-up results [32].

External urethrotomy

There are few indications for this operation but it has a place in complicated strictures (Fig. 30.29). The stricture is slit open through a perineal incision: an inert tube is left indwelling while the skin is closed loosely over it [33]. The stricture is then managed by regular intermittent self-dilatation.

Excision and end-to-end anastomosis

This method was not new when Marion described it in 1936 [34]. The urethra is exposed through a midline incision, the strictured part is cut out, and the spatulated ends are sewn together over a catheter (Fig. 30.30). It is useful in short strictures of the bulbar urethra and is the operation of choice for strictures of the membranous urethra following a type I fractured pelvis.

When the stricture follows undisplaced fracture of the pelvis, the bulbar urethra is mobilized (Fig. 30.31). The upper end is found by cutting down on a bougie introduced through the suprapubic cystostomy (Fig. 30.32). A wide oval opening is made into the urethra through the scar

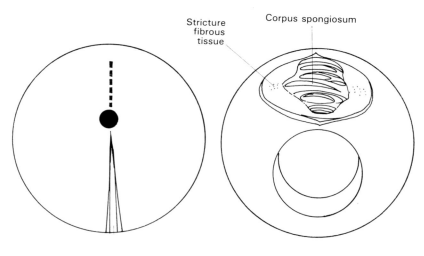

Stricture fibrous tissue

Corpus spongiosum

Sachse knife blade

Fig. 30.27 Optical urethrotomy. The knife must cut right through all the scar tissue.

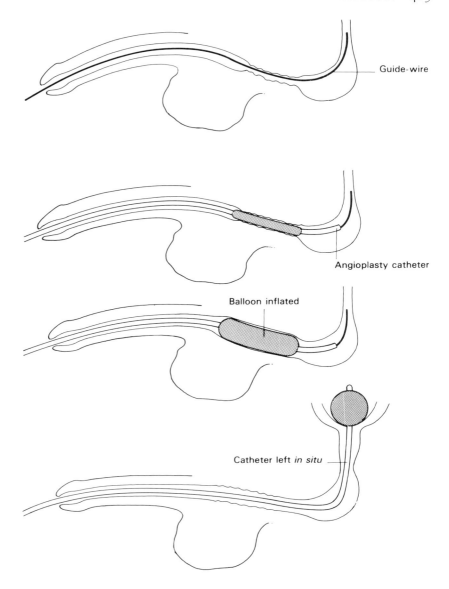

Fig. 30.28 Balloon used
to dilate a urethral
stricture.

tissue and the spatulated bulbar urethra is then
anastomosed to it [35].

When the fracture of the pelvis has led to
much dislocation of the bones there is a longer
gap between the ends of the urethra. The corpora
cavernosa must be separated in the midline and
retracted laterally to expose the lower part of the
symphysis which is always unusually broad because of the malunited fracture (Fig. 30.33).

After scraping the periosteum from the symphysis, a generous window is cut out from its
inferior border (Fig. 30.34). An oscillating bone
saw is used which does not cut the periosteum
on the pelvic surface of the bone. A bougie
introduced through the suprapubic cystostomy
is now felt through the periosteum (Fig. 30.35).
An ellipse is cut out from the anterior lower part

of the symphysis, and an end-to-end anastomosis
made after spatulating the urethra [36]. An alternative technique removes the entire symphysis
and enwraps the anastomosis in omentum to
prevent scar formation [37].

Meatoplasty

For strictures at the tip of the glans penis a
simple ∩-shaped flap of skin is let into the
opened meatus [38] (Fig. 30.36): it gives a trum-
pet-shaped external meatus and the patient must
be warned that he may spray when he urinates.
When the stenosis extends further down the
urethra a pedicled flap of prepuce or penile skin
may give a better result (Fig. 30.37).

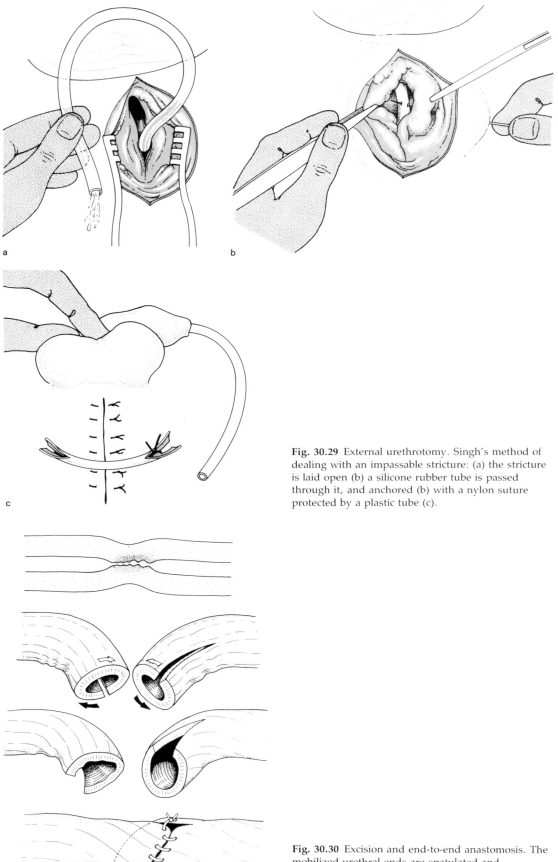

Fig. 30.29 External urethrotomy. Singh's method of dealing with an impassable stricture: (a) the stricture is laid open (b) a silicone rubber tube is passed through it, and anchored (b) with a nylon suture protected by a plastic tube (c).

Fig. 30.30 Excision and end-to-end anastomosis. The mobilized urethral ends are spatulated and anastomosed as an ellipse.

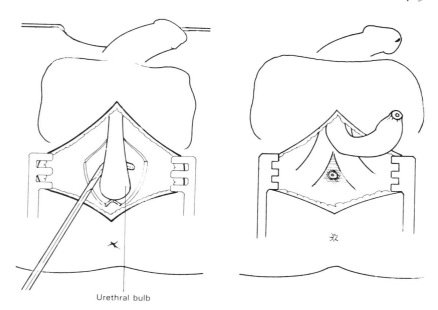

Fig. 30.31 The bulbar urethra is mobilized.

Urethral bulb

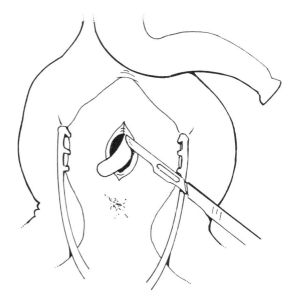

Fig. 30.32 The upper end of the prostatic urethra is found by cutting down onto a bougie passed down through the suprapubic cystostomy.

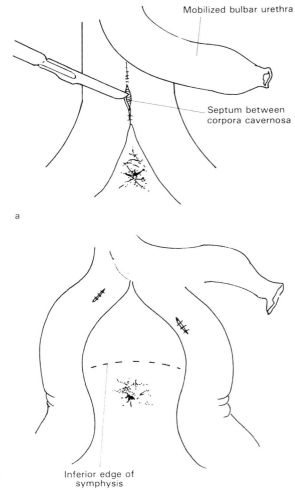

Mobilized bulbar urethra

Septum between corpora cavernosa

a

Inferior edge of symphysis

b

Fig. 30.33 (a) The corpora cavernosa are separated in the midline to (b) reveal the lower edge of the malunited symphysis pubis.

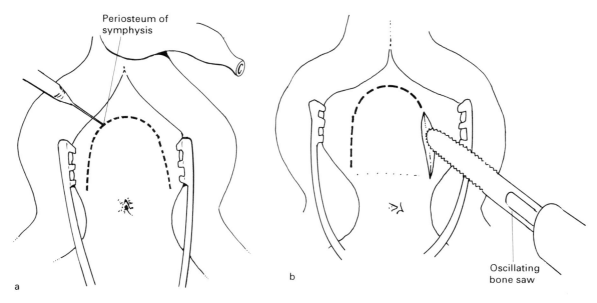

Fig. 30.34 (a) The periosteum of the symphysis is incised with diathermy and scraped away. (b) An arch is cut out using an oscillating bone saw.

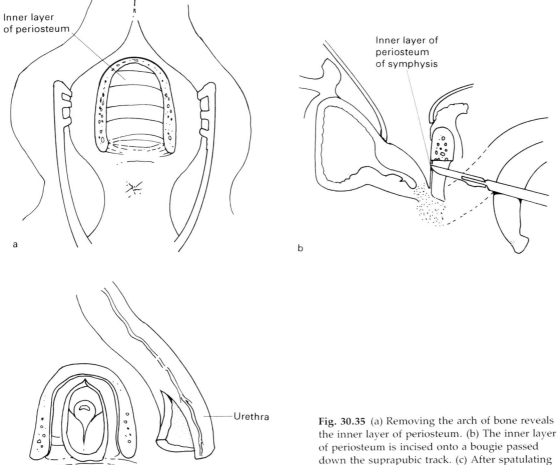

Fig. 30.35 (a) Removing the arch of bone reveals the inner layer of periosteum. (b) The inner layer of periosteum is incised onto a bougie passed down the suprapubic track. (c) After spatulating the prostatic and bulbar urethra they are anastomosed.

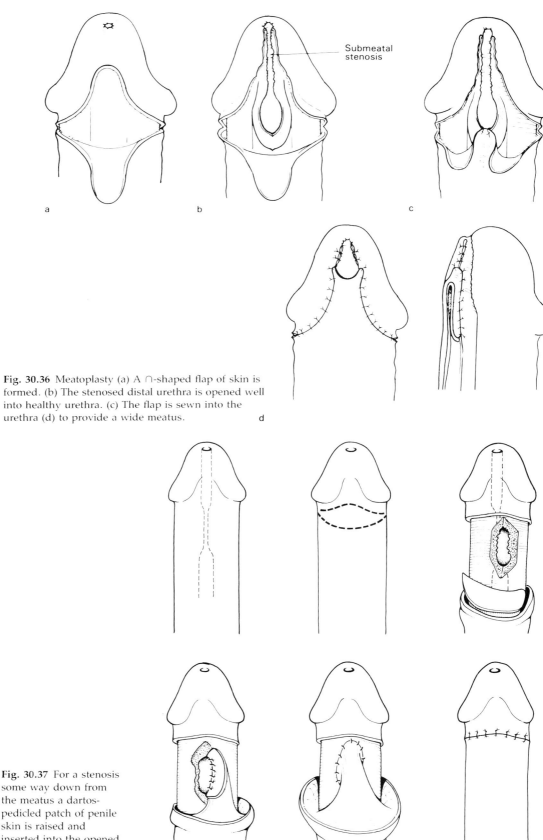

Fig. 30.36 Meatoplasty (a) A ∩-shaped flap of skin is formed. (b) The stenosed distal urethra is opened well into healthy urethra. (c) The flap is sewn into the urethra (d) to provide a wide meatus.

Fig. 30.37 For a stenosis some way down from the meatus a dartos-pedicled patch of penile skin is raised and inserted into the opened up stricture.

Pedicled skin patches

For strictures in the distal few centimetres of the urethra a skin graft may be taken from the prepuce (if available) or the penile shaft. Dissecting in the plane between the dartos muscle and the dermis provides the patch of skin with a vascular pedicle which promotes its survival [39] (Fig. 30.38).

The longer the segment of urethra to be patched, the longer must be the vascular pedicle, and so the less reliable the graft: nevertheless such pedicled preputial skin patches have been used to reach right up to the verumontanum. The preputial skin has the advantage that it does not grow hair [40,41].

Patches of skin from the scrotum, with a dartos pedicle, have an even more reliable blood supply and are very versatile [42,43]; only 1% undergo necrosis [19].

Island patch urethroplasty

For the usual bulbar stricture an ∩-shaped incision (Fig. 30.39) is made in the loose skin of the scrotum which is reflected down to expose the bulbospongiosus muscles, assisted by a weighted retractor (Fig. 30.40). These are separated from the urethra and divided in the midline (Fig. 30.41). The strictured zone is opened, and the bleeding edges of the corpus spongiosum are oversewn with fine absorbable suture material to control bleeding [36] (Fig. 30.42).

Using the foil from a catgut package as a template, the size of patch needed to enlarge the urethra is estimated and outlined on the apex of the scrotal flap (Fig. 30.43). The plane of cleavage between the skin and the dartos is now developed with scissors, so that the island of skin is provided with its own 'mesentery' of dartos to supply it with blood.

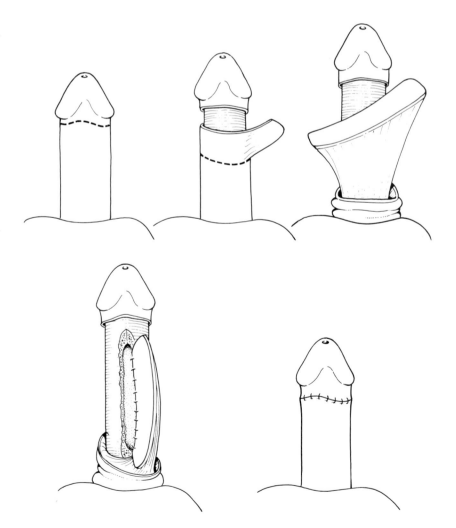

Fig. 30.38 For a longer penile stricture a pedicled graft from the shaft of the penis is raised on a dartos pedicle and inserted into the stricture.

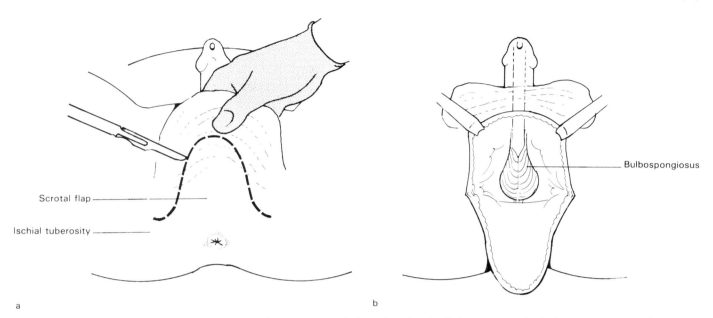

Scrotal flap

Ischial tuberosity

Bulbospongiosus

a

b

Fig. 30.39 (a) A scrotal flap is raised and allowed to drop back (b) to expose the bulbospongiosus muscle and urethra.

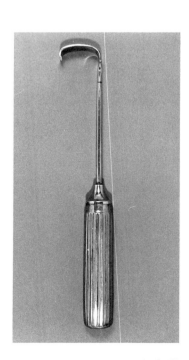

Fig. 30.40 A weighted retractor greatly facilitates the exposure.

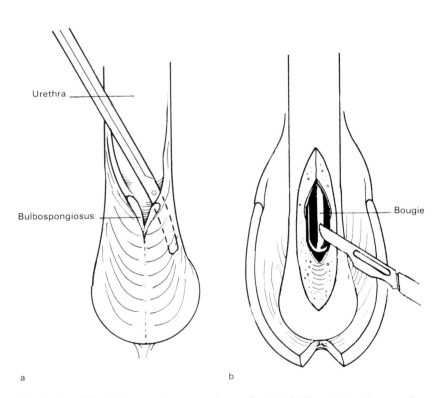

Urethra

Bulbospongiosus

Bougie

a

b

Fig. 30.41 (a) The bulbospongiosus muscle is reflected. (b) The stricture is opened.

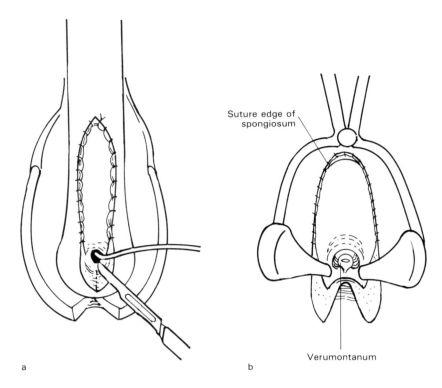

Suture edge of
spongiosum

Verumontanum

Fig. 30.42 The corpus spongiosum is (a) opened, and (b) oversewn to stop bleeding.

a   b

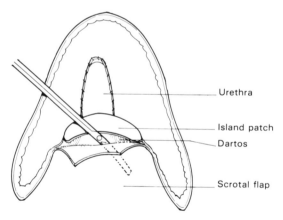

Urethra

Island patch

Dartos

Scrotal flap

Fig. 30.43 A patch of skin is prepared from the tip of the scrotal flap by dissecting in the plane between skin and dartos.

The patch is sewn into the slit-up urethra with absorbable sutures over an appropriate catheter which is left in for 14 days (Fig. 30.44).

For longer strictures a second patch can be taken from the anterior edge of the scrotum (Fig. 30.45), and when the skin has been scarred by old fistulae, an identical patch can be raised from the side of the scrotum. The principles are the same.

For strictures in the penile urethra the operation can be modified to avoid a fistula. Make a transverse incision in the scrotum. Dissect in the midline down onto the penis, and by blunt dissection extract the penis from its sheath of skin — much as you pull your foot out of a sock (Fig. 30.46). This avoids making an incision in the penile skin, and the risk of a fistula afterwards.

After opening up the stricture in the penile urethra (Fig. 30.47), a patch is measured off and the dartos pedicle designed with its base to one or other side so that it will not be angulated when the patch of skin is applied to the urethra.

The skin patch is sewn in position and the penis returned to its sheath of skin.

In cases where the entire penile urethra has been destroyed — as in hypospadiac cripples — the skin patch can be formed into a tube like a cigarette paper and used to replace the missing urethra (Fig. 30.48).

Complications

Any skin which is used to patch the urethra, may develop complications when it comes into contact with urine.

1 Eczema. A kind of eczema may affect scrotal or preputial skin.

2 BXO may develop in the skin and shrink to cause a return of the stricture.

3 Scrotal skin continues to grow hair: when the hairs mature they are usually carried away in the stream of urine, but when there is dilatation or

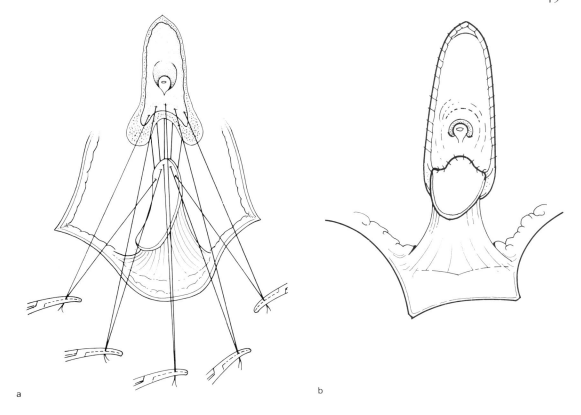

a

b

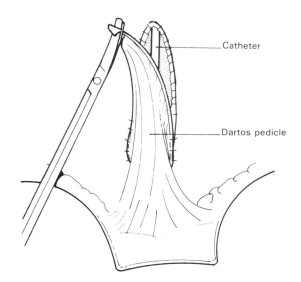

Catheter

Dartos pedicle

c

Fig. 30.44 (a) After placing sutures, the patch of skin (b) is (c) sewn into the defect in the urethra.

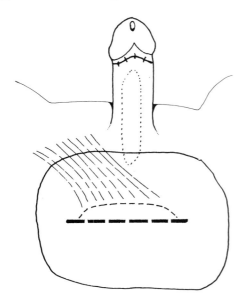

Fig. 30.45 A patch can be taken from the anterior edge of the incision in the scrotum.

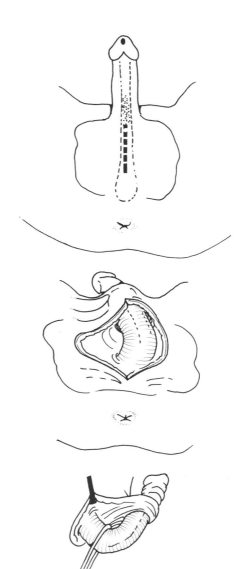

Fig. 30.46 For a stricture in the penile urethra, first the penis is withdrawn from its sleeve.

Fig. 30.47 (a) The stricture is opened up, the edge oversewn for haemostasis, and an anterior patch of skin raised on a dartos pedicle. (b) The patch is sewn into the stricture. (c) The penis is returned to its sleeve.

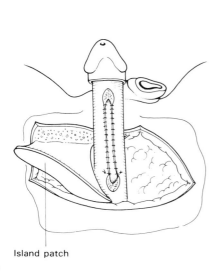

Island patch

a

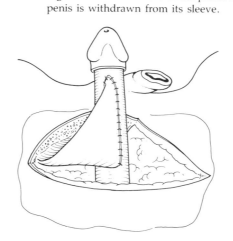

b

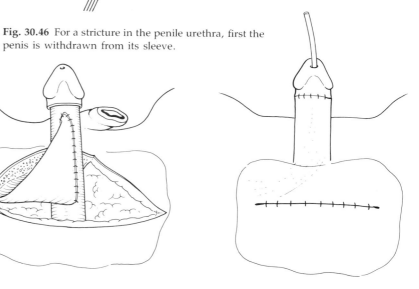

c

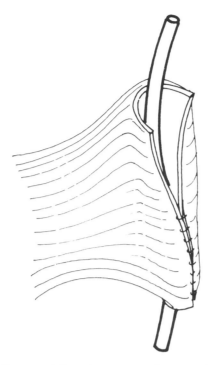
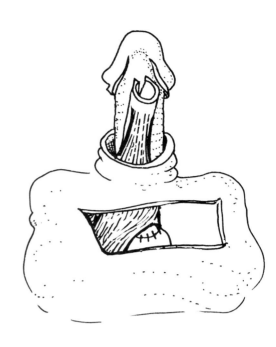

Fig. 30.48 Where the entire urethra has to be replaced the dartos-pedicled patch of skin can be formed into a tube like cigarette paper.

obstruction the hairs accumulate and give rise to a hairball calculus (Figs 30.49 & 30.50).

4 The skin patch may enlarge to form a pouch (Fig. 30.51): this may take place upstream or downstream of a stenosis (Fig. 30.52). Very occasionally such a pouch acts as a valve to cause obstruction (Fig. 30.53).

5 Restenosis is seen in about 10% of scrotal skin urethroplasties in a follow-up of 10 years: usually at one or other end of the skin graft—but also (for no obvious reason) half way along (Fig. 30.54) [19,44].

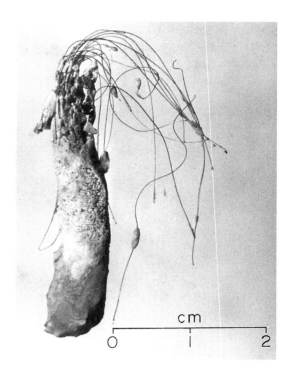

Fig. 30.49 Hairs growing in the urethra on endoscopy. Most of these will be shed and pass out in the urine.

Fig. 30.50 Hairs may act as the nucleus for a calculus.

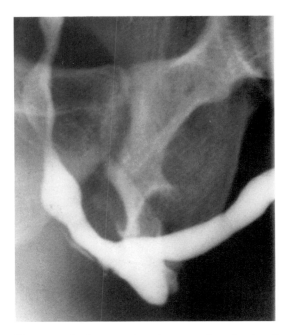

Fig. 30.51 Urethrogram showing a pouch at the site of urethroplasty.

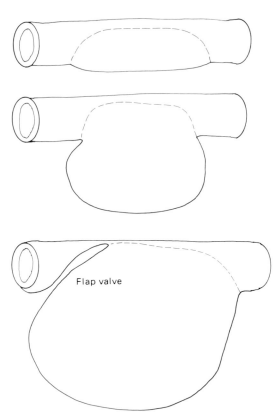

Fig. 30.53 A pouch is apt to form in a skin urethroplasty in the presence of incontinence and can act as a valve to cause obstruction.

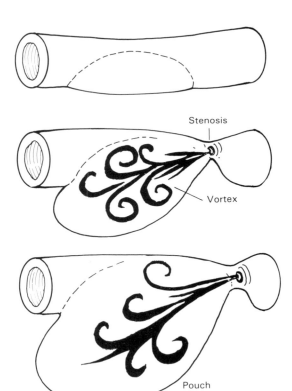

Fig. 30.52 A pouch may form upstream or downstream of a restenosis.

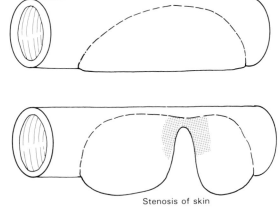

Fig. 30.54 Restenosis may occur at either end of the skin graft or in the middle.

6 Recurrent urinary infection is very common, probably from chronic infection in the dilated prostatic ducts upstream of the stricture. It is often complicated by epididymitis [19].

Free skin grafts

Free skin grafts of various thickness have been used to enlarge the urethra [45]. In such a mobile organ, where urine and infection are always present, free skin grafts do not always survive. One method uses a free skin graft wrapped round a catheter — raw side out — which is placed in the urethra after urethrotomy in the hope that the skin will adhere to the urethrotomy incision and provide a permanent patch [46,47] (Fig. 30.55). No long-term results have ever been published.

A more certain way of using split skin is that of Schreiter. First the urethra is laid open and meshed split skin from a hairless donor area is applied to the perineal wound to give a broad hairless strip of skin the length of the strictured area (Fig. 30.56). At a second stage, several months later, the hairless skin strip is rolled up to form a new urethra [48] (Fig. 30.57).

Bladder mucosa

Strips of mucosa from the bladder seem to offer an ideal substitute for the urethra. So far, most experience has been in children with hypospadias where bladder mucosa takes well but, if it is exposed at the meatus, it becomes inflamed [49,50] and there is a theoretical risk of inducing ectopic bone in the underlying tissues [51].

Tunica vaginalis

When performing urethroplasty the testicle often intrudes on the operative field offering the tunica vaginalis as an attractive patch for the urethra. The results are disappointing [52].

Buccal mucosa

In repairing the urethra of the hypospadiac cripple, free grafts from the mucosa on the inside of the lip appear to take well and give promising short-term results.

Artificial urethras

Every known synthetic material has been tried as an experimental stent, substitute or patch for

Fig. 30.55 A patch of split skin is wrapped round a catheter, raw side out, and inserted after urethrotomy with the intention that the graft will adhere to the raw surface at the urethrotomy.

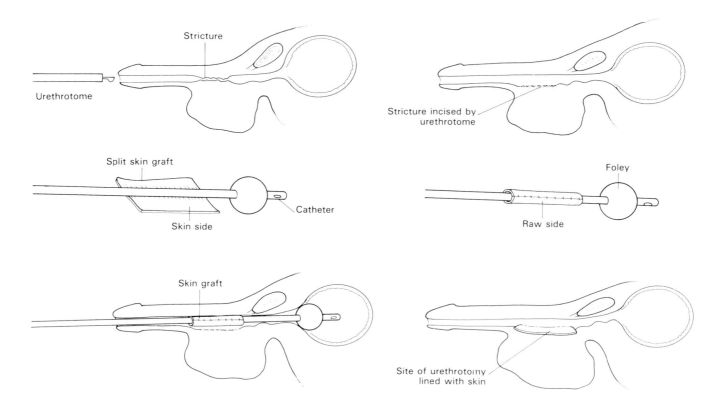

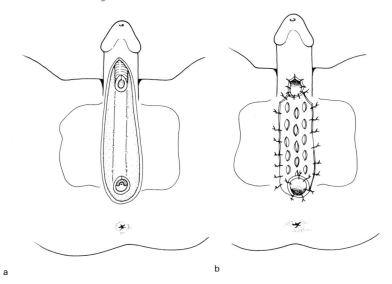

Fig. 30.56 Schreiter's urethroplasty: first stage. (a) The stricture is excised.(b) A meshed split-skin graft is applied to the defect.

a   b

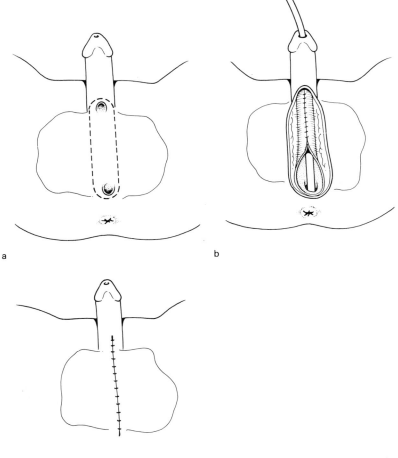

a   b

c

Fig. 30.57 Schreiter's urethroplasty: second stage. (a) After about 6 weeks a new urethra is outlined using the hairless grafted skin. (b) It is closed over a catheter (c) The scrotum is closed over the new urethra.

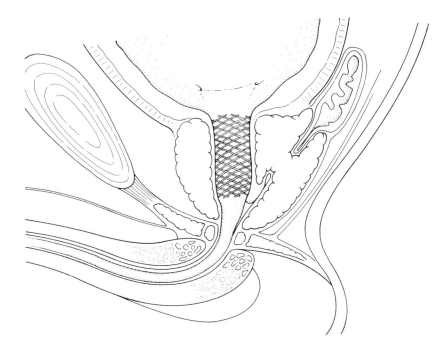

Fig. 30.58 Wallstent — an expanded inert metal mesh here shown in the prostate, may be inserted after urethrotomy. It is lined with granulation tissue and then epithelializes.

the urethra but calculus always forms on the foreign substance. A number of ingenious urethral stents made from relatively inert expansile wire coils or mesh are now under trial [53]. The urethra is slit or dilated and the stent inserted. Granulations grow between the gaps in the mesh and it is hoped that they will become relined with epithelium (Fig. 30.58). This does not always happen: they may form calculi or become obliterated by scar tissue. Removing them requires excision and reconstruction of the urethra [54,55].

References

1 Oates JK (1983) Venereal disease: genital herpes. *Br J Hosp Med* 28: 13.
2 Marx JL (1989) Circumcision may protect against the AIDS virus. *Science* 245: 470.
3 Fink AJ (1987) A possible explanation for heterosexual male infection with AIDS. *New Engl J Med* 316: 1546.
4 Wolach MD, MacDermott JP, Stone AR, deVere White RW (1989) Treatment and complications of Fournier's gangrene. *Br J Urol* 64: 310.
5 Voros D, Pissiotis C, Georgantas D, Katsaragakis S, Antoniou S, Papadimitriou J (1993) Role of early and extensive surgery in the treatment of severe necrotizing soft tissue infection. *Br J Surg* 80: 1190.
6 Sohn M, Kistler D, Kindler J, Lutzeyer W (1989) Fournier's gangrene in hypersensitivity vasculitis. *J Urol* 142: 823.
7 Holmes KK, Mardh P-A, Sparling PF, Wiesner (1984) *Sexually Transmitted Diseases*. New York: McGraw-Hill.
8 Murray WJG, Fletcher MS, Yates-Bell AJ, Pryor JP, Darby AJ, Packham DA (1986) Plasma cell balanitis of Zoon. *Br J Urol* 58: 689.
9 Ridley CM (1993) Genital lichen sclerosus (lichen sclerosus et atrophicus) in childhood and adolescence. *J Roy Soc Med* 86: 69.
10 El-Demiry MIM, Oliver RTD, Hope-Stone HF, Blandy JP (1984) Reappraisal of the role of radiotherapy and surgery in the management of carcinoma of the penis. *Br J Urol* 56: 724.
11 Jamieson NV, Bullock KN, Barker THW (1988) Adenosquamous carcinoma of the penis associated with balanitis xerotica obliterans. *Br J Urol* 58: 730.
12 Tanaka M, Kumazawa J (1993) Diagnosis and management of urethritis. *Curr Opinion Urol* 3: 36.
13 Gupta S, Majumdar B, Tiwari A, Gupta RK, Kumar A, Gujral RB (1993) Sonourethrography in the evaluation of anterior urethral strictures: correlation with radiographic urethrography. *J Clin Ultrasound* 21: 231.
14 Chambers RM (1974) Urethroplasty. *Br J Urol* 46: 118.
15 Symes JM, Blandy JP (1973) Tuberculosis of the male urethra. *Br J Urol* 45: 432.
16 Zaher MF, El Deeb AA (1969) Bilharzial urethritis cystica. *J Urol* 101: 870.
17 Blandy JP, Singh M (1972) Fistulae involving the adult male urethra. *Br J Urol* 44: 632.
18 Blandy JP, Wadhwa S, Singh M, Tresidder GC (1976) Urethroplasty in context. *Br J Urol* 48: 697.
19 Rogers HS, McNicholas TA, Blandy JP (1992) Long-term results of one-stage scrotal patch urethroplasty. *Br J Urol* 69: 621.
20 von Garrelts B (1972) Measurement of micturition parameters and its clinical use. *Proc Roy Soc Med* 65: 132.
21 McAninch JW, Laing FC, Jeffrey RB (1988) Sonourethrography in the evaluation of urethral strictures:

a preliminary report. *J Urol* 139: 294.

22 Das S (1992) Ultrasonographic evaluation of urethral stricture disease. *Urology* 40: 237.

23 Pott P (1779) *The Chirurgical Works of Percivall Pott*, vol. 1, p. 343. London: Lowndes.

24 Phillips CVJ (1849) *Operations qui se Pratiquent sur les Organes Genito-urinaires. Atlas des Journal des Connaissainces Medico-chirugicales.* Reprinted by ICI, Liege, 1992.

25 Newman LH, Stone NN, Chircus JH, Kramer HC (1990) Recurrent urethral stricture disease managed by clean intermittent self-catheterization. *J Urol* 144: 1142.

26 Robertson GCM, Everitt N, Lamprecht JR, Brett M, Flynn JT (1991) Treatment of recurrent urethral strictures using clean intermittent self-catheterisation. *Br J Urol* 68: 89.

27 Matouschek E (1978) Internal urethrotomy of urethral stricture under vision: a 5-year report. *Urol Res* 6: 147.

28 Sachse H (1974) Zur Behandlung der Harnrohrenstriktur. Die transurethrale Schlitzung unter Sight mit scharfen Schnitt. *Fortschr Med* 92: 12.

29 Johnston SR, Bagshaw HA, Flynn JR, Kellett MJ, Blandy JP (1980) Visual internal urethrotomy. *Br J Urol* 52: 542.

30 Daughtry JD, Rodan BA, Bean WJ (1988) Balloon dilatation of urethral strictures. *Urology* 31: 231.

31 Mohammed SH (1989) Retrograde balloon dilatation of urethra. *Urology* 33: 257.

32 Turek PJ, Malloy TR, Cendron M, Cariniello VL, Wein AJ (1992) KTP-532 laser ablation of urethral strictures. *Urology* 40: 330.

33 Singh M (1967) Emergency treatment of impassable urethral strictures in the tropics. *Proc Roy Soc Med* 60: 871.

34 Marion G (1936) *Traité dUrologie*, vol. 2, 3rd edn, pp. 1110–18. Paris: Masson.

35 Glass RE, Flynn JT, King JB, Blandy JP (1978) Urethral injury and fractured pelvis. *Br J Urol* 50: 578.

36 Blandy JP (1986) *Operative Urology*, 2nd edn, pp. 231–3. Oxford: Blackwell Scientific Publications.

37 Turner-Warwick RT (1976) The use of omental pedicle graft in urinary tract reconstruction. *J Urol* 116: 341.

38 Blandy JP, Tresidder GC (1967) Meatoplasty. *Br J Urol* 39: 633.

39 Quartey JKM (1983) One-stage penile preputial cutaneous island flap urethroplasty for urethral stricture: a preliminary report. *J Urol* 129: 284.

40 Mundy AR, Stephenson TP (1988) Pedicled preputial patch urethroplasty. *Br J Urol* 61: 48.

41 Quartey JKM (1985) One stage penile/preputial island flap urethroplasty for urethral stricture. *J Urol* 134: 474.

42 Leadbetter GW (1960) A simplified urethroplasty for strictures of the bulbous urethra. *J Urol* 83: 54.

43 Orandi A (1967) One-stage urethroplasty: 4 year follow-up. *J Urol* 107: 977.

44 Mundy AR (1995) The long term results of skin inlay urethroplasty. *Br J Urol* 75: 59.

45 Brannan W, Ochsner MG, Fuselier HA (1976) Free full thickness skin graft urethroplasty for urethral stricture: experience with 66 patients. *J Urol* 115: 677.

46 Petterson S, Asklin B, Bratt CC (1978) Endourethral urethroplasty: a simple method for treatment of urethral strictures by internal urethrotomy and primary split-skin grafting. *Br J Urol* 50: 259.

47 Chiou RK (1988) Endourethroplasty in the management of complicated posterior urethral strictures. *J Urol* 140: 607.

48 Schreiter F (1984) Mesh-graft-Urethroplastik. *Aktuel Urol* 15: 173.

49 Keating MA, Cartwright PC, Duckett JW (1990) Bladder mucosa in urethral reconstruction (review). *J Urol* 144: 980.

50 Ehrlich RM, Reda EF, Koyle MA, Kogan SJ, Levitt SB (1989) Complications of bladder mucosal graft. *J Urol* 142: 2, 626.

51 Blandy JP, McDonald JH (1961) Heterotopic ossification in uroepithelial regeneration on grafts of ileum and colon. *Surg Forum* 12: 498.

52 Khoury AE, Olson ME, McLorie GA, Churchill BM (1989) Urethral replacement with tunica vaginalis: a pilot study. *J Urol* 142: 628.

53 Milroy EJG, Chapple CR, Eldin EA, Wallsten H (1989) A new stent for the treatment of urethral strictures. a preliminary report. *Br J Urol* 63: 392.

54 Krah H, Djamilian M, Seabert J, Allhoff EP, Stief C, Jonas U (1992) Significant obliteration of the urethral lumen after Wallstent implantation. *J Urol* 184: 1901.

55 Verhamme L, Van Poppel H, Van de Voorde W (1993) Total fibrotic obliteration of urethral stent. *Br J Urol* 72: 389.

Chapter 31: Urethra and penis — neoplasms

Urethral cancer

In males

Aetiology

Viruses

Some carcinomas of the urethra may start off as benign papillomas [1], caused by a papilloma-virus and gradually become more malignant until they metastasize. These are essentially the same as the condylomata acuminata that occur on the glans penis, foreskin and vulva. These carcinomas are particularly active in immuno-suppressed patients.

Implantation

Most tumours of the urethra are transitional cell carcinomas downstream of a recurrent bladder tumour, probably implanted onto slight abrasions of the urethra. It is possible that the same carcinogenic influences which give rise to the original bladder cancer may continue to act on the urethra: for this reason the urethra should always by removed at cystectomy for recurrent multifocal bladder cancer [2,3].

Upstream of stricture

Although rare in the West, squamous cell carcinoma of the urethra associated with urethral stricture is common in Africa [4] where *Schistosoma* infection may play a role. Squamous metaplasia is often present in the urethra upstream of a chronic stricture and may not only involve the bladder, but a previous cystostomy track.

Pathology

Benign tumours of the urethra

Condylomata acuminata in the urethra resemble those on the penis and vulva (Fig. 31.1).

Benign 'polypi' occur from time to time near the verumontanum and may cause obstruction (Fig. 31.2). Capillary haemangioma has been described as a rare cause of bleeding [5].

Fig. 31.1 (a) Condyloma acuminatum at the external meatus; (b) histology of condyloma acuminatum (courtesy of Dr J.K. Oates).

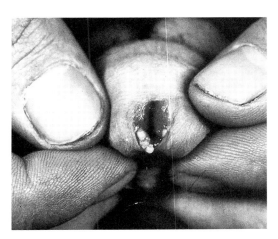

a

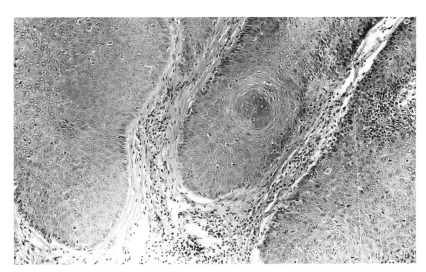

b

499

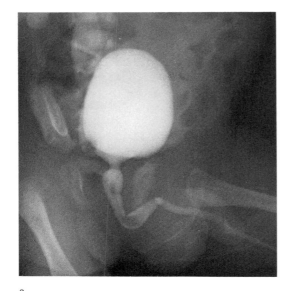

a

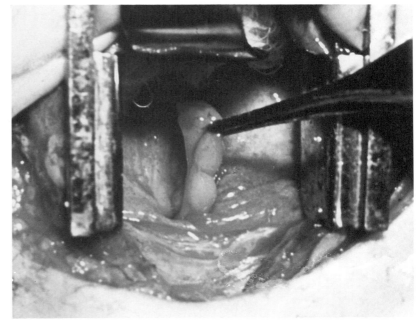

b

Malignant tumours of the urethra

Primary

Squamous cell cancer may arise without any previous stricture, usually in the bulb. Melanoma has been described in the urethra from time to time [6].

Secondary

In addition to the transitional cell cancers implanted from a primary in the bladder, carcinoma of the prostate may occasionally spread along the urethra and produce multiple rounded fleshy tumours.

Spread of tumours of the urethra

Only a thin epithelium separates the urethra from the corpus spongiosum, which drains into the inguinal lymphatics as well as the systemic veins. The inguinal nodes are involved early in this disease. Systemic spread is occasionally seen in patients whose local disease has been controlled.

Clinical features

When a long-standing stricture is complicated by a watering-can perineum one should always

suspect cancer of the urethra (Fig. 31.3). A urethral cancer may present with symptoms of outflow obstruction, mimicking enlargement of the prostate and be discovered only on endoscopy. More often, the malignant stricture leads to a periurethral 'abscess' pointing in the perineum which must be incised and it is only when tissue from the wall of the 'abscess' is examined that the diagnosis is made.

Fig. 31.2 (a) Cysto-urethrogram in 2-month-old boy showing a filling defect extending from the verumontanum down the bulbar urethra. (b) At operation the polyp was drawn up into the bladder and removed (courtesy of Mr J.H. Johnston).

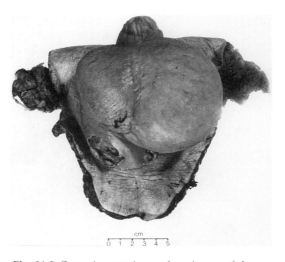

Fig. 31.3 Operation specimen of carcinoma of the urethra presenting as a watering-can perineum (courtesy of Mr P.R. Riddle).

Investigations

When recurrence is suspected after cystectomy the diagnosis may be made using a brush or soluble swab (Fig. 31.4) but usually a biopsy is obtained at urethroscopy.

Fine needle aspiration cytology of palpable inguinal lymph nodes, or pelvic nodes that are discovered in the computerized tomography (CT) scan will help in giving accurate staging.

Treatment

Condyloma acuminatum

For intraurethral condylomas, intraurethral instillation of Thiotepa, 5-fluouracil or Mitomycin is effective, but it may be quicker to coagulate them with diathermy or the neodymium-yttrium aluminium garnet (YAG) laser. Occasionally, they are so widespread and profuse that the only way to deal with them is to lay open the urethra [7].

Urethral cancer

Loop resection is avoided because it may open up venous sinuses and allow cancer cells to escape. The author has seen one case where within a few weeks of resecting such a tumour the inguinal nodes became involved.

There is a difference in the natural history of cancer of the urethra associated with stricture, and that which presents without any previous urethral disease. Cancer occurring in a long-standing stricture, subject to many urethro-tomies, dilatations, and perhaps a urethroplasty, can be cured by local excision of the affected urethra, combined with radiation therapy. None of the author's seven cases have developed metastases in a follow-up extending to 15 years. It may be that the good results in this group of patients results from the inflammatory fibrosis which acts as a barrier to the spread of cancer cells, much as it appears to do in bladder cancer developing in schistosomiasis.

In contrast, new tumours occurring in the bulbar urethra have such a poor outlook that a combination of chemotherapy and radiotherapy should be the first line of treatment and only then is the residual tumour removed surgically.

Resection of urethral cancer in males

Make a ∩-shaped scrotal approach (Fig. 31.5). Excise the affected part of the urethra and check with frozen section that the margins of excision are clear (Fig. 31.6). The resultant defect in the urethra is usually too long to be bridged by end-to-end anastomosis but a pedicled patch of scrotal skin may be formed into a tube and let into the gap (Fig. 31.7). The follow-up must be very careful, for stricture tends to occur after the previous radiotherapy.

When there are positive inguinal nodes, one should consider very carefully whether the chance of getting a cure by block dissection justifies the dreadful swelling of the lower limb which always follows. But this radical surgery offers a cure to about half the patients [8].

When tumour recurs after a conservative resection, or when the upper margin of the

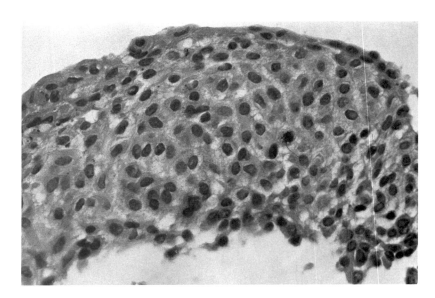

Fig. 31.4 Cytological specimen of transitional cell neoplasm from the urethra.

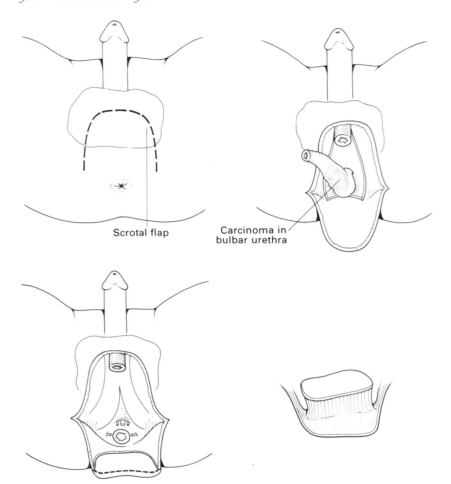

Scrotal flap

Carcinoma in bulbar urethra

Fig. 31.5 To expose the urethra a scrotal flap is formed.

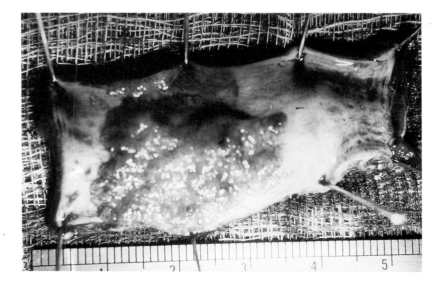

Fig. 31.6 Specimen of carcinoma of the urethra excised by partial urethrectomy.

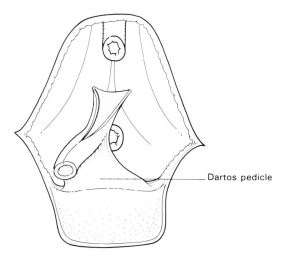

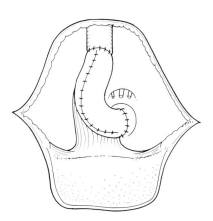

Fig. 31.7 The gap in the urethra is replaced with a tube of dartos pedicled scrotal skin.

tumour encroaches on the prostate, radical removal offers the only hope of saving the patient. The operation is so severe that one must make sure before embarking on it that there are no inguinal or distant metastases. The inguinal nodes should be dissected at a preliminary stage and sent for frozen section.

Radical resection of the urethra

Make a midline incision from above the umbilicus, skirting the penis, to within 2 cm of the anus (Fig. 31.8). All the tissues except the testicles are dissected from lateral to medial towards the midline. When the symphysis is exposed a 4 cm segment is removed with an oscillating bone saw (Fig. 31.9). A block dissection of the common external and internal iliac lymph nodes is performed on each side. The bladder is mobilized in the method usual in cystectomy, and the whole mass is removed *en bloc* (Fig. 31.10). The two ureters and rectum remain in the empty pelvis (Fig. 31.11).

The ureters are led into an ileal conduit (see p. 321). The large gap in the pelvis is bridged by bringing together the local tissues but a ventral hernia is inevitable. Its permanent repair should be deferred for at least 6 months to give time for distant metastasis to appear. The defect can be repaired with a sheet of non-absorbable synthetic mesh.

In females

Urethral tumours in women can be classified as in Table 31.1.

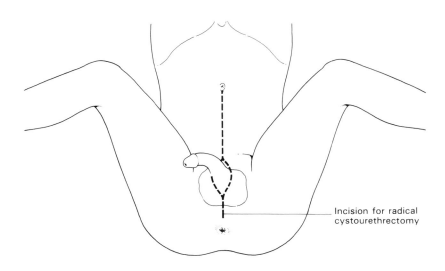

Fig. 31.8 Incision for radical resection of carcinoma of the urethra.

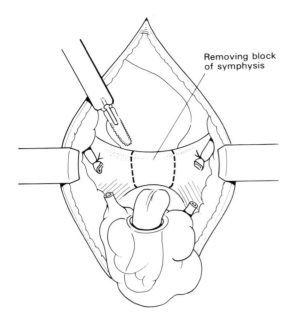

Fig. 31.9 The symphysis is removed *en bloc* with the bladder and urethra.

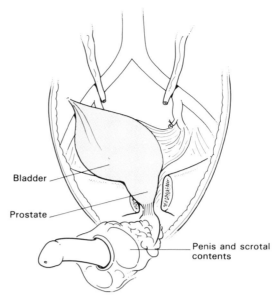

Fig. 31.10 The lymph nodes of the pelvis are dissected with the specimen.

Benign

The expression 'caruncle' — which simply means fleshy lump — is probably best avoided since it applies to a whole range of different conditions.

Prolapse of urethral mucosa

Most of the so-called caruncles are innocent prolapses of the urethral mucosa, analogous to haemorrhoids (Fig. 31.12) and like haemorrhoids,

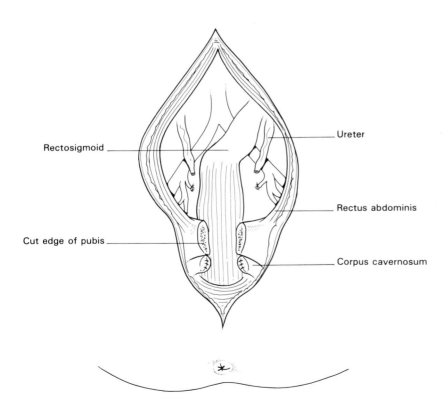

Fig. 31.11 The empty pelvis after radical cystourethrectomy.

Table 31.1 Classification of urethral tumours in female patients

Benign (caruncle)
   Prolapse of urethral mucosa
Thrombosis of urethral vein
   Oedema of the mucosa — polypi
   Condyloma acuminatum (venereal wart)
   Haemangioneurofibroma
Malignant
   Squamous cell cancer of the urethra
   Adenocarcinoma of the urethra
   Transitional cell carcinoma
   Malignant melanoma

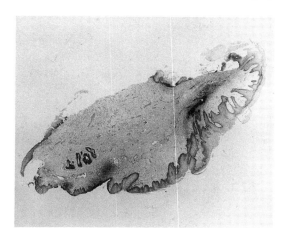

Fig. 31.13 Oedema in a simple urethral polypus.

equally complicated by thrombosis of veins which give rise to painful lumps as big as a cherry.

Oedematous polypi

Infection in the urethra and its surrounding glands may cause oedematous polypi to protrude from the external meatus (Fig. 31.13).

Venereal warts, condyloma acuminatum

Warts caused by papillomavirus are common in and around the urethra.

Haemangioneurofibroma

This rare but characteristic condition gives rise to a painful bright red swelling with a characteristic histology (Fig. 31.14).

To distinguish one of these swellings from another requires a biopsy.

Malignant

Squamous cell cancers present as a painful swelling in the urethra, with frequency and discomfort on urination for which there is no obvious cause. It is all too easy to dismiss such a case with the meaningless label 'urethral syndrome' and to treat it with equally meaningless urethral dilatation. The cancers are easily seen on urethroscopy using the flexible or 0° rigid telescope which should be as routine a part of endoscopy in the female as it is in the male.

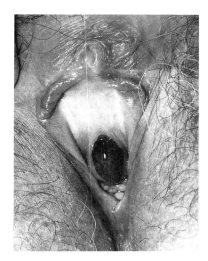

a

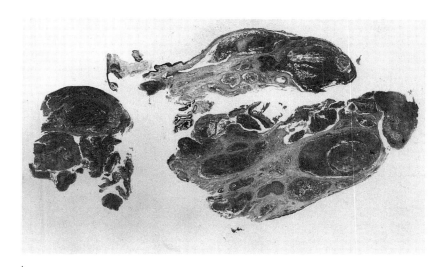

b

Fig. 31.12 Thrombosis in submucosal veins of urethra (a) naked eye appearance, and (b) histology.

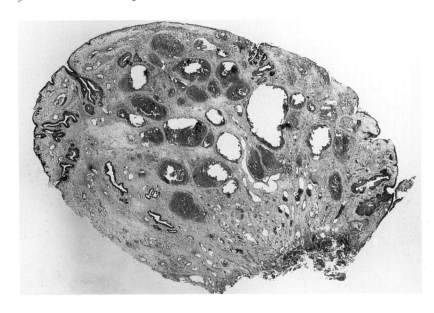

Fig. 31.14 Haemangio-neurofibroma (courtesy of Dr E.A. Courtauld).

Unfortunately, these cancers are often discovered only when they have already metastasized [9,10].

Adenocarcinomas occur at the upper end of the urethra, probably in paraurethral glands. They may arise in a urethral diverticulum [10].

Transitional cell cancers of the urethra are usually secondary to carcinoma of the bladder and their diagnosis and treatment follow the principles used in bladder cancer.

Primary malignant melanoma of the female urethra is rare. It presents with pain and haematuria. Endoscopy shows a friable dark brown mass. Its treatment is sadly ineffective [11].

Spread of urethral cancer in women

Cancer of the external meatus metastasizes to the inguinal nodes, that of the rest of the urethra to the internal iliac nodes.

Staging

Staging requires CT scanning supplemented by fine needle aspiration biopsy of suspicious nodes. Several systems of staging have been proposed. The Union Internationale Cóntre le Cancer (UICC) scheme [10] is as follows:
- **Tis** Carcinoma *in situ*.
- **T1** Invasion of subepithelial connective tissue.
- **T2** Invasion of corpus spongiosum, prostate, periurethral muscle.
- **T3** Invasion of corpus cavernosum, beyond prostatic capsule, vagina or bladder neck.
- **T4** Invasion of other organs.

Treatment

In practice, treatment follows first principles [12,13].

Some tumours respond to irradiation with interstitial radioactive gold grains, tantalum, iridium or radium needles and nothing is lost by trying this first, especially for squamous cell cancers arising at the urethral orifice. If it fails, the urethra can still be excised: a further biopsy is taken 6 weeks after completing radiotherapy [9].

Excision of the female urethra

For tumours at the lower end of the urethra a wide local excision, taking surrounding vaginal mucosa as well, may give a cure without loss of continence (Fig. 31.15). Bilateral block dissection of the inguinal nodes may be added to this procedure, but is only justified when the nodes are known to be positive.

For those involving the middle third of the urethra, it is possible to resect the whole urethra, and reconstruct it with a tube of pedicled skin from the labium minus of the vagina and still retain continence (Fig. 31.16).

Cancers at the upper end of the urethra, and those arising from a diverticulum, do so badly that the first line of treatment is a combination of radical radiotherapy and chemotherapy. Cysto-urethrectomy is reserved for those tumours which remain, and have not metastasized. The results are no better than 36% 3-year survival [9,12].

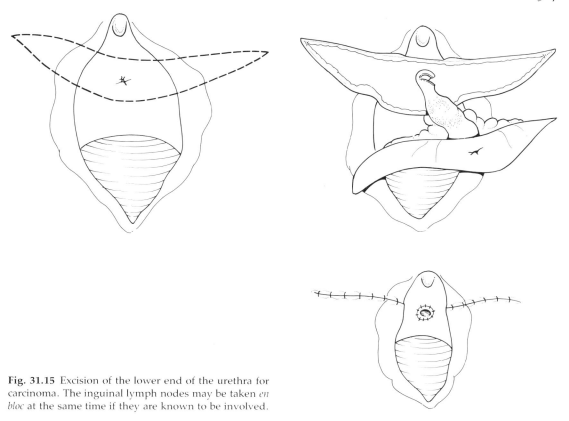

Fig. 31.15 Excision of the lower end of the urethra for carcinoma. The inguinal lymph nodes may be taken *en bloc* at the same time if they are known to be involved.

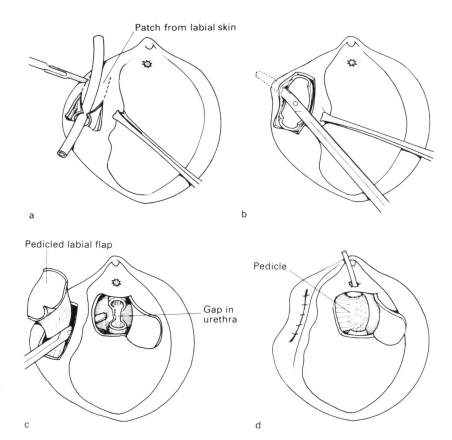

Fig. 31.16 (a) Labial patch marked out and (b) the plane between dartos and skin developed to provide a patch with a pedicle. (c) The tube replaces the defect left by excision of the urethra and (d) the vagina is closed over it.

Neoplasms of the penis

Aetiology

Cancer of the penis has been known through recorded time: its incidence varies so greatly from one place and one race to another, that it is impossible to separate genetic from environmental causes. Several of these are of possible importance.

1 Circumcision. Cancer of the penis is unknown in Jews ritually circumcised on the eighth day [14]. This may be because circumcision removes the prepuce, prevents balanitis and virus infections, or eliminates the carcinogenic action of smegma [15,16].

2 Viruses. There is a spectrum from the benign infective venereal wart (condyloma acuminatum) caused by a papillomavirus, through the intermediate Buschke−Loewenstein 'giant' condyloma in which the virus can be identified in early cases, but not later on when invasive cancer has developed, and it is seldom identifiable in most advanced cases [1,17].

3 Smoking. Circumstantial evidence links smoking with penile cancer but the figures are disputed [18,19].

4 Soft chancre, herpes. Infections with Ducrey's bacillus and herpesvirus are often noted in men with penile cancer [20].

5 Personal hygiene. Carcinoma of the penis has always been a disease of poverty and lack of hygiene [21].

6 Wives of men with penile cancer are more prone to cancer of the cervix [22,23].

7 A history of previous balanitis xerotica obliterans is found in about one in five cases of cancer of the penis [24].

Table 31.2 Classification of tumours of the penis

Benign
   Condyloma acuminatum
   Pearly papillary processes
Precarcinomatous changes
   Buschke−Loewenstein tumour
   Erythroplasia of Queyrat
   Balanitis xerotica obliterans
Malignant
   Squamous cell carcinoma
   Basal cell carcinoma
   Sarcoma
   Fibrosarcoma
   Angiosarcoma — Kaposi's tumour
   Melanoma
Secondary carcinoma, lymphoma, etc.

Age incidence

In Britain cancer of the penis is rare under 50 years of age: in India it is most common between 45 and 55 [21] but elsewhere, e.g. in Russia, one-third of the patients are under 40 [15].

Pathology

Tumours of the penis are classified as in Table 31.2.

Benign

Condyloma acuminatum

Usually transmitted by sexual intercourse, these are caused by a family of viruses of which several strains may be present in the same wart [17]. They present as typical warts on the prepuce, shaft, glans or meatus (Fig. 31.17). Occasionally, especially in immunosuppressed individuals, they form a confluent carpet of tumour that extends along the entire length of the urethra.

The diagnosis is so clear that it is seldom necessary to obtain a biopsy. Since these warts are exceedingly infectious, the patient's sexual partner should be examined: neglected condylomas in women can be very difficult to treat.

Condylomas respond to almost any form of local treatment: a drop of 10% podophyllin (which must be confined to the lesion), usually results in death of the wart within 10 days. Diathermy or the carbon dioxide or neodymium-YAG laser will coagulate them but in the urethra the scarring which follows these methods of treatment in the urethra may result in a stricture (see p. 478).

Pearly penile processes

These normal processes around the corona glandis are occasionally so prominent that they attract the notice of the worried adolescent bent on finding something wrong with himself: they need no treatment [25].

Precarcinomatous changes

Buschke−Loewenstein tumour

These look like very large condylomas (Fig. 31.18) and in the early stages contain papillomaviruses [26,27]. For many years they were believed to be benign, and therefore only to need local removal

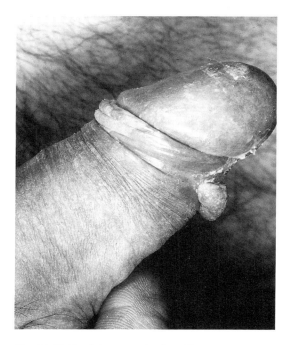

Fig. 31.17 Condyloma on the foreskin.

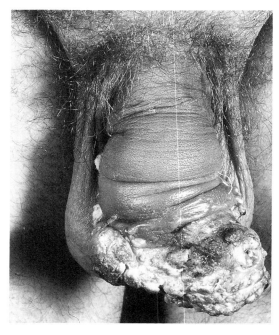

Fig. 31.18 Buschke–Loewenstein tumour of the penis.

but invasive carcinoma usually develops after local removal, therefore they should be treated as if they were carcinomas from the beginning [28,29].

Erythroplasia of Queyrat

This condition was clearly described by Paget in 1874 [30]. Only 37 years later did Queyrat report four cases with a red weeping patch on the glans penis which developed a frankly invasive cancer [31]. Circumcised patient have a painless dry scaly red patch on the penis (Fig. 31.19). In uncircumcised patients the lesion is weeping, red and inflamed. Neither can be distinguished from simple balanitis or balanitis of Zoon, and a biopsy must always be taken [32].

Histology shows every gradation from normal squamous epithelium through carcinoma *in situ* to invasive cancer (Fig. 31.20).

An identical carcinoma *in situ* is seen on the shaft of the penis where it is called Bowen's disease and may be the signal of occult gastro-intestinal cancer [33].

Erythroplasia of Queyrat may respond to topical 5% 5-fluorouracil cream applied twice daily for a month [34,35] and coagulation by the carbon dioxide or neodymium-YAG laser. Whatever method is used the patient must be followed up carefully because late relapse is common.

Cancer of the penis

Pathology

Cancer of the penis presents in one of three macroscopic forms — a papillary cauliflower out-growth, an ulcer or a nodular infiltrating mass (Fig. 31.21).

Microscopically, more than 99% are squamous cell cancers. Basal cell carcinoma occurs in less than 0.5% [19,36]. Most of the squamous cell cancers are well differentiated and erode the local tissues extensively before they metastasize.

There are three grades of malignancy [37], but of more importance than grade is the pattern of growth [38]

1 The solid pattern with large rounded clumps and sheets has an excellent prognosis.

2 The cord pattern where smaller cell masses form cords of cells has a poor prognosis [37] (Fig. 31.22).

Carcinoma of the penis spreads by direct invasion, creeping upwards in the soft tissues of the lower abdominal wall to form a continuous cuirasse. Spread to the inguinal lymph nodes is relatively late. Lymphangiography shows that the tumour may skip them and reach the pelvic nodes [39] or the so-called 'sentinel' lymph node in the fossa ovalis of the deep fascia of the thigh [40,41] (Fig. 31.23).

Cancer of the penis can spread up the mucosa

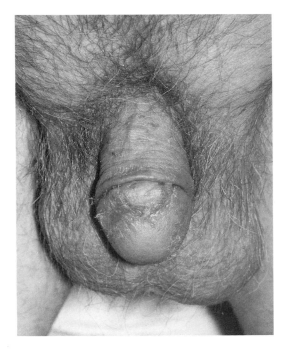

Fig. 31.19 Erythroplasia of Queyrat.

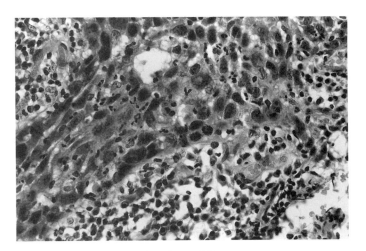

Fig. 31.20 Histology of erythroplasia of Queyrat (courtesy of Dr Suhail Baithun).

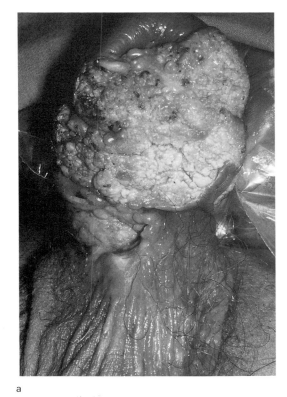

a

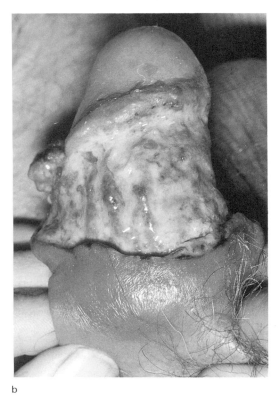

b

Fig. 31.21 (a) Papillary form of carcinoma of the penis. (b) Ulcerative form of carcinoma of the penis.

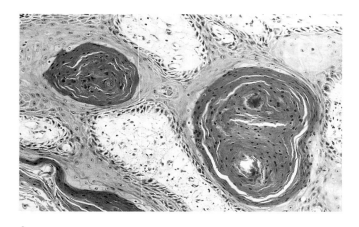

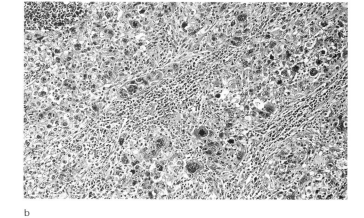

a

b

Fig. 31.22 (a) Well-differentiated solid carcinoma (b) Undifferentiated carcinoma of the penis.

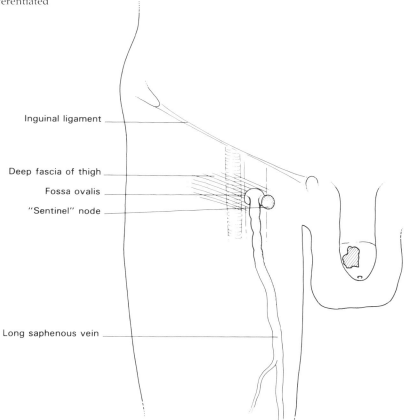

Inguinal ligament

Deep fascia of thigh

Fossa ovalis

"Sentinel" node

Long saphenous vein

Fig. 31.23 The 'sentinel' node where the saphenous vein joins the femoral vein.

of the urethra and great care is needed to ensure a clear margin when performing amputation.

Clinical features

Early carcinoma of the penis may present as a small red patch on the glans, a persistent shallow ulcer in the coronal sulcus or a warty excrescence (Fig. 31.24). In practice, most are only reported when they are advanced and there is a large fungating mass beneath a prepuce inflamed by secondary infection which is oozing pus (Fig. 31.25). Still later on, the entire penis may be eroded leaving only a flat ulcer that is flush with the scrotum (Fig. 31.26).

It is difficult to evaluate the regional lymph nodes at first, because of secondary infection: palpable nodes may only be inflamed, but if lymph nodes are felt when there is no local infection then they are likely to be invaded by cancer and should be investigated by aspiration biopsy [42].

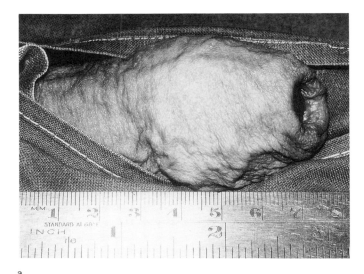

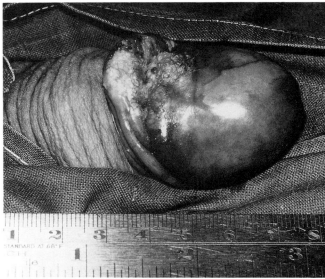

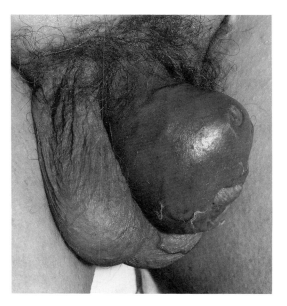

Fig. 31.25 Common presentation: huge infected mass with cellulitis of prepuce.

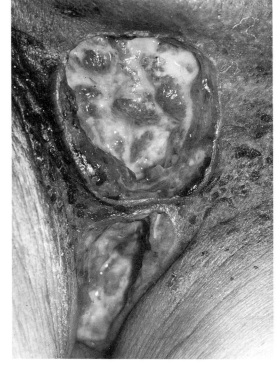

Fig. 31.24 (a) Early carcinoma of penis presenting as a preputial discharge. (b) When the foreskin is retracted the carcinoma is found usually at the corona.

Fig. 31.26 The entire penis is eroded (courtesy of Mr G.C. Tresidder).

Clinical staging

Staging is of use only if it helps to determine treatment. In carcinoma of the penis, the UICC TNM system is as follows [10]:

- **Tx** Cannot be assessed.
- **T0** No evidence of primary tumour.
- **Tis** Carcinoma *in situ*.
- **Ta** Non-invasive verrucous cancer.
- **T1** Invasion of subepithelial connective tissue.
- **T2** Invasion of corpus spongiosum or cavernosum.

- **T3** Invasion of urethra or prostate.
- **T4** Invasion of other adjacent structures.

In clinical practice, the simple staging system of Jackson is more useful [43] (Fig. 31.27):

- **Stage 1** Tumour limited to prepuce or glans.
- **Stage 2** Invasion of the shaft of the penis.

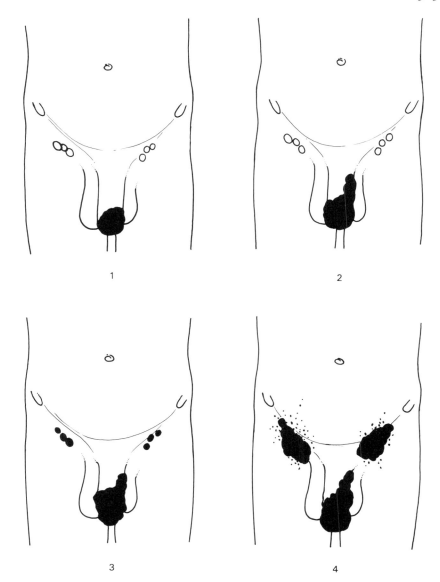

Fig. 31.27 Jackson's system of staging of carcinoma of the penis.

1

2

3

4

- **Stage 3** Inguinal nodes positive but operable.
- **Stage 4** Invasion of scrotum, fixed nodes.

The first step in staging or treatment is circumcision, at which as much of the tumour is removed as possible. This allows infection to be treated, and then the lymph nodes are reassessed about 2 weeks later with CT scanning and aspiration biopsy.

Management

Stage 1

If the cancer is confined to the prepuce, circumcision alone may be curative. When the glans is involved, the tumour may be cured either by local radiotherapy or partial amputation with equally good results.

Irradiation. There are several methods. A plastic mould armed with radioactive iridium$_{192}$ wire [42] may be placed over the penis for a specified time (Fig. 31.28). This method is only feasible when the patient is reasonably intelligent and dexterous. In the older man with failing eyesight and understanding, it may be better to implant radium or tantalum needles, or give teletherapy with ^{60}cobalt or the linear accelerator [43,44].

In stage 1 penile cancer, radiation gives a 5-year cure of 100%, but careful follow-up is essential because about 25% will develop late recurrence and need late partial amputation [42].

Partial amputation for carcinoma of the penis. The margin of resection particularly at the edge of the urethra must be shown to be free by frozen section. Loss of blood is prevented by applying a

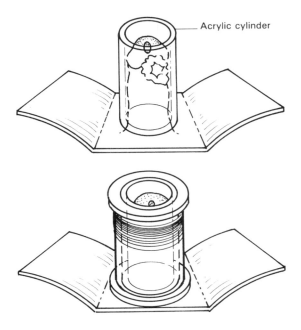

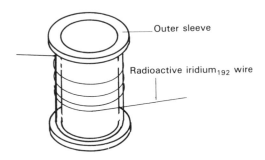

Fig. 31.28 Iridium method for irradiation of carcinoma of the penis.

soft clamp or tourniquet to the base of the penis. A racquet-shaped incision is made with an ∩-shaped tongue of skin on the inferior side of the penis (Fig. 31.29). The corpus spongiosum is cut across about 5 mm distal to the corpora cavernosa. The specimen is sent for frozen section to confirm that the margin — especially of the urethra — is clear (Fig. 31.30).

If the deep arteries of the corpus cavernosum can be identified, they should be suture ligated. The tunica albuginea and Buck's fascia are closed with strong catgut leaving a stump over which the spatulated urethra is attached, and an elliptical anastomosis is made to the ∩-shaped tongue of skin. This technique avoids stricture which was formerly such a common complication of amputation of the penis [45−47].

Stage 2

When carcinoma has invaded the corpora, it is still worth trying preliminary radiotherapy so long as the patient understands that it is successful in only half of the cases, and partial amputation is needed when treatment fails. Even if it fails to effect a cure, preliminary radiation improves the chance of long-term survival [42].

Stage 3

A cancer which has reached the scrotum may still not have involved the inguinal lymph nodes. Preliminary radiation might improve the results,

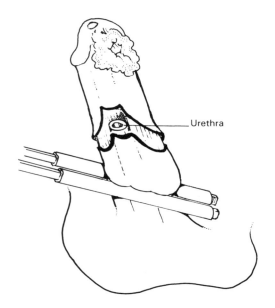

Fig. 31.29 Partial amputation of the penis. Racquet-shaped incision.

but these patients present so late and are in such a sorry state the main objective is to get rid of the stinking mass.

Radical resection of penile cancer. This operation was devised for palliation in the usual elderly man with advanced cancer for whom preserving the testicles was not an issue [47].

The large infected primary tumour is enclosed in a rubber glove before the area is cleaned. The operation is covered with antibiotics.

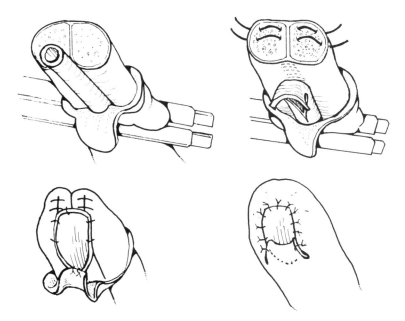

Fig. 31.30 Partial amputation of the penis. The corpus spongiosum is left long, spatulated and attached over the closed corpora cavernosa. The ∩-shaped flap of skin prevents stricture.

Make a racquet incision around the base of the penis well away from the tumour. Continue it down in the middle line and make a ∩-shaped flap which will expose the bulb of the urethra (Fig. 31.31). Divide both spermatic cords. Expose the bulbar urethra by reflecting the bulbo-spongiosus muscles (Fig. 31.32). Free the urethra from the corpora cavernosa for about 5 cm and

cut it across. Clear the soft tissues from the external ring and symphysis. Cut the suspensory ligament. Clamp and divide the corpora cavernosa close to the rami, and oversew them with catgut (Fig. 31.33). Spatulate the urethra and suture it to the symphysis. Sew the ∩-shaped flap of scrotum into the spatulated urethra to make a long elliptical anastomosis. Cover the raw area with the flaps of scrotal skin and close the wound with drainage. This technique prevents urethral stricture and leaves the perineum resembling a vulva (Fig. 31.34).

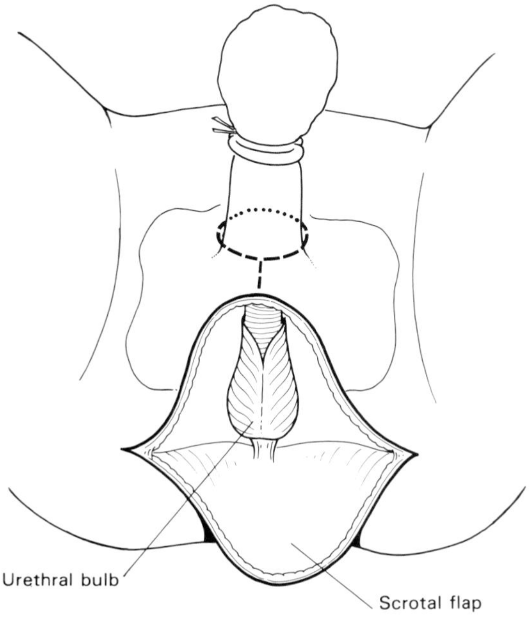

Urethral bulb

Scrotal flap

Fig. 31.31 Radical amputation of the penis. The incision encircles the base, well clear of tumour, and is continued down to form a large ∩-shaped flap.

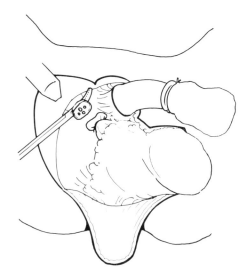

Fig. 31.32 Both spermatic cords and the suspensory ligament are divided.

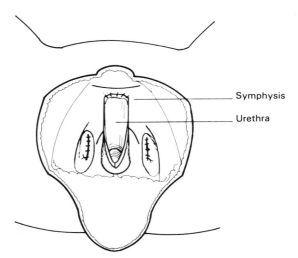

Fig. 31.33 Both corpora cavernosa are divided and oversewn. The urethra is spatulated and attached to the symphysis.

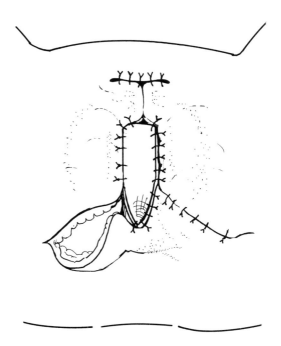

Fig. 31.34 The long elliptical anastomosis of the urethra prevents a stricture.

Results. Although rarely indicated this operation is justified by its long-term results: seven of eight of the author's cases have survived free of recurrence — unusual for an operation whose original purpose was palliation [42].

Stage 4

When inguinal nodes are involved, the control of the local disease is no longer the main issue.

Radical inguinal node dissection is sometimes performed in early cases as a prophylactic measure, but is seldom successful when the nodes are positive and the patient always pays a high price in terms of oedema of the lower limb [44,48,49].

The management of inguinal lymph nodes has changed with the introduction of adjuvant radiotherapy and chemotherapy. Preoperative radiotherapy with parallel and opposed megavoltage fields is first given to the pelvis and inguinal nodes whilst taking care to shield the rectum using a tumour dose of 4500 cGy in 20 daily fractions over 4 weeks. If the CT scan and fine needle aspiration of the pelvic nodes show that these are involved as well, combination chemotherapy is added [50].

Salvage inguinal node dissection. If the inguinal nodes fail to resolve or relapse, block dissection is performed. Great care is taken to achieve primary healing: the penalty for failure is horrific — the groin becomes a huge area of necrosis, beneath which the femoral vessels, softened by bacterial infection, may burst [47].

If the iliac nodes are not enlarged in the CT scan, the dissection may be confined to the groin. Through a long oblique incision parallel with the inguinal ligament the tissues are dissected down to the deep fascia of the femoral triangle (Fig. 31.35). The saphenous vein is removed *en bloc*: the femoral nerve is dissected cleanly and the femoral vessels are denuded (Fig. 31.36). To protect them, the sartorius muscle is detached

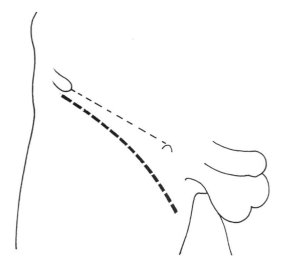

Fig. 31.35 Salvage inguinal node dissection. Long oblique incision.

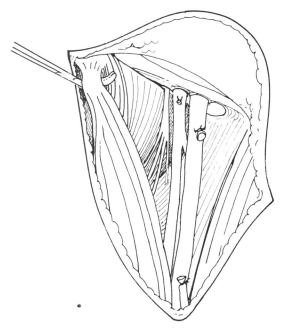

Fig. 31.36 The contents of the femoral triangle are dissected cleanly.

from the anterior superior spine, and swung medially over the femoral vessels (Fig. 31.37). The skin is closed with fine interrupted sutures

tied loosely. Suction drainage is provided. The lower limb is bandaged and kept elevated to prevent oedema.

If the CT scan shows that the iliac lymph nodes are enlarged, an extraperitoneal node dissection may be performed at the same time. The skin and fat of the abdominal wall are dissected off the rectus muscle (Fig. 31.38) for about 10 cm. A muscle cutting oblique incision is made above the inguinal ligament and the peritoneum retracted off the external iliac vessels (Fig. 31.39). With suitable retraction, the vessels are exposed to the bifurcation of the aorta and the sleeve of lymph nodes dissected off the common and external iliac vessels. In view of the risk of infection, the abdominal wound should be closed with an absorbable suture (Fig. 31.40).

Sarcoma of the penis

Several types of sarcomas may affect the penis [51,52]. Most arise near the frenulum. Some are malignant haemangiomas [53,54] arising in erectile tissue and presenting with priapism [54]. Kaposi's sarcoma involving the penis is being reported more frequently [55,56]. Leiomyosarcoma [57], fibrosarcoma, epithelioid sarcoma

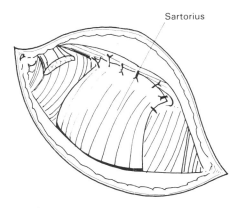

Fig. 31.37 To protect the femoral vessels the sartorius is detached from its origin and brought medially.

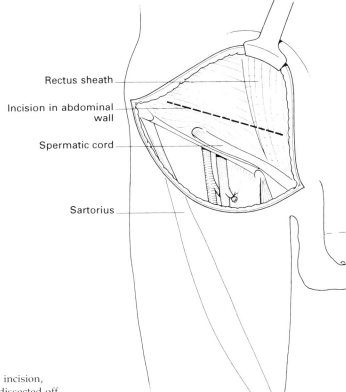

Fig. 31.38 Through the same long oblique incision, the skin and fat of the abdominal wall are dissected off the rectus for about 10 cm.

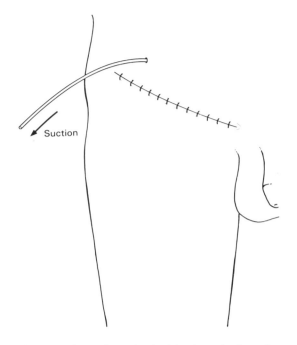

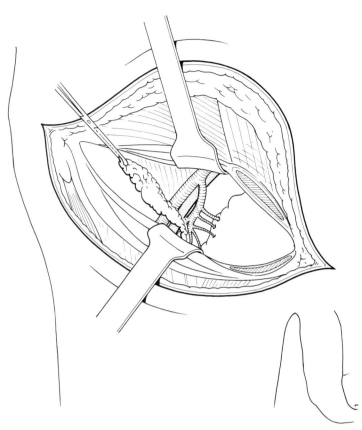

Fig. 31.39 A muscle cutting incision is made above the inguinal ligament and the iliac vessels exposed by retracting the peritoneum.

Fig. 31.40 The lymph nodes are dissected off the vessels from the bifurcation of the aorta down to the inguinal ligament.

[58] and angiomyolipoma [59] are all recorded: local excision is usually combined with radiotherapy.

Melanoma has been reported as a great rarity: the outlook is no predictable than for melanomas elsewhere, with the occasional unexpected long-term survivor [60–62].

Secondary cancer of the penis

Metastases from any primary tumour may occur in the penis, those arising from the prostate and bladder are most common and mimic Peyronie's disease. Others present with priapism especially in children with leukaemia [63]. In general secondary tumours in the penis carry a very poor prognosis [64].

Carcinoma of the scrotum

Percivall Pott named this chimney sweeper's cancer [65]. Later, Curling questioned why it was seen in London, but not in France or North America: was it because a different kind of coal was used, or was it (as he surmised) because of the 'inhuman practice of employing climbing

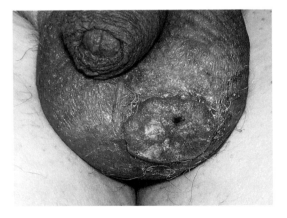

Fig. 31.41 Carcinoma of the scrotum.

boys'? [66] Today, this occupational cancer is very rare (Fig. 31.41). It is usually a well-differentiated squamous cancer and provided local excision is performed with a clear margin the prognosis is excellent, unless the lymph nodes are already involved [67,68].

References

1 Bunney MH (1986) Viral warts: a new look at an old problem. *Br Med J* 293: 1045.

2 Beahrs JR, Fleming TR, Zincke H (1984) Risk of local urethral recurrence after radical cystectomy for bladder cancer. *J Urol* 131: 264.

3 Stockle M, Gokcebay E, Riedmiller H, Hohenfellner R (1990) Urethral tumor recurrences after radical cystoprostatectomy: the case for primary cystoprostatourethrectomy. *J Urol* 143: 41.

4 Levine RL (1980) Urethral cancer. *Cancer* 45: 1965.

5 Sharma SK, Reddy MJ, Joshi VV, Bapna BC (1981) Capillary haemangioma of male urethra. *Br J Urol* 53: 277.

6 Rashid AMH, Williams RM, Horton LWL (1993) Malignant melanoma of penis and male urethra. *Urology* 41: 470.

7 Kesner KM (1993) Extensive condylomata acuminata of male urethra: management by ventral urethrotomy. *Br J Urol* 71: 204.

8 Dinney CPN, Johnson DE, Swanson DA, Babaian RJ, von Eschenbach AC (1994) Therapy and prognosis for male anterior urethral carcinoma: an update. *Urology* 43: 506.

9 Garden AS, Sagars GK, Delclos L (1993) Primary carcinoma of the female urethra: results of radiation therapy. *Cancer* 71: 3102.

10 Hermanek P, Sobin LH (1992) (eds) *UICC International Union against Cancer TNM Classification of Malignant Tumours*, 4th edn, 2nd revision. Berlin: Springer.

11 Katz JI, Grabstald H (1976) Primary malignant melanoma of the female urethra. *J Urol* 116: 454.

12 Skinner EC, Skinner DG (1988) Management of carcinoma of the female urethra, in: Skinner DG, Lieskovsky G (eds) *Diagnosis and Management of Genitourinary Cancer*. Philadelphia: WB Saunders.

13 Woodhouse CRJ, Flynn JT, Blandy JP (1980) Urethral diverticulum in females. *Br J Urol* 52: 305.

14 Paymaster JC, Gangadharan P (1967) Carcinoma of the penis in India. *J Urol* 97: 110.

15 Shabad AL (1964) Some aspects of etiology and prevention of penile cancer. *J Urol* 92: 696.

16 Editorial. (1964) Circumcision and cervical cancer. *Br Med J* 2: 397.

17 Malek RS, Goellner JR, Smith TF, Espy MJ, Cupp MR (1993) Human papillomavirus infection and intraepithelial, *in situ*, and invasive carcinoma of penis. *Urology* 42: 159.

18 Hellberg D, Valentin J, Eklund T, Nilsson S (1987) Penile cancer: is there an epidemiological role for smoking and sexual behaviour? *Br Med J* 295: 1306.

19 Lee PN (1988) Penile cancer and smoking. *Br Med J* 296: 210.

20 Staubitz WJ, Lent MH, Oberkircher OJ (1955) Carcinoma of the penis. *Cancer* 8: 371.

21 Reddy DJ, Indira C (1963) Some aspects of the pathology of carcinoma penis. *J Indian Med Ass* 41: 277.

22 Graham S, Priore R, Graham M, Browne R, Burnett W, West D (1979) Genital cancer in wives of penile cancer patients. *Cancer* 44: 1870.

23 Steinitz R (1967) Uterine cancer. *Lancet* i: 447.

24 Jamieson NV, Bullock KN, Barker THW (1988) Adenosquamous carcinoma of the penis associated with balanitis xerotica obliterans. *Br J Urol* 58: 730.

25 Ackerman AB, Kornberg R (1973) Pearly penile papules. *Arch Derm Chicago* 108: 673.

26 Buschke A (1896) *Neisser's Stereoskopischer Medizinisher Atlas*. Leipzig: Fischer.

27 Loewenstein LW (1939) Carcinoma-like condylomata acuminata of the penis. *Med Clin N Am* 23: 789.

28 Rohde T, Jensen KME, Hoyer S, Colstrup H (1993) Apparent Bushke—Loewenstein tumour of the penis. *Br J Urol* 71: 755.

29 Alfthan O (1970) Condyloma acuminatum giganticum: Buschke—Loewenstein tumour. *Scand J Urol Nephrol* 4: 71.

30 Paget J (1874) On disease of the mammary areola preceding cancer of the mammary gland. *St Barts Hosp Rep* 10: 87.

31 Queyrat L (1911) Erythroplasie du gland. *Bull Soc Franc Derm Syphil* 22: 378.

32 Graham JH, Helwig EB (1973) Erythroplasia of Queyrat: a clinico-pathologic and histochemical study. *Cancer* 32: 1396.

33 Mostofi FK, Price EB (1973) *Tumors of the Male Genital System*, pp. 205—83. Washington DC: Armed Forces Institute of Pathology.

34 Mikhail GR (1980) Cancers, precancers and pseudo-cancer on the male genitalia: a review of clinical appearances, histopathology and management. *J Dermatol Surg Oncol* 6: 1027.

35 Goette DK, Carson TE (1976) Erythroplasia of Queyrat: treatment with topical 5-fluouracil. *Cancer* 38: 1498.

36 Fegen JP, Beebe D, Persky L (1970) Basal cell carcinoma of the penis. *J Urol* 104: 864.

37 Salaverria JC, Hope-Stone HF, Paris AMI, Molland EA, Blandy JP (1979) Conservative treatment of carcinoma of the penis. *Br J Urol* 51: 32.

38 Frew IDO, Jefferies JD, Swinney J (1967) Carcinoma of penis. *Br J Urol* 39: 398.

39 Riveros M, Garcia R, Cabanas R (1967) Lymphangiography of the dorsal lymphatics of the penis. *Cancer* 20: 2026.

40 Cabanas RM (1977) An approach for the treatment of penile carcinoma. *Cancer* 39: 456.

41 Perinetti E, Crane DB, Catalona WJ (1980) Unreliability of sentinel lymph node biopsy for staging penile carcinoma. *J Urol* 124: 734.

42 El-Demiry MIM, Oliver RTD, Hope-Stone HF, Blandy JP (1984) Reappraisal of the role of radiotherapy and surgery in the management of carcinoma of the penis. *Br J Urol* 56: 724.

43 Jackson SM (1966) The treatment of carcinoma of the penis. *Br J Surg* 53: 33.

44 Ravi R (1993) Correlation between the extent of nodal involvement and survival following groin dissection for carcinoma of the penis. *Br J Urol* 72: 817.

45 Krieg RM, Luk KH (1981) Carcinoma of the penis. Review of cases treated by surgery and radiation therapy 1960—1977. *Urology* 18: 149.

46 Gursel EO, Georgountzos C, Uson AC (1973) Penile cancer: clinicopathologic study of 64 cases. *Urology* 1: 569.

47 Blandy JP (1986) *Operative Urology*, 2nd edn. Oxford: Blackwell Scientific Publications.

48 Johnson DE, Lo RK (1984) Management of regional

lymph nodes in penile carcinoma: five year results following therapeutic groin dissections. *Urology* 24: 308.

49 Catalona WJ (1988) Modified inguinal lymph-adenectomy for carcinoma of the penis with preservation of saphenous veins: technique and preliminary results. *J Urol* 140: 306.

50 Blandy JP, Hope-Stone HF, Oliver RTD (1989) Carcinoma of the penis and urethra, in: Oliver RTD, Blandy JP, Hope-Stone HF (eds) *Urological and Genital Cancer*, p. 258. Oxford: Blackwell Scientific Publications.

51 Abeshouse BS, Abeshouse GA, Goldstein AE (1962) Sarcoma of the penis: a review of the literature and a report of a new case; and a brief consideration of melanoma of the penis. *Urol Int* 13: 273.

52 Dehner LP, Smith BH (1970) Soft tissue tumors of the penis. A clinicopathologic study of 46 cases. *Cancer* 25: 1431.

53 Maiche AG, Grohn P, Makinen J (1986) Malignant penile haemangioendothelioma. *Br J Urol* 58: 232.

54 Hodgins TE, Hancock RA (1970) Hemangio-endothelial sarcoma of the penis: report of a case and review of the literature. *J Urol* 104: 867.

55 Linker D, Lieberman P, Grabstald H. (1975) Kaposi's sarcoma of genitourinary tract. *Urology* 5: 684.

56 McNutt NS, Fletcher V, Conant MA (1983) Early lesions of Kaposi's sarcoma in homosexual men. An ultrastructural comparison with other vascular proliferations in skin. *Am J Pathol* 111: 62.

57 Isa SS, Almaraz R, Magovern J (1984) Leomyo-sarcoma of the penis. Case report and review of the literature. *Cancer* 54: 939.

58 Huang DJ, Stanisic TH, Hansen KK (1992) Epithelioid sarcoma of the penis. *J Urol* 148: 1370.

59 Chaitin BA, Goldman RL, Linker DG (1984) Angio-myolipoma of penis. *Urology* 23: 305.

60 Cascinelli N (1969) Melanoma maligno del pene. *Tumori* 55: 313.

61 Bracken RB, Diokno AC (1974) Melanoma of the penis and the urethra. *J Urol* 111: 198.

62 Wheelock MC, Clark PJ (1943) Sarcoma of the penis. *J Urol* 49: 478.

63 Brunetti A (1969) Sulla metastasi del Pene: contri-buto cassistico. *Archiv Ital Urol Nefrol* 42: 409.

64 Powell BL, Craig JB, Muss HB (1985) Secondary malignancies of the penis and epididymis: a case report and review of the literature. *J Clin Oncol* 3: 110.

65 Pott P (1774) *Chirurgical Works*. London: Lowndes, Johnson, Robinson, Cadell, Evans, Fox, Bew and Hayes. Vol 3: 225−229.

66 Curling TB (1843) *A Practical Treatise on the Diseases of the Testis, and of the Spermatic Cord and Scrotum*, pp. 531−3. London Longman, Brown, Green and Longman.

67 Ray B, Whitmore WF (1977) Experience with carcinoma of the scrotum. *J Urol* 117: 741.

68 Burmer GC, True LD, Krieger JN (1993) Squamous cell carcinoma of the scrotum associated with human papillomaviruses. *J Urol* 149: 374.

Chapter 32: Urethra and penis — disorders of function

Impotence

Psychogenic

Down the centuries poets and pornographers have raised so many associations with erection that it is hardly surprising that its failure should have many causes. Few of them have anything to do with the surgeon. Impotence is common in endogenous depression, and is a side effect of many of the drugs given to relieve it.

Neuropathic

Failure in the nervous links between the brain and the penis may follow demyelination in the spinal cord, diabetic nephropathy or trauma from fractures of the pelvis, radical pelvic surgery and transurethral or open resection of the prostate [1,2].

Vascular

Arterial

Blockage of the aorta reduces the blood flow in its terminal branches and impotence is a feature of the Leriche syndrome. It is seen when the internal iliac artery is used for renal transplantation but more often it is the smaller vessels — the deep arteries of the corpora cavernosa which are blocked by atheroma or diabetic arteriopathy.

Venous

In the rigid phase of erection, the venous outflow from the penis is shut off by nervous stimulation and kinking of the veins as they pass through the tunica albuginea (see p. 438). When this final occlusion of the venous outflow fails to take place there is a 'venous leak'.

Local causes

In Peyronie's disease, part of the spongy tissue is replaced by fibrous tissue which prevents filling, and makes the penis so crooked that penetration is difficult. Organization of thrombus after priapism may prevent the sinuses in the corpora from being properly filled.

Hormonal causes

Hyperprolactinaemia causing impotence is found in about 5% of men investigated for this condition [3]. Men reporting lack of desire may rarely have low levels of testosterone [4].

Ejaculatory impotence

The mechanism of ejaculation (Fig. 32.1) requires five coordinated functions:
1 The seminal vesicles contract rhythmically to pump up.
2 Peristaltic contractions of the vas deferens eject a small volume of semen containing sperm through the common ejaculatory ducts.
3 This is followed by contraction of the seminal vesicles which squirt the sperm-rich fraction of semen into the prostatic urethra.
4 At the same time the bladder neck closes and the external sphincter relaxes, preventing the sperm from flowing back and expelling it down the urethra, assisted by the contractions of stage 5.
5 Rhythmical contractions of the bulbospongiosus muscle take place [5−7].

The smooth muscle fibres in the neck of the bladder and seminal vesicles are alpha adrenergic. Diabetic neuropathy, sympathectomy, alpha blocking drugs for hypertension or surgical injury to the sympathetic chain or presacral nerve will prevent contraction of the vesicles and closure of the bladder neck [8−11].

Prostatectomy or bladder neck incision should not affect contraction of the seminal vesicles, but the semen will tend to flow back into the bladder rather than squirt out from the urethra — retrograde ejaculation. Prostatectomy may

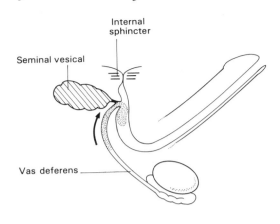

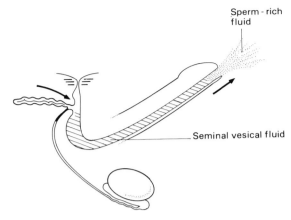

Fig. 32.1 The mechanism of ejaculation.

inadvertently injure and obstruct the common ejaculatory ducts [1].

Urethral strictures are a common cause of obstructed ejaculation.

Investigation of impotence

Clinical history

The first stage is to take a careful and sympathetic history [2,8]. What a patient describes as impotence is often unrealistic expectation — he can no longer make love three times every night. Listening to the history may show that the patient can make love with one partner but not with another. Business potentates obliged to retire — or whose business empires are taken over — may lose their potency with their loss of power. It is not by accident that *potent* means both.

Check what drugs the patient is taking, e.g. antihypertensives, lithium for depression, alcohol, methyldopa and cimetidine [9–11].

Sometimes a patient can masturbate, and ejaculates in his dreams, but has no desire to make love. Often an ambitious professional is exhausted, taking his papers to work on at home and giving no time to his marriage: this condition, all too common, is known as 'barristers' impotence' but is by no means confined to barristers. There is a fine line between want of libido from exhaustion and that which is due to depression.

Some men have a fixed obsession that their penis is too small. Nothing shakes this conviction: they wander from one doctor to another until finally they are offered an operation to make their entirely normal organ bigger. Inevitably, this disappoints the patient: it is never big enough or long enough or just the right colour

and the surgeon gets the blame. Be wary of these people.

Time, patience and willingness to listen may save endless investigations and direct the patient to a psychiatrist who is skilled in psychosexual and marital problems.

Physical examination

Few endocrine causes bring the patient to the surgeon complaining of impotence, for in most endocrine disorders the patient is unaware of what he is missing.

Physical examination nevertheless encompasses the whole patient. Measure the blood pressure and test the urine for glucose [10,11]. Note other evidence of arteriopathy. Note evidence of previous trauma or pelvic surgery. Examine the penis and note its pulses.

A careful decision must now be made whether to pursue the investigations, to refer the patient for appropriate counselling or advise him to put up with his lot. There is no point in pursuing investigations if the patient is not suitable or willing to undergo treatment, e.g. by injections or a prosthesis. Many a borderline patient will be content with reassurance, a dose of yohimbine [12–14] and perhaps a course of exercises [15].

Investigations [2]

Intracorporeal injections

Papaverine or prostaglandin E injected into one corpus cavernosum will relax its arterioles and cause filling of the erectile tissue when the cavernosal arteries are patent. One should start with a very small dose of 7.5 mg of papaverine given through a 25 gauge needle.

Nocturnal penile tumescence

An objective record of nocturnal erection is made with strain gauges fitted around the penis [16] (Fig. 32.2) or a paper strip which records its expansion during sleep [17] (Fig. 32.3). Refinements make it possible to record an increase in length as well as girth of the penis. The normal record shows three or four erections during the period of deep sleep characterized by rapid eye movements (REM), alpha wave activity in the electroencephalogram (EEG) and dreams (Fig. 32.4).

Measurements of arterial blood flow

Ultrasound Doppler studies record the pulse in the arteries of the corpora cavernosa. A small sphygmomanometer cuff allows the blood pressure in the penis to be compared with that in the arm [2,15].

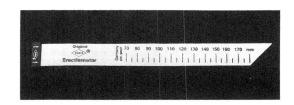

Fig. 32.3 Paper strips can be used to denote expansion of the penis during sleep.

Cavernosography

The pressure in the venous sinuses of the corpora can be recorded during an erection [18]. Two needles are placed in the corpora. Through one needle saline is infused, to which papaverine and contrast medium is added; the second needle measures the pressure (Fig. 32.5). Fluoroscopy shows whether the penile veins are being effectively closed during the phase of rigid erection [19] (Fig. 32.6).

These studies may be made without adding papaverine if the erection is induced by showing the patient an appropriate erogenous videotape.

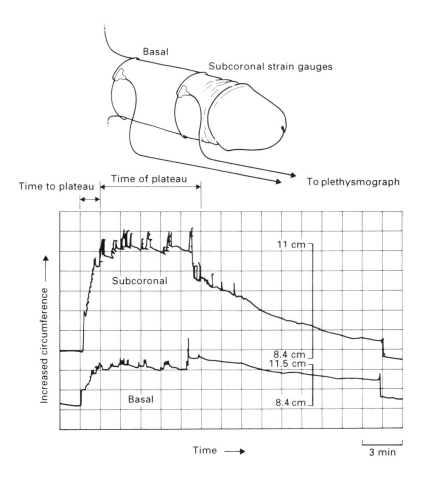

Fig. 32.2 Strain gauges fitted around the penis record nocturnal tumescence (courtesy of Mr Peter Blacklay).

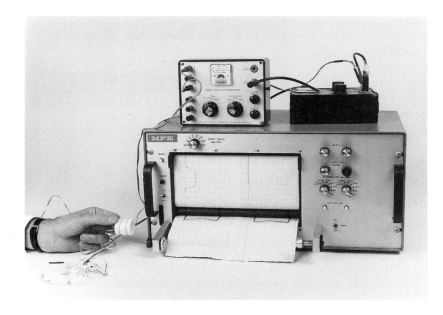

Fig. 32.4 A continuous record is made of expansion and elongation of the penis during sleep.

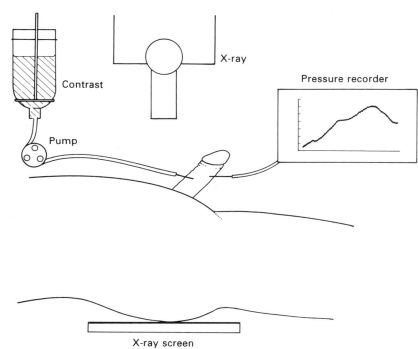

Fig. 32.5 The pressure in the corpora is recorded during erection while fluid is injected under pressure.

The normal record of penile pressure shows a gradual pulsatile rise as the corporeal arteries relax, a more sudden rise as the veins close off and the penis changes from being 'erect' to 'rigid': this does not occur when there is a venous leak [18,19]. Absence of this pressure increase may signify a venous leak.

Tests of autonomic nervous function

Measurements of the rate of conduction in auto-nomic fibres have so far been unhelpful even in diabetic neuropathy [20–22].

Treatment

Yohimbine is an alkaloid similar to reserpine which is found in Rubaceae and other trees. It has had a reputation for improving erections for many years, but has never been taken seriously. Unexpectedly, Morales *et al.* [12] have shown it to have some real action. It is, however, very

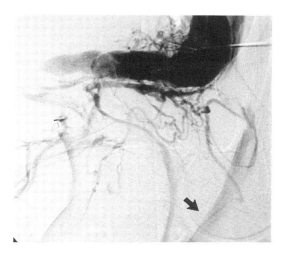

Fig. 32.6 Using radioopaque fluid, leakage of contrast medium during erection can be detected. 120 ml of contrast were injected into one corpus cavernosum at 3 ml/s. The corpora have both filled, but not the corpus spongiosum and glans (normal). Subtracted image towards the end of the injection shows no satisfactory tumescence, due to venous leak from the penile root with numerous veins draining into the right iliac venous system (arrow) (courtesy of Dr Robert Dick).

important not to exceed the usual three times daily dose of 5.4 mg [12,13].

For some patients the experience of a successful erection following a single intracavernosal injection may solve the problem by restoring confidence and after one or two trials, injection is no longer needed. This may be regarded as a short-cut version of psychotherapy, but it is no less valuable for that [23].

Men with a satisfactory blood supply, but a malfunctioning nervous network — from diabetes or injury — find the use of intracorporeal injections a satisfactory remedy.

Regular intracorporeal injections

Many vasoactive substances can be injected into the corpus cavernosum and cause an erection [24−31]. This method is now in widespread use. There is still considerable discussion concerning which combination of drugs is best: some felt that it was better to add phentolamine to the papaverine, others thought it made little difference. The risk of causing fibrosis has made many avoid papaverine in favour of prostaglandin E.

Complications

Priapism

Priapism — erections continuing beyond the desired or appropriate time and accompanied by pain — occurs in up to 18% of patients [32]: it usually resolves if aramine is given promptly, but this may need a continuous infusion over several hours [33] and must be started at once if permanent impotence is to be avoided. All patients undergoing this form of therapy must know whom to telephone in this event [32−36].

Erroneous prescription

Papaveretum has been prescribed in mistake for papaverine with near-fatal results.

Fibrosis

Small areas of fibrosis are seen at the site of injection, similar to Peyronie's disease [35,36]. In monkeys, this occurred with papaverine but not with prostaglandin E1 [37] which is equally effective but more expensive [38,39].

Vasoactive cream

Alternatives to injecting vasoactive drugs are undergoing trial: cream containing amyl nitrite may give an erection, but at the price of headaches for both partners [40,41].

Vacuum devices

Several simple devices consisting of a cylinder from which air is evacuated, suck blood into the penis, which is then surrounded with an elastic band. Available in sex-shops for years, they are said to be effective [42].

Implanted prostheses

Four types of prosthesis are available.
1 Semi-stiff rods that give a permanent erection, with difficulty in adjusting the dress to conceal the erect penis (Fig. 32.7).
2 Hinged rods avoid this difficulty [43,44].
3 The rods may be made bendable by putting in a flexible core of malleable silver wire [45] (Fig. 32.8) or a sophisticated system of plates [46] (Fig. 32.9).
4 Inflatable prostheses are the most ingenious of all (Fig. 32.10). They can be pumped up and

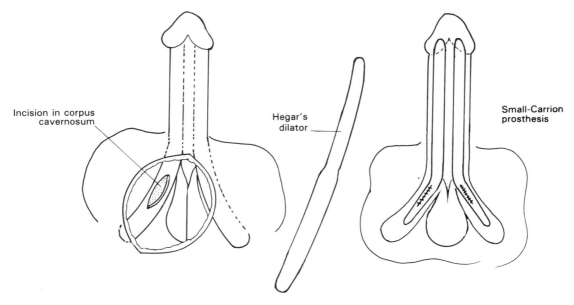

Fig. 32.7 Insertion of semi-stiff silicone Small–Carrion prosthesis into corpora cavernosa.

let down at will. Earlier models required an elaborate system of tubes, reservoir and pump which required a certain manual dexterity on the part of the patient or his partner, and were apt to go wrong from mechanical failure. The latest of these devices is a miracle of bio-engineering (Fig. 23.11). One cylinder is slipped into each corpus cavernosum after dilating the spongy tissue. The tip of the prosthesis is placed in the glans. When an erection is desired, the tip is pinched: valves shunt fluid from one compartment to another within the cylinder changing it from a flaccid to a rigid state. Pinching the tip a second time makes the penis go down [47] (Fig. 32.11).

Complications

These patients need to be followed up carefully. Prostheses are foreign bodies and therefore easily become infected. Obsessional precautions must be taken to avoid infection at the time of their insertion. The foreign bodies may erode into the urethra or glans penis. A second prosthesis can be inserted once the urethral or other fistula has healed.

Relatively few patients with these prostheses actually use them. One reason is the discrepancy between the size of the 'erection' achieved by the device compared with the size and length of a normal one.

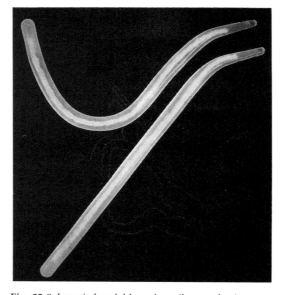

Fig. 32.8 Jonas's bendable rod penile prosthesis.

Impotence in paraplegia

Via direct stimulation of the presacral nerves, using an implanted stimulator worked by radio, erection and ejaculation can be obtained at will [48].

Vascular anastomoses

Many attempts have been made to revascularize the arteries of the penis, stimulated by the success achieved with coronary artery bypass surgery. The early results have been disappointing [49] (Fig. 32.12).

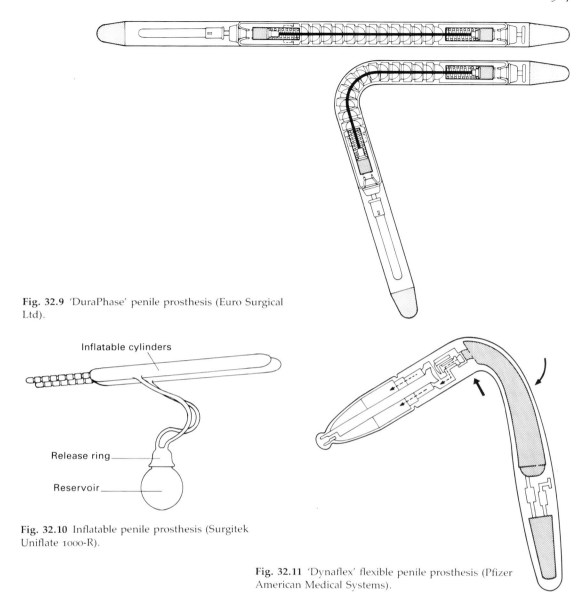

Fig. 32.9 'DuraPhase' penile prosthesis (Euro Surgical Ltd).

Fig. 32.10 Inflatable penile prosthesis (Surgitek Uniflate 1000-R).

Fig. 32.11 'Dynaflex' flexible penile prosthesis (Pfizer American Medical Systems).

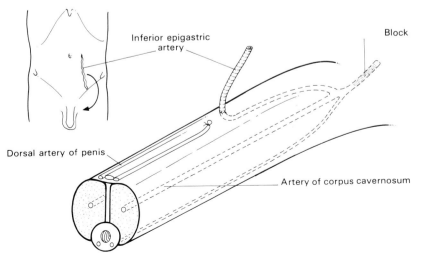

Fig. 32.12 Revascularization of the penile arteries has been attempted in many ways: here the inferior epigastric artery is anastomosed to one of the paired dorsal arteries.

Priapism

Aetiology

Priapism is an unwanted prolongation of erection, long after the appropriate stimulus has stopped: it is usually painful. When it eventually subsides, the erectile mechanism may never work again [50−52]. The aetiology is still a mystery. John Hunter [53] noted that 'in a priapism the blood does not coagulate'. Even after several hours, the blood in the sinuses of the corpora is fluid, though more viscous than normal. Only in very exceptional circumstances does thrombosis take place and may then lead to necrosis [54].

Priapism is seen in sickle-cell anaemia [55−57], leukaemia (where it may be a presenting feature [58]), and in men on haemodialysis who are anticoagulated [59−62].

It occurs with alpha blocking drugs, e.g. prazosin as used for bladder outflow obstruction and hypertension [63−65].

Trauma produces a particular type of high flow priapism [66,67] (Fig. 32.13).

Today it is most commonly seen after self-injection of papaverine or prostaglandin E for impotence.

Pathology

The introduction of the Doppler scanner has made it possible to distinguish between two forms of priapism, high and low flow. In high flow priapism, there is an increased flow of arterial blood into the penis. If the penis is aspirated, the blood shows a high oxygen content, and the fault is in the arterial inflow [66,67]. In low flow priapism, in contrast there is virtually no flow in or out of the penis. The material that is aspirated is thick, dark and venous in oxygen content.

Clinical features

Known predisposing features are the exception. The usual case is a healthy man who has been making love and comes to hospital with a painful erection which is confined to the corpora cavernosa. The glans penis and the corpus spongiosum are flaccid (Fig. 32.14).

Management

When possible a Doppler scan should be obtained to attempt to distinguish between low and high flow conditions. Aspiration and measurement of the Po_2 is an alternative way of confirming the diagnosis. Local intervention is contraindicated when there is leukaemia, sickle-cell disease or the patient is on dialysis.

Plasmaphaeresis has been used successfully in sickle-cell disease, but in most of these cases it is best to provide rest and analgesia and allow the priapism to subside spontaneously [68].

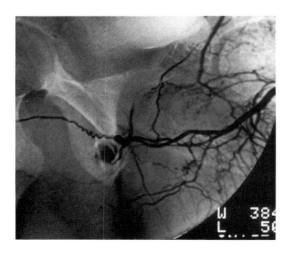

Fig. 32.13 Arteriogram in a case of high flow priapism showing aneurysm of penile artery (courtesy of Dr P. Theodorides and Dr M. Kellett).

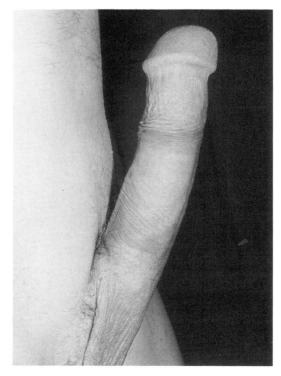

Fig. 32.14 Priapism.

In high flow priapism it may be possible to limit the abnormal inflow by embolization with complete restoration of function [66,67,69].

In the usual cases, an alpha adrenergic agent such as aramine or noradrenaline is injected to close down the arterial inflow and allow the venous outlets to open up [70]; where the cause is self-injection detumescence occurs within minutes.

If this fails a communication is made between the flaccid corpus spongiosum and glans and the erect corpora cavernosa with a knife or biopsy needle [71] (Figs 32.15 & 32.16).

If this fails an elliptical anastomosis is made between the bulb and one or other of the corpora through a small perineal incision — corporo-corporal anastomosis [72–74] (Fig. 32.17).

If this should also fail, the saphenous vein is anastomosed end to side to the corpus caver-nosum. The venous blood flows through the saphenous vein into the femoral vein, and for a time the penis can be made to rise and fall by compressing the vein (Fig. 32.18).

There is a precious window in time during which priapism must be corrected. If delayed, the priapism will eventually subside leaving irreversible changes in the spongy tissue and permanent impotence.

Priapism during operations

An unwanted erection often occurs during trans-urethral resection or urethroplasty. The erection can be immediately reversed by intracavernosal noradrenaline, adrenaline or aramine but the blood pressure must be closely monitored [70].

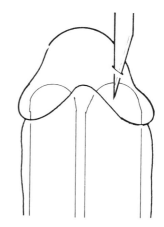

Fig. 32.15 Incision to permit blood to flow from the corpora cavernosa into the glans.

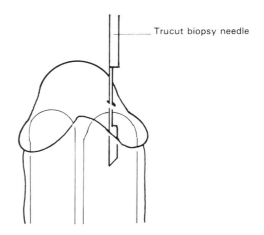

Fig. 32.16 Trucut needle used to make a fistula between the corpora.

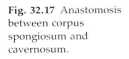

Fig. 32.17 Anastomosis between corpus spongiosum and cavernosum.

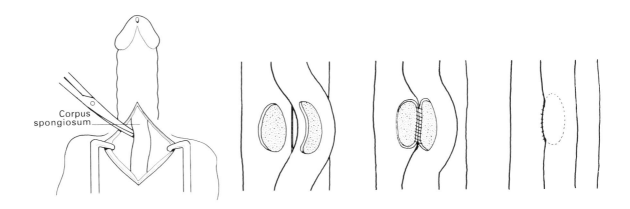

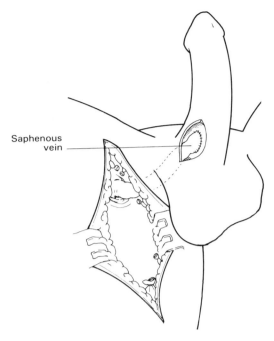

Saphenous
vein

Fig. 32.18 Anastomosis between the saphenous vein
and corpus cavernosum.

Peyronie's disease

Aetiology

Since it was first described by François de la
Peyronie, this curious condition has remained a
mystery [75]. The aetiology is debated. Shearing
forces, during strenuous intercourse, may tear
the attachment of the septa of the venous sinuses
to the inner layer of the fascia of the corpora
causing a haematoma — which heals by fibrosis.
But in practice a history of injury is uncommon.

This does not fully explain the curious relationship between Peyronie's fibrosis in the penis,
Dupuytren's contracture in the fascia of the palms
of the hands and soles of the feet, and the
nodules in the lobes of the ears, features which
are present in about half of the patients [75,76].

Autopsy studies on young soldiers found minor
degrees of fibrosis in the fascia of the corpora
and pectinate septum in 23% [77], suggesting
that this might reflect the prevalence of urethritis
but one would expect the maximum fibrosis
around the corpus spongiosum where it almost
never occurs [78].

Pathology

The fibrous tissue in Peyronie's disease is un-
remarkable. It affects any part of the fascia around

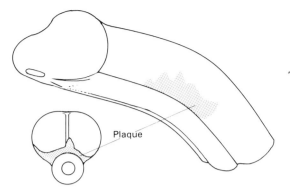

Plaque

Fig. 32.19 Peyronie's disease.

the corpora cavernosa or the septum between
them. When the fibrosis affects one side more
than the other, or the dorsal more than the ventral, the penis bends during erection (Fig. 32.19).
The fibrous tissue may calcify to form ectopic
bone.

Clinical features

At first there is pain on erection. A lump may be
noticed which becomes tender. When the penis
is erect it bends to the side of the lump (Fig.
32.20). Sometimes intercourse may be impossible.
The fibrosis may involve so much of the corpus
that the part distal to it may not fill with blood,
and may remain flaccid. Eventually there may be
erectile impotence.

Investigations

Investigations are seldom necessary or relevant:
the differential diagnosis must always include
metastases from a distant primary cancer and
when in doubt a needle biopsy should be obtained from the tissue of the plaque.

An ultrasound scan or a cavernosogram will
delineate the plaque of fibrous tissue, which is
always larger than appears on clinical palpation.

Medical management

As many methods of treatment have been suggested as there are theories of aetiology in Peyronie's
disease. They include para-aminobenzoic acid,
natulan, vitamin E, ultrasound, short-wave diathermy, radiotherapy, laser therapy, steroids by
injection and inunction, iodine, zinc and mercury.
However, whenever any of these methods are
subjected to controlled trials none are found
to have any advantage and since spontaneous

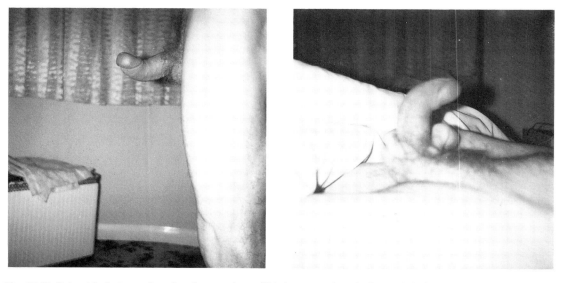

Fig. 32.20 Polaroid photographs taken by a patient of his bent erections in Peyronie's disease.

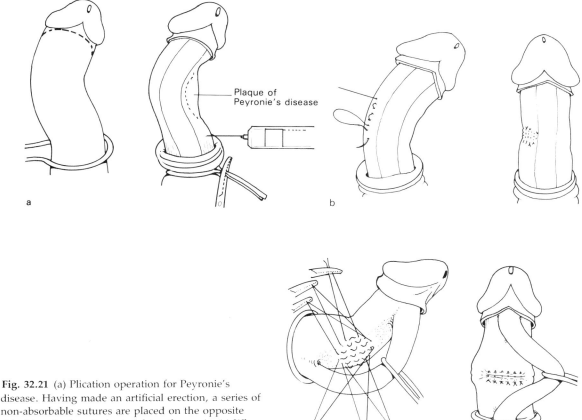

Fig. 32.21 (a) Plication operation for Peyronie's disease. Having made an artificial erection, a series of non-absorbable sutures are placed on the opposite side (b) and when tied, straighten the penis. (c) When there is a dorsal plaque, the sutures are inserted after mobilising the corpus spongiosum.

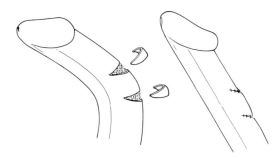

Fig. 32.22 Nesbit's operation for Peyronie's disease. A series of ellipses are removed from the side opposite the plaque.

resolution occurs in half the cases [79], every one of these 'treatments' will produce a cure in a gratifying proportion of cases. The most recent addition to the list is tamoxifen [80].

Surgery

All surgeons instinctively feel that lumps should be cut out. In Peyronie's disease, when the lump is cut out it leaves a gap, and many substances have been used to fill it — dura mater, fascia lata, dermis and innumerable synthetic substances. None of them behave like Buck's fascia, with its unique mixture of elastic and fibrous tissue, and in the end the patches bulge like aneurysms when the penis is erect.

Nesbit suggested taking a reef in the fascia on the side opposite to the bend: an ellipse of fascia can be cut out, or it can be plicated with suitable suture material (Figs 32.21 & 32.22). Whatever method is used great care must be taken not to injure the neurovascular bundle (see p. 432). The reported results are cautiously optimistic, and it is generally recommended only for patients whose married life is incapacitated by the deformity [81,82].

In patients who have impotence as well as a bent penis, a suitable prosthesis may be inserted at the time of plicating the corpus [83].

References

1 Gilling PJ, Wright WL, Gray JM (1988) Factors associated with sexual dysfunction following transurethral resection of the prostate. *New Zeal Med J* 101: 484.
2 Montague DK (1993) Editorial: treatment of erectile dysfunction. *J Urol* 150: 1833.
3 Leonard MP, Nickel CJ, Morales A (1989) Hyperprolactinemia and impotence: why, when and how to investigate. *J Urol* 142: 992.
4 Schiavi RC, Schreiner-Engel P, White D, Mandeli J (1988) Pituitary-gonadal function during sleep in men with hypoactive sexual desire and in normal controls. *Psychosomat Med* 50: 304.
5 Brindley GS, Polkey CE, Rushton DN (1982) Sacral anterior root stimulators for bladder control in paraplegia. *Paraplegia* 20: 365.
6 Brindley GS (1985) *Treatment of Impotence by Intracavernosal Injection of Phenoxibenzamine or Papaverine. Proceedings of the First World Meeting on Impotence*, p. 195. Paris: Editions du CERI.
7 Brindley GS, Sauerwein D, Hendry WF (1989) Hypogastric plexus stimulators for obtaining semen from paraplegic men. *Br J Urol* 64: 72.
8 Newman RJ, Salerno HR (1974) Sexual dysfunction due to methyldopa. *Br Med J* 2: 106.
9 Peden NR, Cargill JM, Browning MCK, Saunders JHB, Wormsley KG (1979) Male sexual dysfunction during treatment with cimetidine. *Br Med J* 280: 659.
10 McCulloch DK, Campbell IW, Wu FC, Clarke B, Prescott RJ (1980) Impotence in diabetic and non-diabetic hospital outpatients. *Br Med J* 281: 1216.
11 Fairburn C (1981) The sexual problems of diabetic men. *Br J Hosp Med* 25: 484.
12 Morales A, Condra M, Owen J, Surridge D, Fenmore D, Harris C (1987) The effectiveness of yohimbine in the treatment of organic impotence. *J Urol* 137: 1168.
13 Schwartz AN, Wang KY, Mack LA *et al.* (1992) Overdose of yohimbine. *Br Med J* 304: 548.
14 Cumming J, Pryor JP (1990) Treatment of organic impotence. *Br J Urol* 67: 640.
15 Claes H, Baert L (1993) Pelvic floor exercises versus surgery in the treatment of impotence. *Br J Urol* 71: 52.
16 Marshall P, Morales A, Surridge D (1982) Diagnostic significance of penile erections during sleep. *Urology* 20: 1.
17 Ek A, Bradley WE, Krane RL (1983) Snap-gauge band: new concept in measuring penile rigidity. *Urology* 21: 63.
18 Dickinson IK, Pryor JP (1989) Pharmacocavernometry: a modified papaverine test. *Br J Urol* 63: 539.
19 Aboseif SR, Breza J, Lue TF, Tanagho EA (1989) Penile venous drainage in erectile dysfunction: anatomical, radiological and functional considerations. *Br J Urol* 64: 183.
20 Parys BT, Evans CM, Parsons KF (1988) Bulbocavernosus reflex latency in the investigation of diabetic impotence. *Br J Urol* 61: 59.
21 Desai M, Dembny K, Morgan H, Gingell JC, Prothero D (1988) Neurophysiological investigation of diabetic impotence. Are sacral response studies of value? *Br J Urol* 61: 68.
22 Fowler CJ, Ali Z, Kirby RS, Pryor JP (1988) The value of testing for unmyelinated fibre, sensory neuropathy in diabetic impotence. *Br J Urol* 61: 63.
23 Kirby RS (1994) Impotence: diagnosis and management of male erectile dysfunction. *Br Med J* 308: 957.
24 Brindley GS (1986) Pilot experiments on the actions of drugs injected into the human corpus cavernosum penis. *Br J Pharmacol* 87: 495.
25 Sidi AA, Cameron JS, Duffy LM, Lange PH (1986) Intracavernous drug-induced erections in the

management of male erectile dsyfunction: experience with 100 patients. *J Urol* 135: 704.

26 Desai KM, Gingell JC (1987) Impotence: treatment by autoinjection of vasoactive drugs. *Br Med J* 295: 922.

27 Williams G (1987) Impotence: treatment by autoinjection of vasoactive drugs. *Br Med J* 295: 1279.

28 Robinette MA, Moffat MJ (1986) Intracorporal injection of papaverine and phentolamine in the management of impotence. *Br J Urol* 58: 692.

29 Nelson RP (1983) Non-operative management of impotence (review). *J Urol* 139: 2.

30 Robinson Q, Stephenson TP (1989) Self injection treatment for impotence. *Br Med J* 299: 1568.

31 Gregoire A (1990) Self injection treatment for impotence. *Br Med J* 300: 537.

32 Hashmat AI, Abrahams J, Fani K, Nostrand I (1991) A lethal complication of papaverine-induced priapism. *J Urol* 145: 146.

33 Zentgraf M, Ludwig G, Ziegler M (1989) How safe is the treatment of impotence with intracavernous autoinjection? *Eur Urol* 16: 165.

34 Buckley JF, Chapple CR, McNicholas T (1989) Continuous infusion of phenylepinephrine in the treatment of papaverine-induced priapism. *Br J Urol* 64: 654.

35 Zorgniotti AW (1986) Corpus cavernosum blockade for impotence: practical aspects and results in 250 cases. *J Urol* 135: 306A.

36 Levine SB, Althoff SE, Turner LA *et al.* (1989) Side effects of self-administration of intracavernous papaverine and phentolamine for the treatment of impotence. *J Urol* 141: 54.

37 Abozeid M, Juenemann KP, Lueo JA, Lue TF, Yen TSB, Tanagho EA (1987) Chronic papaverine treatment: the effect of repeated injections on the simian erectile response and penile tissue. *J Urol* 138: 1263.

38 Lee LM, Stevenson RWD, Szasz G (1989) Prostaglandin E1 versus phentolamine/papaverine for the treatment of erectile impotence: a double-blind comparison. *J Urol* 141: 549.

39 Earle CM, Keogh EJ, Wisniewski ZS *et al.* (1990) Prostaglandin E1 therapy for impotence: comparison with papaverine. *J Urol* 143: 57.

40 Wolfson B, Pickett S, Scott NE, deKernion JB, Rajfer J (1993) Intraurethral prostaglandin E-2 cream: a possible alternative treatment for erectile dysfunction. *Urology* 42: 73.

41 Heaton JPW, Morales A, Owen J, Saunders FW, Fenemore J (1990) Topical glyceryltrinitrate causes measurable penile arterial dilation in impotent men. *J Urol* 143: 729.

42 Broderick GA, Allen G, McClure RD (1991) Vacuum tumescence devices: the role of papaverine in the selection of patients. *J Urol* 145: 284.

43 Finney RP (1977) New hinged silicone penile implant. *J Urol* 118: 585.

44 Finney RP, Sharpe JR, Sadlowski RW (1980) Finney hinged penile implant: experience with 100 cases. *J Urol* 124: 205.

45 Rowe PH, Royle MG (1983) Use of Jonas silicon—silver prosthesis in erectile impotence. *J Roy Soc Med* 76: 1019.

46 Hrebinko R, Bahnson RR, Schwentker FN, O'Donnell WF (1990) Early experience with the Duraphase

penile prosthesis. *J Urol* 143: 60.

47 Mulcahy JJ (1988) The hydroflex self-contained inflatable prosthesis: experience with 100 patients. *J Urol* 140: 1422.

48 Kellett JM (1990) Sexual expression in paraplegia. *Br Med J* 301: 1007.

49 Metz P, Frimodt-Moller C (1983) Epigastrico-cavernous anastomosis in the treatment of arteriogenic impotence. *Scand J Urol Nephrol* 17: 271.

50 Brock G, Breza J, Lue TF, Tanagho E (1993) High flow priapism: a spectrum of disease. *J Urol* 150: 968.

51 Lue TF, Hellstrom WJG, McAninch JW, Tanagho EA (1986) Priapism: a refined approach to diagnosis and treatment. *J Urol* 136: 104.

52 Pohl J, Pott B, Kleinhans G (1986) Priapism: a three phase concept of management according to aetiology and prognosis. *Br J Urol* 58: 113.

53 Hunter J (1812) On priapism, in: *A Treatise on the Blood, Inflammation and Gun-Shot Wounds*, vol. 1, p. 39. London: Cox.

54 Barkley C, Badalament RA, Metz EN, Nesbitt J, Drago JR (1989) Coumarin necrosis of the penis. *J Urol* 141: 946.

55 Rothfeld SH, Mazor D (1971) Priapism in children: a complication of sickle-cell disease. *J Urol* 105: 307.

56 Gillenwater JY, Burros HM, Kornblith PL (1968) Priapism as the first and terminal manifestation of sickle cell disease. *South Med J* 61: 133.

57 Hamre MR, Harmon EP, Kirkpatrick DV, Stern MJ, Humbert JR (1991) Priapism as a complication of sickle cell disease. *J Urol* 145: 1.

58 Stutz FH, Bergin JJ (1970) Priapism in leukemia: a report of two cases. *Milit Med* 135: 44.

59 Eadie DGA, Brock TP (1970) Corpus-saphenous by-pass in the treatment of priapism. *Br J Surg* 57: 172.

60 Port FK, Hecking E, Fiegel P, Kohler H, Distler A (1974) Priapism during regular haemodialysis. *Lancet* ii: 1287.

61 Editorial (1965) Priapism. *Br Med J* 1: 401.

62 Sale D, Cameron JS (1974) Priapism during regular dialysis. *Lancet* ii: 1567.

63 Dawson-Butterworth K (1970) Priapism and phenothiazines. *Br Med J* 2: 118.

64 Bhalla AK, Hoffbrand BI, Phatak PS, Reuben SR (1979) Prazosin and priapism. *Br Med J* 2: 1039.

65 Nakamura N, Takaesu N, Arakaki Y (1991) Priapism in haemodialysis due to Prazosin? *Br J Urol* 68: 551.

66 Gudinchet F, Fournier D, Jichlinski P, Meyrate B (1992) Traumatic priapism in a child: evaluation with colour flow Doppler sonography. *J Urol* 148: 380.

67 Kuwahara M, Fujisaki N, Hakamura K, Ohta K, Hishitani M, Takagi N (1995) High flow priapism after perineal trauma successfully treated by unilateral embolization of the internal pudendal artery. *Jap J Urol* 86: 333.

68 Walker EM, Mitchum EN, Rous SN, Glassman AB, Cannon A, McInnes BK (1983) Automated erythrocytopheresis for relief of priapism in sickle cell hemoglobinopathies. *J Urol* 130: 912.

69 Visvanathan K, Burrows PE, Schillinger JF, Khoury A (1992) Posttraumatic arterial priapism in a 7 year old boy: successful management by percutaneous transcatheter embolization. *J Urol* 148: 382.

70 McNicholas TA, Thomson K, Rogers HS, Blandy JP (1989) Pharmacological management of erections during surgery. *Br J Urol* 64: 435.

71 Winter CC (1978) Priapism cured by creation of fistulas between glans penis and corpora cavernosa. *J Urol* 119: 227.

72 Forsberg L, Mattiason A, Olsson AM (1981) Priapism — conservative treatment versus surgical procedures. *Br J Urol* 53: 374.

73 Blandy JP (1986) *Operative Urology*, 2nd edn, p. 195. Oxford: Blackwell Scientific Publications.

74 Howe GE (1969) Priapism: a surgical emergency. *J Urol* 101: 576.

75 de la Peyronie F (1743) *Memoires de l'Academie Royale de Chirurgie*. 1: p. 318.

76 Gallizia F, Marazzini Z (1959) Triade collageniosica: induratio penis plastica, fibrosi palmare e fibrose della cartilagine auricolare. *Boll Soc Piemont Chir* 28: 679.

77 Ubelhor R (1966) Induratio penis plastica: an international inquiry on the therapy of induratio penis plastica. *Urologia* 33: 113.

78 Smith BH (1969) Subclinical Peyronie's disease. *Amer J Clin Pathol* 52: 385.

79 Williams JL, Thomas GG (1970) The natural history of Peyronie's disease. *J Urol* 103: 75.

80 Ralph DJ, Brooks MD, Bottazzo GF, Pryor JP (1992) The treatment of Peyronie's disease with tamoxifen. *Br J Urol* 70: 648.

81 Bailey MJ, Yande S, Walmsley B, Pryor JP (1985) Surgery for Peyronie's disease: a review of 200 patients. *Br J Urol* 57: 746.

82 Lemberger RJ, Bishop MC, Bates CP (1984) Nesbit's operation for Peyronie's disease. *Br J Urol* 56: 721.

83 Carson CC, Hodge GB, Anderson EE (1983) Penile prosthesis in Peyronie's disease. *Br J Urol* 55: 417.

PART 6
TESTICLE

Chapter 33: Testicle — structure and function

Anatomy

Comparative anatomy

In many mammals the testicles enlarge and shrink with the seasonal rise and fall in testosterone. In man, there is a sudden increase in the size of the testicles with puberty and a slower decline in old age.

There is a wide variation in the location of the testicles in different mammals. In elephants the abdominal testicles are just caudal to the kidneys; in whales they are near the bladder; in hedgehogs at the internal ring; in pigs they are in the superficial inguinal pouch. In sheep and man they hang at the bottom of a pendulous scrotum (Fig. 33.1).

In many mammals the testis is intra-abdominal for most of the year, descending into the scrotum only in the mating season. In some primates the testicles move freely in and out of the scrotum but in most of them the testicles lie permanently in the scrotum [1,2].

The epididymis is only found in mammals. Its purpose is not clear. It was once thought to be responsible for giving sperms the capacity to fertilize the ovum just at the time of ovulation, but no difference can be found by immuno-chemical studies between sperms in the vasa efferentia and those in the ejaculate [3,4].

Embryology

The testis develops from the urogenital ridge behind the coelom. This ridge is soon divided longitudinally, the medial part forming the gonad, the lateral part the urinary tract (Fig. 33.2).

In both sexes the germ cells arise in the yolk sac and make an extraordinary journey by amoeboid movement from the yolk sac along the umbilical cord and across the coelom until they reach the gonadal ridge into which they burrow [1].

The Y chromosome contains the gene coding for the HY enzyme. In the fifth week, this causes

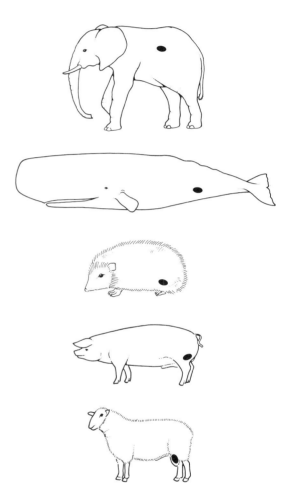

Fig. 33.1 The testicle in varying stages of descent in different mammals: in elephants they are near the kidney; in whales, near the bladder; in hedgehogs at the internal ring; in pigs in the superficial inguinal pouch; in sheep and man at the bottom of a pendulous scrotum (after [1]).

the germ cells to differentiate into gonadocytes or Sertoli cells (Fig. 33.3). The Sertoli cells secrete the Müllerian duct inhibitory factor which causes the Müllerian structures — uterus and fallopian tubes — to vanish [5]. About a week later, the same HY enzyme causes the germ cells to differentiate into Leydig cells whose 17-ketosteroid

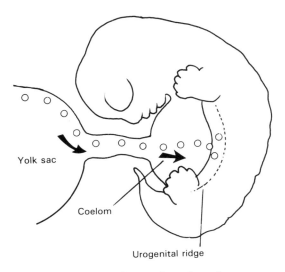

Fig. 33.2 The germ cells pass from the yolk sac across the coelom to the gonadal ridge.

reductase forms testosterone. Among the target tissues for testosterone are the phallic tubercles which contain 5-alpha reductase to convert testosterone to dihydrotestosterone, and the cytosol receptor protein needed to react with dihydrotestosterone to set off the train of events leading to growth and fusion of the phallus, inrolling of the urethral tube, formation of the scrotal sac and downward migration of the testicles. The developing testis makes use of the main mesonephric Wolffian duct for the vas deferens, seminal vesicles and epididymis.

In males the Müllerian duct lingers as two tiny vestiges — the utriculus masculinus in the verumontanum and the appendix testis next door to the appendix epididymis which is a vestige of the Wolffian duct. If there is a congenital deficiency of Müllerian duct inhibitory factor, phenotypical males are born with fallopian tubes and a uterus, found by chance at orchidopexy or hernia repair, and occasionally associated with testicular tumours [5].

Maturation of the testis

The Leydig cells are very numerous just before birth but disappear soon afterwards and are replaced by fibroblasts. With puberty, the Leydig cells reappear, the Sertoli cells become mature and the long-dormant germ cells begin to divide [6].

The normal migration of the testicle

Being part of the gonadal ridge the testicle is retroperitoneal. Under the influence of Leydig cell testosterone the testis moves towards the scrotum. A lump of jelly precedes the testicle like a slug, oozing through the tissues and expanding a track for the testicle to follow: this is the gubernaculum (Fig. 33.4). It contains no muscle, and there is no attachment at the bottom of the scrotum [7]. If the gubernaculum oozes in the wrong direction, e.g. towards the root of the penis or into the thigh, the testicle will follow it into an ectopic position. If it fails to reach the bottom of the scrotum, there will be incomplete descent [8–10] (Fig. 33.5).

As the testicle descends towards the scrotum the peritoneum goes with it, hence the processus vaginalis is always anterior to the testicle. The lumen of the processus is normally obliterated within a few weeks of birth, but it may persist in various forms: a congenital hernia, a hydrocele,

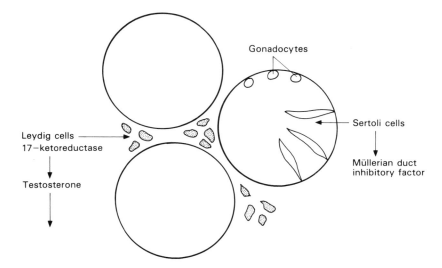

Fig. 33.3 Sertoli cells secrete Müllerian duct inhibitory factor. About a week later Leydig cells secrete testosterone, which is activated to dihydrotestosterone, and causes descent of the testicles and formation of the penis and urethra.

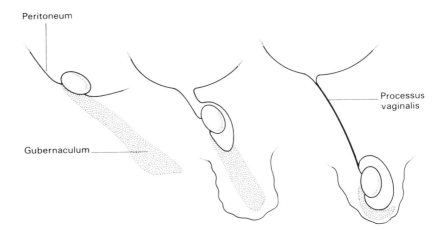

Fig. 33.4 Normal migration of the testicle.

an encysted hydrocele of the cord, an abdomino-scrotal hydrocele and every conceivable variation on these themes [11] (Fig. 33.6).

There is a variation in size of the peritoneal sac that ends up around the testis. When very large, as is often the case is undescended testes, the testicle may be on a stalk which can get twisted — torsion (see p. 569).

Topographical anatomy

The term testicle includes testis and epididymis. The normal adult testicle hangs in the scrotum,

the left usually hanging lower than the right. The left testicle is often larger than the right. The epididymis lies behind the testis.

Testis

The testis is made up of banks of convoluted tubules which empty into the rete testis at the hilum, whence about 12 vasa efferentia cross into the beginning of the long duct which is the epididymis [1] (Fig. 33.7).

Each testicular tubule has a basement membrane, lined by spermatogonia and Sertoli cells.

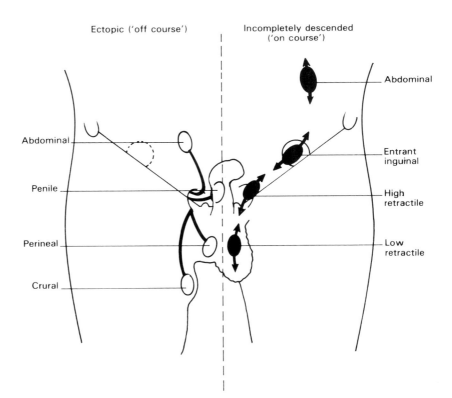

Fig. 33.5 The maldescended testis may be off its normal course of descent (ectopic) or on the normal course (incomplete) descent.

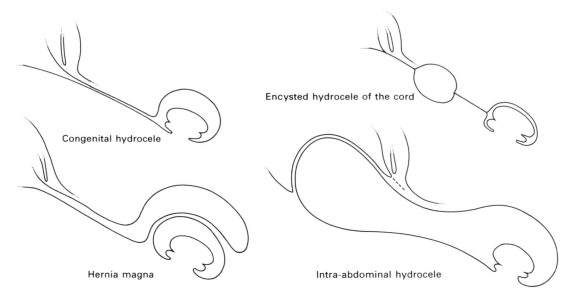

Fig. 33.6 Varieties of hydrocele and hernia.

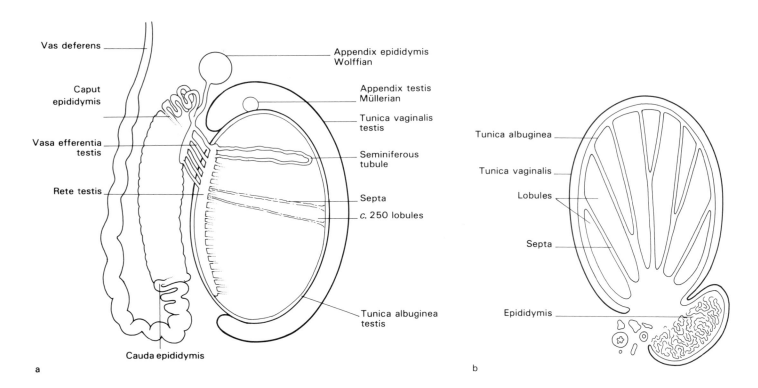

a

b

Fig. 33.7 Diagram of the anatomy of the testicle (a) lateral (b) cross section.

Outside the tubules are connective tissue spaces with blood and lymphatic vessels and interstitial or Leydig cells (Fig. 33.8).

In the fetal testis the tubules contain germ cells and immature Sertoli cells: between the tubules the Leydig cells become particularly abundant just before birth, but disappear afterwards to be replaced by fibroblasts. With puberty pituitary luteinizing hormone stimulates the Leydig cells to reappear, the Sertoli cells to become mature [6], and the dormant germinal cells to spring into activity. The spermatogonia divide by mitosis, some progeny will become spermatocytes, others continue as stem cells. Each spermatocyte divides by meiosis to produce haploid secondary spermatocytes, which eventually become spermatozoa. These changes pass along the testicular tubules in waves so that a biopsy of the adult testis will show several different phases in the sequence of division and maturation from spermatogonia to mature sperms (Fig. 33.9). A testicular biopsy must therefore include several tubules to give a useful picture of spermatogenesis [12].

Coverings of the testicle

The tough outer fibrous tissue around the testicle is the tunica albuginea. The covering of peritoneum provided by the processus vaginalis is called the tunica vaginalis. In the space between them is a small quantity of fluid — enough to permit the testicle to slip freely within its sac.

Blood supply

Arteries

The testis receives its main blood supply from the testicular artery, which leaves the aorta just below the renal artery. An insignificant blood supply comes from the long artery of the vas which anastomoses with a branch from the testicular artery to the epididymis (Fig. 33.10).

Veins

The testicle has a profuse venous drainage arranged in three layers between the external spermatic fascia, the cremaster muscle and the internal spermatic fascia. There are plentiful anastomoses between the veins of the spermatic cord, scrotum and thigh (Fig. 33.11).

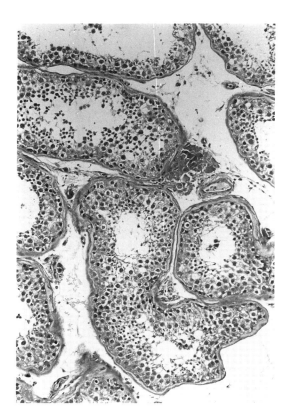

Fig. 33.8 Normal histology of testis (courtesy of Dr Suhail Baithun).

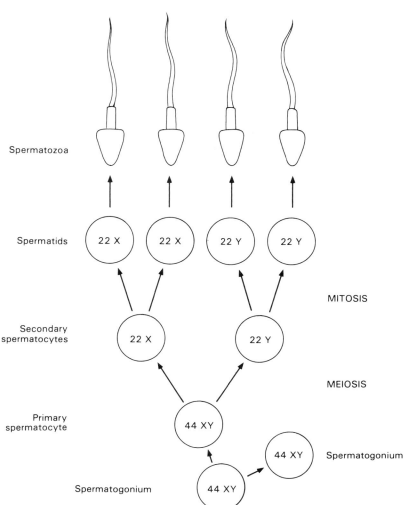

Fig. 33.9 (*right*) Spermatogenesis.

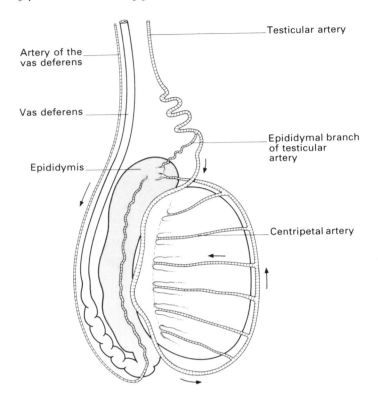

Fig. 33.10 Blood supply to the testis.

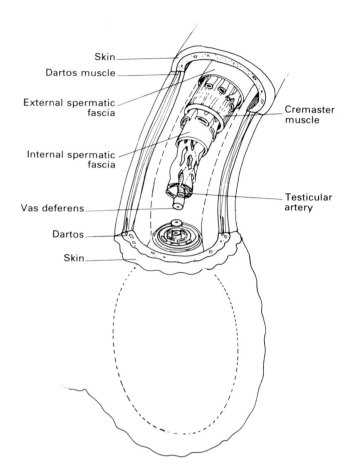

Fig. 33.11 The veins of the testicle and the coverings of the cord.

Lymphatics

The lymphatics of the testis arise in the spaces between the tubules, and flow through the testicular hilum into the cord. They retrace the testicular artery to the para-aortic lymph nodes around the origin of the testicular and renal arteries.

Nerves of the testicle

'The testis, being a visceral organ, receives only visceral afferent and efferent fibres and lacks somatic nerves' [1]. The superior spermatic nerve arises from the spermatic ganglion, which receives fibres from the coeliac and intermesenteric plexuses, as well as the lumbar and thoracic splanchnic nerves and the vagus.

From the spermatic ganglion the nerves run with the internal spermatic artery as a discrete nerve which accompanies the artery to the testis. The tunica albuginea has an abundant sensory nerve supply which is quite distinct from the innervation of the scrotum. The role of the autonomic motor nerves to the testicle is unknown [1].

Epididymis

The tube of the epididymis is said to be 3–4 m long when unravelled [3,13,14]. It is arranged in three parts — head, body and tail. In most mammalian species as well as man it has the shape of a dumb-bell with a distinct waist (Fig. 33.12). Between the epididymis and testis is a sulcus which forms a pocket facing laterally — a useful guide for the surgeon when replacing the testicle after a scrotal operation. The epididymis is lined by columnar ciliated epithelium, with an ultramicroscopic structure typical of secretory epithelia (Fig. 33.13). The cilia of the epididymis closely resemble the cilia of the bronchioles, with which they share the structure of a dynein arm as well as a susceptibility to poisoning with mercury salts [14–17]. The lumen of the epididymis becomes progressively wider as it goes from head to tail, where muscle begins to surround the tubule which continues on as the vas deferens [18].

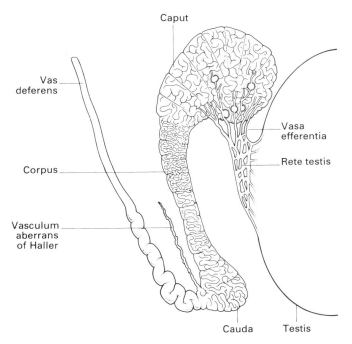

Fig. 33.12 Anatomy of the epididymis (after [17]).

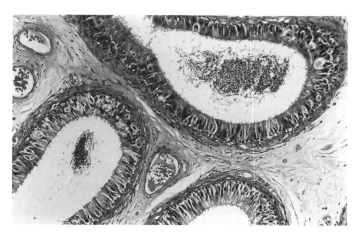

Fig. 33.13 Cross-section through epididymis showing the cilia of the epithelium (courtesy of Dr Suhail Baithun).

and in the adult each may hold up to 2−10 ml of fluid [21] in a convoluted hollow sac with a strong muscular coat (Fig. 33.16) and a columnar epithelium with folds like a honeycomb (an appearance noted by Hippocrates) (Fig. 33.17). Its secretion was tasted and found to be sweet by John Hunter: today we know it is rich in fructose. The common ejaculatory ducts emerge in the prostatic urethra either side of the verumontanum.

Blood supply

The blood supply of the epididymis comes from a branch of the testicular artery which enters the caput epididymis, runs down the epididymis and anastomoses with the terminal branch of the artery of the vas (a branch of the inferior vesical artery) which runs alongside the vas inside its connective tissue sheath.

Vas deferens

The vas deferens is a firm cord with a tiny lumen and a thick wall of smooth muscle. The vas is convoluted at each end (Fig. 33.14). It is lined with a tall columnar epithelium with 'stereocilia' which are not motile and resemble structures in the ependyma of the canal of the spinal cord, and the tympanic cavity [19] (Fig. 33.15).

The vas deferens runs lateral to the inferior epigastric artery, follows the inside of the pelvis, over the ureter to follow the cleft between inner and outer zones of the prostate. Just before it enters the prostate the vas gives off a diverticulum — the seminal vesicle.

Seminal vesicle

The embryology of the seminal vesicle has been meticulously studied [20]. Starting as a modest pouch of the vas deferens it enlarges in puberty

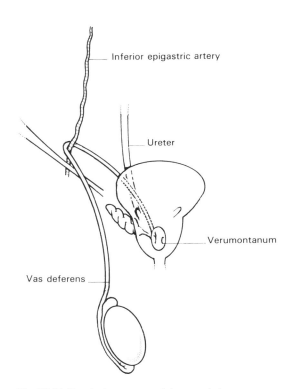

Fig. 33.14 Surgical anatomy of the vas deferens.

Verumontanum

In amphibians such as the toad and frog the verumontanum is the organ of intromission [22]. In man it still contains spongy tissue resembling that of the corpora of the penis. Its summit contains the utriculus masculinus — vestige of the lower ends of the Müllerian ducts: on either side are the ejaculatory ducts (Fig. 33.18).

Spermatic cord

The spermatic cord has four layers, each representing one component of the abdominal wall (see Fig. 33.11). The core of the spermatic cord is the vas deferens, the testicular artery and one or more veins. This core is surrounded by the peritoneum in infants, but in adults the peritoneal layer has shrivelled to a thin strip — the processus vaginalis.

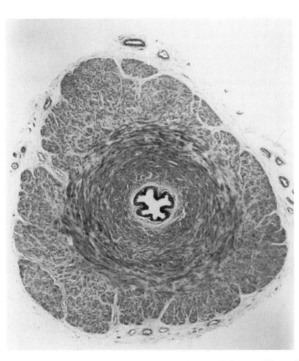

Fig. 33.15 Histological section through vas deferens. The tall columnar epithelium is fringed with non-motile 'stereocilia' of unknown function (courtesy of Dr Suhail Baithun).

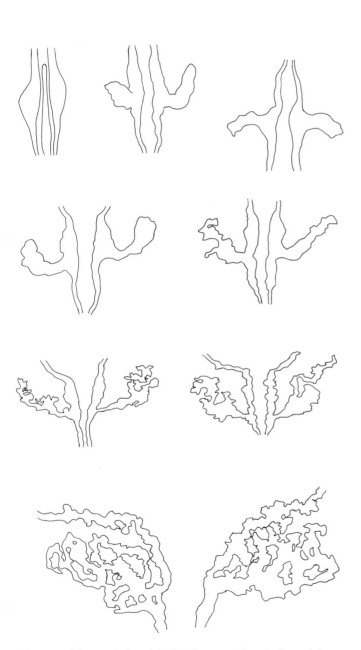

Fig. 33.16 The seminal vesicle develops as a diverticulum of the ejaculatory duct (after [20]).

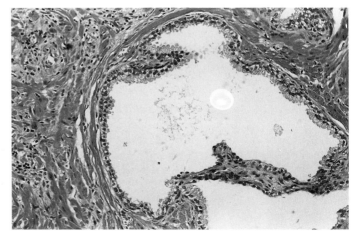

Fig. 33.17 Histological section through the seminal vesicle (courtesy of Dr Suhail Baithun).

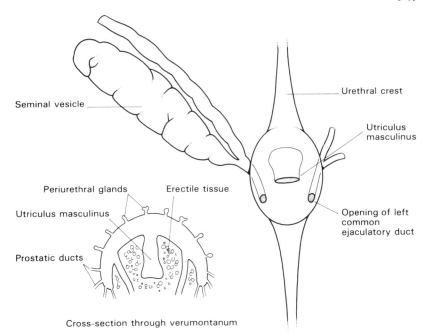

Fig. 33.18 Structure of the verumontanum. Note the presence of erectile tissue.

Cross-section through verumontanum

Outside the layer of peritoneum is a thin layer derived from the transversalis fascia — the internal spermatic fascia. This is surrounded by muscle fibres continuous with the internal oblique muscle of the abdominal wall — the cremaster muscle — which covers the entire testicle. Outside the cremaster, the external spermatic fascia is a continuation of the external oblique aponeurosis.

Serial measurements of the size of the seminal vesicles by transrectal ultrasound show that they progressively enlarge from the age of 20, reaching a peak in the decade 40–50 and thereafter gradually shrink [23].

Physiology

Formation of spermatozoa

Each spermatogonium divides by mitosis to form another spermatogonium and a primary spermatocyte. Each primary spermatocyte divides again by meiosis to form a pair of secondary (haploid) spermatocytes. These give rise to spermatids, which are then moulded by the Sertoli cells into the mature spermatozoa. These are then shed into the lumen of the tubule [24].

The progression from germinal cell to spermatozoon does not take place evenly but in cohorts in each tubule — each generation joined together by loose intercellular bridges — and as a result, a given testicular biopsy gives several single snapshots in time of one part of the complete cycle of spermatogenesis in adjacent tubules [25] (Fig. 33.19).

There may be a complete absence of spermatogonia and spermatocytes, and only Sertoli cells are found within the testicular tubule. Sometimes there appears to be a hold up in the normal cycle of maturation — spermatogenic arrest [24].

Leydig cells

The Leydig cells (Fig. 33.20), in the interstitial spaces between the tubules, secrete testosterone which has to be converted by 5-alpha reductase to dihydrotestosterone, before it can react with a cytosol receptor in a target cell.

Sertoli cells

Sertoli cells [26] have four known functions (Fig. 33.21):
1 In the fetus they release the Müllerian duct inhibitory factor in the seventh week of fetal life.
2 Later they form the barrier between blood and testis [27].
3 They secrete inhibin, which stops the pituitary from secreting luteinizing hormone [28].
4 They act in the final stages of spermatogenesis, converting spermatids to spermatozoa.

Epididymis

Relatively little is known of the physiology of the epididymis [29]. Although it requires testosterone

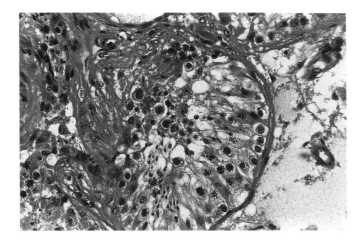

Fig. 33.19 Histology from a testicular biopsy showing tubules in different stages of maturation (courtesy of Dr Suhail Baithun).

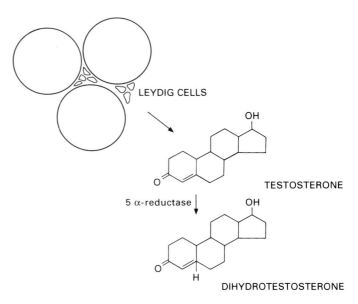

Fig. 33.20 Diagram of function of Leydig cells.

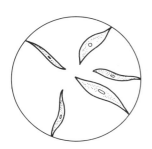

● Müllerian duct inhibitory factor

● Blood–testis barrier

● Inhibin→regulates pituitary secretion of luteinizing hormone

● Convert spermatids to spermatozoa

Fig. 33.21 Diagram of function of Sertoli cells.

and can convert it to dihydrotestosterone no cytosol receptor has so far been found. Possibly some antigenic material is added to sperms in the waist of the epididymis [30] although this is disputed [31,32]. Its main function is thought to be to make the sperm capable of fertilizing the ovum [33] — capacitation. Sperms from the head of the epididymis may produce half as many pregnancies as those in the tail [33]. Capacitation occurs at different levels in the epididymis in different mammals. In man the critical region is about 1 cm from the cauda. Pregnancies have, however, been obtained on rare occasions by sperms taken from the head.

The cilia of the epididymis closely resemble the cilia of the bronchioles with which they share common antigens and a susceptibility to mercury poisoning [34–38].

In some mammals the epididymis is an important store for sperm, but in man storage occurs in the convoluted parts of the vasa deferentia. The sperm is carried passively along the epididymis in the current of seminal plasma, but during this journey its flagellum becomes stiffer, making it a more efficient propeller [39].

Vas deferens

Cineradiological studies show that the vas deferens is capable of active peristaltic contraction during ejaculation.

Seminal vesicle

The function of the seminal vesicles remains an enigma. From the days of the earliest microscopes it was known that they contained sperms: indeed motile sperms can be recovered as long as 82 h after death [40]. Its fluid makes up about 80% of the volume of the semen and contains three to four times as much fructose as there is glucose in the blood [41]. On ejaculation cineradiography shows that the sperms stored in the convoluted ampulla of the vas are ejected first, so that the first fraction of semen is the richest in sperm. Meanwhile, the seminal vesicles have made between seven and 10 muscular contractions before suddenly expelling their contents out through the ejaculatory duct, squirting before them the ampullary sperm-rich fraction [42] (see p. 522).

Verumontanum

It is not known what if any part the erectile tissue of the verumontanum plays in human ejaculation.

Spermatic cord

The complex system of veins of the spermatic cord have been seen as a heat-exchange mechanism, designed to cool the testicle. This concept is widely understood to justify operating on varicoceles for infertility (see p. 571).

References

1 Setchell BP (1978) *The Mammalian Testis*. London: Elek.

2 Hill WCO (1953–1966) *Primates. Comparative Anatomy and Taxonomy*, 6 vols. Edinburgh: Edinburgh University Press.

3 Moore HDM (1990) The epididymis, in: Chisholm GD, Fair WR (eds) *Scientific Foundations of Urology*, 3rd edn, pp. 399–410. Oxford: Heinemann.

4 Partizio P, Bronson R, Silber SJ, Ord T, Asch RH (1992) Testicular origin of immunobead-reacting antigens in human sperm. *Fertil Steril* 57: 183.

5 Eastham JA, McEvoy K, Sullivan R, Chandrasoma P (1992) A case of simultaneous bilateral nonseminomatous testicular tumors in persistent Müllerian duct syndrome. *J Urol* 148: 407.

6 Neville AM, Grigor KM (1976) Structure function and development of the human testis, in: Pugh RCB (ed.) *Pathology of the Testis*. Oxford: Blackwell Scientific Publications.

7 Heyns CF, Hutson JM (1995) Historical review of theories of testicular descent. *J Urol* 153: 754.

8 Wensing CJG (1986) Testicular descent in the rat: a comparison of this process in the rat with that of the pig. *Anat Rec* 214: 154.

9 McLoughlin PVA (1980) Pubic ectopic testicle. *Br J Urol* 52: 1640.

10 Whitaker RH (1992) Undescended testis — the need for a standard classification (review). *Br J Urol* 70: 1.

11 Klin B, Efrati Y, Mor A, Vinograd I (1992) Unilateral hydroureteronephrosis caused by abdominoscrotal hydrocele. *J Urol* 148: 384.

12 Johnsen SG (1970) Testicular biopsy score count — a method for registration of spermatogenesis in human testis: normal values and results in 335 hypogonadal males. *Hormones* 1: 1.

13 Baumgartnen HG, Holstein AF, Rosengren E (1971) Arrangement, ultrastructure and adrenergic innervation of smooth musculature of the ductuli efferentes, ductus epididymis and ductus deferens in man. *Z Zellforsch Mikrosk Anat* 120: 39.

14 Turner TT, Howards SS (1978) Factors involved in the initiation of sperm motility. *Biol Reprod* 18: 571.

15 Editorial (1979) Abnormal cilia. *Br Med J* ii: 1663.

16 Pedersen H, Mygind N (1976) Absence of axonemal arms in nasal mucosa cilia in Kartagener's syndrome. *Nature* 262: 494.

17 Hendry WF, Levison DA, Parkinson MC, Parslow JM, Royle MG (1990) Testicular obstruction: clinicopathological studies. *Ann Roy Coll Surg Engl* 72: 396.

18 Moore HDM, Pryor JP (1981) The comparative ultrastructure of the epididymis in monkeys and man: a search for suitable animal model for studying primate epididymal physiology. *Amer J Primatol* 2: 231.

19 Last RJ (1978) *Anatomy, Regional and Applied*, 6th edn. Edinburgh: Churchill Livingstone.

20 Nillson S (1962) The human seminal vesicle. *Acta Chir Scand Suppl* 296.

21 Boreau J (1953) *L'etude Radiologique des Voies Séminales normales et Pathologiques*. Paris: Masson.

22 Mansell-Moullin CW (1892) *The Operative Treatment of Enlargement of the Prostate*. London: Bale.

23 Terasaki T, Watanabe H, Kamoi K, Naya Y (1993) Seminal vesicle parameters at 10 year intervals measured by transrectal ultrasonography. *J Urol* 150: 914.

24 Skakkebaek NE, Berthelsen JG (1990) Spermatogenesis, in: Chisholm GD, Fair WR (eds) *Scientific Foundations of Urology*, 3rd edn, pp. 399–410. Oxford: Heinemann.

25 Hendry WF, Somerville IF, Hall RR, Pugh RCB (1973) Investigation and treatment of the subfertile male. *Br J Urol* 45: 684.

26 Sertoli E (1865) Dell'esistenza di particolari cellule ramificati nei canalicoli seminiferi del testiculo humano. *Morgagni* 7: 31.

27 Fawcell DW, Leak LV, Hediger PM (1970) Electron microscopic observations on the structural components of the blood—testis barrier. *J Reprod Fertil* 10 (suppl): 105.

28 Hodgson Y, Robertson DM, De Kretser DM (1989) The regulation of testicular function. *Int Rev Physiol* 27: 275.

29 Moore HDM (1990) The epididymis, in: Chisholm GD, Fair WR (eds) *Scientific Foundations of Urology*, 3rd edn, pp. 399–410. Oxford: Heinemann.

30 Turner TT, Howards SS (1978) Factors involved in the initiation of sperm motility. *Biol Reprod* 18: 571.

31 Partizio P, Bronson R, Silber SJ, Ord T, Asch RH (1992) Testicular origin of immunobead-reacting antigens in human sperm. *Fertil Steril* 57: 183.

32 Smith CA, Hartman TD, Moore HDM (1968) A determinant of Mr 34000 expressed by hamster epididymal epithelium binds specifically to spermatozoa in co-culture. *J Reprod Fertil* 18: 337.

33 Moore HDM, Hatman TD, Holt WV (1984) The structure and epididymal maturation of the spermatozoon of the common marmoset (*Callithrix bacchus*). *J Anat* 138: 227.

34 Pedersen H, Rebbe H (1975) Absence of arms in the axoneme of immobile human spermatozoa. *Biol*

Reprod 12: 541.

35 Henry WF, A'Hern RP, Cole PJ (1993) Was Young's syndrome caused by exposure to mercury in childhood? *Br Med J* 307: 1579.

36 Jequier AM, Homes SC (1984) Aetiological factors in the production of obstructive azoospermia. *Br J Urol* 56: 540.

37 Hadelsman DJ, Conway AJ, Boylan LM, Turtle JR (1984) Young's syndrome: obstructive azoospermia and chronic sinopulmonary infections. *New Engl J Med* 310: 3.

38 Kartagener M, Stucki P (1962) Bronchiectasis with situs inversus. *Archiv Ped* 79: 193.

39 Calvin HI, Bedford JM (1971) Formation of disulphide bonds in the nucleus and accessory structures of mammalian spermatozoa during maturation in the epididymis. *J Reprod Fertil* 13 (suppl): 65.

40 Robin CP, Cadiat L (1875) (Robin's) *J. de l'Anatomie et de la Physiologie Normales et pathologiques de l'Homme et des Animaux*, vol. 11, pp. 83 & 105.

41 Mann TRR (1964) *Biochemistry of Semen and the Male Reproductive Tract*. London: Methuen.

42 Brindley GS, Sauerwein D, Hendry WF (1989) Hypogastric plexus stimulators for obtaining semen from paraplegic men. *Br J Urol* 64: 72.

Chapter 34: Testicle — congenital abnormalities

Absence of the testicle

If the entire urogenital ridge fails to develop there is no kidney, ureter, testis or vas deferens on one side [1].

Aplasia may be limited to the gonadal ridge, the kidney and ureter develop, but there is no vas deferens, epididymis or testis (Fig. 34.1). If the Müllerian duct inhibiting factor fails to be secreted by the Sertoli cells, then the male child has fallopian tubes and uterus, with a gonad of indeterminate kind, often presenting in a hernia [2].

In practice, the most likely cause for absence of the testis from the scrotum is cryptorchidism.

It is common to find a vas and an imperfectly formed epididymis but no testis: the kidney and ureter being present: in such cases it is thought

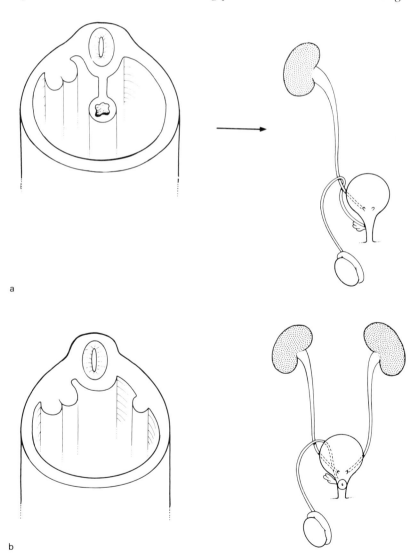

Fig. 34.1 (a) If one complete genitourinary ridge fails to develop there is no kidney, testis, vas or Müllerian system on one side. (b) If only the gonadal ridge fails to develop then there is no testis, epididymis or vas on one side.

549

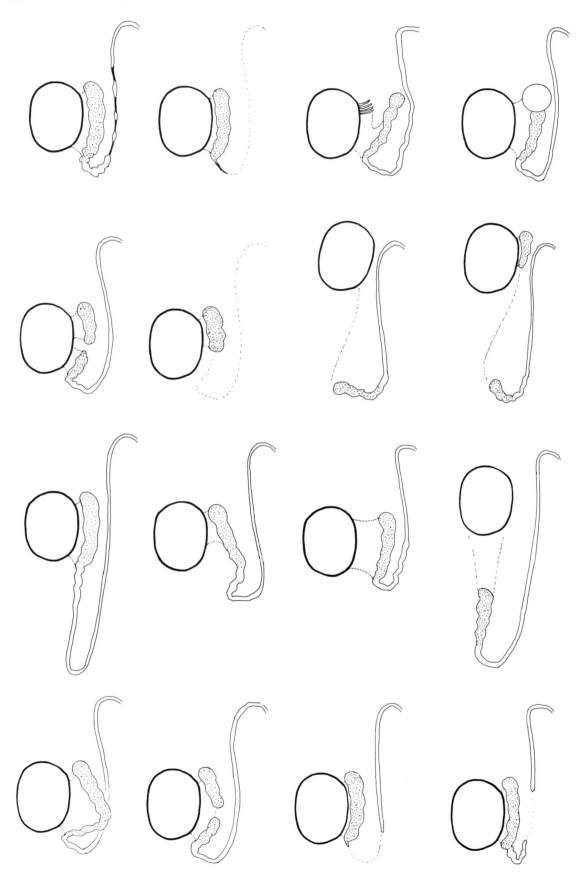

Fig. 34.2 Types of abnormal junctions between the gonad and the Wolffian duct component (vas, vesicle and epididymis) (after [5]).

that the testicle may have undergone torsion *in utero*.

When the testis is present, the vas deferens may be partly or completely absent from one or both sides. There is a wide variety of such defects in the vas or its junction with the epididymis causing obstructive azoospermia [3–8]. They are often seen in association with undescended testes and represent errors in the union of gonad with Wolffian duct (Fig. 34.2).

Duplex testis

Duplication of the testis on one or both sides is so rare that it calls for exploration to rule out cancer [9–11] (Fig. 34.3). Equally rare is duplication of the vas deferens with a single testis: it can cause failure of vasectomy when the surgeon fails to notice the additional vas.

Cryptorchidism

Unilateral cryptorchidism has been seen in twins, brothers, fathers and sons [12]. It is part of the prune-belly syndrome [13] and the Beckwith–Wiedemann syndrome (exopthalmos, macroglossia, gigantism, macrostoma, hemi-hypertrophy, hypoglycaemia and multilobulated kidneys [14]).

There are two main categories of cryptorchidism: (a) incomplete descent, where the testis is held up somewhere along the normal course of descent; and (b) ectopia where the testis has gone off course.

Incomplete descent

When the testis is held up along its normal pathway of descent it may be malformed. Abdominal cryptorchid testicles may amount to no more than a flat streak on the lateral wall of the pelvis. The others all have a certain range of movement, and are defined according to how far they can go up or down (Fig. 34.4): entrant inguinal, inguinal (in the canal), emergent (at the external ring), 'high retractile' (which cannot be coaxed to the bottom of the scrotum) and 'low retractile' testis (which can). The last is an innocent variation of the normal: it sometimes lies at the bottom of the scrotum and sometimes near the external ring, but with warm hands and gentleness it can usually be coaxed down to the normal position at the bottom of the scrotum, but it may take a general anaesthetic for this to happen. Such a testis always achieves the normal position at puberty [15,16]. More sophisticated classifications take into account where the testicle is actually found at operation [17,18].

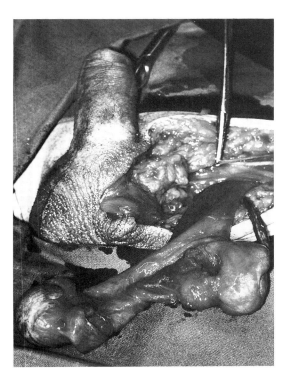

Fig. 34.3 Polyorchism (courtesy of Mr G.C. Tresidder).

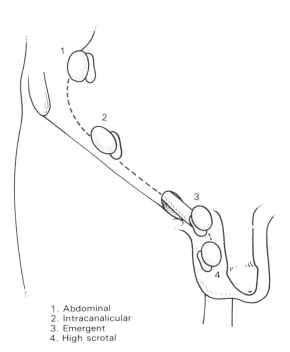

1. Abdominal
2. Intracanalicular
3. Emergent
4. High scrotal

Fig. 34.4 Types of maldescent of testis on normal course of descent (courtesy of Mr R.H. Whitaker).

Since the testicle descends to the scrotum around the time of birth, incomplete descent is more common in premature babies [19]. By the end of the first year, 1% of testicles are undescended and this figure does not change thereafter [20,21].

Ectopia

In ectopia the testis lies in one of several unusual positions, guided there by an errant gubernaculum [21]:

1 In the fat of the abdominal wall above the external ring — the superficial inguinal ectopic pouch.
2 At the root of the penis [22].
3 In the perineum near the midline.
4 'Crural' in the fat of the thigh over the adductor muscles (Fig. 34.5) where it may form part of the so-called popliteal pterygium syndrome [23].

Crossed ectopia has been described, where the testis from one side is found in the hemiscrotum on the other side.

Complications

Hernia

The cryptorchid testis is often accompanied by a patent processus vaginalis in which strangulation is apt to occur, especially in infancy [21].

Torsion

Because their processus vaginalis is unusually

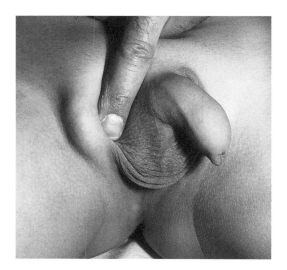

Fig. 34.5 Ectopic testicle — perineal testis (courtesy of Mr R.H. Whitaker).

voluminous the testis may twist within it mimicking a strangulated hernia (see p. 571).

Cancer

About 10% of all testicular cancers are associated with cryptorchidism, but of these about 10% occur in the normally descended gonad. There are various estimates of the increased risk of cancer in a cryptorchid testis: from 1 in 40 to a 50-fold increase [24]. Carcinoma *in situ* is found on biopsy in 1–8% of undescended testes [25,26].

Infertility

In the adult cryptorchid testis a single layer of spermatogonia is present among the Sertoli cells (see p. 543). In bilateral maldescent infertility is over 70% rising to 100% in cases where the testicle was impalpable before orchiopexy. In unilateral cryptorchidism, fertility is also slightly impaired [27–32]. It is widely believed that orchiopexy performed within the first 18 months of birth, may prevent infertility but the evidence is inconclusive. Orchiopexy may prevent damage to the contralateral normally descended testis [33].

If the testis is not placed in the scrotum by the age of 5, there are irreversible changes on light microscopy: electron microscopy detects them at the age of 2 [30,31].

Biopsy of the undescended testis frequently shows a decreased number of germ cells, and an absence of progression beyond the formation of spermatocytes in the testicular tubules. As if in compensation Leydig cells are abundant. Biopsy of both testes at the time of orchiopexy is sometimes advocated to predict future fertility and rule out carcinoma *in situ*.

Management

In infancy

About 90% of testes are in the scrotum by the time of birth: the next 9% descend over the next 12 months and by the end of the first year the incidence of cryptorchidism is the same 1% found in adults [4,18]. A low retractile testicle may rarely rise up again later on and need orchiopexy [34].

Whenever there is a clinical suspicion of a hernia, the infant must be operated on as soon as possible in view of the risk of strangulation. When there is no hernia, orchiopexy should be performed between 12 and 24 months. The operation should be done in a unit which deals with large numbers of babies and by experienced surgeons otherwise there is an unacceptable risk of damage to the testicular artery or vas deferens [20]. The operation should not be an occasional exercise for the surgeon whose practice is mostly with adults. To detect undescended testes at this age requires special expertise in the screening of babies [35—37].

In the prepubertal boy

Ectopic testes

If the testicle is ectopic it will never get into the scrotum and ought to be put there. These ectopic testicles usually have a long spermatic cord and the operation is not difficult.

Imperfect descent

Impalpable testis

In the past it was difficult to find an impalpable testis. Today, computerized tomographic (CT) scanning and laparoscopy has made it possible to find an abdominal testicle. As a rule it is then removed laparoscopically, but an alternative is to perform the first stage of the Fowler—Stephens procedure [38—40].

Inguinal, emergent and high retractile testis

An attempt at orchiopexy should be made: probably the testicle will never produce sperm, but it will produce testosterone and if it undergoes malignant change, will be easy to feel. In general, the younger the age of the patient when the operation is done the better.

Doubtful 'low retractile' testicles

In the past chorionic gonadotrophin was given. It caused oedema of the testis, precocious sexual behaviour and premature fusion of epiphyses. Gonadotrophins only worked for low retractile testicles, and merely hastened a process that would happen naturally. When genuine doubt remains, it is better to proceed to orchiopexy: under anaesthesia some testicles will very obviously be seen to be fully descended. There is a chance however that in this group there may be some impairment of fertility [41].

Orchiopexy

The incision is in the crease of the groin, centred over the midinguinal point (Fig. 34.6). Slit up the external oblique muscle taking care of the genito-femoral nerve. Separate the cremaster muscle fibres to expose the internal spermatic fascia which is deliberately incised to reveal the processus vaginalis which usually envelopes the cord (Fig. 34.7). It is carefully dissected from the cord: separating the peritoneum is the key to successful orchiopexy [15] (Fig. 34.8).

Once the processus has been separated, continue to develop the plane behind the peritoneum right up behind the colon using a long thin retractor or nasal speculum. Gently sweep the testicular vessels medially to straighten them, and divide the arcuate bands of tough fibrous tissue under vision (Fig. 34.9). Only a small further gain in length can be obtained by dissecting fibrous strands within the cord. Very occasionally, the vas deferens is the limiting factor, and it then helps to divide the inferior epigastric vessels.

Make a pocket for the mobilized testis between the skin and the dartos muscle in the scrotum (Figs 34.10 & 34.11). This pocket should be large enough to receive the testis. A buttonhole is made in the dartos to allow the testicle to be

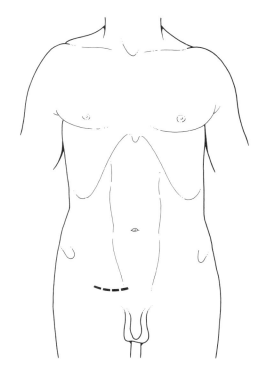

Fig. 34.6 Crease incision for orchiopexy.

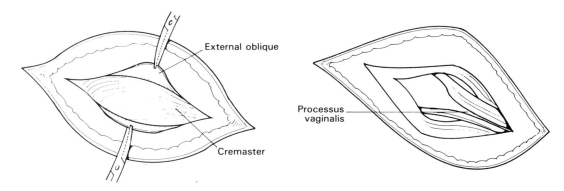

Fig. 34.7 The cremaster is split along its fibres revealing the processus vaginalis.

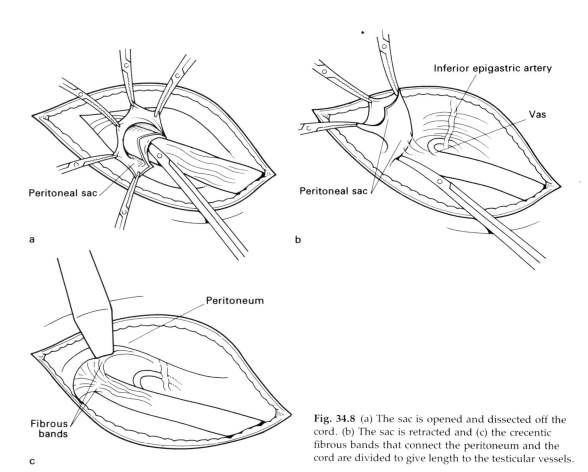

Fig. 34.8 (a) The sac is opened and dissected off the cord. (b) The sac is retracted and (c) the crecentic fibrous bands that connect the peritoneum and the cord are divided to give length to the testicular vessels.

brought through. Close the skin with fine catgut [42,43].

Two-stage orchiopexy

If the testicular vessels are so short that the testicle will not reach easily to the scrotum, after this retroperitoneal dissection, it may be left just outside the external ring. When a second stage is performed some 2 years later, the testicular vessels will be found to have elongated, and the second orchiopexy surprisingly easy [44].

Alternatives to two-stage orchiopexy have been proposed. Fowler and Stephens [45] suggested dividing the testicular artery as a first stage, and hope that the testicle would receive an

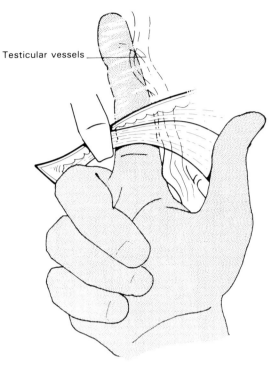

Testicular vessels

Fig. 34.9 Retroperitoneal mobilization of the cord medially is assisted by a finger.

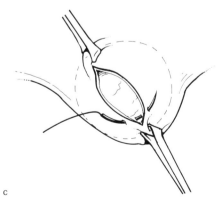

Loop of vas

Fig. 34.10 The testicle is mobilized and brought down to the scrotum, taking care not to injure a long loop of vas which is often present distal to the testis.

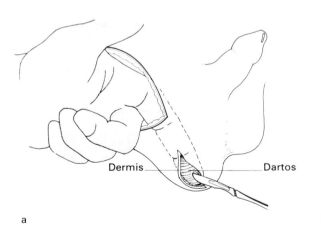

Dermis — Dartos

a

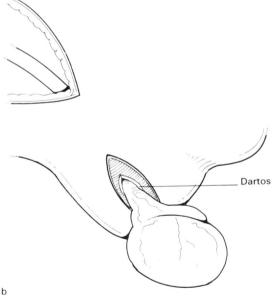

Dartos

b

c

Fig. 34.11 (a) A pocket is made for the testicle by dissecting between the dartos and skin of the scrotum. (b) The testicle is brought through a buttonhole in the dartos. (c) The skin is closed with sutures that just catch the tunica albuginea testis.

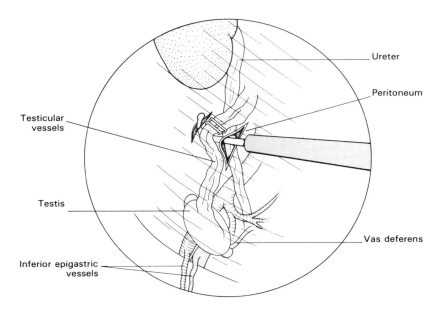

Testicular vessels

Testis

Inferior epigastric vessels

Ureter

Peritoneum

Vas deferens

Fig. 34.12 Laparoscopic division of the testicular artery as the first stage of the Fowler—Stephens manoeuvre.

adequate blood supply from the artery of the vas. If great care is taken to preserve the collateral vessels of the vas and cremaster, isotope studies show that the testicle can remain well vascularized [46] and this manoeuvre can now be done at laparoscopy (Fig. 34.12). It is still very doubtful, however, whether any of these testes ever produce sperm.

Using microsurgical techniques, it is possible to anastomose the testicular artery to the inferior epigastric with preservation of viability in the testicle: an exercise that is not pointless when both testes are undescended [47–49].

References

1 Bobrow M, Gough MH (1970) Bilateral absence of testes. *Lancet* i: 366.

2 Eastham JA, McEvoy K, Sullivan R, Chandrasoma P (1992) A case of simultaneous bilateral non-seminomatous testicular tumors in persistent Müllerian duct syndrome. *J Urol* 148: 407.

3 Rubin S-O (1975) Congenital absence of the vas deferens. *Scand J Urol Nephrol* 9: 94.

4 Hall S, Oates RD (1993) Unilateral absence of the scrotal vas deferens associated with contralateral mesonephric duct anomalies resulting in infertility: laboratory physical and radiographic findings, and therapeutic alternatives. *J Urol* 150: 1161.

5 Gill B, Kogan S, Starr S, Reda E, Levitt S (1989) Significance of epididymal and ductal anomalies associated with testicular maldescent. *J Urol* (2) 142: 556.

6 Lingardh G, Domellof L, Eriksson S, Fahraeus B (1975) Dysplasia of the testis and epididymis. *Scand J Urol Nephrol* 9: 1.

7 Koff WJ, Skaletsky R (1990) Malformation of the epididymis in undescended testis. *J Urol* 143: 340.

8 Hendry WF, Parslow JM, Stedronska J (1983) Exploratory scrototomy in 168 azoospermic males. *Br J Urol* 55: 785.

9 Farrer JH, Walker AH, Rajfer J (1985) Management of the postpubertal cryptorchid testis: a statistical review. *J Urol* 134: 1071.

10 Westcott JW, Dykhuizen RF (1967) Polyorchism. *J Urol* 98: 497.

11 Singh A, Sobti MK (1988) Polyorchidism. *Br J Urol* 98: 458.

12 Corbus BL, O'Conor VJ (1922) The familial occurrence of undescended testis: report of six brothers with testicular anomalies. *Surg Gynecol Obstet* 34: 237.

13 Woodhouse CRJ, Ransley PG, Innes-Williams D (1982) Prune belly syndrome — a report of 47 cases. *Arch Dis Child* 57: 856.

14 Taylor WN (1981) Urological implications of the Beckwith—Wiedermann syndrome. *J Urol* 125: 439.

15 Browne D (1943) Treatment of undescended testes. *Proc Roy Soc Med* 42: 643.

16 Puri P, Nixon HH (1977) Bilateral undescended testes — subsequent effects on fertility. *J Pediatr Surg* 12: 563.

17 Whitaker RH (1992) Undescended testis — the need for a standard classification. *Br J Urol* 70: 1.

18 Cendron M, Huff DS, Keating MA, Snyder HM, Duckett JW (1993) Anatomical, morphological and volumetric analysis: a review of 759 cases of testicular maldescent. *J Urol* 149: 570.

19 Morley R, Lucas A (1987) Undescended testes in low birthweight infants. *Br Med J* 295: 753.

20 Saw KC, Earldey I, Dennis MJS, Whitaker RH (1992) Surgical outcomes of orchiopexy. I. Previously unoperated testes. *Br J Urol* 70: 90.

21 Johansen TEB (1988) The anatomy of gubernaculum testis and processus vaginalis in cryptorchidism. *Scand J Urol Nephrol* 22: 101.

22 McLoughlin PVA (1980) Pubic ectopic testicle. *Br J Urol* 52: 1640.

23 Cunningham LN, Keating MA, Snyder HM, Duckett JW (1989) Urological manifestations of the popliteal

pterygium syndrome. *J Urol* 141: 910.

24 Martin DC (1984) Malignancy in the cryptorchid testis. *Urol Clin N Am* 9: 371.

25 Giwercman A, Bruun E, Frimodt-Moller C, Skakkebaek NE (1989) Prevalence of carcinoma *in situ* and other histopathological abnormalities in testes of men with a history of cryptorchidism. *J Urol* 142: 998.

26 Ozen H, Ayhan A, Esen A *et al.* (1989) Histopathological changes in adult cryptorchid testes. *Br J Urol* 63: 520.

27 Bramble FJ, Eccles S, Houghton AL, O'Shea A, Jacobs HS (1974) Reproductive and endocrine function after surgical treatment of bilateral cryptorchidism. *Lancet* ii: 311.

28 Hargreave TB, Elton RA, Webb JA, Busuttil A, Chisholm GD (1984) Maldescended testes and fertility: review of 68 cases. *Br J Urol* 56: 734.

29 Okuyama A, Nonomura N, Nakamura M *et al.* (1989) Surgical management of undescended testis: retrospective study of potential fertility in 274 cases. *J Urol* 142: 749.

30 Johansen TEB (1988) *Therapeutic Basis in Cryptorchidism: A Clinical and Experimental Study*. Oslo.

31 Huff DS, Hadziselimovic F, Snyder HM, Duckett JW, Keating MA (1989) Postnatal testicular maldevelopment in unilateral cryptorchidism. *J Urol* 142 (2): 546.

32 Puri P, O'Donnell B (1990) Semen analysis in patients operated on for impalpable testes. *Br J Urol* 66: 646.

33 Hadziselimovic F, Hecker E, Herzog B (1984) The value of testicular biopsy in cryptorchidism. *Urol Res* 12: 171.

34 John Radcliffe Hospital Cryptorchidism Study Group (1986) Boys with late descending testes: the source of patients with 'retractile' testes undergoing orchidopexy. *Br Med J* 293: 789.

35 Morecroft JA, Brereton RJ (1992) Preschool screening for cryptorchidism. *Br Med J* 305: 424.

36 London NJM, Joseph HT, Johnstone JMS (1987) Orchidopexy: the effect of changing patterns of referral and treatment on outcome. *Br J Surg* 74: 636.

37 Hadziselimovic F, Herzog B (1987) Cryptorchidism. *Pediatr Surg Int* 2: 132.

38 Glickman MG, Weiss RM, Itzchak Y (1977) Testicular venography for undescended testis. *Am J Roentgenol* 129: 67.

39 Perovic S, Janic N (1994) Laparoscopy in the diagnosis of non-palpable testis. *Br J Urol* 73: 310.

40 Cortes D, Thorup JM, Lenz K, Beck BL, Nielsen OH (1995) Laparoscopy in 100 consecutive patients with 128 impalpable testes. *Br J Urol* 75: 281.

41 Rasmussen TB, Ingerslev HJ, Hestrup H (1988) Bilateral spontaneous descent of the testis after the age of 10: subsequent effects on fertility. *Br J Surg* 75: 820.

42 Brown S, Mackinnon AE (1979) The scrotal pouch operation for undescended testis. *Ann Roy Coll Surg Engl* 61: 377.

43 Bellinger MF, Abramowitz H, Brantley S, Marshall G (1989) Orchiopexy: an experimental study of the effect of surgical technique on testicular histology. *J Urol* 142 (2): 553.

44 Reece-Smith H, Moisey CU (1984) The undescended testicle: a continuing failure. *Br Med J* 288: 1653.

45 Fowler R, Stephens FD (1959) The role of testicular vascular anatomy in the salvage of the high undescended testes. *Aust New Zeal J Surg* 29: 92.

46 Ransley PG, Vordermark JS, Caldamone AA *et al.* (1984) Preliminary ligation of the gonadal vessels prior to orchidopexy for the intraabdominal testicle. *World J Urol* 2: 266.

47 Martin DC, Salibian AH (1988) Orchiopexy using microvascular surgical technique. *J Urol* 123: 435.

48 Corbally MT, Quinn FJ, Guiney EJ (1993) The effect of two-stage orchiopexy on testicular growth. *Br J Urol* 72: 376.

49 Gough MH (1989) Cryptorchidism. *Br J Surg* 76: 109.

Chapter 35: Testicle — trauma and inflammation

Closed injury to the testicle in sport or industry may tear the tunica albuginea and blood will collect around the testis — haematocele (Fig. 35.1). A notorious trap is to fail to notice that the injury has ruptured a testicular tumour. With so-called conservative management there is a strong chance that the haematoma will enlarge and compress the testis into a thin atrophic shell.

All these cases should be explored, the haematoma evacuated and the tunica albuginea repaired: this gives the best chance of preserving testicular size and function [1—4].

When the scrotum and perineum is particularly bruised, ultrasound scanning can be very useful in showing where the testicles are, and what has happened to them [5—7].

Traumatic arteritis

Traumatic arteritis which causes infarction of the testicle has been described in tractor drivers: its cause is still obscure, and was attributed to vibration [8]. More recently, inexplicable pain in the testicles has been shown to be the result of segmental infarction, the diagnosis being made by colour Doppler ultrasound [9].

Injection of grease

Accidental injection of grease into the scrotum by means of an industrial grease-gun may cause an oleogranuloma [10].

Inflammatory diseases of the testicle

Acute inflammation

Acute orchitis

Inflammation of the testicle may involve the testis, epididymis or both. Most inflammation of the epididymis will eventually involve the testis. The epididymis is relatively soft and expands to form a tender mass behind the testis. The rigid tunica albuginea cannot expand and the increased pressure inside the tunica may cause ischaemia of the testis. Inflammation in either testis or epididymis will lead to a secondary hydrocele comparable with the free fluid in the peritoneal cavity in peritonitis.

Pyogenic orchitis may follow bacteraemia: usually the illness is severe and rapidly followed by an abscess. If masked by antibiotics the condition may resemble a tumour and require orchiectomy (Fig. 35.2).

Virus orchitis

Mumps and other viruses can cause an acute orchitis which is sometimes bilateral. Mumps

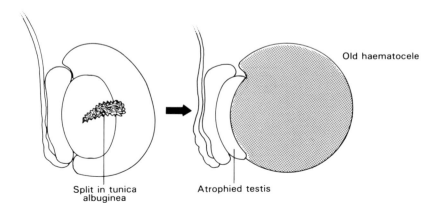

Old haematocele

Split in tunica albuginea   Atrophied testis

Fig. 35.1 To prevent testicular atrophy occurring from pressure by the haematoma, the testicle should be explored, the blood clot evacuated and the tear in the tunica albuginea repaired.

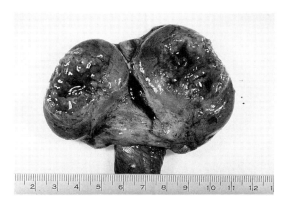

Fig. 35.2 Blood-borne staphylococcal abscess of the testicle — removed in mistake for a tumour.

orchitis only occurs after puberty [11]. There has usually been parotitis a few days previously but not always [12]. During an epidemic gamma globulin will prevent orchitis [13]. Mumps vaccine will prevent this complication which is serious not only because it is so painful, but sterility or permanent impairment of Leydig cell function follows in up to 50% of adults who get mumps orchitis, from ischaemia within the tunica albuginea [14,15]. Incision of the tunica instantly relieves pain, restores the colour of the ischaemic testis and preserves its size [16].

Hydrocortisone does not prevent atrophy and risks septic complications [17].

Many other viruses cause acute orchitis: Coxsackie [18], infectious mononucleosis [19], hepatitis B [20], herpesvirus 2, bat salivary gland virus and dengue [21,22]. Since they all present as acute inflammation without evidence of trauma or infection, they demand exploration to rule out torsion. If the testicle is found to be uniformly inflamed, the tunica albuginea should be incised to relieve pressure: this will also allow a biopsy to be taken.

Acute epididymoorchitis

Acute epididymitis used to be so common after urological operations that 30 years ago vasectomy was always performed before prostatectomy.

The cause is usually a urine-borne coliform [23,24], but blood-borne infection may involve the testicle, where it forms a lump indistinguishable from cancer. Epididymoorchitis is still a serious complication of operations that need a urethral catheter: it occurs in patients with urethral stricture. Occasionally, there is a clear history of urethral discharge [23–25].

Acute epididymitis may occur without urinary infection. Sometimes there has been heavy exertion prior to the onset of the epididymitis, and reflux of urine down the vas is thought to be responsible for a chemical epididymitis [26].

Aspiration of the epididymis may show *Chlamydia*: some of the cases attributed to reflux of urine may have been undiagnosed examples of this condition [25,27–29]. Recently, *Candida* has been recovered from needle aspirates of the epididymis [30] and may be more common than previously supposed.

Clinical features

There is the rapid onset of a painful red swelling: at first it can be seen to involve the epididymis but within hours the secondary hydrocele, oedema of the scrotum and extreme tenderness make it impossible to distinguish testis from epididymis.

Rectal examination may show tenderness in the prostate and vesicles, and on transrectal ultrasound the seminal vesicles may be swollen and distended with pus [31].

Differential diagnosis

The main question that arises is whether it is torsion, for if torsion cannot be safely ruled out the scrotum must be explored (see p. 569). One must always ask — what else could it be? In babies, idiopathic oedema — a kind of streptococcal cellulitis — may affect the fat of the scrotum [32,33]. The appearances are typical: but the risk of torsion demands exploration in a third of the cases.

A similar appearance is seen in children with fat necrosis perhaps arising from hypothermia, giving rise to an inflammation of the scrotum: if correctly diagnosed it can be treated conservatively [34].

Mumps never causes orchitis before puberty [11]. When in doubt, it is better to explore a testis because even if the diagnosis proves to be mumps orchitis the opportunity can be taken to prevent atrophy by decompressing the tunica [16].

^{99m}Technetium pertechnate may be selectively taken up by an inflamed epididymis, but not by the ischaemic testis in torsion [35]. Ultrasound and Doppler scanning though widely advocated, are not completely reliable and none of these sophisticated investigations should ever be allowed to delay intervention. Let them be done 'on the way to the theatre' — it is easy to cancel the operation for torsion but delay can be disastrous [35–38] (see p. 571).

Tuberculous epididymitis may have a surprisingly acute onset: it is still a sound rule always to exclude tuberculosis when there is no evidence of urinary infection.

Treatment

Usually the diagnosis of acute epididymoorchitis is obvious. Systemic antibiotic therapy is given with bed rest. With improvement a scrotal support is comforting. Acute epididymoorchitis takes weeks to resolve during which heavy exertion may cause it to relapse.

The main concern of the surgeon is to relieve ischaemia where this threatens the testis. In very severe forms of epididymitis there may be obstruction of the spermatic veins and the condition may be relieved by incision of the external oblique to relax the external ring [39].

Complications

An abscess in the testicle may form a fluctuating swelling which discharges pus. When this occurs, it usually means the underlying testis has undergone ischaemic necrosis. The 'abscess' discharges necrotic testicular tubules — 'fungus testis' — which necessitates orchiectomy (Fig. 35.3).

Chronic inflammation

Relapsing bacterial epididymitis

From time to time a straightforward acute epididymitis fails to resolve. A few weeks later there is another acute attack, and another, and so on. When the source of infection is clearly from the urinary tract it may help to stop the succession of attacks by dividing the vasa. Unfortunately, this is not always successful: even after vasectomy the inflammation of the epididymis may grumble on and require epididymectomy. The specimen usually shows granulomatous epididymitis [40].

Granulomatous epididymitis

Extravasation of spermatozoa into the epididymis provokes a chronic granuloma with features suggestive of tuberculosis, probably because the acid-fast helmet of the spermatozoon — the galea

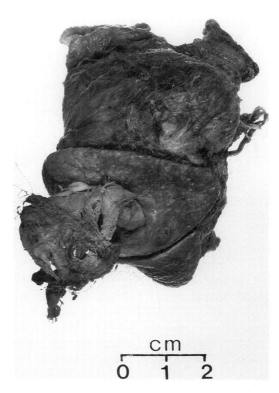

Fig. 35.3 'Fungus testis' — ischaemic necrosis of the testis following acute inflammation. The necrotic tubules fungate through the skin.

capitis — is antigenically similar to the envelope of the tubercle bacillus [40]. Around these acid-fast particles there are foreign body giant cells and macrophages but no caseation (Fig. 35.4).

Granulomatous epididymitis occurs after prolonged inflammation in which sperms are extravasated. Today, this condition has become much more common as a delayed complication of vasectomy.

Granulomatous orchitis

This seminal granuloma is different from another chronic granuloma in the testis which follows repeated urinary infections (Fig. 35.5). It forms a firm mass in the testicle which cannot be distinguished from cancer and demands orchiectomy. Histologically, there is chronic inflammatory tissue and fibrosis [41,42].

Tuberculous epididymitis

Blood-borne tubercle bacilli may lodge in the caput epididymis to form a tuberculoma: urine-borne infection (the usual type) travels along the vas deferens and fetches up in the cauda epi-

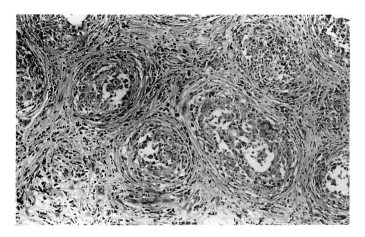

Fig. 35.4 Granulomatous epididymoorchitis — a granuloma formed in response to extravasation of highly antigenic spermatozoa.

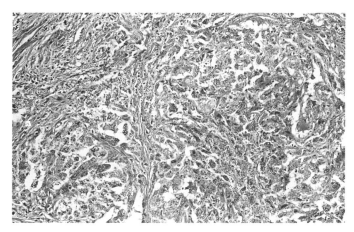

Fig. 35.5 Seminal granuloma: a chronic granuloma of the testis which follows repeated urinary infections. The firm mass in the testis cannot be distinguished from a cancer.

didymis [43]. In either situation they may provoke an acute inflammatory response which is followed by a chronic phase in which the caseating tuberculoma of the epididymis forms a chain of bead-like swellings continuing up the vas and involving the seminal vesicle (Fig. 35.6).

Complications

A small abscess may point to the skin of the scrotum and break down to form a sinus from which tubercle bacilli may be recovered.

When there is no evidence of tuberculosis elsewhere in the urinary tract the diagnosis is difficult and may require a biopsy. Modern treatment for tuberculosis is so harmless and effective that it may be preferable to give a short course of treatment as a therapeutic trial.

When only the epididymis is involved it may be removed (see below) but often the testicle is also involved and orchiectomy is necessary.

Bilharzial epididymitis

Chronic granulomatous inflammation of the vas and testicle can be caused by infection with *Schistosoma*. The vas deferens and seminal vesicles may be outlined in the plain abdominal X-ray with thin lines of calcification. The inflammation of the testis is complicated by vascular obstruction by the worms and ova and ischaemia is part of the pathological process [44]. The mass is indistinguishable from a tumour [45–47].

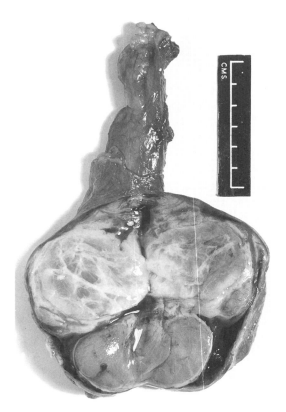

Fig. 35.6 Tuberculosis of the testicle.

Malacoplakia

Malacoplakia is a chronic granuloma in which histiocytes contain specific calcified and laminated microspheres — the Michaelis–Guttmann bodies. In the testicle it gives rise to a hard mass indistinguishable from cancer [48–50].

Actinomycosis

Actinomycosis of the testicle produces a complex of sinuses leading down to the chronically inflamed mass. The characteristic 'sulphur grains' formed by the fungal mycelia may help in the diagnosis of this exceptionally rare disease. The treatment is orchiectomy along with all the sinuses under tetracycline cover [51].

Brucellosis

Brucellosis is equally rare, except in the Middle East. It forms a hard mass in the testicle, and only when the testicle has been removed on suspicion of cancer is the diagnosis questioned, and then confirmed by immunological tests [52–54].

Behçet's disease

Up to 6% of patients with Behçet's disease have involvement of the epididymis [55].

Syphilis

Gumma of the testis was common during the nineteenth-century epidemic of syphilis and much was made of the clinical distinction between gumma and cancer. Gumma was said to feel 'light'; a tumour felt 'heavy'. Gumma is still reported from time to time, but is impossible to distinguish from cancer. The testicle is useless and the treatment orchiectomy [56].

Other causes of epididymoorchitis

These include coccidiomycosis [57], cytomegalovirus [58] (after immunosuppression), sarcoidosis [59,60], filariasis — which causes acute inflammation at first before it goes on to elephantiasis of the scrotum and hydrocele with a chronic granuloma in the testicle. Perhaps the rarest of all causes of epididymitis is leprosy [61].

Treatment

Epididymectomy

The indications for this operation are few. It is seldom that the epididymis is involved alone in tuberculosis: for sperm granuloma after vasectomy epididymectomy usually fails to cure the symptoms. Deliver the testicle through a transverse scrotal incision. Locate the vas and

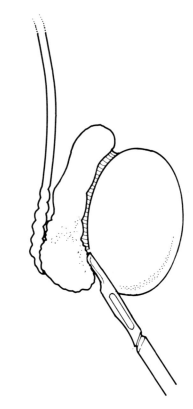

Fig. 35.7 Epididymectomy: a little branch of the testicular artery supplies the epididymis.

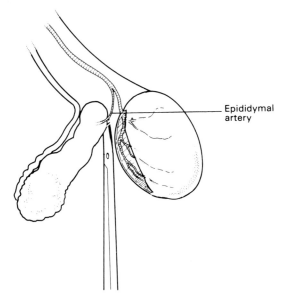

Epididymal artery

Fig. 35.8 Epididymectomy: the epididymis is removed, sparing the main testicular artery.

trace it down to the epididymis. The blood supply to the epididymis comes from a small branch of the testicular artery near the caput epididymis (Fig. 35.7). The only difficult part of the operation is to find this little vessel without injuring the main artery of the testis. Locate the vas and trace it down to the testis. Separate the epididymis at the hilum of the testis; seal tiny vessels with bipolar diathermy. Special care is needed when dissecting off the head of the epididymis: by pulling it laterally the main testicular artery is preserved (Fig. 35.8).

References

1 Gross M (1969) Rupture of the testicle: the importance of early surgical treatment. *J Urol* 101: 196.

2 Del Villar RG, Ireland GW, Cass AS (1972) Early exploration in acute testicular conditions. *J Urol* 108: 887.

3 MacDermott JP, Gray BK, Stewart PAH (1988) Traumatic rupture of the testis. *Br J Urol* 62: 179.

4 Pohl DR, Johnson DE, Robison JR (1968) Bilateral testicular rupture: report of a case. *J Urol* 99: 772.

5 Corriere JN (1992) Lower urinary and genital tract trauma. *Curr Opinion Urol* 2: 202.

6 Urarte R, Spaedy M, Coss AS (1990) Diagnosis of rupture after blunt testicular trauma. *Urology* 36: 253.

7 Corrales JG, Corbel L, Cipolla B *et al.* (1993) Accuracy of ultrasound diagnosis after blunt testicular trauma. *J Urol* 150: 1834.

8 Clarke JV (1967) Tractor accidents. *Br Med J* 1: 237.

9 Kramolowsky EV, Beauchamp RA, Milby WP (1993) Color Doppler ultrasound for the diagnosis of segmental testicular infarction. *J Urol* 150: 972.

10 O'Rourke MGE (1967) Lipogranulomata of male genitalia. *Br J Urol* 39: 426.

11 Sparks JP (1971) Torsion of the testis. *Ann Roy Coll Surg Engl* 49: 77.

12 Manson AL (1990) Mumps orchitis. *Urology* 36: 355.

13 Scott LS (1960) Mumps and male fertility. *Br J Urol* 32: 183.

14 Werner CA (1950) Mumps orchitis and testicular atrophy: occurrence. *Ann Int Med* 32: 1066.

15 Adamopoulos DA, Lawrence DM, Vassilopoulos P, Contoyiannis PA, Swyer GIM (1978) Pituitary—testicular interrelationships in mumps orchitis and other viral infections. *Br Med J* 1: 1177.

16 Craighead JE, Mahoney EM, Carver DH, Nafiey K, Fremont-Smith P (1962) Orchitis due to Coxsackie virus group B, type 5: report of a case with isolation of the virus from the testis. *New Engl J Med* 267: 498.

17 Smith IM, Bishir JW (1958) Treatment of mumps orchitis with ACTH and cortisone. *New Engl J Med* 258: 120.

18 Freij L, Norrby R, Olsson B (1970) A small outbreak of Coxsackie B5 infection with two cases of cardiac involvement and orchitis followed by testicular atrophy. *Acta Med Scand* 187: 177.

19 Ralson LS, Saiki AK, Powers WT (1960) Orchitis as a complication of infectious mononucleosis. *J Am Med Assoc* 173: 1348.

20 Molitor PJA, Warrens AN (1985) Acute orchitis associated with hepatitis B infection. *Br Med J* 291: 940.

21 Deture FA, Drylie DM, Kaufman HE, Centifanto YN (1976) Herpesvirus type 2: isolation from seminal vesicles and testes. *Urology* 1: 541.

22 Riggs S, Sanford JP (1962) Viral orchitis. *New Engl J Med* 266: 990.

23 Barker K, Raper FP (1964) Torsion of the testis. *Br J Urol* 36: 35.

24 Mittemeyer BT, Lennox KW, Borski AA (1966) Epididymitis: a review of 610 cases. *J Urol* 95: 390.

25 De Jong Z, Pontonnier F, Plante P *et al.* (1988) The frequency of *Chlamydia trachomatis* in acute epididymitis. *Br J Urol* 62: 76.

26 Badenoch AW (1953) Vaso-epididymal reflux syndrome. *Proc Roy Soc Med* 46: 847.

27 Grant JBF, Costello CB, Sequeira PJL, Blacklock NJ (1987) The role of *Chlamydia trachomatis* in epididymitis. *Br J Urol* 60: 355.

28 Pearson RC, Baumber CD, McGhie D, Thambar IV (1988) The relevance of *Chlamydia trachomatis* in acute epididymitis in young men. *Br J Urol* 62: 72.

29 Robinson AJ, Grant JBF, Spencer RC, Potter C, Kinghorn GR (1990) Acute epididymitis: why patient and consort must be investigated. *Br J Urol* 66: 642.

30 Docimo SG, Rukstalis DB, Rukstalis MR, Kang J, Cotton D, DeWolf WC (1993) *Candida* epididymitis: newly recognized opportunistic epididymal infection. *Urology* 41: 280.

31 Krishnan R, Heal MR (1991) Study of the seminal vesicles in acute epididymitis. *Br J Urol* 67: 632.

32 Nicholas JL, Morgan A, Zachary RB (1970) Idiopathic edema of scrotum in young boys. *Surgery* 87: 847.

33 Najmaldin A, Burge DM (1987) Acute idiopathic scrotal oedema: incidence, manifestations and aetiology. *Br J Surg* 74: 634.

34 Ong TH, Solomon JR (1973) Fat necrosis of the scrotum. *J Ped Surg* 8: 919.

35 Stage KH, Schoenvogel R, Lewis S (1981) Testicular scanning: clinical experience with 72 patients. *J Urol* 125: 334.

36 Brereton RJ (1981) Limitations of the Doppler flow meter in the diagnosis of the 'acute scrotum' in boys. *Br J Urol* 53: 380.

37 Abu-Sleiman R, Ho JE, Gregory JG (1979) Scrotal scanning. *Urology* 13: 326.

38 King H, Whelan P (1984) Treatment of acute scrotal pain. *Br Med J* 288: 1576.

39 Costas S, Van Blerk PJP (1973) Incision of the external inguinal ring in acute epididymitis. *Br J Urol* 45: 555.

40 Glassy FJ, Mostofi FK (1956) Spermatic granulomas of the epididymis. *Am J Clin Pathol* 26: 1303.

41 Lynch VP, Eakins D, Morrison E (1968) Granulomatous orchitis. *Br J Urol* 40: 451.

42 Cruickshank B, Stuart-Smith DA (1959) Orchitis associated with sperm-agglutinating antibodies. *Lancet* i: 708.

43 Ferrie BG, Rundle JSH (1983) Tuberculous epididymo-orchitis. A review of 20 cases. *Br J Urol* 55: 437.

44 Joshi RA (1967) Total granulomatous infarction of the testes due to *Schistosoma haematobium*. *J Clin Pathol* 20: 273.

45 Mitry NF, Satti MB, Tamimi DM, Metawaa B (1986) Testicular schistosomiasis. *Br J Urol* 58: 721.

46 Mikhail NE, Tawfic MI, Hadi AA, Akl M (1988)

Schistosomal orchitis simulating malignancy. *J Urol* 140: 147.

47 Elbadawi A, Khuri FJ, Cockett ATK (1979) Polypoid granulomatous and sclerosing endophlebitis of spermatic cord. *Urology* 13: 309.

48 Green WO (1968) Malakoplakia of the epididymis without testicular involvement. *Arch Pathol* 86: 438.

49 Shaba JK, Black WA (1971) Malakoplakic granuloma of the testis. *J Urol* 105: 687.

50 Gonzales RD, Palacios JJN, Usera G, Castillo RG, Montalban MA, Borobia V. (1982) Testicular malakoplakia. *J Urol* 127: 325.

51 Scorer CG (1952) Actinomycosis of the testis. *Br J Surg* 40: 244.

52 Rothenburg RC (1933) Undulant fever: a fatal case. *Ann Int Med* 6: 1275.

53 Reisman EM, Colquitt LA, Childers J, Preminger GM (1990) Brucella orchitis: a rare cause of testicular enlargement. *J Urol* 143: 821.

54 Afsar H, Baydar I, Sirmatel F (1993) Epididymo-orchitis due to brucellosis. *Br J Urol* 72: 103.

55 Kirkali Z, Yigitbasi O, Sasmaz R (1991) Urological aspects of Behçet's disease. *Br J Urol* 67: 638.

56 Persaud V, Rao A (1977) Gumma of the testis. *Br J Urol* 49: 142.

57 Bodner H, Howard AH, Kaplan JH (1959) Coccidiomycosis of the spermatic cord: roentgen therapy. *J Int Coll Surg* 32: 530.

58 McCarthy JM, McLoughlin MG, Shackleton CR *et al.* (1991) Cytomegalovirus epididymitis following renal transplantation. *J Urol* 146: 417.

59 Winnacker JL, Becker KL, Katz S, Matthews MJ (1967) Recurrent epididymitis in sarcoidosis: report of a patient treated with corticosteroids. *Ann Int Med* 66: 743.

60 Longcope WT, Fisher AM (1942) Involvement of the heart in sarcoidosis or Besnier—Boeck—Schaumann's disease. *J Mt Sinai Hosp* 8: 784.

61 Pareek SS, Tandon RC (1985) Epididymal lesion in tuberculoid leprosy. *Br Med J* 291: 313.

Chapter 36: Testicle — benign swellings

Hydrocele

A hydrocele is a collection of fluid between the layers of the tunica vaginalis. It has been recognized since ancient times: perhaps its most eminent sufferer was Gibbon — author of *The Decline and Fall of the Roman Empire* who was incapacitated by hydrocele in his later years and died when it was tapped [1,2].

Congenital hydrocele follows late or patchy closure of the processus vaginalis testis, associated with late maturation of the lymphatics of the cord. The processus may close above and below a short segment, resulting in an 'encysted hydrocele of the cord'; or a hydrocele may be associated with a hernial sac, with obliteration of the intervening processus. Rarely, a hydrocele may extend through the internal ring to cause a retroperitoneal swelling [3] (Fig. 36.1).

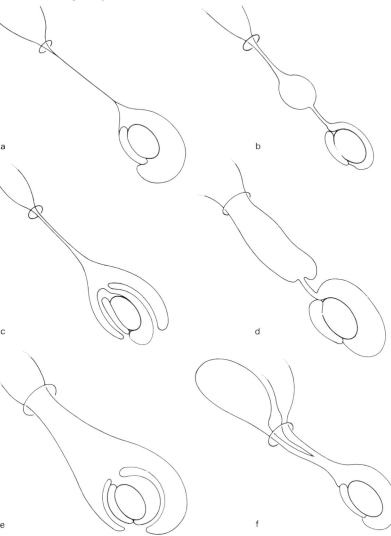

Fig. 36.1 Various types of hernia and hydrocele. (a) Common hydrocele, (b) encysted hydrocele of the cord, (c) 'double' hydrocele, (d) hernia and hydrocele, (e) 'hernia magna' (f) abdominoscrotal hydrocele.

Primary or idiopathic hydrocele

The fluid in primary hydrocele is lymph. The lymphatic drainage of the testis is of great interest, since the testicular tubules are immunologically deprived sites, keeping the haploid gametes safe from the immune defences of the body. Between the tubules, the lymphatic capillaries drain into the lymphatics of the cord: when these are obstructed, the intertubular spaces expand not the lumina of the tubules.

There is always a little fluid between the layers of the tunica vaginalis. In primary hydrocele in the adult, there is decreased absorption of the fluid from the sac [4,5] but why this occurs is not known. Hydrocele is seen in ascites and heart failure, and in men who have undergone radical retroperitoneal node dissection or radical removal of the kidney for cancer.

Secondary hydrocele

Secondary effusion into the peritoneal sac of the tunica vaginalis is analogous to the secondary pleural or peritoneal effusion seen with almost any disease in the pleural or peritoneal cavities. So it occurs with epididymitis, orchitis and trauma, and can be a rare presenting symptom of cancer. Obstruction of the lymphatics of the cord by the filarial worm *Wuchereria bancrofti* gives rise to hydroceles, sometimes of prodigious size [6,7].

Calcification is sometimes seen in the wall of a hydrocele in very elderly men [8].

Clinical features

There is a translucent sac, fluctuant in two planes, lying anterior to the testis which may be difficult to feel. It is sometimes difficult to distinguish a hydrocele from a collection of cysts of the epididymis (see p. 568) especially when both are present in the same patient. Cysts of the epididymis arise behind the testis and are multilocular.

Investigations

The physical signs are usually conclusive. In children it is important, but often difficult, to make sure there is no hernia. In adults the chief issue is the question of an underlying cancer of the testis. Cancer can usually be excluded by ultrasound scanning (Fig. 36.2): if in doubt the fluid should be aspirated to allow the testis to be

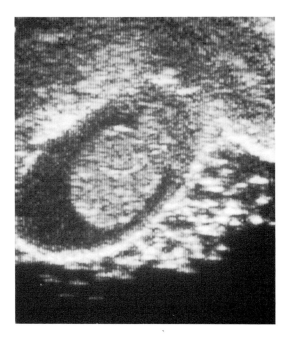

Fig. 36.2 Ultrasound scan of hydrocele (courtesy of Dr W. Hately).

carefully palpated and if the findings are still inconclusive, then the testicle should be explored (see p. 587).

Treatment

Most hydroceles need no treatment. An old rule is to advise treatment if a man's wife or his tailor complain.

Aspiration

Aspiration of the hydrocele demands strict asepsis. Shine a light through the scrotum to avoid the testis and large subcutaneous veins. Inject a drop of local anaesthetic under the skin. Insert an intravenous cannula and withdraw the stylet (Fig. 36.3). Connect a three-way tap and aspirate the hydrocele until it is dry. If a vein is torn, or the tunica albuginea is cut, blood will collect in the vaginal sac (haematocele) and may become infected (pyocele).

Injection

To obliterate the hydrocele sac many fluids have been injected, e.g. brandy, port, sugar, ginger, tincture of iodine, talc and phenol. The technique is rediscovered every few years. It is at best painful and at worst dangerous. The vaginal sac is converted into a honeycomb of little hydroceles

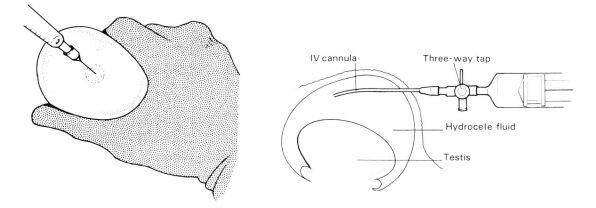

Fig. 36.3 Aspiration of a hydrocele.

which readily become infected and need orchiectomy [1,9,10].

Operations for hydrocele

Make a transverse scrotal incision. Seize and empty the sac to make it easier to deliver the testicle. When the sac is thin, it may be opened, everted and closed behind the testicle [11,12] (Fig. 36.4). An alternative is to plicate the sac [13] (Fig. 36.5). More often the sac is thick and stiff: it is cut away leaving a frill round the epididymis, which must be oversewn with fine catgut to achieve perfect haemostasis (Fig. 36.6).

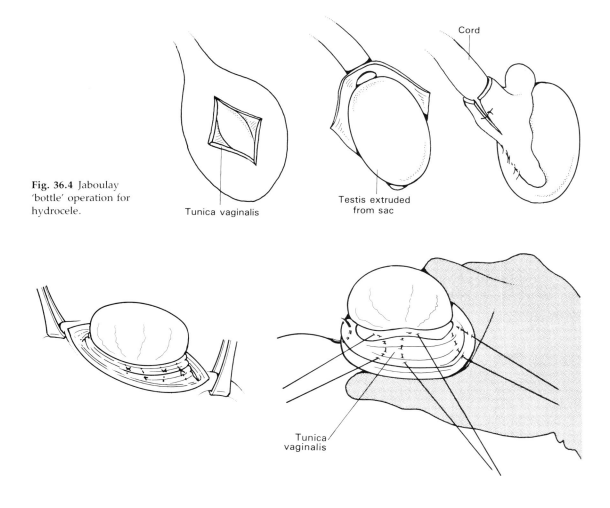

Fig. 36.4 Jaboulay 'bottle' operation for hydrocele.

Fig. 36.5 Lord's plication for hydrocele.

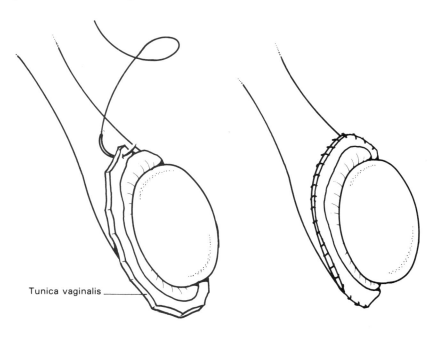

Tunica vaginalis

Fig. 36.6 Radical cure of hydrocele. The surplus tunica vaginalis testis is excised and the edge oversewn to effect haemostasis.

The main complication with these, as with any operations on the testis, is haematoma. Haemostasis at every stage must be perfect: the bipolar diathermy avoids the slight risk of coagulating the vessels of the cord while the dartos and skin are closed with continuous catgut.

Cysts of the epididymis

Cysts of the epididymis arise as diverticula of the vasa efferentia testis (Fig. 36.7). Little attention has been given to their aetiology. They vary in size from a pea to a large apple and are nearly always multilocular.

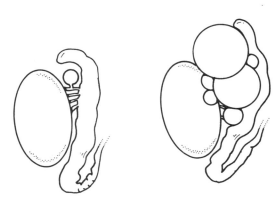

Fig. 36.7 Cysts of epididymis are diverticula of the vasa efferentia testis.

The epididymal cysts lie behind the testis, and the diagnosis is often confused by a coexisting hydrocele. They are translucent. Aspiration withdraws clear watery fluid, sometimes as opalescent as lime-water, sometimes creamy with spermatozoa — hence the common alternative term spermatocele.

Cysts of the epididymis need treatment only when they become so bulky that they bother the patient. Aspiration is futile: they always recur. Claims are frequently made (see p. 566) that aspiration and injection will cure them, but the treatment is painful and seldom effective.

Removal of epididymal cysts

Deliver the testis through a transverse scrotal incision. The cysts are easily dissected from the rest of the epididymis up to the hilum when they burst. It is not necessary to remove them intact. The usual precautions are taken to avoid a haematoma when closing the scrotal incision.

Benign cysts of the testis

These are so rare that it is usually a mistake to consider the diagnosis before the testis has been removed since teratoma is much more likely. Nevertheless, they do occur and improved techniques of ultrasound scanning make it justifiable on rare occasions to explore them with a view to carrying out a conservative operation [14,15] (see p. 583).

Torsion of the testis

Torsion of the testis was first described by Delasiauve (1840) [16]. It occurs at any age, but there is an anatomical distinction between the extravaginal torsion which occurs in the newborn, and the more common intravaginal torsion which is seen in all other ages [17−21].

Extravaginal torsion (Fig. 36.8) usually occurs at the time of birth, and is noticed as a firm mass in the scrotum [22−24], but it has been diagnosed by ultrasound *in utero* [25].

Intravaginal torsion requires a capacious tunica which is the rule with undescended testes, where torsion is a common complication. Since this is a congenital anomaly and is often present on both sides, bilateral torsion occurs in about 10% of cases.

Clinical features

Torsion is more common in childhood [24] and around puberty, but can occur at any age. It is more common in cold weather [21].

There are two distinct clinical pictures. Half have a clear history of warning attacks of testicular pain, relieved spontaneously. The other half have no warning, and may be woken from sleep with pain and swelling in the testis: sometimes accompanied by vomiting and shock. In patients with warning attacks, it may be possible to detect a difference in the way the testicle lies in the scrotum — somewhat more horizontally on one side than on the other. In the acute attack it may be possible to see that one testicle lies more horizontally but usually the testicle is too tender to be palpated with accuracy [18].

Investigations

None of the methods of investigating torsion are completely reliable. If it is possible to obtain a Doppler scan or radioisotope scan *en route* to the operating theatre, this may save the occasional needless exploration of a patient with acute epididymitis [26−28] but must not delay exploration because if the testicle is to be saved the sooner it is untwisted the better.

Differential diagnosis

In infants scrotal haemorrhage [28], fat necrosis [29] and acute idiopathic scrotal oedema [30] are mimics of torsion in children. In older children acute epididymoorchitis can exactly resemble torsion (Figs 36.9 & 36.10), and sometimes it is only the presence of obvious urinary infection which permits the surgeon to refrain from exploring the testicle, though even then it might be wise to operate in order to decompress the tunica albuginea (see p. 558).

About 15% of cancers present with an inflammatory mass — often surprisingly acute.

Mumps and other kinds of viral orchitis can seldom be clearly distinguished from torsion unless there is an epidemic or the patient has had parotitis within the last few days. Again, no harm is likely to follow exploration, for to decompress the ischaemic testis by incision of the tunica albuginea may prevent atrophy (see p. 558). It is worth remembering that mumps does not affect the testicle of prepubertal boys [18].

It is seldom possible to distinguish between torsion of the entire testicle and torsion of one of its appendages unless one can actually see the black swelling of the twisted appendix through the thin skin of the scrotum. This is uncommon but obvious. Much more often the whole testicle and scrotum are so oedematous that no distinct physical signs can be made out and the scrotum has to be explored [31] (Fig. 36.11).

Other causes of acute ischaemia in the testicle should be remembered: they include infarction in sickle-cell disease [32], Henoch−Schoenlein

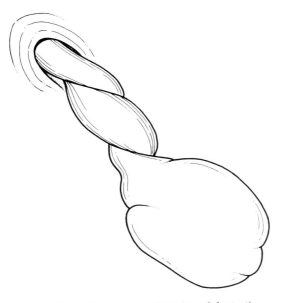

Fig. 36.8 Neonatal extravaginal torsion of the testis.

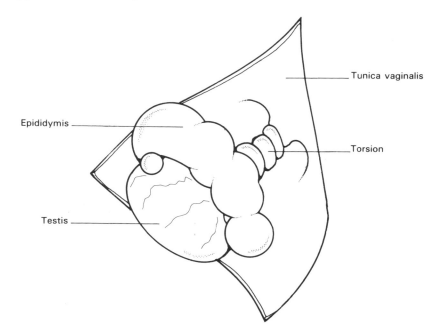

Epididymis

Tunica vaginalis

Torsion

Testis

Fig. 36.9 Intravaginal torsion of the testis.

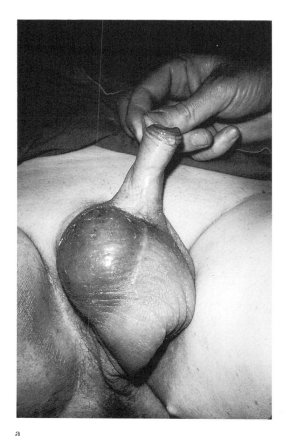

a

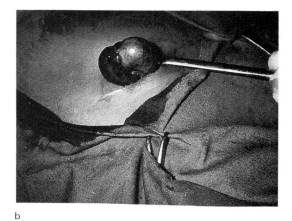

b

Fig. 36.10 (a) The scrotum in torsion of the right testis. (b) Torsion in an undescended testis.

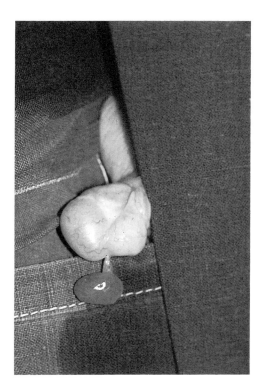

Fig. 36.11 Torsion of the appendix testis.

purpura [33] and coincidental strangulation of a hernia [34].

Treatment

Deliver the testicle through a transverse scrotal incision. Open the tunica. You may find a grossly distended black epididymis and a pale testis. Untwist the stalk. To decide whether or not to remove the testicle incise the tunica albuginea. If it bleeds it means the blood supply is not entirely thrombosed. Complete this incision through the tunica vaginalis to relieve pressure within its closed compartment: it may prevent atrophy.

The precondition for torsion is present on the other side so often that it justifies prophylactic fixation every time. It had been suggested that a twisted testicle not untwisted in time to prevent shrinkage should be removed, lest it cause damage to the contralateral testis. Experimental studies do not confirm this suggestion [35–37].

With prompt exploration, many testes can be untwisted and preserved [38]. Unfortunately, torsion is seldom diagnosed in time even when patients give a history of previous episodes of suggestive pain [39,40]. There is only one rule — to explore every case where the diagnosis of epididymitis is not absolutely certain: investi-

gations such as ultrasound, isotope scanning and Doppler studies of blood flow should not be used to delay the operation, nor should they ever be entirely trusted.

Varicocele

Two systems of veins drain the testicle. The first comprises the internal spermatic vein or veins and flows into the renal vein on the left or the vena cava on the right. The second system drains through the cremasteric vein into the deep epigastric vein [41]. Dilatation of either or both of these groups of veins constitutes a varicocele, but some dilatation is entirely physiological (Fig. 36.12).

In boys between 6 and 19 years of age, varicoceles were never found below the age of 9: after the age of 10 the incidence rose to 16%, occurring nearly always on the left [42]. In healthy recruits, 8% had varicoceles without atrophy of the testis [43].

Pathology

In a very small number of patients a varicocele follows obstruction to the spermatic veins, classically when a carcinoma of the kidney invades and obstructs the left renal vein, but it is also seen with retroperitoneal metastases from a cancer of the testis.

Varicocele and infertility

Varicocele is thought to raise the temperature of the testicle and to cause subfertility and testicular atrophy [44,45]. Biopsies of testicles on the side with the varicocele are said to show increased Leydig cell activity, deoxyribonucleic acid polymerase activity and changes in the endothelium [45,46] and an LHRH stimulation test has been suggested to detect such damage to the testis [47].

In the few controlled studies that have been carried out none show any improvement after varicocelectomy either in pregnancy rates or semen analysis [48–50]. These observations should be borne in mind when considering proposals to operate on varicoceles in normal adolescents [51], and even to do the operation for varicoceles which cannot be seen, but have to be detected by means of a Doppler scan [52,53].

The whole basis of this practice is questioned: 'it is very strange that a unilateral vascular abnormality should produce a bilateral testicular

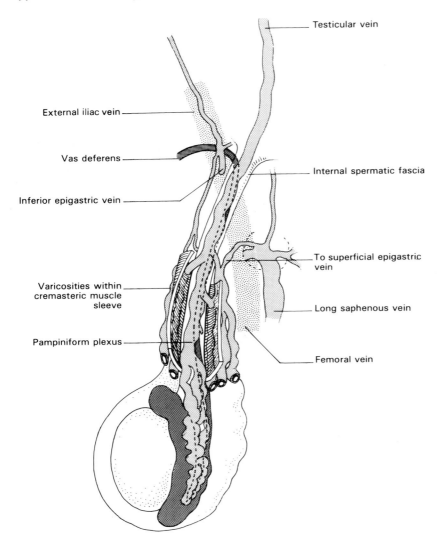

Testicular vein

External iliac vein

Vas deferens

Inferior epigastric vein

Internal spermatic fascia

To superficial epigastric vein

Varicosities within cremasteric muscle sleeve

Long saphenous vein

Pampiniform plexus

Femoral vein

Fig. 36.12 Venous drainage of the testis.

lesion' [54]. So too is the concept of retrograde flow of blood down the testicular veins; 'None of the authors make it clear just where they imagine this retrogradely flowing blood goes to and how a high concentration of hormones in the venous blood reaches the testis. It is to be hoped that they are not advocating a return to pre-Harveian cardiovascular ideas or suggesting that blood can flow from vein to artery against the pressure gradient' [54].

Clinical features

Patients may complain of a swelling or a dragging discomfort in the testicle. Physical examination shows a collection of dilated veins — the classical 'bag of worms' — with a cough impulse. The veins empty when the patient is supine (Fig. 36.13).

Treatment

1 Embolism. The testicular veins may be embolized by injecting them with Gianturco coils or thrombin via an angiographic catheter (Fig. 36.14).

2 Laparoscopic technique. Through a laparoscope the testicular veins may be separated from the artery and clipped near the internal inguinal ring (Fig. 36.15).

3 Through a small crease incision over the internal ring, the external oblique is slit open, the internal oblique and transversus are split in the line of their fibres giving access to the retroperitoneal fat. The testicular vessels are seen just as they curl round the inferior epigastric artery. The testicular artery is carefully dissected from the veins, which are divided between ligatures (Fig. 36.16).

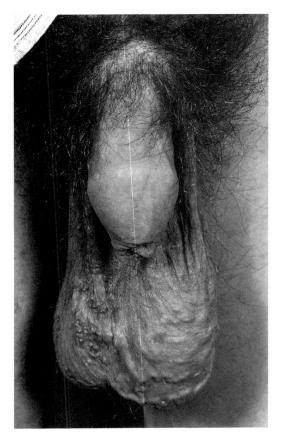

Fig. 36.13 Varicocele.

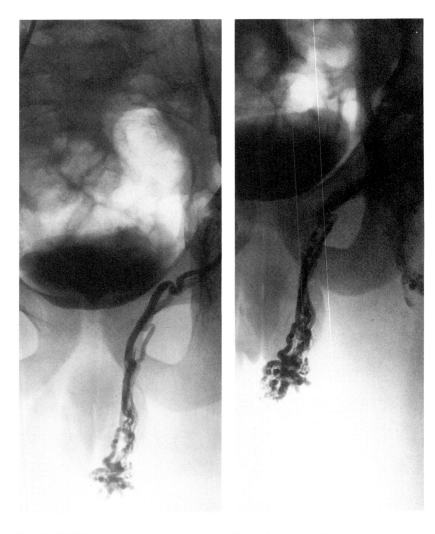

Fig. 36.14 Phlebogram showing retrograde filling of varicocele from spermatic vein.

4 The spermatic cord may be exposed as it emerges from the external ring, and all the veins divided between ligatures outside the internal spermatic fascia, sparing the testicular artery and its immediately adjacent veins (Fig. 36.17).

Varicocelectomy is not entirely without complications: the author has seen two patients where it was followed by infarction of the testis.

Orchialgia

Nux amatoris

This painful condition is sometimes seen in young men who have become sexually excited without the opportunity to ejaculate. On examination the veins of the cord are tender and distended. The condition may be accompanied by so much discomfort in the iliac fossa that a diagnosis of appendicitis is contemplated. The venous congestion is relieved by a warm bath.

Idiopathic

Pain arising from the testicle for no discoverable reason is not uncommon and presents a baffling clinical picture. One must be aware of the possibility of pain referred from a renal calculus or a leaking aortic aneurysm [55], and one can never be too careful to exclude carcinoma. Drugs, e.g. mazindol, have occasionally been implicated, though the mechanism is not understood [56]. All too often some trivial anomaly is found, e.g. a minute cyst of the epididymis or an innocent hydatid of Morgagni, and an unnecessary operation is performed. Frequently, the symptoms

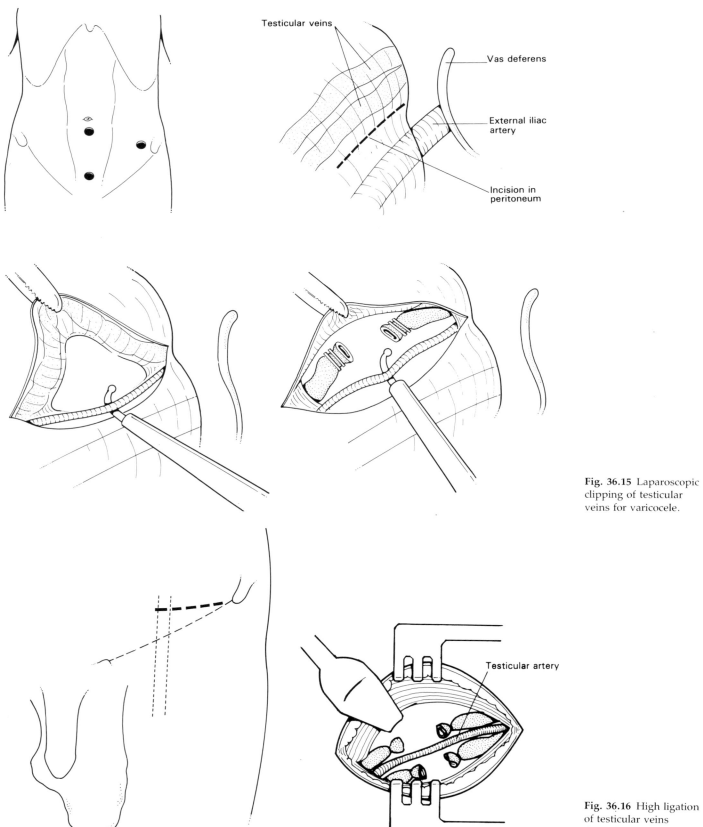

Testicular veins

Vas deferens

External iliac
artery

Incision in
peritoneum

Fig. 36.15 Laparoscopic
clipping of testicular
veins for varicocele.

Testicular artery

Fig. 36.16 High ligation
of testicular veins
through the inguinal
approach.

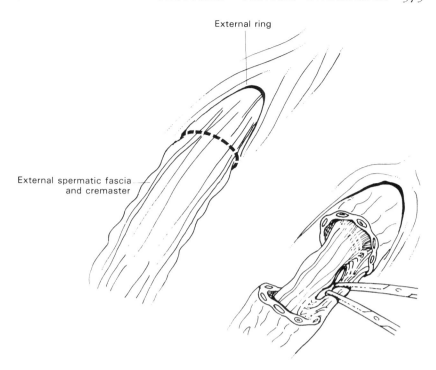

External ring

External spermatic fascia
and cremaster

Fig. 36.17 Low ligation
of testicular veins at the
external ring.

seem to follow vasectomy especially when this
was followed by a haematoma.

However, there remain a small number of
patients with pain of unknown origin. In some
there is a deep-seated psychological disorder,
and any surgical intervention only makes things
worse. Orchiectomy is usually followed by a
return of the pain on the other side [57].

References

1 Landes RR, Leonhardt KO (1967) The history of
hydrocele. *Urol Surv* 17: 135.

2 Wallace AF (1960) Aetiology of the idiopathic
hydrocele. *Br J Urol* 32: 79.

3 Klin B, Efrati Y, Mor A, Vinograd I (1992) Unilateral
hydroureteronephrosis caused by abdominoscrotal
hydrocele. *J Urol* 148: 384.

4 Lascelles PT, Annis D (1969) Transport of intravenously administered ^{131}IRIHSA into primary
hydroceles and the tunical sac of patients undergoing herniorrhaphy. *Br J Surg* 56: 405.

5 Huggins CB, Entz FH (1931) Absorption from tunica
vaginalis testis, hydrocele and spermatocele. *J Urol*
25: 447.

6 Sanjurjo LA (1970) Parasitic diseases of the genito-
urinary system, in: Campbell MF, Harrison JH (eds)
Urology, vol. 1, pp. 480–511. Philadelphia: WB
Saunders.

7 Malik MOA, Ibrahim A (1982) Scrotal swellings in
Sudanese patients: a surgical pathology study. *Int
Surg* 67: 513.

8 Kokotas N, Kontogeorgos L, Kyriakidia A (1983)

9 Calcification of the tunica vaginalis. *Br J Urol* 55:
128.

9 Badenoch DF, Fowler CG, Jenkins BJ, Roberts JV,
Tiptaft RC (1987) Aspiration and instillation of tetra-
cycline in the treatment of testicular hydrocele. *Br
J Urol* 59: 172.

10 Breda G, Giunta A, Gherardi L, Xausa D, Silvestre
P, Tamai A (1992) Treatment of hydrocele: randomised prospective study of simple aspiration and
sclerotherapy with tetracycline. *Br J Urol* 70: 76.

11 Jaboulay M (1902) *Chirurgie des Centres Nerveuses
des Visceres et des Membres*. vol. 2, p. 192. Lyons:
Storck.

12 Andrews EW (1907) The 'bottle' operation for the
radical cure of hydrocele. *Ann Surg* 46: 915.

13 Lord PH (1964) A bloodless operation for the radical
cure of idiopathic hydrocele. *Br J Surg* 51: 914.

14 Dmochowski RR, Rudy DC, Weitzner S, Corriere
JN (1989) Simple cyst of the testis. *J Urol* 142: 1078.

15 Shapeero LC, Vorderkark JS (1993) Epidermoid cysts
of testes and role of sonography. *Urology* 41: 75.

16 Delasiauve LJF (1840) Descente tardive du testicule
gauche, prise pour une hernie stranglée. *Rev Med
Franc Etrang* 1: 363.

17 Chapman RH, Walton AJ (1972) Torsion of the
testis and its appendages. *Br Med J* 1: 164.

18 Sparks JP (1971) Torsion of the testis. *Ann Roy Coll
Surg Engl* 49: 77.

19 Dennis MJS, Fahim SF, Doyle PT (1987) Testicular
torsion in older men. *Br Med J* 294: 1680.

20 Creagh TA, McDermott TE, McLean PA, Walsh A
(1988) Intermittent torsion of the testis. *Br Med J*
297: 525.

21 Shukla RB, Kelly DG, Daly L, Guiney EJ (1982)
Association of cold weather with testicular torsion.

Br Med J 285: 1495.

22 Anderson JB, Williamson RCN (1988) Testicular torsion in Bristol: a 25 year review. *Br J Surg* 75: 988.

23 Das S, Singer A (1990) Controversies of perinatal torsion of the spermatic cord: a review. *J Urol* 132: 231.

24 Brown SM, Casillas VJ, Montalvo B, Albores-Saavedra J (1990) Intrauterine spermatic cord torsion in the newborn: sonographic and pathologic correlation. *Radiology* 177: 755.

25 Macnicol MF (1974) Torsion of the testis in childhood. *Br J Surg* 61: 905.

26 Brereton RJ (1981) Limitations of the Doppler flow meter in the diagnosis of the 'acute scrotum' in boys. *Br J Urol* 53: 380.

27 Burks DD, Markey BJ, Burkhard TK, Balsara ZN, Haluszka MM, Canning DA (1990) Suspected testicular torsion and ischemia: evaluation with color Doppler sonography. *Radiology* 175: 815.

28 Fenner MN, Roszhart DA, Texter JH (1991) Testicular scanning: evaluating the acute scrotum in the clinical setting. *Urology* 38: 237.

29 Ong TH, Solomon JR (1973) Fat necrosis of the scrotum. *J Ped Surg* 8: 919.

30 Najmaldin A, Burge DM (1987) Acute idiopathic scrotal oedema: incidence, manifestations and aetiology. *Br J Surg* 74: 634.

31 Dix VW (1931) On torsion of the appendages of testis and epididymis. *Br J Urol* 3: 245.

32 Urwin GH, Kehoe N, Dundas S, Fox M (1986) Testicular infarction in a patient with sickle cell trait. *Br J Urol* 58: 340.

33 Eadie DGA, Higgins PM (1964) Apparent torsion of the testicle in a case of Henoch–Schoenlein purpura. *Br J Surg* 51: 634.

34 Sturdy DE (1960) Incarcerated inguinal hernia in infancy with testicular gangrene. *Br J Surg* 48: 210.

35 Turner TT (1987) On unilateral testicular and epididymal torsion: no effect on the contralateral testis. *J Urol* 138: 1285.

36 Anderson JB, Williamson RCN (1990) Fertility after torsion of the spermatic cord. *Br J Urol* 65: 225.

37 Sade M, Amato S, Buyuksu C, Mertan S, Canda MS, Kalanoglu N (1989) The effect of testicular torsion on the contralateral testis and the value of various types of treatment. *Br J Urol* 62: 69.

38 Brasso K, Andersen L, Kay L, Wille-Jorgensen P, Linnet L, Egense J (1993) Testicular torsion: a follow up study. *Scand J Urol Nephrol* 27: 1.

39 Bennett S, Nicholson MS, Little TM (1987) Torsion of the testis: why is the prognosis so poor? *Br Med J* 294: 824.

40 Kiely EM (1987) Torsion of the testis: why is the prognosis so poor? *Br Med J* 294: 1552.

41 Hanley HG, Harrison RG (1962) The nature and surgical treatment of varicocele. *Br J Surg* 50: 64.

42 Oster J (1971) Varicocele in children and adolescents. *Scand J Urol Nephrol* 5: 27.

43 Clarke BG (1966) Incidence of varicocele in normal men and among men of different ages. *J Am Med Assoc* 198: 1121.

44 Tulloch WS (1955) Varicocele in subfertility: results of treatment. *Br Med J* 2: 356.

45 Hadziselimovic F, Herzog B, Liebundgut B, Jenny P, Buser M (1989) Testicular and vascular changes in children and adults with varicocele. *J Urol* 142: 583.

46 Fujisawa M, Yoshida S, Matsumoto O, Kojima K, Kamidono S (1988) Deoxyribonucleic acid polymerase activity in the testes of infertile men with varicocele. *Fertil Steril* 50: 795.

47 Kass EJ, Freitas JE, Bour JB (1989) Adolescent varicocele: objective indications for treatment. *J Urol* 142: 579.

48 Nilsson S, Edvinsson A, Nilsson B (1979) Improvement of semen and pregnancy rate after ligation and division of the internal spermatic vein: fact or fiction? *Br J Urol* 51: 591.

49 Vermeulen A, Vandeweghe M (1984) Improved fertility after varicocele correction: fact or fiction? *Fertil Steril* 42: 249.

50 Baker HWG, Burger HG, de Kretser DM, Hudson B, Rennie GC, Straffon WGE (1985) Testicular vein ligation and fertility in men with varicoceles. *Br Med J* 291: 1678.

51 Steckel J, Dicker AP, Goldstein M (1993) Relationship between varicocele size and response to varicocelectomy. *J Urol* 149: 769.

52 Okuyama A, Nakamura M, Namiki M et al. (1988) Surgical repair of varicocele at puberty: preventive treatment for fertility improvement. *J Urol* 139: 562.

53 Bsat FA, Masabni R (1988) Effectiveness of varicocelectomy in varicoceles diagnosed by physical examination versus Doppler studies. *Fertil Steril* 50: 321.

54 Setchell BP (1978) *The Mammalian Testis*, pp. 420–1. London: Elek.

55 Cawthorn SJ, Giddings AEB, Taylor RS, Thomas MH (1991) Isolated testicular pain: an unrecognised symptom of the leaking aortic aneurysm. *Br J Surg* 78: 886.

56 McEwen J, Meyboom RHB (1983) Testicular pain caused by mazindol. *Br Med J* 287: 1763.

57 Costabile RA, Hahn M, McLeod DG (1991) Chronic orchialgia in the pain-prone patient: the clinical perspective. *J Urol* 146: 1571.

Chapter 37: Testicle — neoplasms

History

The distinction between solid tumours of the testicle (lethal) and cystic (innocent) ones was known to the Romans. William Harvey advised ligature of the testicular artery as a safer alternative to castration; Astley Cooper researched the lymphatic drainage of the testicle — and the method of tumour spread [1]. The crucial biological difference between the two main histological types of testicular tumour was discovered by Chevassu who coined the terms seminoma and teratoma [2].

Kocher was the first to attempt to cure testicular cancer by radical node dissection: both his patients were far advanced and both died [3]. In 1926, Cairns reviewed these attempts and concluded that they were futile [4]. Within a few years radiotherapy replaced surgery for lymph nodes in some centres: in others the morbidity caused by overdoses of radiation discredited it. So, for the next 50 years a rather meaningless contest began between radical node dissection versus radiation [1] — meaningless because advocates of either method were always comparing tumours that were classified by different systems and staged by different criteria. Eventually, the argument was overtaken by the introduction of the tumour markers, combination chemotherapy and a better understanding of the natural history of these tumours.

Aetiology

Incidence

In England and Wales about 900 new cases of testicular tumour are registered each year, with only 157 deaths — a crude death rate of 6.5 and incidence of 37.5 per million. This is less than 1% of all cancers in males, but in the age group 15–50 it is 10 times more common than any other cancer except of the skin [5].

The incidence has been rising over the last century [6] in Denmark [7,8] Scotland [9],

Connecticut [10] and the UK [11] (Fig. 37.1). Not only are there more cases but they occur in younger men. Fortunately the death rate is falling (Fig. 37.1b).

The age incidence of testicular cancer has always been unlike most cancers, which increases with age. Testicular cancer is a disease of youth: rare before puberty, peaking around the age of 20 for teratomas and about the age of 30 for seminomas [1] (Fig. 37.2).

Genetic influences affect the incidence of testicular cancer. It is virtually unknown in black men in Africa, the West Indies and America [12–14] and when it occurs, it seems to have a better prognosis [12].

Cancer is associated with some human leucocyte antigens (HLA) and has been reported in families [15–22].

One in every 10 testicular tumours occur in men with an undescended testicle. In these cryptorchid men the cancer affects the descended testicle in about 10%. The higher the undescended testicle the more likely it is to become malignant [10]. Cryptorchidism is not the only congenital anomaly associated with cancer: inguinal hernia, torsion, hypospadias, ectopic and duplex kidney and intersex are also associated. Indeed dysgenetic gonads are so prone to cancer that they must always be removed (see p. 442). Mumps is also a possible aetiological factor [5,17].

Trauma

A previous history of trauma is common in men with testicular tumour, and trauma might precipitate the malignancy, but it is never possible to be sure that the injury did not bring a hitherto unnoticed lump to the attention of the patient [5].

Hormones may be implicated in the aetiology of testis cancer: stilboestrol in pregnancy increases the risk of maldescent and testis cancer in the offspring [23] and it is suggested that high levels of natural oestrogens may be equally important [14,17,24].

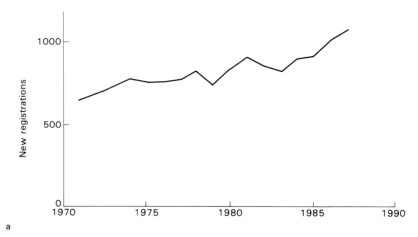

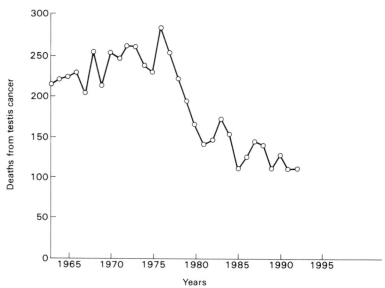

Fig. 37.1 (a) Number of new cases of testicular cancer reported in England and Wales, and (b) deaths from testis cancer (from the Registrar General, Office of Population Census and Surveys). Note that although the number of new cases continues to rise, the death rate has fallen rapidly.

A common theme behind these aetiological factors may be failure of germ cell differentiation leading to carcinoma *in situ* [5].

Pathology

Any tissue in the testicle may undergo malignant change. Most arise from germ cells (gonadocytes), and as a group are referred to as germ cell tumours (Fig. 37.3).

The former confusion of classification has now been largely resolved [25–27]. The entire spectrum of germ cell tumours may arise from the gonadocyte. There may be only one kind of tissue in the tumour but more often there is a mixture, and the prognosis depends on how malignant are each of the tissues present in the mixture, and how much there is of each [26–28].

The variety of these tissues recalls the amazing embryological journey of the germ cells from the yolk sac, across the coelom, to the gonadal ridge (see p. 538) where they differentiate into Leydig, Sertoli and more germ cells. The germ cells continue to divide to form diploid primary spermatocytes, haploid secondary spermatocytes and finally spermatozoa from which may arise every cell that may occur in the fetus, yolk sac or placenta, in benign or malignant variations.

Germ cells have clear cytoplasm full of glycogen and stain for placental alkaline phosphatase (PLAP). If held up in their journey from yolk sac to gonadal ridge, they may give rise to extragonadal germ cell tumours in the para-aortic region, mediastinum or pineal gland [25]. If they arise in streak gonads in intersex they are called dysgerminomas (Fig. 37.4). The primordial germ cells, the atypical cells found in seminiferous tubules and seminoma cells are probably identical [26].

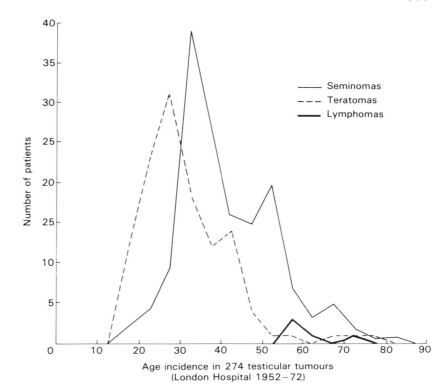

Fig. 37.2 Age incidence of germ cell tumours.

Age incidence in 274 testicular tumours
(London Hospital 1952–72)

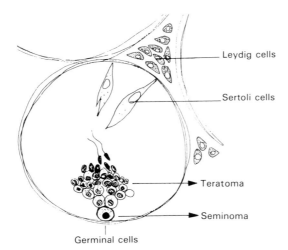

Fig. 37.3 Cellular origin of germ cell tumours.

Seminoma

When germ cells are the only element present, the tumour is called a seminoma. There is a peak age incidence at about 30 — a decade later than other germ cell tumours. Macroscopically, it forms a pinky-grey lobulated swelling (Fig. 37.5). Microscopically, sheets of glycogen-filled cells, staining for placental alkaline phosphatase (PLAP), are interspersed with lymphocytes.

Seminomas are part of a continuum. At one extreme is the well-differentiated spermatocytic seminoma of older men, whose cells resemble spermatocytes [25] (Fig. 37.6). They rarely metastasize [29,30] and are highly chemosensitive [31]. At the other extreme is the anaplastic seminoma (Fig. 37.7) with nuclear pleomorphism, scanty lymphocytes and giant cells resembling syncytiotrophoblast which stain for beta human chorionic gonadotrophin (HCG) and raise the serum HCG [28,31,32] — verging with embryonal carcinoma [26].

Embryonal carcinoma

In embryonal carcinoma the macroscopic appearance is even more blotchy. Microscopically, among sheets of cells and embryoid bodies there are areas with papillary and pseudoglandular patterns arranged in single or double layers of cells which stain for alpha fetoprotein (AFP), betraying their yolk sac origin [25–27] (Fig. 37.8).

Yolk sac tumours

Pure yolk sac tumours are found in infants. In adults, yolk sac tissue is often found in mixed tumours. AFP can be detected in the tissue by immunoperoxidase staining and in the serum is a useful marker of response to treatment [25–27] (Fig. 37.9).

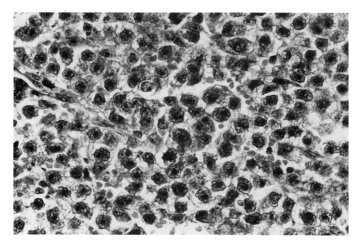

Fig. 37.4 Dysgerminoma.

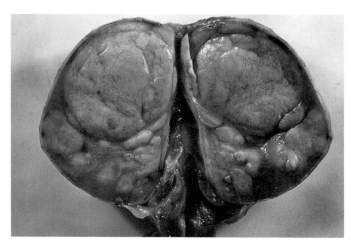

Fig. 37.5 Cut surface of seminoma.

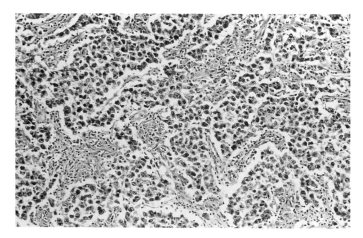

Fig. 37.6 Differentiated seminoma.

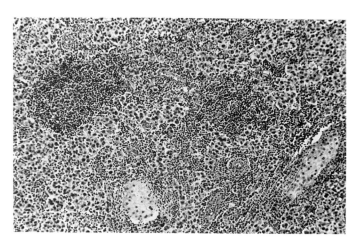

Fig. 37.7 Anaplastic seminoma.

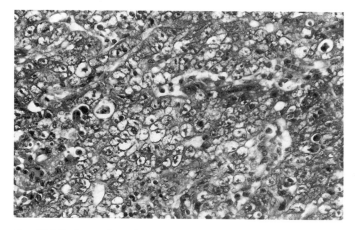

Fig. 37.8 Embryonal carcinoma.

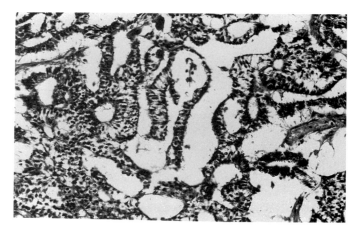

Fig. 37.9 Yolk sac tumour (courtesy of Dr Suhail Baithun).

Epidermoid cyst

This is very rare and probably benign. Clinically, it presents as a hard discrete lump in the testicle. The author has performed one segmental resection (with a clear margin) at the patient's insistence but does not know the long-term follow-up. Clinically, it is impossible to distinguish from mature teratoma and the safest course is usually to perform an orchiectomy [28].

A very rare benign tumour, thought to be of Müllerian duct origin, can arise in the epididymis [39] (Fig. 37.14).

Teratocarcinoma

In teratocarcinoma the tissues are similar to those of the developing fetus and have a spectrum of appearances from the most benign to the most malignant. When only mature tissue is present, the tumour is referred to as mature teratoma (Fig. 37.10). Of the malignant tissues the worst is choriocarcinoma: it may be the only tissue present, but is more often present as part of a mixture (Fig. 37.11).

Non-germ cell tumours

In addition to germ cell tumours, benign and malignant tumours can arise in any of the other tissues present in the testis, epididymis or their coverings.

Leydig cell tumours

These are composed of normal looking interstitial cells and secrete testosterone. Before puberty they give rise to precocious sexual development: after puberty they cause feminization with gynaecomastia [33,34] (Fig. 37.12).

Sertoli cell tumours

These are even more rare. They occasionally metastasize and occasionally cause gynaecomastia [34–36] (Fig. 37.13).

Connective tissue tumours

Connective tissue tumours from the tissues in and around the testis can give rise to angioma, fibroma or neuroma. The tunica albuginea often forms benign fibromatous nodules: rarely it may form mesothelioma or even fibrosarcoma, most often in children [37,38].

Classification

Given the wide variety of tissues which can arise from germ cells the permutations that are possible in a given tumour make classification difficult (Table 37.1). Many systems have been proposed in the past. The classification adopted by the World Health Organization (WHO) is based on that of the US Armed Forces Institute of Pathology [41]. British surgeons are more familiar with that of the Institute of Urology [43].

More important than nomenclature is to understand the natural history of the various components in these mixtures since the behaviour of a given tumour largely depends on how much of each is present and how malignant it is. For example, pure seminoma is very sensitive to radiation and chemotherapy but metastasizes early to lymph nodes. Choriocarcinoma invades vessels, spreads rapidly through the body and is resistant to chemotherapy and radiotherapy.

Tumour markers [44]

Alpha fetoprotein

In fetal life AFP is the second most common protein next to albumen [25,45,46]; it is made by the endodermal layer of cells in the yolk sac. Its function is not known, but it allows yolk sac elements to be identified by immunoperoxidase staining histologically. It is present in many teratomas, some seminomas, but not in 'pure' seminoma or choriocarcinoma. Normal adults have a serum level of less than 20 μg/l. It has a half-life of a week. The rise and fall of serum AFP provides a useful marker for the response of metastases to chemotherapy or surgery.

Human chorionic gonadotrophin (HCG)

HCG is made by the syncytiotrophoblast of the placenta. The normal level is less than 1 ng/ml, and its half-life 1 day. Its molecule is similar to growth hormone and other messenger hormones, with a common body and two arms like a lobster (alpha and beta). These arms differ in the details of the last dozen amino acids on the beta arm. The beta arm (beta HCG) can be detected by immunoperoxidase staining in fixed tissue. HCG is always raised in choriocarcinoma, often in embryonal carcinoma and in about 10% of so-called pure seminoma [27,44].

Table 37.1 Comparative table of histological classifications of testis tumours.

Friedman & Moore 1946 [42]	Institute of Urology 1976 [43]	WHO 1977 [41] *Tumours of one histological type*	WHO 1977 [41] *Tumours of more than one histological type*	Friedman 1988 [26]
				Germinoma in situ
Seminoma	Seminoma	Seminoma		Germinoma
		Spermatocytic seminoma		
Teratoma	Teratoma differentiated	Teratoma mature		Teratoma
Teratocarcinoma	Malignant teratoma intermediate	{ Teratoma mixed / Teratoma with malignant transformation	Embryonal carcinoma and teratoma (teratocarcinoma)	Teratocarcinoma
Embryonal carcinoma	Malignant teratoma undifferentiated	{ Embryonal carcinoma / Yolk sac tumour (embryonal carcinoma, infantile type, endodermal sinus tumour) / Polyembryoma		{ Embryonal carcinoma / Yolk sac tumour
Choriocarcinoma	Malignant teratoma trophoblastic	Choriocarcinoma	Choriocarcinoma and any other type (specify) / Other combinations (specify)	Choriocarcinoma

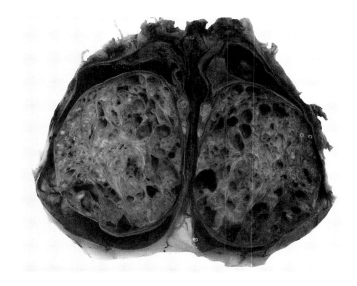

Fig. 37.10 Mature teratoma, macroscopic view.

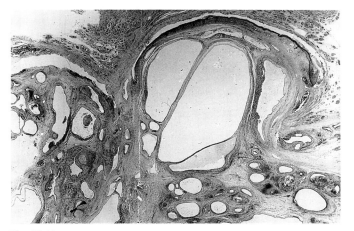

Fig. 37.11a

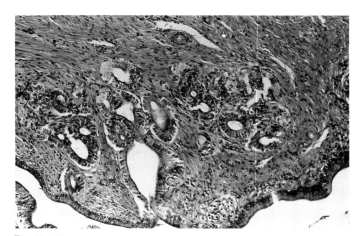

Fig. 37.11b

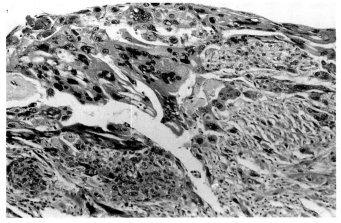

Fig. 37.11c

Fig. 37.11 Variations in the histological appearance of non-seminomatous germ cell tumours. (a) Teratocarcinoma. (b) Immature teratoma with occasional organoid changes. (c) Trophoblastic teratoma showing cyto- and syncytiotrophoblast.

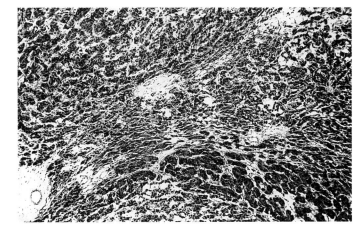

Fig. 37.12 Leydig cell tumour.

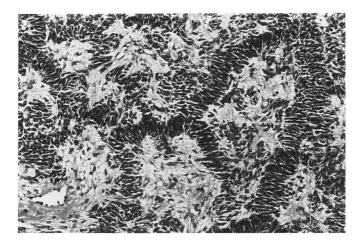

Fig. 37.13 Sertoli cell tumour (courtesy of Dr Suhail Baithun).

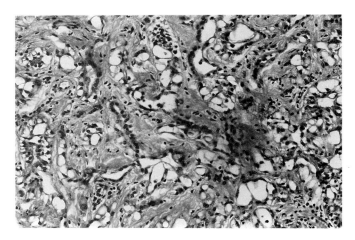

Fig. 37.14 Epididymal tumour (courtesy of Dr Suhail Baithun).

Placental alkaline phosphatase (PLAP)

PLAP is another placental enzyme which is present in the cytoplasm of germ cells and seminoma cells, and in the serum of men with seminoma [27]. It is a useful marker in the treatment of seminoma.

Method of spread

Direct spread

Germ cell tumours spread by direct invasion from the testicular tubules into the surrounding interstitial spaces, through the rete testis into the epididymis, and finally through the tunica albuginea into the scrotum. They invade the connective tissue and veins of the spermatic cord. The extent of local invasion determines the T element of the TNM system of classification of the stage of the tumour.

Lymphatic spread

The lymphatics of the testis arise between the tubules and drain along the spermatic cord to the primary regional lymph nodes around the origin of the testicular arteries — the first lymph nodes to be involved in testicular cancer [47,48]. Secondary lymph node spread occurs upwards from the para-aortic nodes to the mediastinum, and enters the systemic circulation via the thoracic duct. There may also be secondary spread downwards to the lymph nodes of the pelvis (Fig. 37.15).

Haematogenous spread

Testicular tumours with trophoblastic elements erode veins and spread via the bloodstream at an early stage. Choriocarcinoma is notorious for this — haemoptysis from lung metastases being a classic presenting symptom.

Clinical features

Lump

The most common and important symptom and sign is a lump in the body of the testis: all lumps in the testis demand exploration. For all practical purposes there are no benign hard lumps in the testicle [1,46].

Palpation of a lump in the testicle is difficult when it is surrounded by normal testicular tissue or arises near the epididymis (Fig. 37.16). Either case calls for an ultrasound scan, measurement of tumour markers and follow-up examination [46]. If there is still any doubt, the testis must be explored (see below).

Inflammation

About 15% of tumours have physical signs of inflammation — the testicle is swollen, red and warm — features suggesting epididymoorchitis, or possibly neglected torsion (Fig. 37.17). What makes a testicular cancer inflamed is not clear, perhaps haemorrhage into the tumour [1,46]. Unless the diagnosis of epididymitis is certain beyond any doubt the testicle should be explored.

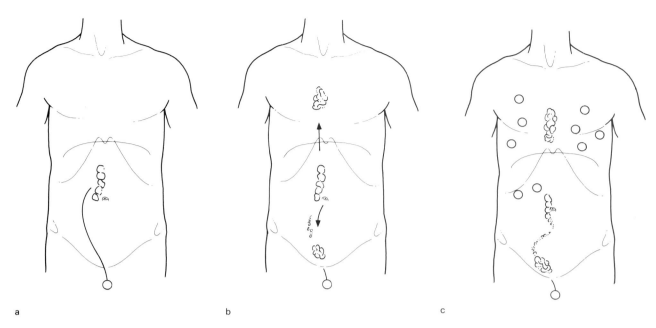

a   b   c

Fig. 37.15 Spread of testis tumours. (a) By lymphatics to the ipsilateral para-aortic lymph nodes (b) Secondary lymphatic spread to the mediastinum and pelvic nodes (c) Haematogenous spread to lungs, etc.

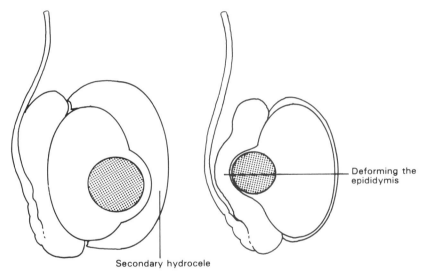

Fig. 37.16 It is difficult to feel a lump in the testicle when it is surrounded by healthy tissue or situated near the epididymis.

Deforming the epididymis

Secondary hydrocele

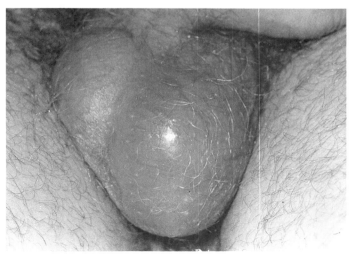

Fig. 37.17 About 15% of testis tumours present with the features of acute inflammation.

Inflammation in an abdominal cryptorchid testicle may present as an acute abdomen [47].

Trauma

Trauma brings another 10% of patients to the doctor. Every case of serious trauma to the testis demands exploration (see p. 558) but one must always be on the alert for coexisting cancer and should warn the patient that orchiectomy may be necessary: at the very least a biopsy must be taken from any suspicious tissue [1,48].

Hydrocele

A small secondary hydrocele is always present when there is a cancer in the testis: very rarely it may be the presenting feature. Larger tumours may be concealed by a thick-walled hydrocele containing turbid fluid through which light will not shine. A hydrocele in a young male always calls for confirmation of the diagnosis by ultrasound, tumour markers and, when in doubt, exploration [46,48].

Other testicular trivia

Beware the young man with vague discomfort in the testicle or the sensation of a lump. Do not be reassured with the finding of a mere varicocele or dismiss his discomfort as adolescent neurosis until you have carefully examined the testicle. Always insist on an ultrasound scan and tumour markers [48]. Varicoceles are very common: testicular tumours are rare; but to miss even one is a tragedy.

Shrinking testis

Sometimes the tumour eats through the testis, leaving behind a scar that shrinks as it heals (Fig. 37.18). The patient notices that his testicle is getting smaller. A small primary tumour may be entirely replaced by a scar, leaving a normal testicle even though the tumour has metastasized widely [46–49].

Gynaecomastia

Gynaecomastia from release of chorionic gonadotrophin can be the first symptom of a testicular tumour. Every young man with swollen breasts must have his testicles carefully examined and his tumour markers measured [1,46].

Backache

When a fit young man complains of vague backache, metastases from a testicular tumour should be excluded even when the testes appear normal. It takes no trouble to scan the testes and abdomen by ultrasound, and to measure the tumour markers [1,46–51].

Investigations

Ultrasound scanning

Ultrasound scanning is non-invasive, quick and cheap [51–53] (Fig. 37.19). It may give false positive findings, and lead to unnecessary exploration but this is better than missing a testicular tumour at a stage when it is small and curable. It

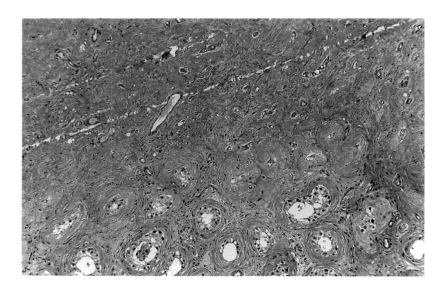

Fig. 37.18 Azzopardi tumour: as the tumour spreads through the testis it leaves a healed scar behind it, and the testicle appears to be shrinking (courtesy of Dr Suhail Baithun).

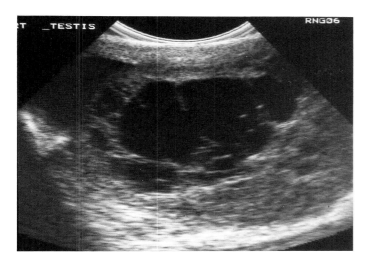

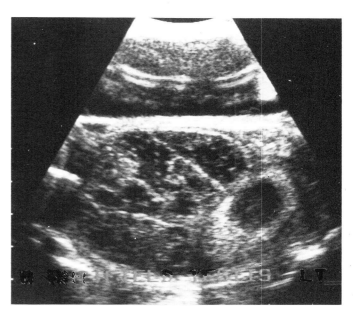

Fig. 37.19 Ultrasound of (a) seminoma of testis and (b) cystic teratoma of testis (courtesy of Dr W. Hately).

is possible to obtain a fine needle biopsy under ultrasound control, though it remains to be seen whether this technique is truly without hazard [53].

Tumour markers

The serum levels should be measured of HCG, AFP and perhaps PLAP and LDH. A 'pregnancy test' is a cheap and readily available way of detecting elevated levels of HCG.

Orchiectomy

The most important investigation is the histological examination of the testis and cord. An incision in the scrotum risks implanting cancer in the scrotal tissues (Fig. 37.20) and may allow lymphatic spread to occur to the inguinal nodes which are otherwise never involved [54]. This risk has recently been discounted by those who have not seen this disaster but those with more experience take every precaution not to seed tumour into the scrotum. This remains a concern in respect of needle biopsies.

Through an inguinal incision, open the external oblique. Place a vascular clamp across the cord at the internal ring to prevent tumour cells escaping as you deliver the testicle from the scrotum (Fig. 37.21). If a patient has a very large tumour it is better to carry the inguinal incision into the neck of the scrotum rather than risk bursting the tumour.

Chevassu's manoeuvre

Once the testis is examined there is usually no doubt about the diagnosis: if uncertainty remains,

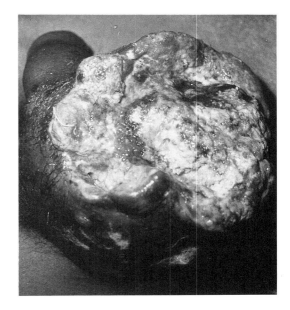

Fig. 37.20 Fungation into the wound after scrotal incision for an inflammatory cancer of the testis (courtesy of Dr A.K. Sharma and the Editor of *Surgical Journal of North India*).

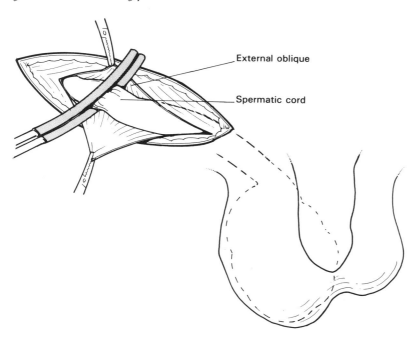

Fig. 37.21 Orchiectomy for testicular tumour. A clamp is placed on the cord before delivering the testis.

isolate the field and slice open the testis along its antimesenteric border with a large knife blade (Fig. 37.22). If the naked eye appearance is still doubtful, send tissue for frozen section. If the lump proves benign the tunica albuginea may be closed with continuous 3−0 catgut. The testicle survives: by 6 months it will be impossible to tell which side has been operated on [2].

If the testicle is obviously the seat of a cancer transfix and ligate the cord above the clamp (Fig. 37.23). Haemostasis must be perfect before closing the wound because infection in a haema-

toma may postpone adjuvant radiotherapy or chemotherapy.

Staging the tumour

A computerized tomography (CT) scan of the lung fields, mediastinum and abdomen is routine (Fig. 37.24): it can detect lymph nodes over 1 cm in diameter [55] and has replaced lymphangiography and urography. Retroperitoneal lymph node dissection is even more accurate as a method of staging the tumour, since it can detect met-

Fig. 37.22 (a) Chevassu's manoeuvre. Isolate the field, and slice the testis along the antimesenteric border. (b) The naked eye appearance is usually diagnostic but if necessary this may be confirmed by frozen section.

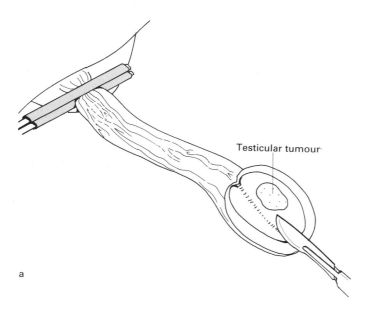

a

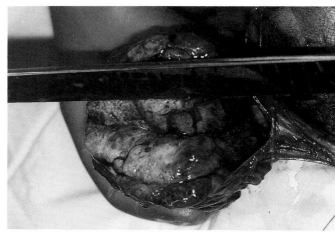

b

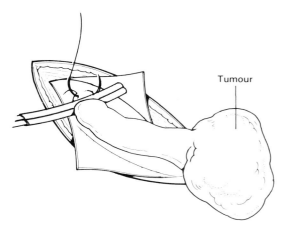

Fig. 37.23 The cord is transfixed and ligated above the clamp.

astases in lymph nodes that are less than 1 cm in diameter. By taking care to preserve the sympathetic chain, ejaculation is usually preserved — formerly the chief objection to this procedure. Staging node dissection is not only diagnostic, but will suffice to cure patients who only have microscopic metastases and excuse them unnecessary chemotherapy [55], but at the price of all the risks of major abdominal surgery.

When comparing different methods of treatment it is necessary to take account of the way the tumour was staged. Where retroperitoneal

node dissection is the routine practice, then lymph node metastases will be detected that would have been missed in the CT scan, and so invalidate the comparison.

The TNM system [56]

The entire surgical specimen, including the cut edge of the cord, must be examined (Fig. 37.25) otherwise the tumour must be classified Tx.

- **pTx** Primary tumour cannot be assessed.
- **pT0** No evidence of primary tumour or scar.
- **pTis** Intratubular tumour.
- **pT1** Limited to testis, including rete.
- **pT2** Spread beyond tunica albuginea or into epididymis.
- **pT3** Spread into spermatic cord.
- **pT4** Spread into scrotum.

N stage

- **N1** Single node less than 2 cm diameter.
- **N2** Single node more than 2–5 cm, but less than 5 cm.
- **N3** Nodes more than 5 cm diameter.

When CT scanning is used to evaluate the regional nodes in the para-aortic region N1 indicates enlargement of the nodes below the diaphragm and N2 nodes in the mediastinum or supra-clavicular group. It would be better to make a

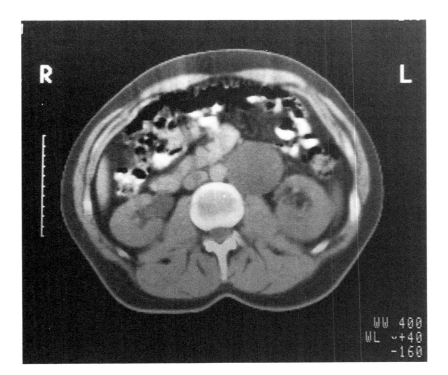

Fig. 37.24 CT scan showing para-aortic metastases.

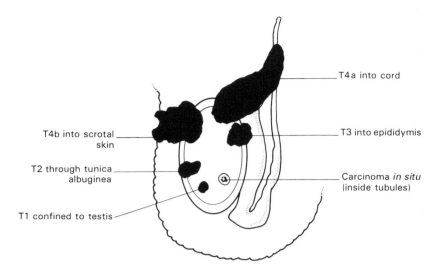

Fig. 37.25 T staging of tumour of the testis.

distinction between N1 (based on CT scanning) and pN1 based on pathological examination of the tissue removed at node dissection.

M stage

In the TNM system M1 signifies systemic metastases in the lungs or liver, etc.

Royal Marsden system

This system is relevant to staging by CT scanning. Stage I equals T1N0M0, but must include a number with microscopic metastases that would be classified as pN2 if node dissection had been used to stage the tumour. Stage II is subdivided into IIa where the nodes detected by the CT below the diaphragm are less than 2 cm in diameter and IIb where they are more than 2 cm in diameter. Stage III includes those in the mediastinum (N2) and stage IV haematogenous metastases [57] (Fig. 37.26).

Other commonly used staging systems are those of the Walter Reed Army Hospital [58] Skinner [59] and O'Donohue [60]. Table 37.2 compares these five systems.

Differential diagnosis

Every solid lump in the testis is a cancer until proven otherwise by Chevassu's manoeuvre or orchiectomy. With features of inflammation, the differential diagnosis rests between torsion, tumour and epididymoorchitis. So for an inflammatory mass, if the diagnosis is torsion the only hope is to untwist it. If a tumour is found it calls for orchidectomy. If the mass proves to be epididymoorchitis, ischaemia should be relieved by incision of the tunica albuginea (see p. 559).

Unless the inflammation is clearly confined to

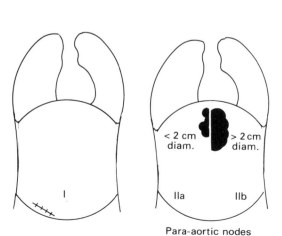

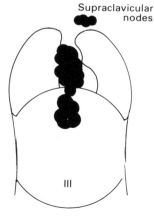

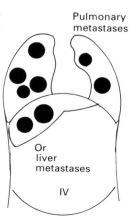

Fig. 37.26 The Royal Marsden Hospital system of staging of testis tumours.

Table 37.2 Staging of testis tumours

	Rowland & O'Donohue 1991 [60] Clinical	Rowland & O'Donohue 1991 [60] Pathological	Walter Reed Hospital 1973 [58]	Skinner 1969 [59]	Royal Marsden Hospital 1989 [61]	UICC 1992 [56]
Tumour limited to testis alone	A	A	Ia Clinical, X-ray	A Negative node dissection	I No evidence of mets IM Marker elevation after orchidectomy: no detectable metastatic disease	pT Classified after radical orchidectomy: otherwise Tx pT x Cannot be assessed o No evidence for primary tumour, or scar is Intratubular tumour pT1 Limited to testis, including rete pT2 Beyond tunica albuginea or into epididymis pT3 Into spermatic cord pT4 Into scrotum
Involvement of retroperitoneal lymph nodes	B1 <2 cm (CT) B2 >2–6 cm (CT) B3 >6 cm	B1 1–6 nodes + B2 >6 cm or gross nodal involvement B3 >6 cm	Ib Mets at node dissection in iliac or para-aortic II Mets below diaphragm; no spread to viscera III Palpable mass >5 cm	B1 <6 positive nodes B2 >6 nodes ± extension into fat; any node >2 cm B3 Bulky mass >5 cm	II Infradiaphragmatic node involvement IIa <2 cm diameter (CT) IIb 2–5 cm diameter (CT) IIc >5 cm diameter (CT)	N1 Single <2 cm N2 Single >2–5 cm; multiple <5 cm N3 >5 cm
Above diaphragm or involving abdominal solid organs	C	C	III Disease above diaphragm or spread to other organs (clinical, X-rays)	C Mets above diaphragm or liver mets	III Supradiaphragmatic node involvement IIIM+ Mediastinal nodes IIIN+ Neck nodes IV Lung involvement IV1 <3 small mets IV2 >3 mets <2 cm diameter IV3 Multiple large mets	Mo No distant mets M1 Distant mets

the epididymis there is no excuse for not exploring every 'inflamed' testicle. Other solid lumps in the testis may prove to be benign: benign dermoid cysts are exceedingly rare — and it is seldom possible to be sure that they are benign until they have been removed and examined histologically. Testicles destroyed by syphilis, tuberculosis, bilharziasis, malacoplakia, brucellosis or actinomycosis are all best treated by orchiectomy.

Serious trauma may present a difficult problem in diagnosis. Since most injured testicles ought to be explored, then, so long as surgeons are aware that cancer may be present no harm will be done.

Management

Stage I germ cell cancer

In germ cell tumours without CT evidence of lymph node or distant metastases and where, after orchiectomy the tumour markers fall according to their expected half-life in the following week, management depends on the histology of the tumour and the T stage of the specimen.

For well-differentiated tumours, which have not invaded the epididymis or cord, there are four alternative courses of action: (a) surveillance, i.e. wait and see; (b) prophylactic para-aortic node dissection; (c) chemotherapy; or (d) radiotherapy.

Retroperitoneal lymph node dissection

This ought to detect patients with microscopic metastases who will relapse under a policy of surveillance. By preserving the sympathetic chain, ejaculatory failure is avoided and surgical removal of any nodes that are involved may be curative.

Surveillance

Until about 10 years ago routine prophylactic treatment by radical node dissection or prophylactic radiation therapy gave equally excellent results [1]. Then it was pointed out that with either method about 80% were undergoing unnecessary treatment and it was suggested that such patients should be kept under strict surveillance, and treatment only given when there was evidence of relapse.

Surveillance is only possible in a well-equipped unit with ready access to CT scanning and prompt measurement of tumour markers. The patient must understand the need for strict cooperation and repeated follow-up, and it assumes that treatment of any tumour that appears during surveillance will be successful.

Seminoma

From the start there was a difficulty with seminoma, for in stage I 'pure' seminoma, a small dose of prophylactic radiation therapy gave 100% 5-year survival [1]. Tentative trials of surveillance were made for seminomas but the rate of relapse was very high and this policy was abandoned [62,63].

Most centres give a short course of 200 cGy radiation therapy to the retroperitoneal nodes, protecting the other testicle and the kidneys. Equally effective is a short course of single agent chemotherapy [64].

Non-seminoma

In the early studies of surveillance there was a 15–20% relapse rate [65,66]. Unfavourable features associated with a relapse were invasion of the veins or lymphatics of the testis and cord (T4a), an absence of yolk sac elements and the presence of undifferentiated cells [66].

In another large series of patients treated by surveillance, five out of the 27 who relapsed under surveillance died whose small metastases might have been detected or cured by diagnostic retroperitoneal node dissection [67]. As a result of these studies those with unfavourable histological features are now treated by prophylactic chemotherapy even in centres which favour a policy of surveillance, and this has been shown to reduce the relapse rate from 16 to 5% [67,68].

Staging retroperitoneal node dissection

In experienced hands prophylactic retroperitoneal lymph node dissection has a low morbidity. By preserving one sympathetic chain and its pre-aortic nerve fibres, ejaculation can be protected. The specimen provides histological evidence of staging and identifies microscopic metastases that would be too small to be detected by CT scan. If the specimen is free from tumour, the patient is cured, needs no chemotherapy and is spared the anxiety of surveillance [69].

If cancer is present and is anaplastic, or contains trophoblastic tissue, then the patient can be offered chemotherapy.

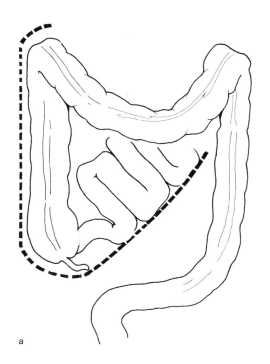

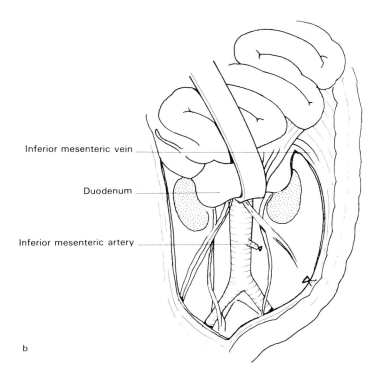

Inferior mesenteric vein

Duodenum

Inferior mesenteric artery

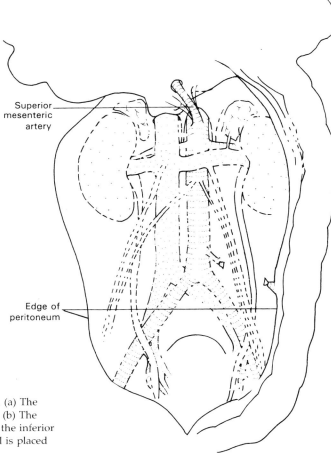

Superior mesenteric artery

Edge of peritoneum

Fig. 37.27 Retroperitoneal node dissection. (a) The small bowel and right colon are mobilized. (b) The inferior mesenteric artery and, if necessary the inferior mesenteric vein, are divided. (c) The bowel is placed on the chest.

Technique

Through a long midline incision the peritoneal reflection is divided along the ascending colon and medial edge of the mesentery to mobilize the entire bowel. The ligament of Trietz and inferior mesenteric vein are divided to expose the left renal vessels (Fig. 37.27).

A template of tissue is removed according to the side of the primary tumour aiming to remove all the lymph node catchment system, but to spare the opposite sympathetic chain and the presacral nerve. The tissues around the aorta and cava are considered as forming four wedges [69] (Fig. 37.28).

For a right-sided tumour, the tissues in front of the inferior vena cava are split from the right common iliac artery to the renal veins (Fig. 37.29). The right testicular artery and vein are divided and the complete lateral wedge of tissue between the vena cava and ureter is removed along with the testicular vessels down to the internal ring (Fig. 37.30). As the vena cava is rolled over, the lumbar veins are carefully divided between pairs of ligatures or clips.

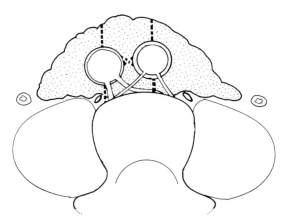

Fig. 37.28 The para-aortic tissues form four 'wedges' of tissue.

A second split is made along the tissues in the midline in front of the aorta (Fig. 37.31). The inferior mesenteric artery is divided between ligatures (Fig. 37.32). The anterior wedge of tissue is removed by rolling the aorta over, and dividing its pairs of lumbar arteries between clips or ligatures (Fig. 37.33).

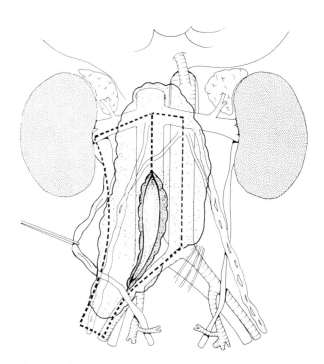

Fig. 37.29 For a right-sided tumour, the tissues are split along the front of the inferior vena cava from the common iliac artery up to the renal veins.

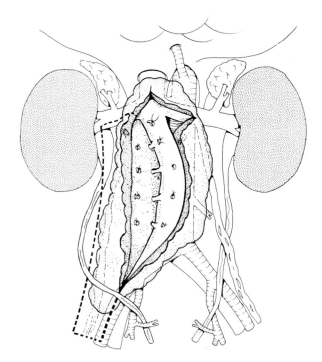

Fig. 37.30 The vena cava is rolled over and all its lumbar veins divided between ligatures or clips. All the tissues between the cava and the ureter form the right lateral wedge.

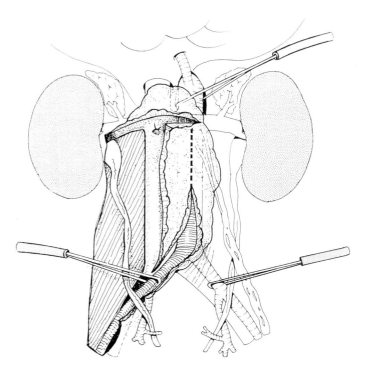

Fig. 37.31 The right lateral wedge has been removed: the anterior wedge is formed by splitting the tissues along the midline in front of the aorta.

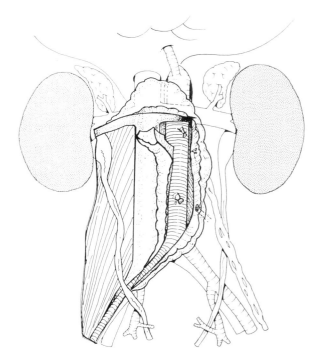

Fig. 37.32 The inferior mesenteric artery is divided.

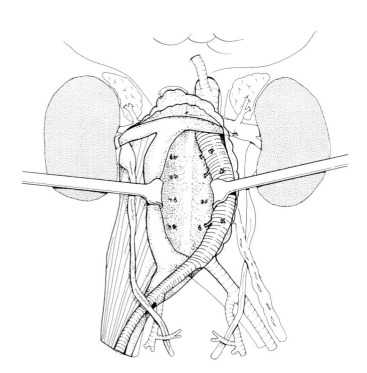

Fig. 37.33 The anterior wedge has been removed. The aorta is now mobilized and rolled over by dividing all its lumbar arteries.

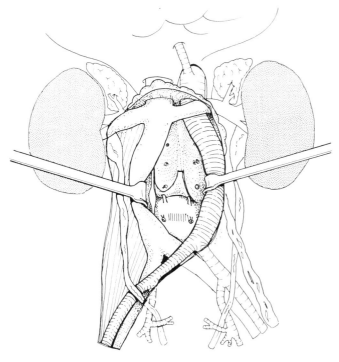

Fig. 37.34 The posterior wedge is removed taking all the lumbar vessels again. The left sympathetic chain and its fibres passing in front of the aorta are avoided.

The aorta and vena cava are now lifted up, to allow the posterior wedge of tissue to be dissected off the anterior intervertebral ligament, dividing again the pairs of lumbar arteries and veins (Fig. 37.34). The left sympathetic chain and its fibres crossing in front of the bifurcation of the aorta are carefully preserved (Fig. 37.35).

For a left-sided tumour the template of tissue to be removed includes the left, anterior and posterior wedges, but leaving the wedge on the right of the vena cava and the right sympathetic chain untouched [69] (Fig. 37.36).

Stage II germ cell cancer

Stage TNM N1 (Marsden IIa)

If the CT scan shows only very small nodes, many centres will perform retroperitoneal node dissection and if only a small number of nodes are found, chemotherapy is omitted [59,69]. In centres where staging is based on CT scanning only, all patients are given a full course of combination chemotherapy. Radiation therapy is sometimes given for pure seminoma.

Stage TNM N2 (Marsden IIb)

When the nodes are over 2 cm in diameter, combination chemotherapy is the first line of treatment in all centres, whatever the histology of the primary tumour [70]. This requires skill, dedication and teamwork, to avoid morbidity [71], the detail of which is beyond the scope of this book. However, surgeons must remember that bleomycin is toxic for the lungs, vinblastine for bone marrow, and cisplatin for the kidneys. Smokers tend to develop drug-resistant tumours [72].

Stage TNM N3 (Marsden III, IV)

Bulky and metastatic tumours are given combination chemotherapy. If the mass found on CT scanning disappears completely it has been shown that subsequent lymph node dissection virtually never reveals tumour, and such a dissection is no longer performed [73].

When a mass remains after two or three cycles of treatment, it may be merely fibronecrotic tissue without any cancer cells, it may be mature teratoma, or it may contain active cancer. It is impossible to tell these apart until the mass has been removed by so-called 'salvage' node dis-

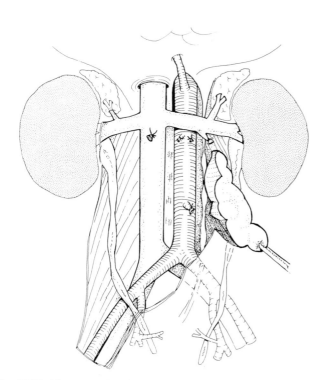

Fig. 37.35 After removing the posterior wedge the right sympathetic chain (shown here) has usually been taken with the lymphatics.

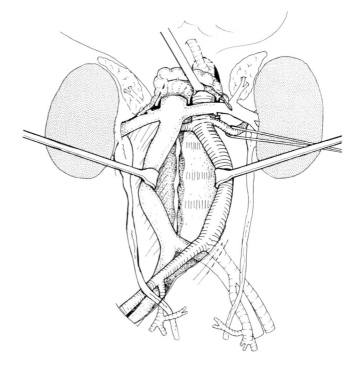

Fig. 37.36 For a left-sided tumour the left lateral and both anterior and posterior wedges are taken, but the right lateral wedge and the sympathetic chain and pre-aortic nerves are, if possible, preserved.

section. If mature teratoma is not removed, it will return within 3 years in a form which may be resistant to chemotherapy in up to 30% of cases [74,75]. Removing small islands of active cancer can give long-term survival without further chemotherapy although in general if active cancer is found, further second-line chemotherapy is usually given [76].

For the same reasons, masses remaining in the lungs or mediastinum should be removed.

Technique of salvage node dissection

This follows the same steps as prophylactic node dissection described above, but one must be ready to deal with major complications on the table including repair or reconstruction of the aorta and cava, and resection of damaged bowel [76,77]. The mass usually conceals the aorta and cava, but the operation follows the same four steps, aiming to divide the mass into four wedges by splitting and rolling the great vessels away from the mass. An attempt should be made to preserve at least one sympathetic chain and pre-sacral nerve, but this may be impossible when there is tumour between the bifurcation of the aorta [76].

Small masses of tumour behind the crura can be removed through the abdominal approach, if necessary by incising the crura to improve access (Fig. 37.37).

Removal of the wedge on the opposite side to the main bulk of the tumour can sometimes be achieved without sacrifice of the sympathetic chain, and it is well worth making this effort [78, 79] (Fig. 37.38).

When bulky tumour is shown in the CT scan behind the crura of the diaphragm a thoraco-abdominal approach gives a more secure approach [80].

The greatest difficulty is found with residual masses of seminoma which are particularly densely adherent but it is still worth making the attempt to remove them [79].

Prognosis

With the combination of radical surgery and chemotherapy one expects to cure nearly every patient with a cancer of the testis. The continuing tragedy is that so many of these young men still come up so late in the course of their disease [81]. In children the long-term follow-up calls for particular care [82].

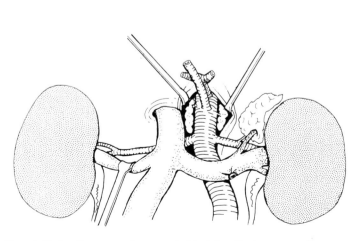

Fig. 37.37 Small masses of tumour behind the diaphragm can be removed by retracting or dividing the crura.

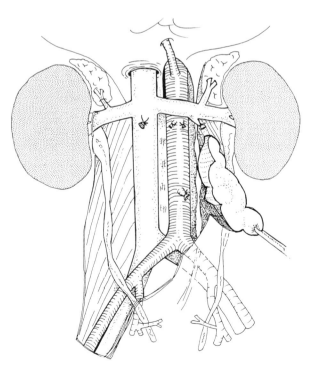

Fig. 37.38 Even in a salvage lymphadenectomy it is sometimes possible to remove the contralateral wedge and still preserve one sympathetic chain.

References

1 Blandy JP (1970) History of the surgery of testicular tumours, in: Blandy JP, Hope-Stone HF, Dayan AD (eds) *Tumours of the Testicle*, pp. 1–11. London: Heinemann.

2 Chevassu M (1906) *Tumeurs du Testicule*. Thèse de Paris, No. 193, Steinheil.

3 Kocher P (1883) cited by Chevassu (1906) *Tumeurs du Testicule*. Thèse de Paris, No. 193, Steinheil.

4 Cairns HWB (1926) Neoplasms of the testicle. *Lancet* i: 845.

5 Forman D (1991) Aetiology of testicular tumours, in: Alderson AR, Oliver RTD, Hanham IWF, Bloom HJG (eds) *Urological Oncology: Dilemmas and Developments*, pp. 269–82. Chichester: Wiley.

6 Davies JM (1981) Testicular cancer in England and Wales: some epidemiological aspects. *Lancet* i: 928.

7 Clemmesen J (1968) A doubling in mortality from testis carcinoma in Copenhagen 1943–62. *Acta Pathol Microbiol Scand* 72: 348.

8 Osterlind A (1986) Diverging trends in incidence and mortality of testicular cancer in Denmark 1943–1982. *Br J Cancer* 53: 501.

9 Forman D, Pike MC, Davey G et al. (1994) Aetiology of testicular cancer: association with congenital abnormalities, age at puberty, infertility and exercise. *BMJ* 308: 1393.

10 Brown LM, Pottern LM, Hoover RN, Devesa SS, Aselton P, Flannery JT (1986) Testicular cancer in the United States: trends in incidence and mortality. *Int J Epidemiol* 15: 164.

11 Mead GM (1992) Testicular cancer and related neoplasms. *Br Med J* 304: 1426.

12 Daniels JL, Stutzman RE, McLeod DG (1981) A comparison of testicular tumors in black and white patients. *J Urol* 125: 341.

13 Onuigbo WIB (1977) Relevance of race in management of testicular tumours. *Br Med J* 1: 22.

14 Sherman FP, Ciavarra VA, Cohen MJ (1973) Testis tumors in Negroes. *Urology* 2: 318.

15 Oliver RTD, Stephenson CA, Parkinson MC et al. (1986) Germ cell tumours of the testicle. A model for MHC influence on human malignancy. *J Immunogen* 13: 85.

16 Swerdlow AJ, Huttly SRA, Smith PG (1987) Prenatal and familial associations of testicular cancer. *Br J Cancer* 55: 571.

17 Forman D (1989) Epidemiology of testis cancer, in: Oliver RTD, Blandy JP, Hope-Stone HF (eds) *Urological and Genital Cancer*. Oxford: Blackwell Scientific Publications.

18 Stewart JR, Bagshaw MA (1965) Malignant testicular tumors appearing simultaneously in identical twins. *Cancer* 18: 895.

19 Durig JC, Kandzari SJ, Milam DF (1975) Primary extratesticular seminoma in non-twin brothers. *J Urol* 114: 412.

20 Gawande AS (1980) Histologically similar testicular neoplasms occurring in brothers. *J Urol* 123: 963.

21 Silber SJ, Cittan S, Friedlander G (1972) Testicular neoplasm in father and son. *J Urol* 108: 889.

22 Raghavan D, Jelihovsky T, Fox RM (1980) Father–son testicular malignancy: does genetic anticipation occur? *Cancer* 45: 1005.

23 Depue RH, Pike MC, Henderson BE (1983) Estrogen exposure during gestation and risk of testicular cancer. *J Natl Canc Inst* 71: 1151.

24 Bernstein L, Pike MC, Depue RH, Ross RK, Moore JW, Henderson BE (1988) Maternal hormone levels in early gestation of cryptorchid males: a case–control study. *Br J Cancer* 58: 379.

25 Oliver RTD (1994) Testicular cancer (Review). *Curr Opin Oncol* 6: 285.

26 Friedman NB (1988) Pathology of testicular tumors, in: Skinner DG, Lieskovsky G (eds) *Diagnosis and Management of Genitourinary Cancer*, pp. 215–34. Philadelphia: WB Saunders.

27 Jacobsen GK (1989) Pathology and cytochemistry of germ cell tumours, in: Oliver RTD, Blandy JP, Hope-Stone HF (eds) *Urological and Genital Cancer*, pp. 322–58. Oxford: Blackwell Scientific Publications.

28 Stevens MJ, Norman AR, Fisher C, Hendry WF, Dearnaley DP, Horwich A (1994) Prognosis of testicular teratoma differentiated. *Br J Urol* 73: 124.

29 Janssen M, Johnston WH (1978) Anaplastic seminoma of the testis: ultrastructural analysis of three cases. *Cancer* 41: 538.

30 Weitzner S (1976) Spermatocytic seminoma. *Urology* 7: 646.

31 Talerman A (1980) Spermatocytic seminoma. *Cancer* 45: 2169.

32 Schoborg TW, Whittaker J, Lewis CW (1980) Metastatic spermatocytic seminoma. *J Urol* 124: 739.

33 Percarpio B, Clements JC, McLeod DG, Sorgen SD, Cardinale FS (1979) Anaplastic seminoma: an analysis of 77 patients. *Cancer* 43: 2510.

34 Davis S, Di Martino NA, Schneider G (1981) Malignant interstitial cell carcinoma of the testis: report of two cases with steroid synthetic profiles, response to therapy and review of the literature. *Cancer* 47: 425.

35 Ober WB, Kabakow B, Hecht H (1976) Malignant interstitial cell tumor of the testis: a problem in endocrine oncoloby. *Bull NY Acad Med* 52: 561.

36 Cantu JM, Rivera H, Ocampo-Campos R et al. (1980) Peutz–Jeghers syndrome with feminizing Sertoli cell tumor. *Cancer* 45: 223.

37 Morin LJ, Loening S (1975) Malignant androblastoma (Sertoli cell tumor) of the testis: a case report with a review of the literature. *J Urol* 114: 476.

38 Lioe TF, Biggart JD (1993) Tumours of the spermatic cord and paratesticular tissue. A clinicopathological study. *Br J Urol* 71: 600.

39 Williams GB, Banerjee R (1969) Paratesticular tumours. *Br J Urol* 412: 332.

40 Orozco RE, Murphy WM (1993) Carcinoma of the rete testis: case report and review of the literature. *J Urol* 150: 974.

41 Mostofi FK, Sobin LH (1977) *Histological Typing of Testis Tumours. International Histological Classification of Tumours No. 16*. Geneva: World Health Organisation.

42 Friedman NB, Moore RA (1946) Tumors of the testis: a report on 922 cases. *Milit Surg* 99: 573.

43 Pugh RCB (1976) *Pathology of the Testis*. Oxford: Blackwell Scientific Publications.

44 Javadpour N (1980) The role of biologic tumor markers in testicular cancer. *Cancer* 45: 1755.

45 Donohue JP, Roth LM, Zachary JM, Rowland RG,

Einhorn LH, Williams SG (1982) Cytoreductive surgery for metastatic testis cancer: tissue analysis of retroperitoneal masses after chemotherapy. *J Urol* 127: 1111.

46 Oliver RTD (1985) Factors contributing to delay in diagnosis of testicular tumours. *Br Med J* 290: 356.

47 Awad RM, Shetty SD, Ibrahim A (1987) Intra-abdominal seminoma presenting as acute abdomen: report of a case. *Ann Saudi Med* 8: 290.

48 Richie JP (1988) Diagnosis and staging of testicular tumors, in: Skinner DF, Lieskovsky G (eds) *Diagnosis and Management of Genitourinary Cancer*, pp. 498–507. Philadelphia: WB Saunders.

49 Azzopardi JG, Hoffbrand AV (1965) Retrogression in testicular seminoma with viable metastases. *J Clin Pathol* 18: 135.

50 Sgelov E, Cox KM, Raghavan D, McNeil E, Lancaster L, Rogers J (1993) The impact of histological review on clinical management of testicular cancer. *Br J Urol* 71: 736.

51 Richie JP (1982) Ultrasonography as a diagnostic adjunct for the evaluation of masses in the scrotum. *Surg Gynecol Obstet* 154: 695.

52 Vogelzang RL (1985) Real-time scrotal ultrasound with a water bath: comparison of results using 5 and 8 mHz transducers. *J Urol* 134: 687.

53 Heikkila R, Heilo A, Stenwig AE, Fossa SD (1993) Testicular ultrasonography and 18 G Biopty biopsy for clinically undetected cancer or carcinoma *in situ* in patients with germ cell tumours. *Br J Urol* 71: 214.

54 Sharma AK, Mathur RK (1992) Fungating testicular tumour — a successful outcome. *Surg J N India* 8: 62.

55 McLeod DG, Weiss RB, Stablein DM *et al.* (1991) Staging relationships and outcome in early stage testicular cancer: a report from the testicular cancer inter-group study. *J Urol* 145: 1178.

56 Hermanek P, Sobin LH (eds) (1992) *UICC International Union Against Cancer TNM Classification of Malignant Tumours*, 4th edn, 2nd revision. Berlin: Springer.

57 Peckham MJ, Barrett A, Liew KH (1983) The treatment of metastatic germ-cell testicular tumours with bleomycin, etoposide and cis-platin (BEP). *Br J Cancer* 47: 613.

58 Maier JG, Sulak MH (1973) Proceedings: radiation therapy in malignant testis tumors. II. Carcinoma. *Cancer* 32: 1212.

59 Skinner DG (1969) Non-seminomatous testis tumors: a plan of management based on 96 patients to improve survival in all stages by combined therapeutic modalities. *J Urol* 115: 65.

60 Rowland RG, O'Donohue JP (1991) Scrotum and testis, in: Gillenwater JY, Grayhack JT, Howards SS, Dunckett JW (eds) *Adult and Pediatric Urology*, 2nd edn, pp. 1565–98. St Louis: CV Mosby.

61 Bellamy EA, Husband JE (1989) CT scanning and ultrasound in the diagnosis and assessment of testicular tumours, in: Oliver RTD, Blandy JP, Hope-Stone HF (eds) *Urological and Genital Cancer*, pp. 44–59. Oxford: Blackwell Scientific Publications.

62 Peckham MJ, Hamilton CR, Horwich A, Hendry WF (1987) Surveillance after orchidectomy for stage I seminoma of the testis. *Br J Urol* 59: 343.

63 Oliver RTD (1987) Limitations to the use of surveillance as an option in the management of stage I

seminoma. *Int J Androl* 10: 263.

64 Oliver RTD, Lore S, Ong J (1990) Alternatives to radiotherapy in the management of seminoma. *Br J Urol* 65: 61.

65 Oliver RTD, Freedman LS, Parkinson MC, Peckham MJ (1987) Medical options in the management of stages 1 and 2 (No−3,Mo) testicular germ cell tumors. *Urol Clin N Am* 4: 721.

66 MRC Testicular Tumour Working Party (1984) Report on prognostic factors in advanced non-seminomatous testicular germ cell tumours. *Lancet* i: 8.

67 Donohue JP, Einhorn LH, Perez JM (1978) Improved management of non-seminomatous testis tumours. *Cancer* 42: 2903.

68 Oliver RTD, Raja MA, Gallagher CJ (1992) Pilot study to evaluate impact of a policy of adjuvant chemotherapy for high risk stage I malignant teratoma on overall relapse rate of stage I cancer patients. *J Urol* 148: 1453.

69 Donohue JP, Thornhill JA, Foster RS, Rowland RG, Bihrle R (1993) Retroperitoneal lymphadenectomy for clinical stage A testis cancer (1965–1989): modifications of technique and impact on ejaculation. *J Urol* 149: 237.

70 Mead GM, Stenning SP, Parkinson MC *et al.* (1992) The second Medical Research Council study of prognostic factors in nonseminomaous germ cell tumours. *J Clin Oncol* 10: 85.

71 Oliver RTD, Blandy JP, Hendry WF, Pryor JP, Williams JP, Hope-Stone HF (1983) Evaluation of radiotherapy and/or surgico-pathological staging after chemotherapy in the management of metastatic germ cell tumours. *Br J Urol* 55: 764.

72 Smith RB (1988) Testicular seminoma, in: Skinner DG, Lieskovsky G (eds) *Diagnosis and Management of Genitourinary Cancer*, pp. 508–15. Philadelphia: WB Saunders.

73 Hendry WF, A'Hern RP, Hetherington JW, Peckham MJ, Dearnley DP, Horwich A (1993) Para-aortic lymphadenectomy for metastatic non-seminomatous germ cell tumours: prognostic value and therapeutic benefit. *Br J Urol* 71: 208.

74 Oliver RTD, Blandy JP, Hope-Stone HF (1989) Modern management of germ cell tumours, in: Oliver RTD, Blandy JP, Hope-Stone HF (eds) *Urological and Genital Cancer*, pp. 358–81. Oxford: Blackwell Scientific Publications.

75 Loehrer PJ, Williams SD, Clark SA *et al.* (1983) Teratoma following chemotherapy for non-seminomatous germ cell tumours (NSGCT): a clinico-pathologic correlation. *Proc Am Soc Clin Oncol* 12: 139.

76 Williams SN, Jenkins BJ, Baithun SI, Oliver RTD, Blandy JP (1989) Radical retroperitoneal node dissection after chemotherapy for testicular tumours. *Br J Urol* 63: 641.

77 Blandy JP, Jenkins BJ, Badenoch DF, Fowler CG, Oliver RTD (1991) *Radical Retroperitoneal Node Dissection After Chemotherapy for Testicular Tumours. EORTC Genitourinary Group Monograph 10: Urological Oncology: Reconstructive Surgery, Organ Conservation and Restoration of Function*, pp. 399–401. New York: Wiley–Liss.

78 Hendry WF, A'Hern RP, Hetherington JW, Peckham MJ, Dearnaley DP, Horwich A (1993) Para-aortic

lymphadenectomy after chemotherapy for metastatic non-seminomatous germ cell tumours: prognostic value and therapeutic benefit. *Br J Urol* 71: 208.

79 Blandy JP, Jenkins BJ, Oliver RTD (1992) Preservation of sexual function after salvage retroperitoneal node dissection following chemotherapy for testicular tumors. *World J Urol* 10: 59.

80 Hoeltl W, Aharinejad S (1990) Surgical approach to the retrocrural lymph nodes. *Br J Urol* 66: 523.

81 Wishnow KI, Johnson DE, Preston WL, Tenney DM, Brown BW (1990) Prompt orchiectomy reduces morbidity and mortality from testicular carcinoma. *Br J Urol* 65: 629.

82 Bruce J, Gough DCS (1991) Long-term follow-up of children with testicular tumours: surgical issues. *Br J Urol* 67: 429.

Chapter 38: Male infertility

It is said that about four out of five couples will conceive within a year of starting unprotected intercourse, and in the couples who do not conceive a male factor is present in half, while in a third some contributing factor is found in both partners. Both should be investigated. At the outset it is wise to point out that there is still much that is not known about human fertility, e.g. why the sperm count seems to have declined, in the West, in the last 50 years [1].

Pathology

Defective spermatogenesis

Genetic defects

Genetic defects may cause infertility. In Klinefelter's syndrome (XXY) azoospermia is the rule, resulting from hyalinization of the tubules and absence of spermatogenesis. Other genetic anomalies are also associated with deficient spermatogenesis [2].

Toxins

Toxins thought to impair spermatogenesis include pesticides, alcohol, cimetidine, heavy metals, e.g. lead, cadmium, manganese and iron, including that which is accumulated in haemochromatosis [3–5]. Radiation impairs spermatogenesis but may be reversible if only a low dose has been received.

Inflammation

The testicles may have been damaged by inflammation, e.g. mumps orchitis [6] and hepatitis B [7] (see p. 558).

Cryptorchidism

In cryptorchidism there is failure of spermatogenesis, the tubules having only a single layer of germ cells among the Sertoli cells. Fertility has been variously estimated at from as low as 7% to as high as 48% [8,9] in men who underwent bilateral orchiopexy in childhood.

Hormonal

A pituitary tumour may lead to a deficiency of circulating pituitary gonadotrophin or an excess of prolactin. Corticosteroids used in treatment and androgens taken by athletes to cheat may suppress pituitary function.

Defects in transport

Congenital defects in the seminal tract

There are many congenital anomalies in the Wolffian duct derivatives. There may be a complete absence of one or both vasa deferentia, atresia, a failure of union between the vas and the epididymis, or a hiatus in the epididymis itself. Many of these congenital anomalies occur in association with maldescent. Other conditions, especially those affecting the seminal vesicles, are being diagnosed by transrectal ultrasound scanning [10–15].

Inflammatory obstruction

Infection may cause a stenosis of the vas deferens or the tail of the epididymis [10].

The ejaculatory ducts may be obstructed by inflammatory scarring — to cause one form of Müllerian duct cyst that may be cured by incision of the obstructed duct [10].

Young's syndrome

Here there is a history of long-standing bronchitis and obstruction in the epididymes [16]. An interesting trail of circumstantial evidence led Hendry to suggest that this was caused by mercurous chloride given as 'teething powders'. In this syndrome, the epithelial cells of the ductuli efferentes in the caput epididymis contain an excess of lipid, probably causing the seminal fluid (and bronchial mucus) to become abnormally viscous [10]. Mercury is known to cause permanent damage to other enzyme systems, an effect which may be partly reversed by carbocisteine.

Retrograde ejaculation

If the bladder neck has been cut or paralysed by sympathectomy or alpha blocking drugs, then ejaculation forces the semen back into the bladder. This condition is rarely seen in men who have not undergone any previous treatment or surgery. (Fig. 38.1). After orgasm sperms may be recovered from the urine (see p. 608).

Previous surgery

The vas deferens is easily injured during operations for hernia repair in infancy either from inadvertent division of the vas or diathermy injury.

Investigations

A careful physical examination must be performed first, taking note of the distribution of pubic hair and gynaecomastia. In Klinefelter's syndrome the caricature long limbs are not always present but the testicles are always very small.

Look carefully for the scars of previous hernia surgery and feel the cords for the characteristic absence of the vasa deferentia. The testicles are measured using a set of beads of appropriate size.

The presence of a varicocele should be noted in the standing position. A cough impulse is said to be an important sign and the Doppler scan is often used to confirm this (see p. 572).

Semen analysis

After a 72-h period of abstinence semen is collected by masturbation into a clean plastic container. It coagulates within a few seconds and liquifies again within the next 10 min. Semen analysis should be performed as soon as possible thereafter. The usual criteria of normality have been subjected to much criticism in the light of careful studies which show a very wide range of normal in all the usual factors that are measured [17−19].

Semen volume

There is a wide range of normal volume from 1 to 8 ml. The most common cause for a low volume is inept collection of the specimen, although it may reflect disease of the seminal vesicles (see p. 615).

Sperm density and motility

Using conventional haemocytometer or Makler chamber methods (Fig. 38.2) for counting sperm, there is a very wide coefficient of variation when different technicians count the same sample [17] and it is hardly surprising that different figures

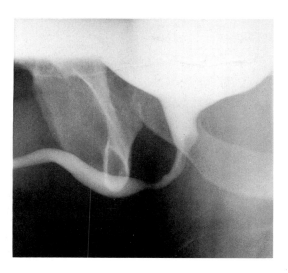

Fig. 38.1 Congenital dilatation of the bladder neck, leading to retrograde ejaculation of semen.

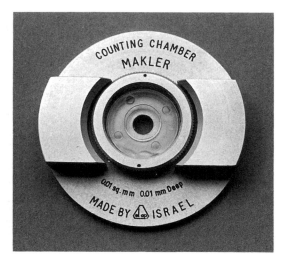

Fig. 38.2 Makler chamber for semen counting (courtesy of Mr D.F. Badenoch).

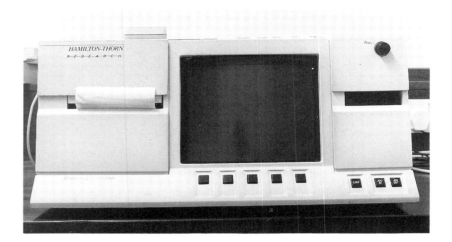

Fig. 38.3 Hamilton—Thorn system for measuring sperm density and velocity (courtesy of Mr D.F. Badenoch).

have been taken for the lower limit of normal sperm density [18,19].

When a more accurate and reproducible computer system is used to measure sperm density [19,20] (Fig. 38.3), it is found that normal fertility is compatible with a sperm density as low as $1 \times 10^6/ml$ so long as they swim fast enough [21−23].

Morphology

Light microscopic examination of normal semen reveals a number of odd or immature forms of which much has been made in the past. Electron microscopy shows even more, but there is only a slim correlation between morphological 'abnormalities' and infertility [21,22] (Fig. 38.4).

Antibodies

Antibodies to both the head and the tail of the human spermatozoon can be found in blood and seminal plasma, as well as in the mucus of the female cervix [23].

Postcoital tests

If the cervical mucus is examined immediately after coitus in most women many actively motile

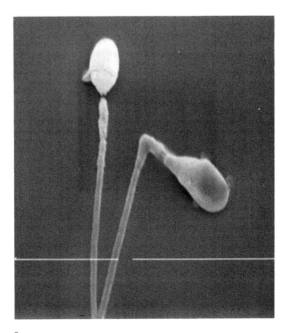

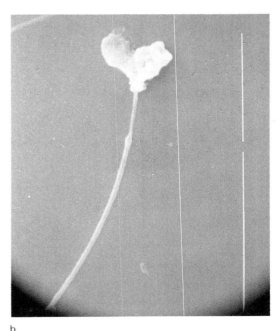

a

b

Fig. 38.4 (a) Scanning electron microscopy (b) reveals many morphological 'abnormalities', but these have little to do with fertility (courtesy of Mr D.F. Badenoch).

sperms are to be seen. In others, they are still. The factors that stop the sperms from swimming are not all known: some may be immunological [24].

Egg penetration tests

The ideal test would be to take sperms, lead them to a human egg and see if they can achieve fertilization. Until recently this was not feasible, and recourse was had to the eggs of hamsters. Much was made of the 'hamster ova penetration test' but it has since been discredited [25].

With the more recent development of techniques of artificial insemination a number of spare human eggs have become available for experiments which suggest that sperms from infertile males do not stick to the cells normally surrounding the human egg as readily as those from fertile men [26]. It seems unlikely that this test will come into routine use, but it is of great theoretical interest.

Luteinizing hormone (LH) and follicle-stimulating hormone (FSH) estimations

Measurement of the serum LH and FSH is now routine. If spermatogenesis is absent, the level of these hormones is elevated. If spermatogenesis is proceeding normally, but the seminal tract is blocked, they are not elevated. For practical purposes this is a useful test, since raised levels of LH and FSH make it futile to proceed to a testicular biopsy [27].

Testis biopsy

The standard method is to expose the testis through a 1 cm incision, incise the tunicae and allow a tuft of testicular tubules to extrude (Fig. 38.5). They are snipped off cleanly with fine sharp scissors and at once put into Bouin's fixative — a mixture of formalin, alcohol and picric acid which prevents cellular distortion and gives a better picture of the testicular tubule than if the biopsy is put into the usual formalin fixative. The nick in the tunica albuginea is closed with a fine catgut suture as is the incision in the skin.

In many centres the biopsy is taken with a Biopty needle using local anaesthetic.

Because spermatogenesis does not proceed at a uniform rate in every tubule in the testis, but in waves — some actively dividing, others resting — the interpretation of a biopsy makes it necessary that several tubules are present, and

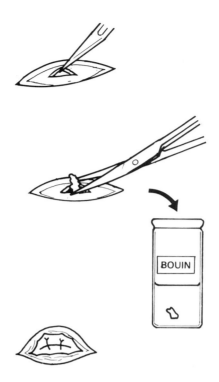

Fig. 38.5 Testis biopsy. A few tubules are snipped off and immersed in Bouin's fluid.

the opinion is based on the proportion of tubules in the biopsy which show each stage in spermatogenesis. This is the Johnsen mean score. At least ten tubules are examined. Each is assigned a score on a scale of 1 to 10: in 1 there are spermatogenic cells at all, in 10 there are healthy spermatids. The normally fertile man has a mean score of $9.38 + 0.24$ [28].

Testicular biopsies show a wide range of appearances (Fig. 38.6). In practice, testicular biopsy is seldom helpful, except in confirming the hopelessness of a given case of azoospermia.

Treatment

Azoospermia

When there are no spermatozoa in the specimen it is wise to repeat the test several times with several weeks' interval to make sure that the cause is not a temporary and reversible one. In the meantime, the serum LH and FSH are measured. If they are elevated, the condition is probably hopeless, i.e. there is a defect in spermatogenesis and no useful purpose will be served by testis biopsy.

If the biopsy shows normal spermatogenesis, and the tubules are distended with sperm, it

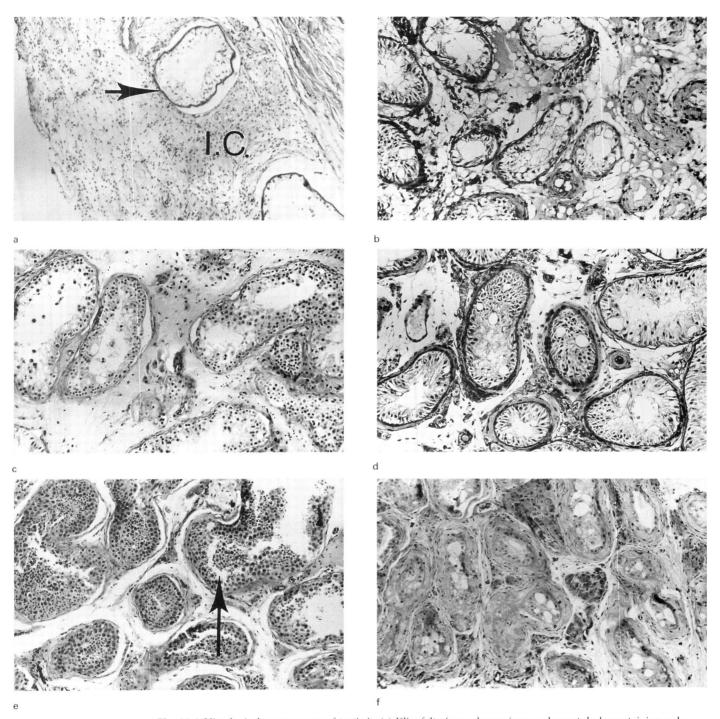

Fig. 38.6 Histological appearances of testis in (a) Klinefelter's syndrome (arrow shows tubule containing only Sertoli cells). IC; interstitial cells. (b) Sertoli-cell-only syndrome (c) Atrophy after mumps (d) Disordered spermatogenesis in cryptorchidism (e) Maturation arrest (arrow shows 'sloughing') immature cells shed into lumen (f) Extensive degeneration and fibrosis — 'end stage testis'.

suggests that there is a block. If it shows maturation arrest it may be possible to restore normal spermatogenesis with Pergonal [10]. Presence of lymphocytes in the biopsy, along with raised antibody titres, tends to confirm a diagnosis of

autoimmunological disorder and strengthens the indication for prednisone treatment.

If the LH and FSH values are normal, then it is likely that there is a block in the seminal tract.

Transrectal ultrasound may reveal dilated

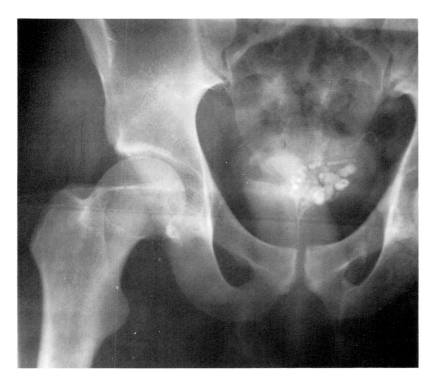

Fig. 38.7 Vasogram.

seminal vesicles or obstructed ejaculatory ducts which can be unblocked by transurethral incision [10]. A vasogram may be performed by cutting down on the vas and injecting contrast up towards the seminal vesicles (Fig. 38.7). This will reveal blocks in the vas or ejaculatory duct.

In most cases it will be necessary to explore the testis. What is then done will depend on what is found.

If the epididymis is empty and there are high serum antibody titres, a prolonged course of prednisolone may cause a return to a normal sperm count. If part or all of the epididymis is found to be distended and its tubules stuffed with sperm, then an anastomosis is made between the vas deferens and the dilated part of the epididymis. This anastomosis is made easier with the help of an operating microscope or

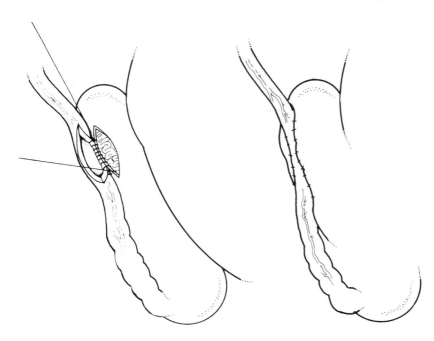

Fig. 38.8 Epididymo-vasostomy.

loupes (Fig. 38.8). In some series, up to 43% of patients have recovered a normal sperm count with pregnancies in up to 30% [10].

In patients who have suffered a block to the vasa either from previous hernia surgery or deliberate vasectomy, successful reunion by vasovasostomy may be obtained in up to 90% of patients with pregnancy achieved in about 30%, depending on the cause of the blockage (see p. 615).

One of the factors which complicate the presence of a block to the seminal tract is extravasation of sperm upstream of the blockage, with resulting antisperm antibodies [29]. When these are present it is worthwhile treating these with prednisone as well as correcting the block surgically [10,29,30].

Antibodies

When antibodies are found either in the patient's serum or in the cervical mucus of his partner, it is well worth giving either or both partners a prolonged course of prednisone 5 mg three times daily. This has replaced the use of hydrocortisone vaginal douches. It may be possible to remove the antibodies by suitably washing the sperms prior to artificial insemination [31].

Oligozoospermia

Nobody should be treated for supposed oligozoospermia — a 'low sperm count' — without the method of measuring the sperm density and motility being very carefully scrutinized: very large errors occur with conventional techniques. Because of these errors, claims that any method of treatment achieves good results must be treated with the greatest scepticism unless there have been adequate controls.

Cooling the testicles

Loose pants, ice packs and cold baths have all been used with the aim of cooling the testicles. Innumerable treatments have been proclaimed to be effective ranging from every known hormone, to arginine and vitamin E: when careful controlled trials have been performed none of them have been shown to be of any value. This is a field of medicine that provides rich pickings for quacks and sharks.

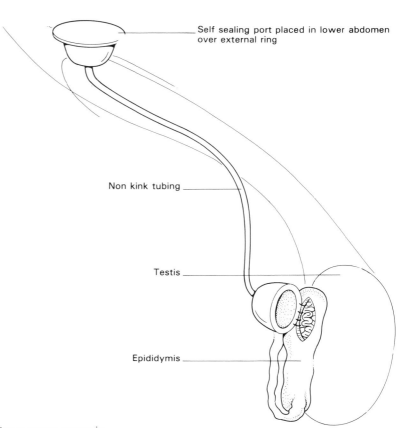

Self sealing port placed in lower abdomen over external ring

Non kink tubing

Testis

Epididymis

Fig. 38.9 One method of forming a sperm reservoir.

Varicocele surgery

Varicocele surgery is not immune from this criticism. Whilst widely practised, its physiological basis is highly questionable (see p. 573) and no controlled trial has so far shown any benefit. Nevertheless, the controversy continues [32−36].

Retrograde ejaculation

It is sometimes possible to get the bladder neck to close by giving alpha adrenergic drugs, e.g. ephedrine 50 mg 30 min before intercourse. This can produce prograde ejaculation in men whose sympathetic chain has been removed for testicular cancer, at the cost of formidable side effects [37].

When this fails, the sperms can be recovered from the urine after ejaculation. First the urine is rendered alkaline by giving the patient sodium bicarbonate 6 g every 4 h for 24 h beforehand. The bladder is emptied, and after ejaculation, the patient can 'urinate' before withdrawing, or the voided urine is centrifuged and placed in a plastic cup over the cervix, or injected into it [37,38].

Artificial insemination using the husband's semen is seldom worthwhile when his sperm is of poor quality, and before embarking on any programme it needs to be understood by everyone involved that it takes an average of 12 attempts before pregnancy is achieved, even with normal semen. The greatest tact and care is necessary when setting up such a service, for the recurring monthly disappointment demands great sympathy.

Sperm reservoirs

For many years surgeons have tried to use sperms aspirated from cysts of the epididymis in artificial insemination. There have been occasional anecdotal reports of success. More recently, attempts have been made to form artificial sperm reservoirs with various implanted devices (Fig. 38.9) and in at least one series the aspirated sperms achieved pregnancy in two out of seven patients [39,40].

If sperms are aspirated from epididymal tubules they can be used to fertilize ova obtained at laparoscopy. Contrary to what is generally believed about the importance of travel through the epididymis to confer the capacity to fertilize the ovum on the sperm, these spermatozoa may be obtained from the head of the epididymis [41].

References

1 Bromwich P, Cohen J, Stewart I, Walker A (1994) Decline in sperm counts an artefact or changed reference range of 'normal'? *Br Med J* 309: 19.

2 Bandmann HJ, Breit R, Perwin D (eds) (1984) *Klinefelter's Syndrome*. New York: Springer.

3 Winder C (1989) Reproductive and chromosomal effects of occupational exposure to lead in the male. *Reprod Toxicol* 3: 221.

4 Gennart JP, Hoet P, Lison D, Lauwerys R, Coche E, Lambert M (1992) Fertility of male workers exposed to cadmium, lead or manganese. *Amer J Epidemiol* 135: 1208.

5 Thrupp LA (1991) Sterilization of workers from pesticide exposure: the causes and consequences of DBCP-induced damage in Costa Rica and beyond. *Int J Health Serv* 21: 731.

6 Manson AL (1990) Mumps orchitis. *Urology* 36: 355.

7 Molitor PJA, Warrens AN (1985) Acute orchitis associated with hepatitis B infection. *Br Med J* 291: 940.

8 Okuyama A, Nonomura N, Nakamura M *et al.* (1989) Surgical management of undescended testis: retrospective study of potential fertility in 274 cases. *J Urol* 142: 749.

9 Bramble FJ, Eccles S, Houghton AL, O'Shea A, Jacobs HS (1974) Reproductive and endocrine function after surgical treatment of bilateral cryptorchidism. *Lancet* ii: 311.

10 Hendry WF, Levison DA, Parkinson MC, Parslow JM, Royle MG (1990) Testicular obstruction: clinicopathological studies. *Ann Roy Coll Surg Engl* 72: 396.

11 Johansen TEB (1987) Anatomy of the testis and epididymis in cryptorchidism. *Andrologia* 19: 565.

12 Heaton ND, Pryor JP (1990) Vasa aplasia and cystic fibrosis. *Br J Urol* 66: 538.

13 Dominguez C (1991) Agenesis of seminal vesicles in infertile males: ultrasonic diagnosis. *Eur Urol* 20: 129.

14 Clements R, Griffiths GJ, Peeling WB, Conn IG. (1991) Transrectal ultrasonography of the ejaculatory apparatus. *Clin Radiol* 44: 240.

15 Pryor JP, Hendry WF (1991) Ejaculatory duct obstruction in subfertile males: analysis of 87 patients. *Fertil Steril* 56: 725.

16 Young D (1970) Surgical treatment of male infertility. *J Reprod Fertil* 23: 541.

17 Jequier AM, Ukombe EB (1983) Errors inherent in the performance of a routine semen analysis. *Br J Urol* 55: 434.

18 Hargreave TB, Elton RA (1983) Is conventional sperm analysis of any use? *Br J Urol* 55: 774.

19 Badenoch DF, Evans SWJ, McCloskey DJ (1989) Sperm density measurement: should this be abandoned? *Br J Urol* 64: 521.

20 Badenoch DF, Moore HDM, Holt WV, Evans PR, Sidhu BS, Evans SJW (1990) Sperm motility, velocity and migration. *Br J Urol* 65: 204.

21 Jequier AM, Holmes SC (1993) Primary testicular

disease presenting as azoospermia oligozoospermia in an infertility clinic. *Br J Urol* 71: 731.

22 Boyle CA (1992) The relation of computer based measures of sperm morphology and motility to male infertility. *Epidemiology* 3: 239.

23 Check JH, Nowroozi K, Bollendorf A. (1991) Correlation of motile sperm density and subsequent pregnancy rates in infertile couples. *Arch Androl* 27: 113.

24 Halim A, Antoniou D, Lane J, Blandy JP (1974) The significance of antibodies to sperm in infertile men and their wives. *Br J Urol* 46: 65.

25 Hargreave TB, Aitken RJ, Elton RA (1988) Prognostic significance of the zona-free hamster egg test. *Br J Urol* 62: 603.

26 Fisch H, Lipshultz LI (1991) Advanced sperm function testing. *Curr Opinion Urol* 1: 156.

27 Bramble FJ, Houghton AL, Jacobs HS (1975) Serum follicle-stimulating hormone estimation in the investigation of azoospermia. *Br J Surg* 62: 159.

28 Johnsen SG, (1970) Testicular biopsy score count. A method for registration of spermatogenesis in human testis: normal values and results in 335 hypogonadal males. *Hormones* 1: 1.

29 Hendry WF (1986) Clinical significance of unilateral testicular obstruction in subfertile males. *Br J Urol* 58: 709.

30 Parslow JM, Royle MG, Kingscott MMB, Wallace DMA, Hendry WF (1983) The effects of sperm antibodies on fertility after vasectomy reversal. *Amer J Reprod Immunol* 3: 28.

31 Grundy CE, Robinson J, Guthrie KA, Gordon AG, Hay DM (1992) Establishment of pregnancy after removal of sperm antibodies *in vitro*. *Br Med J* 304: 292.

32 Hargreave TB (1993) Varicocele — a clinical enigma. *Br J Urol* 72: 401.

33 Vermeulen A, Vandeweghe M (1984) Improved fertility after varicocele correction: fact or fiction? *Fertil Steril* 42: 249.

34 Lynch WJ, Badenoch DF, McAnena OJ (1993) Comparison of laparoscopic and open ligation of the testicular veins. *Br J Urol* 72: 796.

35 Hendry WF (1992) Effects of left varicocele ligation in subfertile males with absent or atrophic right testis. *Fertil Steril* 57: 1342.

36 Gentile DP, Cockett AT (1992) The effect of varicocelectomy on testicular volume in 89 infertile adult males with varicoceles. *Fertil Steril* 58: 209.

37 van der Liaden PJ, Nan PM, te Velde ER, Van Kooy RT (1992) Retrograde ejaculation: successful treatment with artificial insemination. *Obstet Gynecol* 79: 126.

38 Thomas A (1983) Ejaculatory dysfunction. *Fertil Steril* 39: 445.

39 Brindley GS, Scott GI, Hendry WF (1986) Vas cannulation with implanted sperm reservoirs for obstructive azoospermia or ejaculatory failure. *Br J Urol* 58: 721.

40 Miura K, Matsuhashi M, Takanami M, Ishii N, Shirai M (1991) Clinical experience and successful impregnation using an artificial spermatocele. *Urol Int* 47: 149.

41 Oates RD (1991) Microsurgical epididymal sperm aspiration. *Curr Opinion Urol* 1: 160.

Chapter 39: Vasectomy and disorders of seminal vesicles

Vasectomy

Vasectomy is so commonly performed today that it is in danger of being regarded with too little seriousness and yet it is fraught with medicolegal hazards for the surgeon.

Indications

Recurrent epididymitis may be halted by division of the vas, but infection after prostatectomy is now so infrequent that prophylactic vasectomy is no longer performed. Today, most vasectomies are done for sterilization.

Consultation with husband and wife are essential before embarking on vasectomy. The wife may be about to undergo a hysterectomy. Both partners must understand that the procedure is probably irreversible but that the ends may spontaneously rejoin in a very small number of cases (see below). In the current state of the law in England and Wales, it is necessary to obtain the informed consent of the man and his wife before doing the operation.

One must be very cautious: beware of the husband who is being driven to submit to vasectomy to save a failing marriage.

Investigations

Examine the patient carefully before deciding to proceed: it is difficult to do a vasectomy under local anaesthetic in a frightened man with a tight scrotum or when there has been previous scrotal or inguinal surgery.

Shaving

Let the patient shave his own scrotum: it is much more comfortable for him if he does it in the bath at leisure.

Anaesthesia

Local infiltration with 1% lignocaine with or without adrenaline gives excellent anaesthesia which is usually sufficient in the relaxed co-operative patient.

Choice of incision

The operation may be done through a single transverse or vertical scrotal incision, or through two incisions, one over each vas (Fig. 39.1).

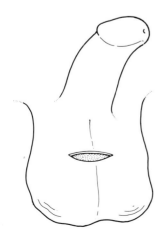
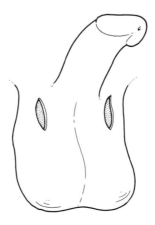

Fig. 39.1 Choice of incision for vasectomy.

Operative technique

There are many techniques for performing vasectomy. Despite confident claims, there is no evidence that any one method is any better than another. The essential steps are that the vas deferens is located by its characteristic feel (Fig. 39.2). The sheath of the vas is incised longitudinally taking care to avoid the artery and veins of the vas. The vas is lifted up out of the sheath. Care is taken not to pull on the vas: this can cause vagal stimulation, bradycardia, fainting and even cardiac arrest.

The vas is doubly clamped and divided. It is usual to keep a small segment of vas from each side, carefully labelled in formalin as medicolegal proof that the right organ was removed, should questions arise afterwards.

How to close the vas is the subject of endless variations, each author convinced that his or her own method is best. One way is to ligate the testicular end of the vas with fine (4−0) chromic catgut, curl the end back on itself into a loop, and tie it again [1]. The other end is ligated and dropped back into the sheath of the vas, which is then closed with a stitch. The looped-back end is left outside the sheath. It is the intention that the fascia of the sheath will prevent the ends coming together again: note that there has never been any proof that this method is better than any other.

Other techniques coagulate the lumen of the vas with diathermy [2]: place metal clips on each end of the vas or use non-absorbable ligatures.

There are as many opinions as to the right length of vas to be removed [3,4]. When the divided ends of the vasa were ligated with stainless steel, and the patients were X-rayed over the next 3−6 months, the ends always came together unless at least 7 cm of vas had been removed [5].

Complications

Every large series of vasectomies records complications: few are severe, but all of them are notoriously apt to generate resentment and litigation [6].

Haematoma is common after vasectomy as after all operations on the scrotum. It usually starts about 30 min after the end of the operation, at which the surgeon was satisfied that haemostasis had been perfect and is generally thought to be due to arterial or venous spasm, caused by handling the vas, and relaxing spontaneously later on [7].

When reactionary haemorrhage occurs and leads to a haematoma it is usual to return the patient to the operating theatre and evacuate the clot under anaesthesia. In practice, it is rare that a single bleeding vessel can be identified, and the blood is usually found between the tissues of the scrotum. After evacuation of the haematoma the swelling may take several weeks to resolve completely. It is common for the patient to complain of pain in the scrotum for some time afterwards. Never is anything found wrong and the cause of the pain remains uncertain.

Infection after vasectomy is rare, but may be very severe with mixed infection resulting in cellulitis. The author has seen two patients in whom an infected haematoma was followed by epididymoorchitis, necrosis and fungus testis, requiring orchiectomy. Infective gangrene leading to septicaemia, cardiac arrest and loss of skin of the entire scrotum have been recorded [8,9].

Sperm granuloma

In up to 33% of patients a painful swelling may develop either at the site of the divided vasa or

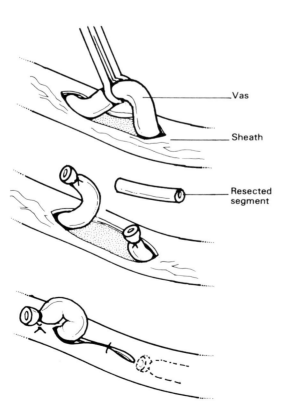

Fig. 39.2 The sheath of the vas deferens is slit open and the vas lifted out. After resecting 1 cm one end is turned back and ligated. A suture closes the sheath.

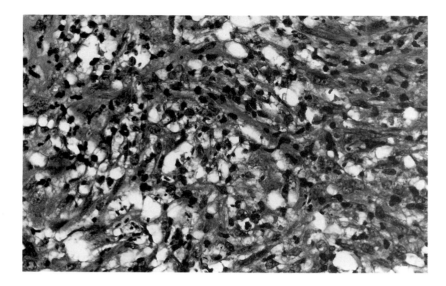

Fig. 39.3 Typical sperm granuloma at the cut end of the vas deferens (courtesy of Dr Suhail Baithun).

in the epididymes [10] (Fig. 39.3). In most cases it resolves spontaneously, but in others it persists and the patient demands treatment. It has been the author's experience that removal of the epididymis may, but does not always, relieve the pain. Histologically, there is a sperm granuloma — a chronic inflammatory response to extravasated sperm [10,11] (Fig. 39.4).

Spontaneous recanalization

The mechanism of spontaneous recanalization seems to be that sprouts of the epithelium lining the vas burrow into the granulation tissue filling the gap between the divided ends of the vasa [12,13]. If the sprouts meet each other, continuity is re-established. For a long time it was believed that this recanalization took place in the first few months after vasectomy, when the granuloma was new, and before scar tissue had contracted to form an impenetrable barrier. Early recanalization was thought to occur in 0.4–0.7% of cases [6,13,14] and would be detected by regular examination of the semen after operation, for the sperms would never completely disappear from the semen.

Very occasional cases were reported where the vasa would reunite years later: they were regarded as an extreme rarity [15,16]. However, whenever spontaneous reunion of the vas results in an unwanted pregnancy, the surgeon is likely to be accused of negligence, and the defence organization may be held liable for the upbringing of the unwanted child — hence the intense medicolegal interest in the issue of 'late' recanalization, i.e. after the semen had been shown to

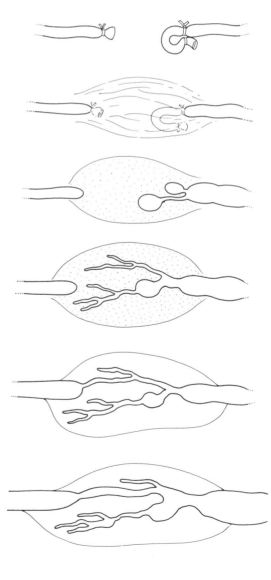

Fig. 39.4 Regeneration of the epithelium of the vas into the granuloma may result in spontaneous recanalization even years after the vasectomy.

be entirely free from spermatozoa in at least two consecutive specimens. In careful studies [17] such late recanalization was found in about 0.04%.

This has to be put into perspective. The present author took part in a series of 6000 vasectomies in which two patients developed cardiac arrest (0.03%) and two developed infective necrosis of the testicle (0.03%).

Few surgeons would think it necessary to warn of complications so rare: but vasectomy is an exception because of the suspicions and ill feeling that are aroused by an unexpected pregnancy years after vasectomy. It is therefore a wise precaution to warn the patient and his wife that this — however rare — can happen.

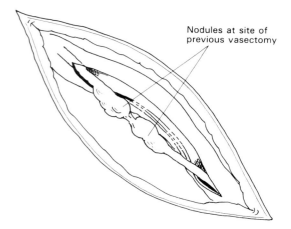

Fig. 39.5 Reversal of vasectomy. The nodules at the site of the previous vasectomy are exposed.

Postoperative semen analysis

After vasectomy the semen is repeatedly examined until two consecutive samples show no sperms in the centrifuged specimen [6]. Many centres have given their patient a 'special clearance' when only a very few non-motile sperms can be found in the ejaculate. Because this takes so long, many centres give a 'special clearance' when only a few immotile sperms can be found [18]. Experience teaches us to be even more cautious: paternity has been proven when not a single sperm can be found [19].

Vasectomy reversal

There are many techniques of reversal of vasectomy. All require patience, time and adequate anaesthesia. Most surgeons use loupes or the operating microscope. The divided ends of the vasa are exposed and sectioned until the lumen is revealed (Fig. 39.5). The ends are anastomosed, some prefer an end-to-end method, others end-to-side [20,21] (Fig. 39.6). Because it is thought that failure may be caused by extravasation of sperm from the suture line it has been suggested that this should be sealed with a tissue glue.

The results of reversal of vasectomy are disappointing. Although sperms reappear in the ejaculate in 80–90%, pregnancy is achieved in only 50% of couples. There are several explanations: first the couples are older, and biologically less likely to conceive. Second, while the sperms are retained in the epididymis, they may leak into the tissues and provoke an immunological reaction which will result in death or immobilization of the sperms [22,23].

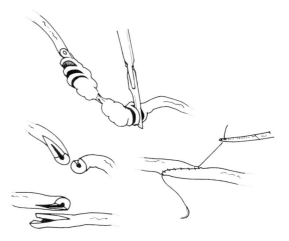

Fig. 39.6 Each end of the vas is sectioned until the lumen is seen. The ends are spatulated and anastomosed with 7–0 non-absorbable suture.

Vasectomy and other diseases

It had been suggested that vasectomy might increase the chance of myocardial infarction. This has not been confirmed [24,25] in a study of over 4000 vasectomized men followed for over 15 years.

More disturbingly it has recently been found in a retrospective study involving over 14 000 vasectomized husbands of nurses, with age-matched controls, and a prospective study of over 10 000 males who had vasectomy compared with over 37 000 who did not, that vasectomy carried a significantly increased risk of prostate cancer [26,27].

Seminal vesicles

For many years the seminal vesicles were something of a mystery to urologists. Recently, with the advent of transrectal ultrasound, we have come to appreciate that they may suffer all the disorders that affect all other hollow organs in the body.

History

Hippocrates noted a paired structure resembling a honeycomb on either side of the base of the bladder. Bold early investigators like Fallopius, de Graaf and John Hunter all found that their secretions tasted sweet. But their function remained a mystery, much as it does today [28].

Until quite recently gonorrhoea was the chief urological disease, and when it went for many years virtually untreated, it could give rise to chronic abscesses in the seminal vesicles. Fuller [29] developed a method for draining them via the perineum. Others injected silver nitrate into them through the vasa deferentia [30]. A more effective treatment was to remove them entirely — especially when they harboured tuberculosis [31]. All this was to disappear with the advent of antibiotics — first the sulphonamides and penicillin, later streptomycin and therapy for tuberculosis. There was no need to operate on the seminal vesicles, and for a generation urologists forgot about them. Today, the ease of providing an image with transrectal ultrasound and computerized tomographic (CT) scanning is reviving interest in these organs.

Anatomy and physiology

Development

The seminal vesicle arises in the third month of fetal life as a diverticulum from the vas deferens just before it joins the ejaculatory duct (see p. 544). Surrounding mesenchyme clothes it with a muscular coat. It remains small until puberty, when it swells and becomes convoluted.

Topographical anatomy

The seminal vesicles lie in the groove between bladder and prostate, inferior to the ampullae of the vasa deferentia. The ureter passes inferior to the vas deferens *en route* to the bladder (see p. 545).

In adult life the vesicle holds from 1.5 to 10 ml of fluid. When unravelled each vesicle consists of a sac about 15 cm long, with one or two side arms. The low columnar mucosa is thrown into ridges and creases to enlarge its surface area (see p. 546). After the age of 40 its mucosa becomes thinner and flatter [32,33].

The seminal vesicles have alpha adrenergic smooth muscle in their wall. Stimulation of the presacral nerve causes them to contract [34,35]. This contraction is inhibited by testosterone [36]. Sympathectomy, e.g. during bilateral retroperitoneal node dissection for testicular cancer is followed by ejaculatory paralysis. If one chain can be preserved ejaculation is normal, though with a reduced volume.

Studies using contrast medium injected into the seminal tract show that the ampullae of the vasa deferentia empty first, and then the seminal vesicles, which function like a syringe to flush out the first sperm-rich fraction of semen.

From puberty onwards, the seminal vesicles normally contain live spermatozoa, and were considered to be reservoirs, but probably the main sperm reservoir is the ampulla of the vasa deferentia. Their secretion makes up about 80% of the ejaculate and is rich in fructose, citric acid, magnesium, ammonium and ascorbic acid [37].

Congenital anomalies

The seminal vesicles may be absent on one or both sides, the ureter may enter the vesicle, and the vesicle may have cysts and diverticula [38−40] (Figs 39.7 & 39.8). Some of these cysts are very large [39] and may contain up to 5l of fluid [41], which may become infected and form stones (Fig. 39.9, 39.10). Cysts of the seminal vesicles must be distinguished from cysts arising from the midline Müllerian duct [42].

Infection

Gonococcal infection of the seminal vesicles is no longer seen today, where once it was common and serious [28]. Occasionally, abscesses are seen [43] and all the causes of chronic infection of the urinary tract, e.g. *Schistosoma*, *Amoeba* and *Trichomonas*, may involve the seminal vesicles.

With the increasing use of transrectal ultrasound it has become possible to identify obstruction of the seminal vesicle complicated by infection (39.11): in one case this was caused by a small calculus lodged in the common ejaculatory duct [44].

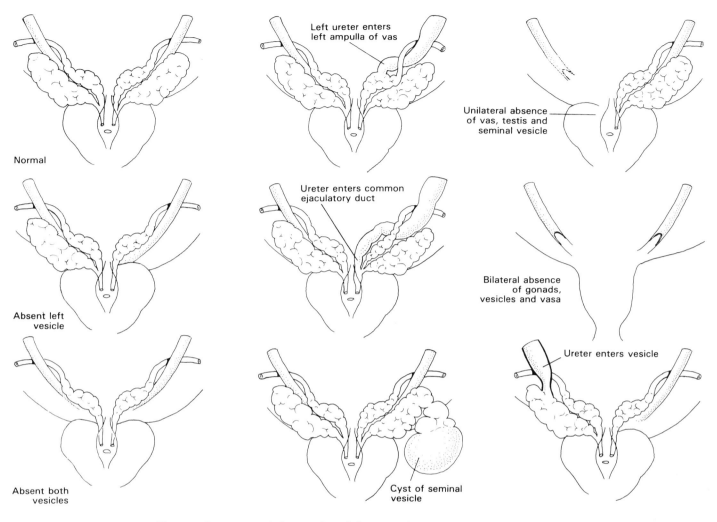

Fig. 39.7 Some congenital anomalies of the seminal vesicles.

Neoplasms

Any cavity lined with mucosa may give rise to adenocarcinoma. The difficulty with the seminal vesicle is that by the time the diagnosis is made it is almost impossible to be sure that the origin of the cancer was in the vesicle [45].

Their spread, like the prostate, is by the Batson's veins to the pelvis and femora, eroding the bone rather than causing sclerosis, but it seems that these metastases may be hormone sensitive. Sarcoma and choriocarcinoma arising from the connective tissue of the seminal vesicle have been reported [46].

Degenerative diseases

Amyloid is seen in the seminal vesicle as a normal feature in old men, and it occurs at an earlier age in diabetics [47,48]. Stones are common in seminal vesicles, though they seldom cause symptoms.

Investigations

Imaging

Transrectal ultrasonographic scans show the vesicles with great clarity, and when there is an obstructed seminal vesicle, it allows aspiration and biopsy to be performed under ultrasound control (Fig. 39.9).

Plain radiographs may show calculi in seminal vesicles (Fig. 39.10) and calcification of the vesicles and vasa is commonly seen in bilharziasis, and may occur in diabetes.

Injection of contrast medium into the vas gives an outline of the vasa, the ampulla and the

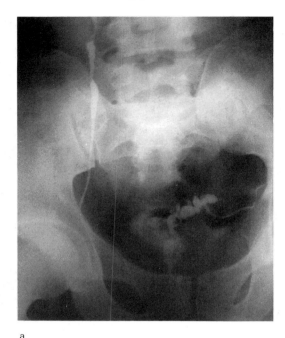

a

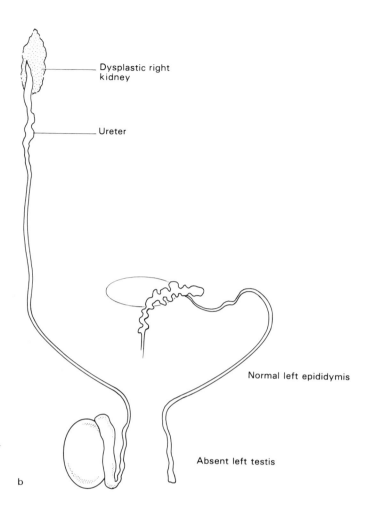

Dysplastic right kidney

Ureter

Normal left epididymis

Absent left testis

b

Fig. 39.8 (a) Radiograph and (b) diagram of an example of a congenital anomaly of the Wolffian system causing infertility. On the right side a dysplastic kidney was connected to the right vas deferens: on the left there was no testis. When the right vas was joined to the left one the patient became fertile.

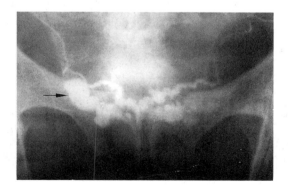

Fig. 39.9 Cyst of right seminal vesicle (arrow).

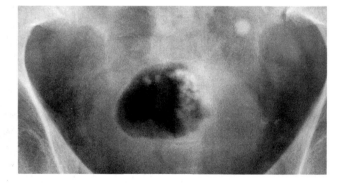

Fig. 39.10 At open prostatectomy the seminal vesicle was found to be full of calculi.

seminal vesicle but the wide range of normal variations makes them difficult to interpret [48,49] (Fig. 39.12). CT and magnetic resonance imaging (MRI) scanning are both useful in imaging of the seminal vesicle, and have been particularly useful in showing invasion of the vesicles by cancer of the prostate [50] (Fig. 39.13).

Semen analysis

The majority of the volume of the semen is derived from the seminal vesicles, as is all the fructose, so that semen of small volume with an absence of fructose generally signifies disease of the vesicles. This is common in diabetics, but also occurs as a result of inflammation.

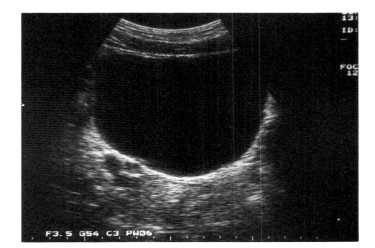

Fig. 39.11 Ultrasound showing absence of the left seminal vesicle and dilatation of the right one (courtesy of Dr W. Hately).

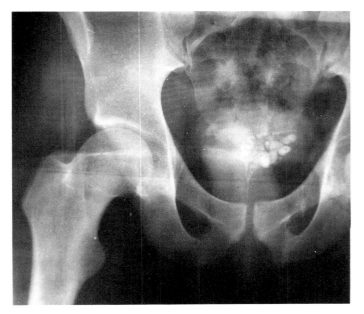

a

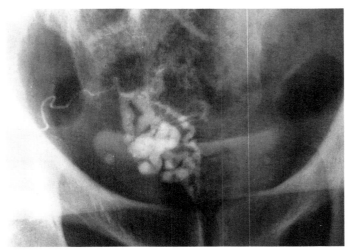

b

Fig. 39.12 (a & b) Normal seminal vesiculograms.

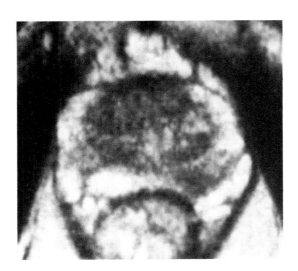

Fig. 39.13 CT showing invasion of the seminal vesicle by cancer of the prostate (courtesy of Dr W. Hately).

Surgical approach to the seminal vesicles

The most simple and direct approach to the vesicles is through an abdominal incision, stripping the peritoneum off the posterior surface of the bladder, and following the vas deferens down on either side. Care must be taken to avoid injury to the ureter which passes under the seminal vesicle.

References

1 Blandy JP (1979) Contemporary surgery: vasectomy. *Br J Hosp Med* 21: 520.

2 Schmidt SS (1973) Prevention of failure in vasectomy. *J Urol* 109: 296.

3 Hanley GH (1968) Vasectomy for voluntary male sterilisation. *Lancet* ii: 207.

4 Kaplan KA, Heuther CA (1975) A clinical study of vasectomy failure and recanalisation. *J Urol* 113: 71.

5 Hallan RI, May ARL (1988) Vasectomy: how much is enough? *Br J Urol* 62: 377.

6 Barnes MN and staff of Margaret Pyke Centre (1973) One thousand vasectomies. *Br Med J* 4: 216.

7 Burch GE, Phillips J (1963) Peripheral vascular diseases — diseases other than atherosclerosis. Spasm of major arteries, in: Hamilton WF, Dow P (eds) *Handbook of Physiology*, vol. 2, section 2, pp. 1263−8. Washington: American Physiological Society.

8 Pryor JP, Yates-Bell AJ, Packham DA (1971) Scrotal gangrene after male sterilization. *Br Med J* 1: 272.

9 Patel A, Ramsay JWA, Whitfield HN (1991) Fournier's gangrene of the scrotum following day-case vasectomy. *J Roy Soc Med* 82: 49.

10 McMahon AJ, Buckley J, Taylor A, Lloyd SN, Deane RF, Kirk D (1992) Chronic testicular pain following vasectomy. *Br J Urol* 69: 188.

11 Glassy FJ, Mostofi FK (1956) Spermatic granulomas of the epididymis. *Amer J Clin Pathol* 26: 1303.

12 Paris AMI, Leedham PW (1973) Histology of the divided vas. *Proc Roy Soc Med* 66: 371.

13 Pugh RCB, Hanely HG (1969) Spontaneous recanalisation of the divided vas deferens. *Br J Urol* 41: 340.

14 Philp T, Guillebaud J, Budd D (1984) Complications of vasectomy: review of 16000 patients. *Br J Urol* 56: 745.

15 Rolnick HC (1924) Regeneration of the vas deferens. *J Urol* 9: 188.

16 O'Conor VJ (1948) Regeneration of the vas deferens after purposeful division for sterility. *J Am Med Assoc* 136: 162.

17 Philp T, Guillebaud J, Budd D (1984) Late failure of vasectomy after two documented analyses showing azoospermic semen. *Br Med J* 289: 77.

18 Davies AH, Sharp RJ, Cranston D, Mitchell RG (1990) The long-term outcome following 'special clearance' after vasectomy. *Br J Urol* 66: 211.

19 Smith JC, Cranston D, O'Brien T, Guillebaud J, Hindmarsh J, Turner AG (1994) Fatherhood without apparent spermatozoa after vasectomy. *Lancet* 344: 30.

20 Schlegel PN, Goldstein M (1993) Microsurgical vasoepididymostomy: refinements and results. *J Urol* 150: 1165.

21 Royle MG, Hendry WF (1985) Why does vasectomy reversal fail? *Br J Urol* 57: 780.

22 Halim A, Antoniou D (1973) Autoantibodies to spermatozoa in relation to male infertility and vasectomy. *Br J Urol* 45: 559.

23 Fisch H, Laor E, Barchama N, Witkin SS, Tolia BM, Reid RE (1989) Detection of testicular endocrine abnormalities and their correlation with serum anti-sperm antibodies in men following vasectomy. *J Urol* 141: 1129.

24 Walker AM, Jick H, Hunter JR, McEvoy J (1983) Vasectomy and non-fatal myocardial infarction: continued observation indicates no elevation of risk. *J Urol* 130: 936.

25 Nienhuis H, Goldacre M, Seagrott V, Gill L, Vessey M (1992) Incidence of disease after vasectomy: a record linked retrospective cohort study. *Br Med J* 304: 743.

26 Giovanucci E, Ascherio A, Rimm EB, Colditz GA, Stampfer MJ (1993) A prospective cohort study of vasectomy and prostate cancer in US men. *J Am Med Assoc* 269: 873.

27 Giovanucci E, Tosteson TD, Spelzer FE, Ascherio A, Vessey MP, Colditz GA (1993) A retrospective cohort study of vasectomy and prostate cancer in US men. *J Am Med Assoc* 269: 878.

28 Gutierrez R (1935) *Surgery of the Seminal Vesicles, Ampullae and Vasa Deferentia*. New York: Oxford University Press.

29 Fuller E (1913) The cure through genitourinary surgery of arthritis deformans and allied varieties of chronic rheumatism. *Med Rec* 84: 691.

30 Kidd F (1923) Vasotomy for seminal vesiculitis. *Lancet* ii: 213.

31 Young HH (1912) A perineal method for excising or draining the seminal vesicles. *Trans Am Assoc Genitourin Surg* 7: 73.

32 Nilsson S (1962) The human seminal vesicle. *Acta Chir Scand Suppl* 296.

33 Riva A, Stockwell RA (1969) Histochemical study of human seminal vesicle epithelium. *J Anat* 104: 253.

34 Learmonth JR (1931) A contribution to the neuro-physiology of the urinary bladder in man. *Brain* 54: 147.

35 Brindley GS (1986) Sacral root and hypogastric plexus stimulators and what these models tell us about autonomic actions on the bladder and urethra. *Clin Sci* 70 (Suppl 14): 41s.

36 Grunt JA, Higgins JR (1960) Seminal vesicle response to androgen with adrenaline, nor-adrenaline, and acetyl-choline. *Amer J Physiol* 198: 15.

37 Mann TRR (1964) *Biochemistry of Semen and the Male Reproductive Tract*. London: Methuen.

38 Young JN (1955) Ureter opening into the seminal vesicle: report of a case. *Br J Urol* 27: 57.

39 Chatterjee SK, Sarkar SK (1973) Retrovesical cysts in boys. *J Urol* 109: 107.

40 Beeby DI (1974) Seminal vesicle cyst associated with ipsilateral renal agenesis: case report and review of literature. *J Urol* 112: 120.

41 Damjanov I, Apic R (1974) Cystadenoma of seminal vesicles. *J Urol* 111: 808.

42 Sheih CP, Liao YJ, Li YW, Yang LY (1993) Seminal vesicle cyst associated with ipsilateral renal malformation and hemivertebra: report of two cases. *J Urol* 150: 1214.

43 Conn IG, Peeling WB, Clements R (1992) Complete resolution of a large seminal vesicle cyst — evidence for an obstructive aetiology. *Br J Urol* 69: 636.

44 Hendry WF, Levison DA, Parkinson MC, Parslow JM, Royle MG (1990) Testicular obstruction: clinico-pathological studies. *Ann Roy Coll Surg Engl* 72: 396.

45 Gohji K, Kamidono S, Okada S (1993) Primary adenocarcinoma of the seminal vesicle. *Br J Urol* 72: 514.

46 Fairey AE, Mead GM, Murphy D, Theaker J (1993)

Primary seminal vesicle choriocarcinoma. *Br J Urol* 71: 756.

47 Novia HJ, Yunis E (1964) Age changes of seminal vesicles and vasa deferentia in diabetics. *Arch Pathol* 77: 126.

48 Boreau J (1953) *L'Étude Radiologique des Voies Seminales Normales et Pathologiques*. Paris: Masson.

49 Singh H, Singh G, Kera KS (1970) Seminal vesiculography as a diagnostic aid in differentiating benign hypertrophy from malignant prostate. *Indian J Surg* 32: 36.

50 Maeda H, Toyooka N, Kinukawa T, Hattori R, Furukawa T (1993) Magnetic resonance images of hematospermia. *Urology* 41: 499.

PART 7
ADRENAL

Chapter 40: Adrenal glands

Anatomy

Embryology

The cortex of the adrenal gland arises from the genitourinary ridge near the developing gonads and kidneys: tiny rests of adrenal cortical tissue are common in the renal cortex, retroperitoneum, and testis as well as the broad ligament near the ovary (Fig. 40.1). The adrenal cortex shares many of the enzymes of gonads — notably those for the synthesis of steroids — so that some inborn errors of metabolism affect them both.

In the seventh week of fetal life neuroblasts from the neural crest invade the developing adrenal cortex to form the medulla. After a week they differentiate into sympathicoblasts and pheochromocytes containing the intracellular catecholamines, adrenalin and noradrenalin.

In fetal life, the adrenals are larger than the kidneys and are still about one-third of their size at birth [1,2].

Topographical anatomy

The adrenal has two distinct parts: (a) the cortex, a busy endocrine gland subordinate to the pituitary; and (b) the medulla, a specialized part of the sympathetic nervous system [3].

Each adrenal gland is shaped like a cocked hat. Its cross-section resembles a triple sandwich: the outermost layer is the yellow zona glomerulosa, next the zona fasciculata, and third, the brown zona reticularis. Finally, there is a vascular filling — the medulla. (Fig. 40.2). The triple layer of cortex is only a few millimetres thick — hence the term suprarenal capsule.

Each of the three layers of the cortex has a different function. The foamy cells of the outermost zona glomerulosa form aldosterone (Fig.

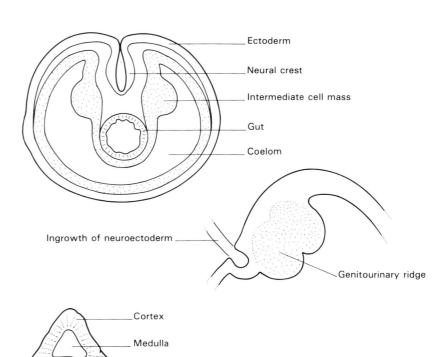

Fig. 40.1 Embryology: the cortex arises in the mesoderm of the 'intermediate cell mass' which later forms the genitourinary ridge. Neuroectodermal cells migrate into it from the neural crest to form the medulla.

623

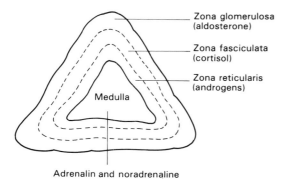

Fig. 40.2 The sandwich structure of the adrenal: zona glomerulosa (aldosterone); zona fasciculata (cortisol); zona reticularis (androgens); and medulla (adrenalin and noradrenalin).

40.3). The zona fasciculata — so called because its cells are lined up in orderly bundles — produces glucocorticoids, mainly cortisol. The zona reticularis produces androgens.

The medulla is made of pheochromocytes surrounded by spongy vascular spaces, rich in sympathetic ganglion cells. The pheochromocytes make the catecholamines adrenalin and noradrenalin. Because these turn brown when oxidized, this is called the chromaffin reaction.

Surgical relations

Above each adrenal (Fig. 40.4) lies the diaphragm; medially are the aorta or the vena cava; laterally is the abdominal wall; inferiorly is the kidney to which the adrenal is so firmly attached that pulling down the kidney is a useful way of bringing the adrenal into a surgical incision. In front are the duodenum and colon: behind the diaphragm, 12th rib and the pleural recess.

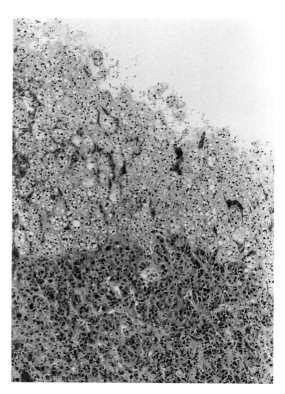

Fig. 40.3 Histological section through the adrenal showing the three zones of the cortex, and the vascular spaces of the medulla (courtesy of Dr Suhail Baithun).

Arterial supply

The adrenal is supplied by small branches of the phrenic, renal and lumbar arteries. Blood leaves the hilum through a single vein which flows into the renal vein on the left side, and the inferior vena cava on the right. These adrenal veins are easily torn: on the right such a tear may lead to daunting haemorrhage from the vena cava.

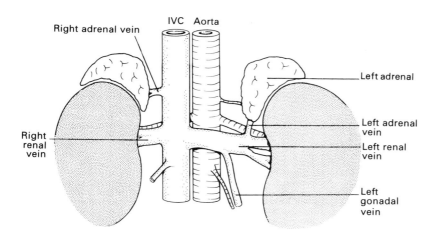

Fig. 40.4 Surgical relations of the adrenal glands.

Nerve supply

A rich plexus of sympathetic nerves enters the adrenal medulla.

Physiology

Adrenal cortex

The cells of the zona glomerulosa make aldosterone — the 18-aldehyde of corticosterone which is released under the action of angiotensin II, and by retaining water and salt in the distal tubules helps to sustain a rise in blood pressure by increasing blood volume.

The zonae fasciculata and reticularis are controlled by adrenocorticotrophic hormone (ACTH) from the anterior pituitary, which in turn responds to ACTH-releasing hormone of the hypothalamus (Fig. 40.5).

The zona fasciculata forms the glucocorticoids cortisol and corticosterone, and the mineralocorticoid deoxycorticosterone. The glucocorticoids — all 17-hydroxycorticosteroids — can be measured in the urine. Cortisol can be measured in the plasma where it rises and falls according to the time of day, usually being lowest in the morning and highest in the evening.

Glucocorticoids are so named because they increase the production of glucose. Many synthetic glucocorticoids are available, e.g. prednisone, prednisolone, betamethasone and dexamethasone, which all vary in the relative strength of their effects on inflammation and sodium retention.

The zona reticularis forms a little testosterone, and more of the androgen precursors dihydroepiandrosterone and androstenedione, which are converted into testosterone in tissue. The metabolic end-product of all these androgens appears in the urine as the 17-ketosteroids. The androgens stimulate growth and the appearance of male secondary sexual hair.

Adrenal medulla

The medulla secretes the catecholamines dopamine, noradrenalin and adrenalin which are in turn metabolized to normetanephrin and metanephrin. Their common metabolic end-result in the urine is vanillyl mandelic acid (VMA) (Fig. 40.6).

Noradrenalin raises the blood pressure by increasing peripheral resistance without changing the cardiac output. Adrenalin increases cardiac output by raising pulse rate and systolic pressure, without increasing peripheral vascular resistance.

Congenital disorders of the adrenals

Haemorrhage into the adrenals on one or both sides may follow a difficult labour or childbirth asphyxia. The diagnosis is usually made post-

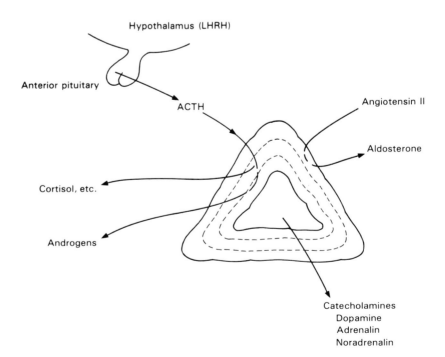

Fig. 40.5 Hormonal control of the layers of the adrenal: the zona glomerulosa secretes aldosterone under the influence of angiotensin II. The hypothalamus secretes LHRH, which stimulates the anterior pituitary to secrete ACTH, which stimulates the zona fasciculata to secrete the corticoids, and the zona reticularis to secrete androgens. The medulla secretes the catecholamines dopamine, adrenalin and noradrenalin.

Hypothalamus (LHRH)

Anterior pituitary

ACTH

Angiotensin II

Aldosterone

Cortisol, etc.

Androgens

Catecholamines
Dopamine
Adrenalin
Noradrenalin

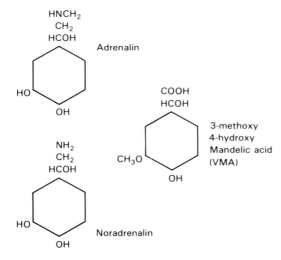

Fig. 40.6 Biochemistry of adrenalin, noradrenalin and VMA.

mortem, the child having died of exsanguination and hypoadrenalism [1]. Sometimes Gerota's fascia will tamponade the bleeding and control it and the child then survives with a mass which displaces the kidney downwards and may calcify later on. There may be late adrenal insufficiency [2].

Trauma

The adrenal is often torn during nephrectomy, when there may be bleeding from the venous sinuses of the medulla, which may need suture ligature.

Inflammation

Spontaneous haemorrhage into the adrenals occurs in the Waterhouse—Friderichsen syndrome in septicaemic shock. Calcification in the adrenals from old tuberculosis was in former times an important cause of Addison's disease — hypoadrenalism.

Hyperplasia and neoplasia

Each of the three zones of the cortex may undergo hyperplasia or neoplastic change.

Hyperplasia

Hyperplasia of the zonae fasciculata and reticularis follow an oversupply of ACTH usually coming from a basophil adenoma in the pituitary, but sometimes from cancers in other organs — notably

the lung. Cortisol from the zona fasciculata produces Cushing's syndrome: androgens from the zona reticularis cause virilization: catecholamines from the medulla cause hypertension.

Cortisol-producing tumours of the zona fasciculata are usually small and well defined. Zona reticularis tumours which cause virilization are brown, sometimes very large and often malignant [4].

Most carcinomas of the adrenal cortex only secrete inactive precursors of hormones and do not give rise to endocrine syndromes. If they do secrete any hormone it is usually cortisol, and causes Cushing's syndrome — of which they are the usual cause in children. They may also virilize or produce hyperaldosteronism. Carcinomas spread and metastasize like any other retroperitoneal tumour [5,6].

By the time they are diagnosed non-secreting tumours are usually large and have often metastasized [7]. Any non-functioning adrenal tumour over 3.5 cm in diameter is likely to be malignant and should be removed [8].

Whether endocrine-secreting or non-functioning, the treatment of malignant cortical tumours is surgery. Recently chemotherapy and 1,1 dichloro-2-(O-chlorophenyl)-2-(P-chlorophenyl) (OPDDD) ethane has been used, with little benefit. The 5-year survival is 23% [9].

The secreting tumours and hyperplastic glands of the cortex produce three characteristic syndromes, according to whether their chief product is cortisol (Cushing's syndrome), aldosterone (Conn's syndrome) or androgens (virilization).

Cushing's syndrome

Whether caused by hyperplasia, benign adenoma or cancer, the clinical features are the same because they are due to excess of cortisol. Obesity is confined to the trunk. The extremities are wasted. There is a moon face, buffalo hump, striae, acne, hypertension and a pronounced smell. Patients bruise easily; females grow facial hair and stop menstruating (Fig. 40.7).

Investigations. These include the following:
1 Plasma ACTH. When Cushing's syndrome is caused by an adenoma of the pituitary or an ACTH-secreting tumour in another organ, the plasma ACTH may be as much as double its normal level [10]. If caused by an adrenal tumour the plasma level of ACTH is low.
2 Plasma cortisol. When Cushing's syndrome is

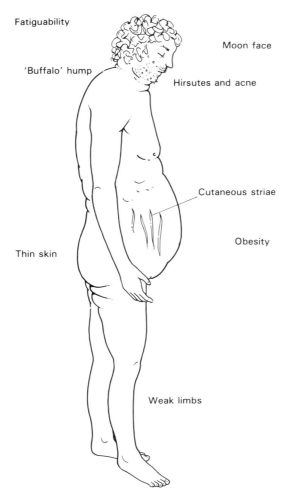

Fatiguability

Moon face

'Buffalo' hump

Hirsutes and acne

Cutaneous striae

Obesity

Thin skin

Weak limbs

Fig. 40.7 Caricature showing the principal clinical features of Cushing's syndrome.

caused by an adrenal cortical tumour, the plasma cortisol does not show the usual diurnal variation, but remains constant, nor does it fall if dexamethasone is given to suppress the pituitary ACTH. Metyrapone inhibits the synthesis of cortisol and if given after ACTH, the change in plasma cortisol helps to distinguish Cushing's

syndrome caused by adrenal tumour from adenoma of the pituitary [10].

3 Glucose tolerance curve. The glucocorticoids elevate the blood glucose and give a diabetic glucose tolerance curve.

4 Imaging. Ultrasound and computerized tomography (CT) scans identify the 20% of cases with an adrenal tumour, but in the remainder they show bilateral hyperplasia [10,11].

Surgery. If investigations show a single small tumour, it is approached through the 12th rib bed with the patient in the usual lateral position, the adrenal being brought down by traction on the kidney. A large tumour may require a thoraco-abdominal approach. The colon and duodenum are reflected medially to give access to the adrenal which is removed after dividing its afferent arteries and its single efferent vein.

For bilateral hyperplasia the adrenals are best approached through a bilateral 12th rib approach with the patient in the prone position [10].

Conn's syndrome: aldosteronism

Hyperplasia is the usual cause of aldosteronism in children [10] but in adults it is usually due to a small benign adenoma of the zona glomerulosa [12]. The hypertrophied zona or adenoma secretes aldosterone, causing sodium retention (hypertension), hypokalaemia (weakness) and polyuria (Fig. 40.8). There is a low level of plasma renin and often a metabolic alkalosis. The tumours are usually small and yellow [12].

The striking clinical symptom is muscle weakness. Hypertension may be the only physical sign: and the only diagnostic clue — hypokalaemia, is easily missed in a patient taking diuretics for hypertension.

The plasma aldosterone is elevated and does not fall when the patient is given 2 l of normal saline. The plasma renin does not rise when the patient is deprived of salt and given frusemide.

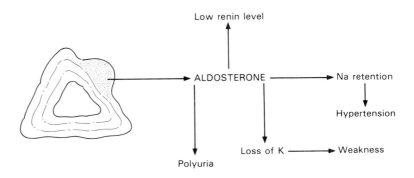

Low renin level

ALDOSTERONE → Na retention

Hypertension

Polyuria

Loss of K → Weakness

Fig. 40.8 Principal features of Conn's syndrome.

It is difficult to localize these small tumours even with CT. Renal vein venography may help (Fig. 40.9) and the level of aldosterone in the adrenal veins may be measured [10]. Even then it may be necessary to explore both adrenals at the same time, as in Cushing's disease.

Virilizing tumours

Virilization is usually caused by a solitary tumour of the adrenal which is often malignant. There are elevated levels of ketosteroids, testosterone and other androgens which do not fall with dexamethasone or rise with ACTH. They can usually be localized with CT scanning: occasionally an angiogram is helpful. Their surgical removal is exactly as for a tumour giving rise to Cushing's syndrome.

Maternal cortical tumours may cause virilization of a female fetus — female pseudohermaphroditism [13] (see p. 441).

Pheochromocytoma

Aetiology (Table 40.1)

Pheochromocytoma may occur in association with hyperparathyroidism, medullary carcinoma of the thyroid, the inherited (type II) form of the multiple endocrine neoplasia (Sipple's syndrome) [14–16], renal cell carcinoma, and von Hippel–Lindau disease — retinal angiomatosis, cerebellar and pancreatic cysts [17–19]. There is some evidence that it is becoming more common [20].

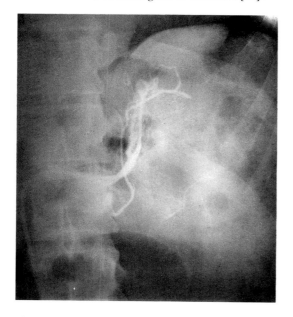

Fig. 40.9 Renal vein phlebogram showing an adrenal adenoma (courtesy of Mr Kenneth Owen).

Table 40.1 Pheochromocytoma — associated syndromes

Sturge–Weber syndrome
  (Multiple endocrine neoplasia type 2a)
  Carcinoma of thyroid
  Hyperparathyroidism
  Pheochromocytoma
  Diagnosis by DNA analysis
von Recklinghausen's disease
  Café au lait patches
  Multiple neurofibromas
von Hippel–Lindau disease
  Angiomatosis of retina
  Haemangioma of cerebellum
  Mental retardation
  Fits

About 10% are bilateral, 10% are extra-adrenal but only about 1% are malignant [3]. Outside the adrenal these chromaffinomas occur in the retroperitoneum near the adrenals, mediastinum, carotid body, organ of Zuckerkandl (at the origin of the inferior mesenteric artery) and bladder, where paroxysmal hypertension occurs with micturition.

Clinical features

Typically, there are paroxysms of hypertension headache, palpitation and sweating, brought on by smoking, sexual intercourse, defaecation, pressure on the abdomen, pregnancy and drugs such as morphine, ACTH and parenteral methyldopa. In practice, many patients have sustained rather than paroxysmal hypertension — classic hypertensive crises are absent in nearly half of patients [20].

Diagnosis

For measurement of urine VMA, normetanephrine, metanephrine and the free catecholamines hydrochloric acid must be added to the container to preserve them. Adrenalin and noradrenalin can be measured in plasma by a radioenzymatic assay [10]: after giving clonidine, which prevents them being released from the normal adrenal (i.e. in essential hypertension) [18].

Once the biochemical diagnosis has been established the tumours must be found. They are usually revealed by CT scanning (Fig. 40.10) which has largely replaced angiography which was diagnostic because of the profuse blood supply of these tumours (Fig. 40.11). If angiography is required, the risk of precipitating an

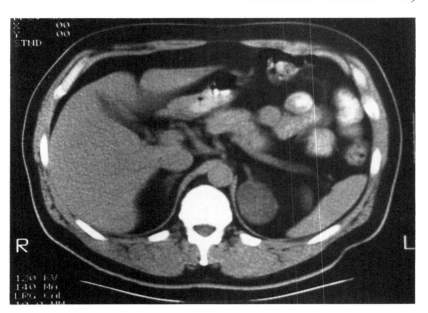

Fig. 40.10 CT scan showing pheochromocytoma (courtesy of Dr W. Hately).

episode of hypertension can be avoided by thorough alpha blockade beforehand.

Isotope scanning with [131]iodine-meta-iodo-benzylguanidine (MIGB) an analogue of noradrenalin gives exact localization especially of those with metastases [21]. It is said that ^{11}C-hydroxyephredrine, which attaches to adrenergic nerve terminals, gives even better localization [22].

Treatment

Full alpha blocking with phenoxybenzamine is given for 2 weeks before the operation. On the table a central venous line monitors the blood pressure. Ample blood is crossmatched in case of a fall in blood pressure after removing the pheochromocytoma.

Except when there is a large tumour, make a transverse or vertical abdominal incision. Display the right adrenal by mobilizing the colon and duodenum, and retracting the liver and gallbladder upwards (Fig. 40.12). On the left side, mobilize the splenic flexure and duodenum downwards and medially (Fig. 40.13). For a very large left tumour a thoracoabdominal approach is used.

Handle the adrenal very gently. Ligate its vein as soon as possible, and preferably before touching the growth. Its arteries, derived from the renal and phrenic, are usually small.

It is difficult to tell the benign from the malignant pheochromocytomas — DNA ploidy may help [23]. They should all be followed up in view of the slight risk of late metastasis.

Neuroblastoma

Neuroblastoma is the most common solid tumour of infancy, making up half of all tumours in this

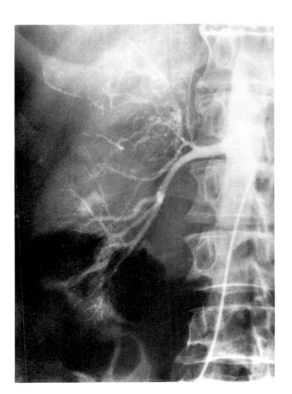

Fig. 40.11 Angiogram of pheochromocytoma (courtesy of Mr Kenneth Owen).

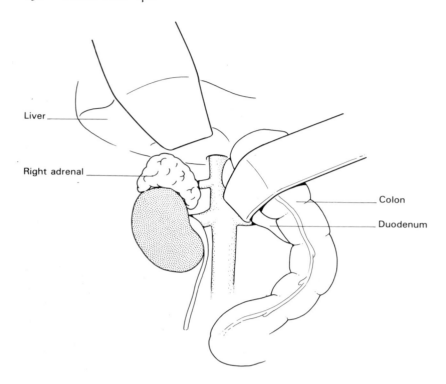

Fig. 40.12 Exposure of the right adrenal in pheochromocytoma. The liver is retracted upwards and the colon and duodenum mobilized medially.

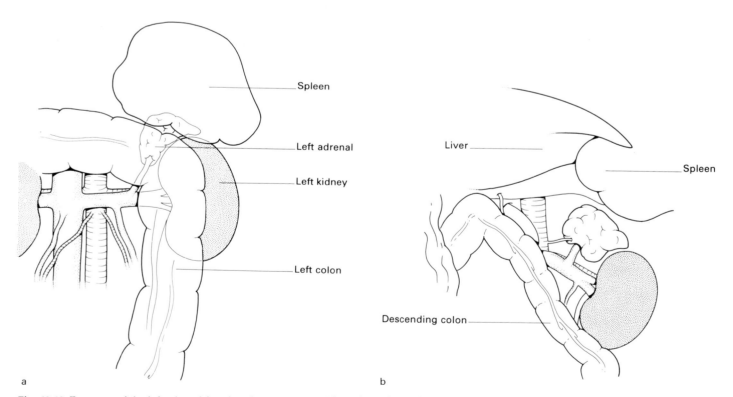

a

b

Fig. 40.13 Exposure of the left adrenal for pheochromocytoma. After taking down the splenic flexure (a) the colon and (b) the duodenum are retracted medially.

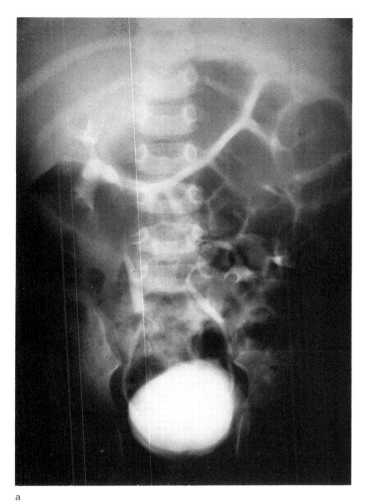

a

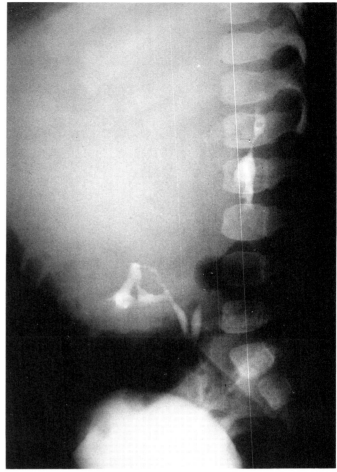

b

c

Fig. 40.14 IVU of a left-sided neuroblastoma displacing the whole kidney downwards. (a) AP; (b) lateral; (c) DMSA scan (courtesy of Dr W. Hately).

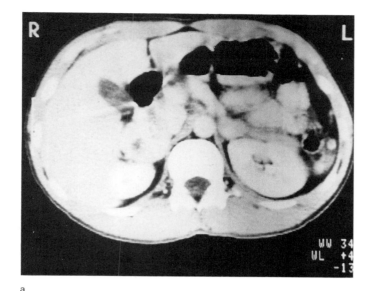

a

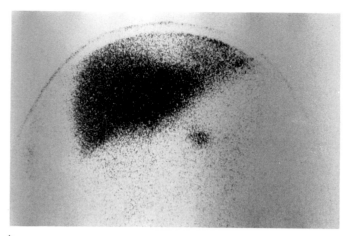

b

Fig. 40.15 (a) CT scan of neuroblastoma; (b) MIGB scan (courtesy of Dr W. Hately).

age group. Most occur below the age of 5 and half below the age of 2. More than half arise in the neural crest tissues of the abdomen, 25% of them in the adrenal, the rest arise anywhere in association with the sympathetic trunk, thorax and neck.

Lymphocytes cytotoxic for neuroblastoma cells may occur in parents and siblings of children with neuroblastoma suggesting a viral origin for this cancer which has been found in more than one member of the same family [24]. The more lymphocytes in the peripheral blood, the better the prognosis.

Nephroblastomas metastasize early and through the bloodstream but sometimes regress spontaneously, especially in the first 6 months of life.

Clinical features

Clinically, 75% of neuroblastomas present as a large fixed nodular lump, usually on the left. One in three under the age of 2 already have metastases causing 'joint pains' and fever, prompting the misdiagnosis of rheumatic fever. Retroorbital metastases cause the classical malignant proptosis. The catecholamines are raised in the urine, and if the tumour occurs *in utero*, it may cause hypertension in the mother.

Investigations

Bleeding into the tumour causes anaemia. Marrow aspiration may show infiltration by tumour. Alpha fetoprotein and carcinoembryonic antigen

are raised — the latter being a useful marker of response to chemotherapy.

Ultrasound and CT scanning confirms the mass (Figs 40.14 & 40.15). The plain radiograph shows scattered calcification, which helps to distinguish this from Wilms' tumour, as does the downward displacement of the kidney in the urogram.

Treatment

The mainstay of treatment is surgical excision. When complete excision is impossible, an attempt is made to debulk the tumour, even if this means opening its capsule and spooning out its soft contents. Before this is attempted the blood supply must be secured otherwise there may be uncontrollable bleeding. Radiotherapy helps shrink the tumour before the operation. Combination chemotherapy may give a dramatic reduction in the size of tumours and metastases, but seldom prolongs life [25].

Miscellaneous disorders of the adrenal gland

Cysts

Cysts in the adrenal may be so large as to be palpable. They rarely occur in infants [1]. They displace the kidney and are easily imaged by ultrasound and CT scanning. True cysts may be lymphangiomatous with milky fluid: pseudocysts are reported from degeneration or haemorrhage in a normal gland or tumour [2].

They are usually detected by chance in adults, but occasionally become infected, or give rise to retroperitoneal haemorrhage [26]. In the tropics they may occasionally be hydatid cysts [27]. Cysts of the adrenal can usually be left alone unless they are causing discomfort by pressure on adjacent organs when they can be aspirated under CT or ultrasound control [28].

Bilateral adrenal masses are nearly always metastases from some other primary cancer [29].

Autotransplantation for Parkinson's disease

Urologists may be called upon to remove the adrenal for the purposes of its autotransplantation to the caudate nucleus in Parkinson's disease. The objective of this as yet somewhat experimental procedure is to supply dopamine to the brain, whose substantia nigra has stopped making it. The procedure is performed in collaboration with the neurosurgical team who localize the target area with CT scanning and a stereotactic system. The patient is then placed prone, and the left adrenal approached through a 12th rib exposure [30].

References

1 Burgige KA (1993) Prenatal adrenal hemorrhage confirmed by postnatal surgery. *J Urol* 150: 1867.

2 Patti G, Fiocca G, Latini T, Celli E, Bellussi A, Nazzicone P (1993) Prenatal diagnosis of bilateral adrenal cysts. *J Urol* 150: 1189.

3 Neville AM, O'Hare MJ (1979) Aspects of structure, function and pathology, in: James VHT (ed.) *The Adrenal Gland*, vol. 2, pp. 52–5. New York: Raven Press.

4 Symington T (1969) *Functional Pathology of the Human Adrenal Gland*. Edinburgh: Churchill Livingstone.

5 Del Gaudio A, Del Gaudio G-A (1993) Virilizing adrenocortical tumors in adult women. *Cancer* 72: 1997.

6 Sullivan M, Boileau M, Hodges CV (1978) Adrenal cortical carcinoma. *J Urol* 120: 660.

7 Weiss LM (1984) Comparative histologic study of 43 metastasizing and nonmetastasizing adrenocortical tumors. *Amer J Surg Pathol* 8: 163.

8 Venkatesh S, Hickery RC, Sellin RV, Fernandez JF, Samaan NA (1989) Adrenal cortical carcinoma. *Cancer* 64: 765

9 Chang SY, Lee SS, Ma CP, Lee SK (1989) Nonfunctioning tumours of the adrenal cortex. *Br J Urol* 63: 462.

10 Donohue JP (1988) Diagnosis and management of adrenal tumors, in: Skinner DG, Lieskovsky G (eds) *Diagnosis and Management of Genitourinary Cancer*, pp. 372–89. Philadelphia: WB Saunders.

11 Hata M, Yanaihara H, Hayakawa K *et al.* (1994) Clinical study on 26 cases of incidental adrenal tumors. *Jap J Urol* 85: 974.

12 Ganguly A, Donohue JP (1983) Primary aldosteronism: pathophysiology, diagnosis and treatment (review). *J Urol* 129: 241.

13 Miyata M, Nishihara M, Tokunaka S, Yachiku S. (1989) A maternal functioning adrenocortical adenoma causing fetal female pseudohermaphroditism. *J Urol* 142: 806.

14 Sipple JH (1961) The association of phaeochromocytoma with carcinoma of the thyroid gland. *Am J Med* 31: 163.

15 Hensle TW, Parkhurst EC (1976) Sipple's syndrome: a urologist's viewpoint. *Urology* 8: 258.

16 Neumann JPH, Berger DP, Sigmund G *et al.* (1995) Pheochromocytomas, multiple endocrine neoplasia Type 2, and von Hippel-Lindau disease. *New Eng J Med* 329: 1531.

17 Lindau A (1926) Studen ueber Kleinhirncysten: Bau, Pathogenese und Beziehungen zur Angiomatosis Retinae. *Acta Path Microbiol Scand Suppl* 1: 1.

18 Ducatman BS, Scheithauer BW, van Heerden JA, Sheedy PF (1983) Simultaneous phaeochromocytoma and renal cell carcinoma: report of a case and review of the literature. *Br J Surg* 70: 415.

19 Bravo EL, Tarazi RC, Fouad FM *et al.* (1981) Clonidine suppression test: a useful aid in the diagnosis of pheochromocytoma. *New Engl J Med* 305: 623.

20 Edwards GA, Smythe GA, Graham PE, Lazarus L (1992) The impact of recent advances in diagnostic technology on the clinical presentation of phaeochromocytoma. *Med J Aust* 156: 153.

21 Ackery DM, Tippett PA, Condon BR, Sutton HE, Wyeth P. (1984) New approach to the localisation of phaeochromocytoma: Imaging with iodine-131-meta-iodobenzylguanidine. *Br Med J* 288: 1587.

22 Shulkin BL, Wieland DM, Schwaiger M *et al.* (1992) PET scanning with hydroxephedrine: an approach to the localization of pheochromocytoma. *J Nuclear Med* 33: 1125.

23 Nativ O, Grant CS, Sheps SG *et al.* (1992) Prognostic profile for patients with pheochromocytoma derived from clinical and pathological factors and DNA ploidy pattern. *J Surg Oncol* 50: 258.

24 Mancini AF (1982) Neuroblastoma in a pair of identical twins. *Med Pediatr Oncol* 10: 45.

25 Duckett JW, Koop CE (1977) Neuroblastoma. *Urol Clin N Am* 4: 285.

26 Pasciak RM, Cook WA (1988) Massive retroperitoneal hemorrhage owing to a ruptured adrenal cyst. *J Urol* 139: 98.

27 Stroujieh AS, Frah GD, Haddad MJ, Abu-Khalaf MM (1990) Adrenal cysts: diagnosis and management. *Br J Urol* 65: 570.

28 Buchino JJ, Dougherty HK, Shearer LT (1985) Adrenal cyst. *Arch Pathol Lab Med* 109: 377.

29 Gibb WRG, Ramsay AD, McNeil NI, Wrong OM (1985) Bilateral adrenal masses. *Br Med J* 291: 203.

30 Skinner EC, Boyd SD, Apuzzo MLJ (1990) Technique of left adrenalectomy for autotransplantation to the caudate nucelus in Parkinson's disease. *J Urol* 144: 838.

Index